Nutrition & Diet Therapy

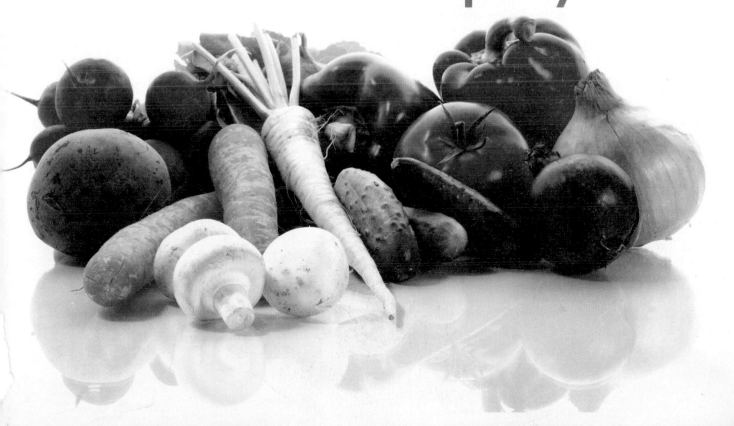

Nutrition & Diet Therapy

Eleventh Edition

Ruth A. Roth, MS, RD

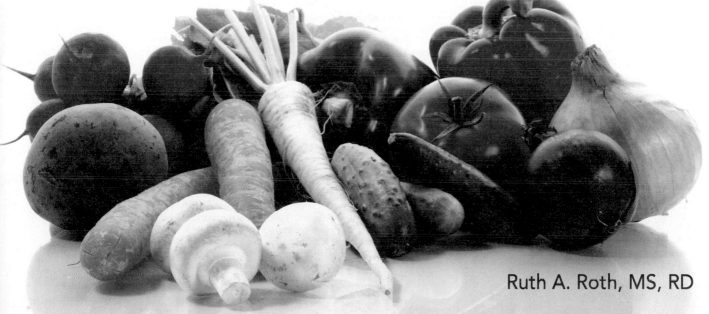

DELMAR
CENGAGE Learning·

Australia   Canada   Mexico   Singapore   Spain   United Kingdom   United States

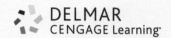

Nutrition and Diet Therapy, 11th edition
Ruth A. Roth, MS, RD

Vice President, Careers & Computing:
  Dave Garza

Publisher, Health Care: Stephen Helba

Director, Development-Careers & Computing:
  Marah Bellegarde

Product Development Manager, Careers:
  Juliet Steiner

Development Editor: Brooke Wilson

Editorial Assistant: Jennifer Wheaton

Brand Manager: Wendy Mapstone

Market Development Manager: Nancy
  Bradshaw

Senior Production Director: Wendy A.
  Troeger

Production Manager: Andrew Crouth

Senior Content Project Manager: Kara A.
  DiCaterino

Senior Art Director: Jack Pendleton

Cover Image: © www.Shutterstock.com

For product information and technology assistance, contact us at
Cengage Learning Customer & Sales Support, 1-800-354-9706

For permission to use material from this text or product,
submit all requests online at **www.cengage.com/permissions.**
Further permissions questions can be e-mailed to
permissionrequest@cengage.com

Library of Congress Control Number: 2012953797

ISBN-13: 978-1-133-96050-8

ISBN-10: 1-133-96050-2

Delmar
5 Maxwell Drive
Clifton Park, NY 12065-2919
USA

Cengage Learning is a leading provider of customized learning solutions
with office locations around the globe, including Singapore, the United
Kingdom, Australia, Mexico, Brazil, and Japan. Locate your local office at:
international.cengage.com/region

Cengage Learning products are represented in Canada by
Nelson Education, Ltd.

To learn more about Delmar, visit **www.cengage.com/delmar**

Purchase any of our products at your local college store or at our
preferred online store **www.cengagebrain.com**

Notice to the Reader

Printed in Canada
1 2 3 4 5 6 7 17 16 15 14 13

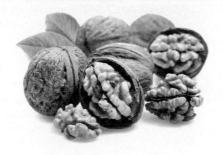

*To my family and friends who love
and support me.*

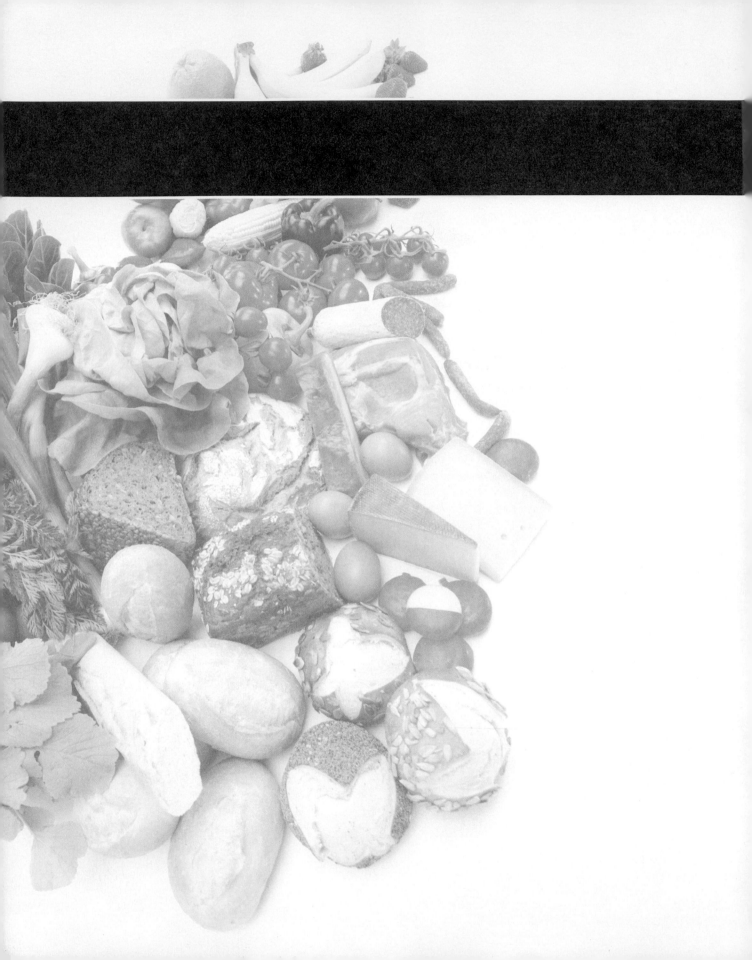

BRIEF **CONTENTS**

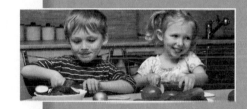

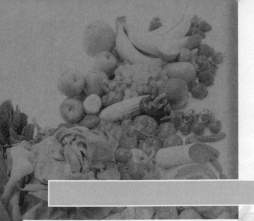

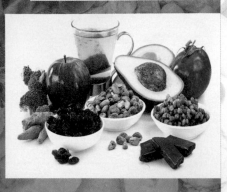
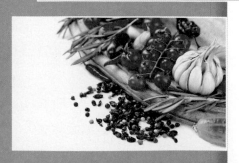

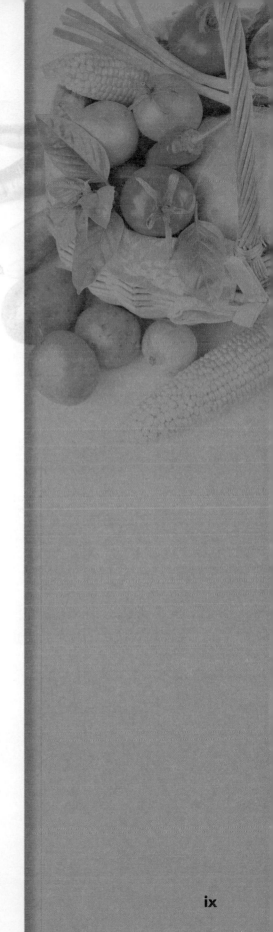

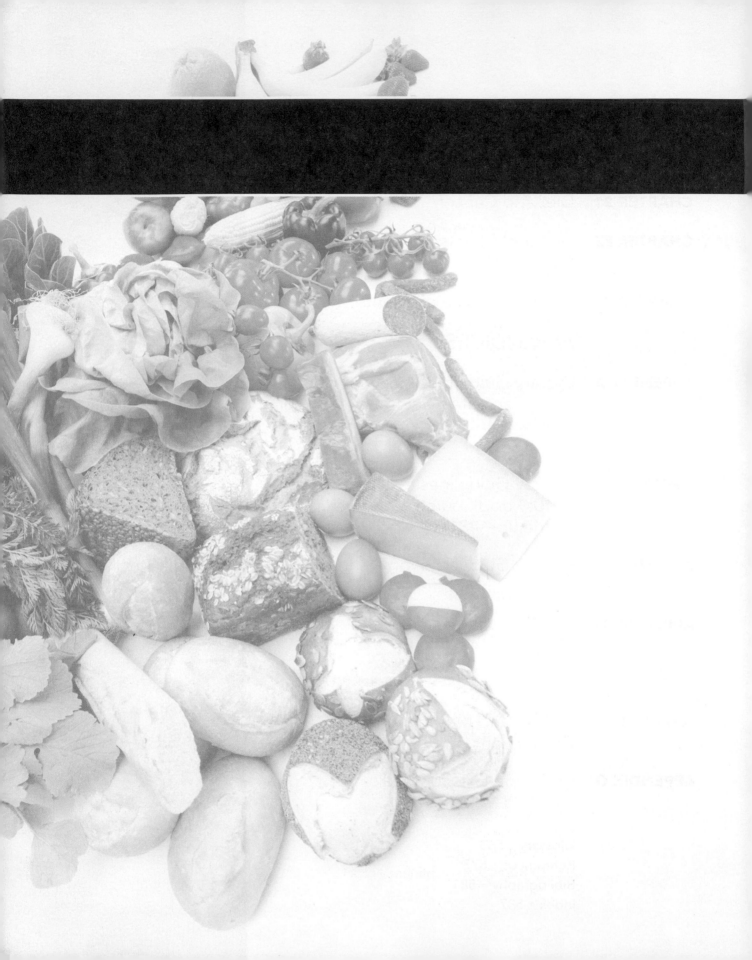

TABLE OF **CONTENTS**

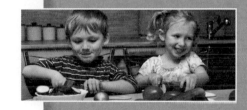

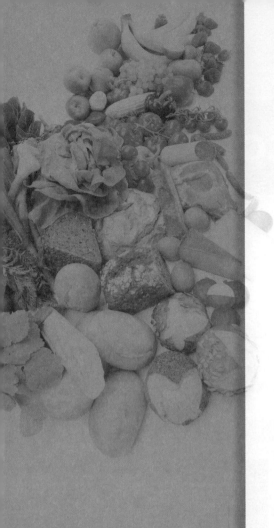

SECTION 2

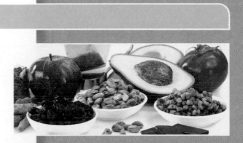

ACHIEVING HEALTH THROUGH GOOD NUTRITION   185

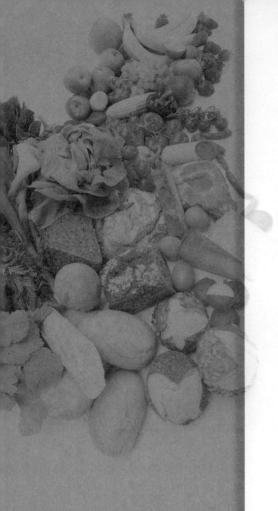

SECTION 3

MEDICAL NUTRITION THERAPY   293

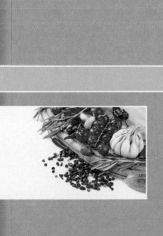

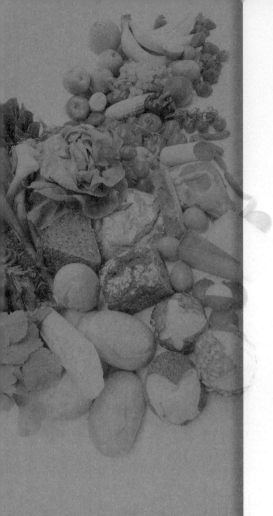

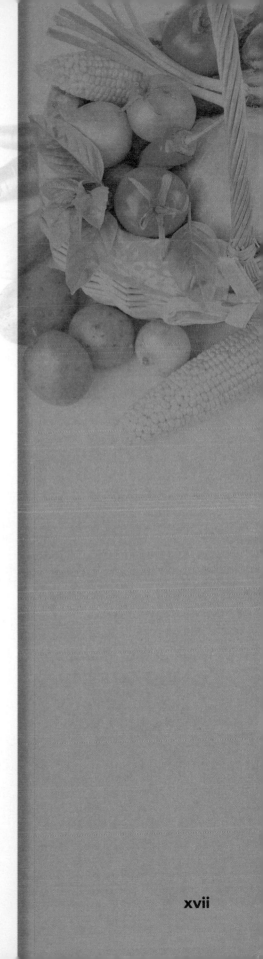

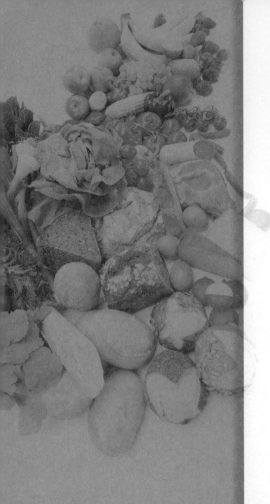

PREFACE

In our health-conscious society, the link between good nutrition and good health is seen everywhere, from magazine and newspaper headlines to television shows and websites. Recipes for low-fat, heart-healthy meals, fad diets, and stories about foods that claim to prevent certain diseases and health ailments abound. This presents a challenge to nurses working with clients to help them focus on improving both their nutrition and their overall health. *Nutrition & Diet Therapy,* 11th edition, provides sound nutritional information based upon fact. It is important that nurses have a solid foundation in the basic principles and concepts of good nutrition; then they can help clients debunk the myths and help them move toward better health through nutritional awareness.

Section 1, **Fundamentals of Nutrition**, includes chapters on the relationship of nutrition and health; planning a healthy diet; digestion, absorption, and metabolism; and chapters on each of the six nutrient groups (carbohydrates, lipids, proteins, vitamins, minerals, and water). Content has been thoroughly revised to embrace the MyPlate guidelines.

Section 2, **Achieving Health Through Good Nutrition**, includes chapters on foodborne illnesses and allergies, nutritional care during the various stages of life from pregnancy and lactation through infancy, childhood, adolescence, young and middle adulthood, and the senior years. This information provides sound knowledge of the changes in nutritional requirements across the lifespan.

Section 3, **Medical Nutrition Therapy**, includes discussion and research for many nutrition-related disorders. It covers the effects of disease and surgery on nutrition and the appropriate uses of diet therapy in restoring and maintaining health. It includes chapters with specific nutritional information for clients requiring help with weight control, diabetes, cardiovascular disease, renal disease, gastrointestinal problems, and cancer. It also discusses the nutritional needs of surgical clients, clients suffering burns and infections including HIV, and clients requiring enteral and parenteral nutrition. There is also a chapter on the general nutritional care of clients.

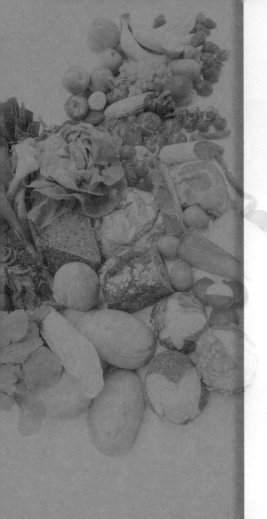

Chapters follow a consistent format to help facilitate and enhance learning:

- **Objectives**—learning goals to be achieved upon completion of the chapter

- **Key Terms**—a list of terms used in text and defined in the margin; these are also included in the master glossary

- **In the Media**—boxes highlighting current trends, events, and fads and the potential impact on clients' health

- **Supersize USA**—boxes highlighting information and current events surrounding the national obesity epidemic

- **Exploring the Web**—directions to Internet resources and websites

- **Spotlight on Lifecycle**—boxes focusing on nutritional concerns for the different stages of life

- **Health and Nutrition Considerations**—recommendations for health care professionals to help clients achieve optimal health through the knowledge of nutrition

- **Summary**—a brief narrative overview of the most important chapter highlights

- **Discussion Topics**—critical-thinking activities that encourage synthesis and application of new concepts

- **Suggested Activities**—creative suggestions on how to implement the knowledge presented in the chapter

- **Review**—study questions to test understanding of content and to help prepare for examinations

- **Case in Point**—reality-based case studies that apply to the chapter topics, followed up by a "Rate This Plate" challenge that asks for evaluation of a proposed meal plan for a client

KEY FEATURES

- **MyPlate** guidelines are recommended and embraced throughout the text.

- **Supersize USA** boxes highlight information and current events pertaining to the national obesity epidemic.

- **Spotlight on Life Cycle** boxes outline nutritional concerns at each stage of life.

- **In the Media** boxes present some of the current events and fads influencing what we know about health and nutrition today.

- **Exploring the Web** boxes provide websites with more depth on chapter topics.

- Two **Case in Point** and **Rate This Plate** features can be found at the end of each chapter. The Case in Points are reality-based case studies that apply to the chapter topics, followed up by a Rate This

Plate challenge that asks for evaluation of a proposed meal plan for a client.

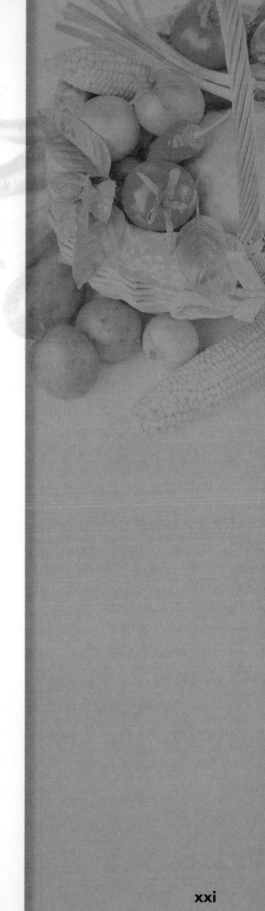

- **Dietary Guidelines for Americans, 2010** are located in the appendix and throughout the chapters.

NEW TO THIS EDITION

- **Chapter 7** *Vitamins* includes new vitamin D_3 recommendations and discusses current research for all ages and the importance of increasing vitamin D_3 intake.

- **Chapter 13** *Nutrition for Children and Adolescents* includes a new look at the diet quality of children in America, new information on ADHD and diet (and which medicines can affect appetite) as well as expanded information on eating disorders, including binge eating disorders in children, and the female athletic triad.

- **Chapter 16** *Weight Management Across the Life Cycle* includes the latest on weight regulation, obesity trends in kids and adults, and health consequences of overweight, especially pre-diabetes. The latest prevention and treatment strategies are discussed including conventional and less conventional methods, with expanded information on bariatric surgery in America.

- **Chapter 17** *Diet and Diabetes Mellitus* includes the most up-to-date statistics on the number of Americans with diabetes, an expanded list of oral medications used to treat diabetes, and a new chart of insulin currently available to treat diabetes. For easier access, the Exchange Lists have been moved from Chapter 17 to Appendix G.

- **Chapter 20** *Diet and Gastrointestinal Problems* includes new information on celiac disease and the growing incidence of gluten sensitivity, as well as new information about Crohn's disease.

- New and refreshed **Case in Point** and **Rate This Plate** features are at the end of each chapter with new scenarios and critical-thinking questions.

- **In the Media** boxes have been refreshed and added throughout the chapters to keep students up to speed on some of the current events and fads in nutrition and health-related topics.

- Updated **Recommended Dietary Allowances (RDA)** and **Daily Recommended Intake (DRI)** can be found in tables throughout the book.

- The new **MyPlate** method replaces MyPyramid and gives guidelines for intake of nutrients with various calorie levels. Information about the new MyPlate method is introduced in Chapter 2, and is referenced throughout the text.

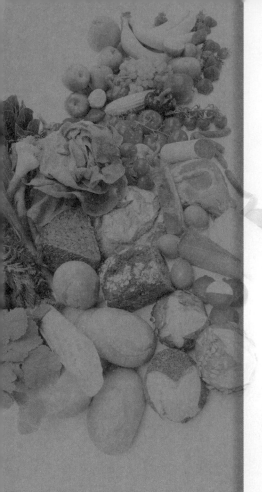

- **Supersize USA** boxes have been refreshed to bring current nutrition concerns to the forefront and to generate discussion in the classroom.
- *Dietary Guidelines for Americans, 2010* has been updated with current recommendations for nutritional intake and exercise.

SUPPLEMENTAL MATERIALS

Free Study Tools and Resources Only Available at CengageBrain.com
Access to FREE book companion resources including:

- Objectives
- Answers to Case Study and Review Questions
- Weblinks
- PowerPoint Presentation

Enter 978-1-133-96050-8 into the search field and follow directions to access your free resources!

Diet Analysis Plus, 10th Edition

The top-rated diet-analysis software and a must-have for success in your nutrition course, DIET ANALYSIS PLUS enables you to track diet and physical activity, and analyze the nutritional value of the food intake! Diet Analysis Plus includes a 20,000+ food database, custom food and recipe features, the latest Dietary References, as well as actual percentages of essential nutrients, vitamins, and minerals. New features include enhanced search functionality with filter option, and resources tab with helpful information. You can create personal profiles based on height, weight, age, sex, and activity level and use this information to adjust diet and gain a better understanding of how nutrition relates to personal health goals. The dynamic interface makes it easy to track the types and serving sizes of the foods consumed from one day to 365 days. DIET ANALYSIS PLUS can help you gain a better understanding of how nutrition relates to, and impacts, your life and the health of your client.

ISBN: Instant Access Code: 978-0-538-49509-7
ISBN: Printed Access Code: 978-0-538-49508-0

WebTutor Advantage Plus

WebTutor™ Advantage Plus is an exciting online ancillary that takes your course beyond the classroom boundaries. WebTutor Advantage Plus provides a content-rich, Web-based teaching and learning environment that reinforces and helps clarify complex concepts. Elements include advance preparation, objectives, overview, class notes, discussion, glossary, multiple-choice questions, and Web links and videos. Rich communication tools for instructors and students include a course calendar, chat, e-mail, threaded discussions, and a whiteboard. The computerized testbank provided on the Instructor Resource can also be found embedded within the WebTutor Advantage Plus for instructor use. WebTutor Advantage Plus is available in both the Angel and Blackboard platforms.

WebTutor Advantage Plus on Blackboard
ISBN: 978-1-133-95989-2

WebTutor Advantage Plus on Angel
ISBN: 978-1-133-95987-8

COURSEMATE

CourseMate complements your textbook with several robust and noteworthy components:

- An interactive eBook, with highlighting, note taking, and search capabilities
- Interactive and engaging learning tools including, flashcards, quizzes, videos, games, PowerPoint presentations, and much more!
- Engagement Tracker, a first-of-its-kind tool that monitors student participation and retention in the course.

To access CourseMate content:

- Go to www.cengagebrain.com.
- For an Instant access code: ISBN: 978-1-133-95977-9
- For a Print access code: ISBN 978-1-133-95975-5

Instructor Companion Website

This instruction companion website is accessible via Cengage.com through an instructor account. This provides a complete customizable resource for the instructor. Contents include an Instructor's Manual that contains teaching strategies, answers to text questions, listings of additional resources, and critical-thinking exercises that can be done in small groups or as a whole class; an 800-slide PowerPoint presentation correlating to each chapter of the text; and a computerized test bank with over 1,000 questions offered in a variety of types such as multiple choice, short answer, true and false, and matching to customize exams and quizzes.

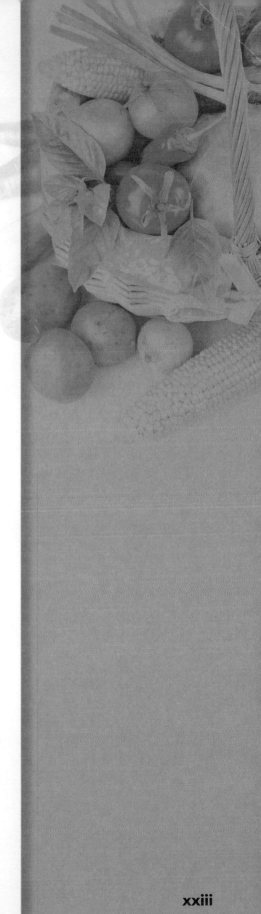

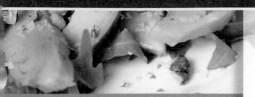

ACKNOWLEDGMENTS

The author wishes to express her appreciation to the following people:

Delia Uherec
Brooke Wilson
Monica Ohlinger
Lauren Mullins
Kathy Wehrle
Leigh Ann Brooks
Jamie Lovejoy
Troy Wietfeldt

Contributor to Case in Point Features
Leigh Ann Brooks RN, RD, CDE
Certified Diabetes Educator

Contributor to Weight Management and additional writing throughout text
Kathy Wehrle, RD
Certified Weight Management Specialist

Cynthia Blanton, PhD
Assistant Professor
Division of Health Sciences, Dietetic Programs
Idaho State University
Pocatello, Idaho

Kathy Carter MS, RD/LD
Instructor
Athens Technical College
Elberton, Georgia

Sherri Comfort, RN
Practical Nursing Instructor
Holmes Community College
Goodman, Mississippi

Catherine Hutcheson, RN, BSN
Associate Professor of Nursing
Mineral Area College
Park Hills, Missouri

Judy Kitson, RN, MSN, FNP-BC, LPN
LPN Program
Dalton State College
Dalton, Georgia

Cheryl Pratt
National Director of Academic Standards and Quality
Rasmussen College
Mankato, Minnesota

HOW TO **USE THIS TEXT**

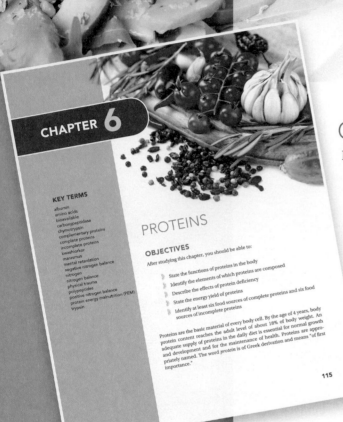

OBJECTIVES

Read the chapter Objectives before reading the chapter content to set the stage for learning. Return to the Objectives when the chapter study is complete to see which entries you can respond to with, "Yes, I can do that."

KEY TERMS

Glance over this list of terms before you tackle the chapter. Flip through the pages to check the definitions in the margins and make a list of those terms that are unfamiliar.

SUPERSIZE USA

Obesity has become a national health epidemic. Read over these boxes to find out why and also for suggestions on what you, as a consumer and as a nurse, can do to help curb this trend.

Supersize **USA**

I was having dinner with a friend who was expecting a baby and when she picked up the menu she said, "I am eating for two now!" I looked at her and proceeded to tell her that she was misinformed. In the first trimester, a woman needs no additional calories. In the second and third trimesters, calorie needs increase only by about 300 calories per day. Three hundred calories is equal to ½ a chicken sandwich, or ¼ cup of dried fruit plus ¼ cup of nuts. You need extra nutrients though, which means you need to eat smarter while you are pregnant. Choosing healthy, nutrient-dense snacks over junk food or calorie-dense foods is a better alternative for the mother and growing baby. There are too many empty calories in soda and other junk food—80 oz of soda equals 1,000 calories. Increasing whole grains, fiber, fruits, vegetables, and milk intake will help provide the additional calories and nutrients needed throughout the pregnancy.

SPOTLIGHT ON LIFE CYCLE

Nutritional concerns and needs will change at each stage of life. Test your knowledge of the needs of children, adolescents, pregnant women, and the elderly.

IN THE MEDIA

Which of these "hot topics" do you already know something about? Check here for current trends, events, and fads and understand the potential impact on clients' health.

EXPLORING THE WEB

Be sure to visit these websites for more depth on chapter topics. These are also excellent sources for information to make care plans and teaching guides.

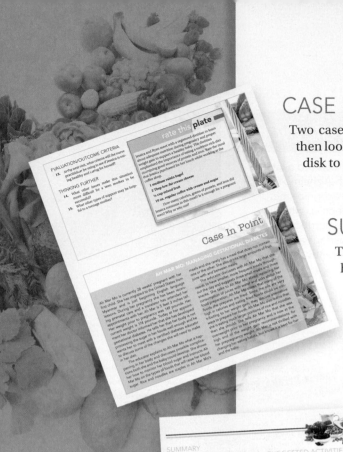

CASE IN POINT

Two case studies conclude each chapter. Read these real-life stories, then look at the sample diet and **Rate This Plate.** Visit the StudyWARE™ disk to see how your answers match up to those of the experts.

SUMMARY

This brief narrative overview of the most important chapter highlights is ideal for testing your grasp of the chapter material. Always start your study sessions with a quick glance at the Summary to refresh your memory on the basics of the chapter.

DISCUSSION TOPICS

Critical thinking is key to your success as a nurse. Use these activities to synthesize and apply what you have read and learned.

SUGGESTED ACTIVITIES

Put your knowledge to the test; see how many of these activities you can successfully complete once you finish studying the chapter. Make a list of any areas needing additional attention.

REVIEW

These study questions are in multiple-choice format, perfect for preparing for your nursing examinations.

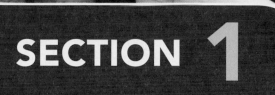

SECTION 1

FUNDAMENTALS OF NUTRITION

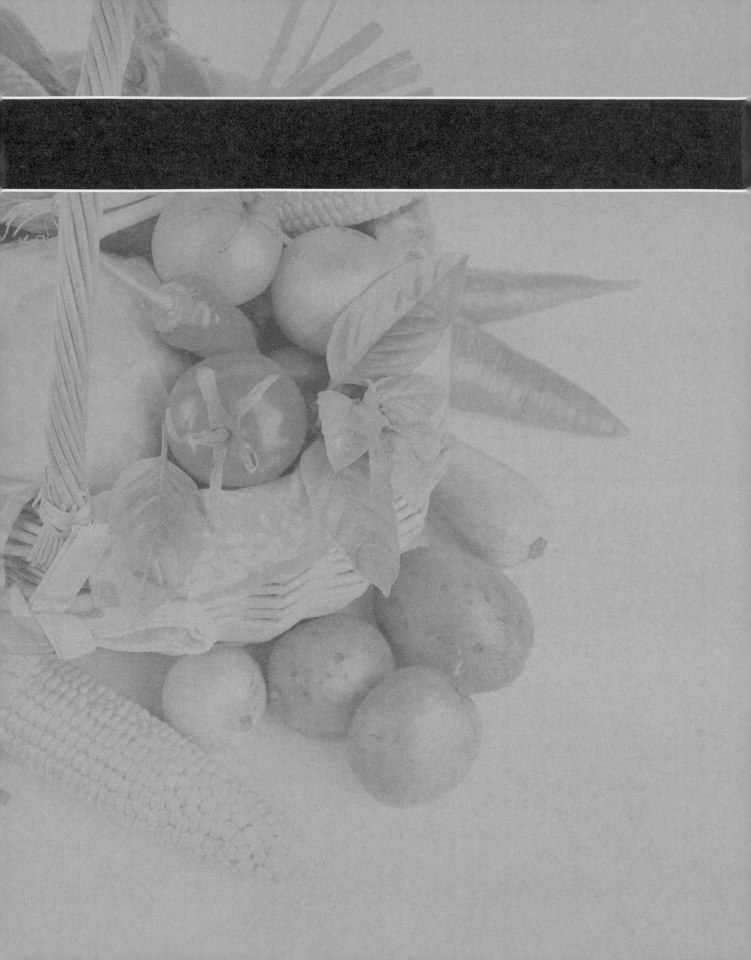

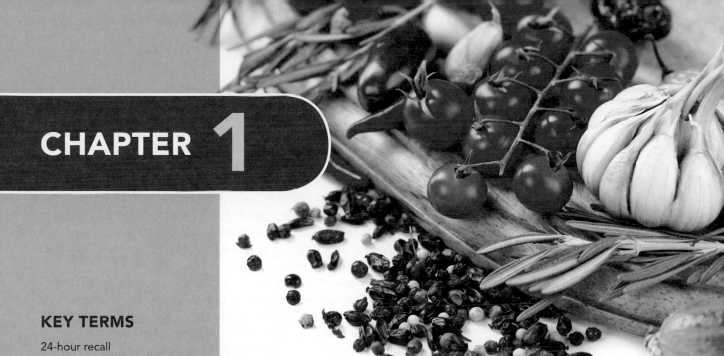

CHAPTER 1

KEY TERMS

24-hour recall
anthropometric measurements
atherosclerosis
biochemical tests
caliper
carbohydrates (CHO)
circulation
clinical examination
cumulative effects
deficiency diseases
dietary-social history
dietitian
digestion
elimination
essential nutrients
fats (lipids)
food diary
goiter
iron deficiency
malnutrition
minerals
nourishing
nutrient density
nutrients
nutrition
nutrition assessment
nutritional status
nutritious
obesity
osteomalacia
osteoporosis
peer pressure
proteins
respiration
rickets
vitamins
water
wellness

THE RELATIONSHIP OF NUTRITION AND HEALTH

OBJECTIVES

After studying this chapter, you should be able to:

- Name the six classes of nutrients and their primary functions
- Recognize common characteristics of well-nourished people
- Recognize symptoms of malnutrition
- Describe ways in which nutrition and health are related
- List the four basic steps in nutrition assessment

The United States was historically referred to as the "melting pot" because it represented people of many nationalities who immigrated to this country in hopes of finding a better life. The individuals in this country bring all their cultural diversities with them, including their cuisine. Many choose to assimilate immediately by learning the language and trying the foods of their new country; others may favor the foods and customs of their country of origin. The diet that individuals follow will determine, to a large extent, their health, growth, and development. It has never been more imperative that active measures be taken to make our social, cultural, political, and economic environment in relation to diet a health-promoting one.

Taking care of one's health is all about prevention. In the past, the focus was on treatment of diseases, with little, if any, attention to prevention. Prevention, however, can often be less costly than treatment and offer a better quality of life for an individual as well as the community. Nutrition and diet choice form a logical starting point for preventive health care measures and education to improve quality of life.

Achieving **wellness** that integrates body, mind, and spirit should be the main goal in life. This can be accomplished through lifestyle changes such as focusing on healthy food choices, not smoking, participating in regular physical activity, and maintaining a healthy weight. Expanding one's mind through continued education, in both nutrition and other areas, and finding a source of inner strength to deal with life changes will all contribute to one's sense of wellness.

Living a long life without major health problems is possible. The younger one is when positive changes are made, the healthier one is throughout the life span.

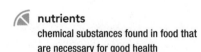

wellness
a way of life that integrates body, mind, and spirit

NUTRIENTS AND THEIR FUNCTIONS

To maintain health and function properly, the body must be provided with **nutrients**. Nutrients are chemical substances that are necessary for life. They are divided into six classes:

nutrients
chemical substances found in food that are necessary for good health

- Carbohydrates (CHO)
- Fats (lipids)
- Proteins
- Vitamins
- Minerals
- Water

The body can make small amounts of some nutrients, but most must be obtained from food in order to meet the body's needs. Those available only in food are called **essential nutrients**. There are about 40 of them, and they are found in all six nutrient classes.

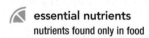

essential nutrients
nutrients found only in food

The six nutrient classes are chemically divided into two categories: organic and inorganic (Table 1-1). Organic nutrients contain hydrogen, oxygen, and carbon. (Carbon is an element found in all living things.) Before the body can use organic nutrients, it must break them down into their smallest components. Inorganic nutrients are already in their simplest forms when the body ingests them, except for water.

Each nutrient participates in at least one of the following functions:

- Providing the body with energy
- Building and repairing body tissue
- Regulating body processes

TABLE 1-1 The Six Essential Nutrients and Their Functions	
ORGANIC NUTRIENTS	**FUNCTION**
Carbohydrates	Provide energy
Fats	Provide energy
Proteins	Build and repair body tissues; provide energy
Vitamins	Regulate body processes
INORGANIC NUTRIENTS	**FUNCTION**
Minerals	Regulate body processes
Water	Regulates body processes

© Cengage Learning 2014

Carbohydrates (CHO), **proteins**, and **fats (lipids)** furnish energy. Proteins are also used to build and repair body tissues with the help of vitamins and minerals. **Vitamins**, **minerals**, and **water** help regulate the various body processes such as **circulation**, **respiration**, **digestion**, and **elimination**.

Each nutrient is important, but none works alone. For example, carbohydrates, proteins, and fats are necessary for energy, but to provide it, they need the help of vitamins, minerals, and water. Proteins are essential for building and repairing body tissue, but without vitamins, minerals, and water, they are ineffective. Eating the antioxidant vitamins such as A, D, E, and K help to enhance your immune system. Foods that contain substantial amounts of nutrients are described as **nutritious** or **nourishing**. Nutrients are discussed in detail in Chapters 4 through 9.

CHARACTERISTICS OF GOOD NUTRITION

Most people find pleasure in eating. Eating allows one to connect with family and friends in pleasant surroundings. This connection creates pleasant memories. Unfortunately, in social situations it is easy for one to make food choices that may not be conducive to good health.

What determines when one needs to eat? Does one wait until the body signals hunger or eat when one sees food or when the clock says it is time? Hunger is the physiological need for food. Appetite is a psychological desire for food based on pleasant memories. When the body signals hunger it indicates a decrease in blood glucose levels that supplies the body with energy. If one ignores the signal and hunger becomes intense, it is possible to make poor food choices. The choices one makes will determine one's nutrition status. A person who habitually chooses to overeat, or not eat, as a way of coping with life's emotional struggles may be suffering from an eating disorder. The various eating disorders will be discussed in Chapter 16.

Once food has been eaten, the body must process it before it can be used. **Nutrition** is the result of the processes whereby the body takes in and uses food for growth, development, and the maintenance of health.

carbohydrates (CHO)
the nutrient class providing the major source of energy in the average diet

proteins
the only one of the six essential nutrient classes containing nitrogen

fats (lipids)
highest calorie-value nutrient class

vitamins
organic substances necessary for life although they do not, independently, provide energy

minerals
one of many inorganic substances essential to life and classified generally as minerals

water
major constituent of all living cells; composed of hydrogen and oxygen

circulation
the body process whereby the blood is moved throughout the body

respiration
breathing

digestion
breakdown of food in the body in preparation for absorption

elimination
evacuation of wastes

nutritious
foods or beverages containing substantial amounts of essential nutrients

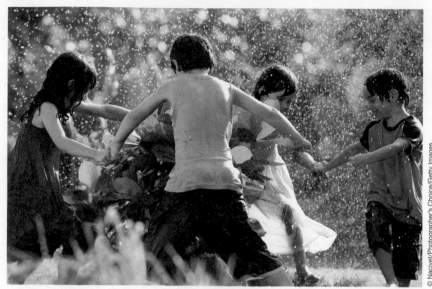
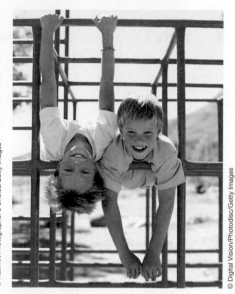

FIGURE 1-1 Good nutrition shows in the happy faces of these children.

nourishing
foods or beverages that provide substantial amounts of essential nutrients

nutrition
the result of those processes whereby the body takes in and uses food for growth, development, and the maintenance of health

nutritional status
one's physical condition as determined by diet

malnutrition
poor nutrition

These processes include digestion, absorption, and metabolism. (They are discussed in Chapter 3.) One's physical condition as determined by the diet is called **nutritional status**.

Nutrition helps determine the height and weight of an individual. Nutrition can also affect the body's ability to resist disease, the length of one's life, and the state of one's physical and mental well-being (Figure 1-1).

Good nutrition enhances appearance and is commonly exemplified by shiny hair, clear skin, clear eyes, erect posture, alert expressions, and firm flesh on well-developed bone structures. Good nutrition aids emotional adjustments, provides stamina, and promotes a healthy appetite. It also helps establish regular sleep and elimination habits (Table 1-2).

MALNUTRITION

Malnutrition can be caused by overnutrition (excess energy or nutrient intake) or undernutrition (deficient energy or nutrient intake). We usually think of malnutrition as a condition that results when the cells do not receive an adequate supply of the essential nutrients because of poor diet or poor utilization of food (Figure 1-2). Sometimes it occurs because people do not or cannot eat enough of the foods that provide the essential nutrients to satisfy body needs. At other times people may eat well-balanced diets but suffer from diseases that prevent normal usage of the nutrients.

Overnutrition has become a larger problem in the United States than undernutrition. Overeating and the ingestion of megadoses of various vitamins and minerals (without prescription) are two major causes of overnutrition in the United States.

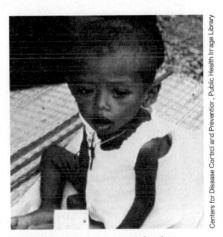

TABLE 1-2   Characteristics of Nutritional Status

GOOD	POOR
Alert expression	Apathy
Shiny hair	Dull, lifeless hair
Clear complexion with good color	Greasy, blemished complexion with poor color
Bright, clear eyes	Dull, red-rimmed eyes
Pink, firm gums and well-developed teeth	Red, puffy, receding gums and missing or cavity-prone teeth
Firm abdomen	Swollen abdomen
Firm, well-developed muscles	Underdeveloped, flabby muscles
Well-developed bone structure	Bowed legs, "pigeon" chest
Normal weight for height	Overweight or underweight
Erect posture	Slumped posture
Emotional stability	Easily irritated; depressed; poor attention span
Good stamina; seldom ill	Easily fatigued; frequently ill
Healthy appetite	Excessive or poor appetite
Healthy, normal sleep habits	Insomnia at night; fatigued during day
Normal elimination	Constipation or diarrhea

© Cengage Learning 2014

Nutrient Deficiency

A nutrient deficiency occurs when a person lacks one or more nutrients over a period of time. Nutrient deficiencies are classified as primary or secondary. Primary deficiencies are caused by inadequate dietary intake. Secondary deficiencies are caused by something other than diet, such as a disease condition that may cause malabsorption, accelerated excretion, or destruction of the nutrients. Nutrient deficiencies can result in malnutrition.

INDIVIDUALS AT RISK FROM POOR NUTRITIONAL INTAKE

Teenagers may eat often but at unusual hours. They may miss regularly scheduled meals, become hungry, and satisfy their hunger with foods that have low nutrient density such as potato chips, cakes, soda, and candy. Foods with low **nutrient density** provide an abundance of calories, but the nutrients are primarily carbohydrates and fats and, except for sodium, very limited amounts of proteins, vitamins, and minerals. A 2010 U.S. Department of Agriculture, Agricultural Research Service survey, included 4,000 teenagers and the results indicated that snack foods accounted for 43% of total sugar intake. Teenagers are subject to **peer pressure**; that is, they are easily influenced by the opinions of their friends. If friends favor foods with low nutrient density, it is difficult for a teenager to differ with them. Fad diets, which unfortunately are common among teens, sometimes result in a form of malnutrition. This condition occurs because some nutrients are eliminated from the diet when the types of foods eaten are severely restricted.

Centers for Disease Control and Prevention , Public Health Image Library

FIGURE 1-2 The poor-quality hair, mottled complexion, dull expression, spindly arms and legs, and bloated abdomen of this baby girl exemplify many signs of malnutrition.

 nutrient density
nutrient value of foods compared with number of calories

peer pressure
pressure of one's friends and colleagues of the same age

Supersize USA

Supersizing in the fast-food industry and large quantities served in restaurants lead to portion distortion. Those growing up in the supersized world may have no concept of what constitutes a normal portion. Children who are encouraged to, or have been made to, eat everything on their plates may feel compelled to finish their supersized meals, easily contributing to obesity and type 2 diabetes.

SPOTLIGHT on Life Cycle

Infants, young children, teenage girls, and adults have risk for iron-deficiency anemia. Full-term infants are born with enough iron stores to last 4 to 6 months. A premature infant is at even greater risk for iron-deficiency anemia. Baby foods and cereals are fortified with iron to help prevent iron deficiency in young children. Underweight teens or teenage girls who have heavy monthly periods are at an increased risk for iron-deficiency anemia. Women of child-bearing age are also at risk. Pregnant women are prone to anemia due to the increased need for iron during pregnancy. A supplement that is higher in iron may be prescribed for pregnant women. Internal bleeding can lead to iron-deficiency anemia due to blood loss. Clients who have undergone kidney dialysis or gastric bypass surgery are also at an increased risk. Treatments include dietary changes and supplements, medicines, and surgery.

(Source: Adapted from *Who Is at Risk for Iron-Deficiency Anemia?* National Heart Lung and Blood Institute; U.S. Department of Health and Human Services. 2011. http://www.nhlbi.nih.gov)

EXPLORING THE WEB

Search the Web to find information on osteomalacia and osteoporosis. What are the leading causes? Should you take a calcium plus vitamin D supplement?

cumulative effects
results of something done repeatedly over many years

atherosclerosis
a form of arteriosclerosis affecting the intima (inner lining) of the artery walls

obesity
excessive body fat, 20% above average

deficiency diseases
diseases caused by the lack of one or more specific nutrients

iron deficiency
intake of iron is adequate, but the body has no extra iron stored

Pregnancy increases a woman's hunger and the need for certain nutrients, especially proteins, minerals, and vitamins. Pregnancy during adolescence requires extreme care in food selection. The young mother-to-be requires a diet that provides sufficient nutrients for the developing fetus as well as for her own still-growing body.

Many factors influence nutrition in the elderly. Depression, loneliness, lack of income, inability to shop, inability to prepare meals, and the state of overall health can all lead to malnutrition. Chapter 15 is another source of information on the elderly.

CUMULATIVE EFFECTS OF NUTRITION

There is an increasing concern among health professionals regarding the **cumulative effects** of nutrition. Cumulative effects are the results of something that is done repeatedly over many years. For example, eating excessive amounts of saturated fats (saturated fats are discussed in Chapter 5) for many years contributes to **atherosclerosis**, which leads to heart attacks. Years of overeating can cause **obesity** and may also contribute to hypertension, type 2 (noninsulin-dependent) diabetes, gallbladder disease, foot problems, certain cancers, and even personality disorders.

Deficiency Diseases

When nutrients are seriously lacking in the diet for an extended period, **deficiency diseases** can occur. The most common form of deficiency disease in the United States is **iron deficiency**, which is caused by a lack of the mineral iron and can cause iron-deficiency anemia, which is discussed further in Chapter 8. Iron deficiency is particularly common among children and women. Iron is a necessary component of the blood and is lost during each menstrual period. In addition, the amount of iron needed during childhood

TABLE 1-3 Nutritional Deficiency Diseases and Possible Causes

DEFICIENCY DISEASE	NUTRIENT(S) LACKING
Iron deficiency	Iron
Iron-deficiency anemia	Iron
Beriberi	Thiamin
Night blindness	Vitamin A
Goiter	Iodine
Kwashiorkor	Protein
Marasmus	All nutrients
Osteoporosis	Calcium and vitamin D
Osteomalacia	Calcium and vitamin D, phosphorus, magnesium, and fluoride
Pellagra	Niacin
Rickets	Calcium and vitamin D
Scurvy	Vitamin C
Xerophthalmia (blindness)	Vitamin A

© Cengage Learning 2014

and pregnancy is greater than normal because of the growth of the child or the fetus.

Rickets is another example of a deficiency disease. It causes poor bone formation in children and is due to insufficient calcium and vitamin D. The same deficiencies cause **osteomalacia** in young adults and **osteoporosis** in older adults. Osteomalacia is sometimes called "adult rickets." It causes the bones to soften and may cause the spine to bend and the legs to become bowed. Osteoporosis is a condition that causes bones to become porous and excessively brittle. Too little iodine may cause a **goiter**, and a severe shortage of vitamin A can lead to blindness.

Examples of other deficiency diseases (and their causes) are included in Table 1-3. Information concerning these conditions can be found in the chapters devoted to the given nutrients.

NUTRITION ASSESSMENT

That old saying, "You are what you eat," is true, indeed; but one could change it a bit to read, "You are *and will be* what you eat." Good nutrition is essential for the attainment and maintenance of good health. Determining whether a person is at risk requires completion of a **nutrition assessment**, which should, in fact, become part of a routine examination done by a registered **dietitian** or other health care professional specifically trained in the diagnosis of at-risk individuals. A proper nutrition assessment includes **anthropometric measurements**, **clinical examination**, **biochemical tests**, and **dietary-social history**.

Anthropometric measurements include height and weight and measurements of the head (for children), chest, and skinfold (Figure 1-3).

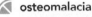

rickets
deficiency disease caused by the lack of vitamin D; causes malformed bones and pain in infants and children

osteomalacia
a condition in which bones become soft, usually in adults because of calcium loss and vitamin D deficiency

osteoporosis
condition in which bones become brittle because there have been insufficient mineral deposits, especially calcium

goiter
enlarged tissue of the thyroid gland due to a deficiency of iodine

nutrition assessment
evaluation of one's nutritional condition

dietitian
professional trained to assess nutrition status and recommend appropriate diet therapy

anthropometric measurements
of height, weight, head, chest, skinfold

clinical examination
physical observation

biochemical tests
laboratory analysis of blood, urine, and feces

dietary-social history
evaluation of food habits, including client's ability to buy and prepare food

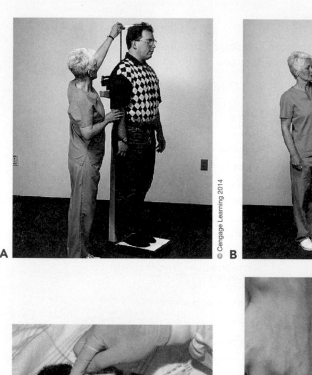

FIGURE 1-3 (A) Height is one anthropometric measurement used in the nutrition assessment. (B) Weight is an anthropometric measurement used in the nutrition assessment. (C) Head circumference is an anthropometric measurement used to assess brain development during the first year of life. (D) Skinfold is an anthropometric measurement used to assess lean muscle mass versus fat.

caliper
mechanical device used to measure percentage of body fat by skinfold measurement

The skinfold measurements are done with a **caliper**. They are used to determine the percentage of adipose and muscle tissue in the body. Measurements out of line with expectations may reveal failure to thrive in children, wasting (catabolism), edema, or obesity, all of which reflect nutrient deficiencies or excesses.

During the clinical examination, signs of nutrient deficiencies are noted. Some nutrient deficiency diseases, such as scurvy, rickets, iron deficiency, and kwashiorkor, are obvious; other forms of nutrient deficiency can be far more subtle. Table 1-4 lists some clinical signs and probable causes of nutrient deficiencies.

Biochemical tests include various blood, urine, and stool tests. A deficiency or toxicity can be determined by laboratory analysis of the samples.

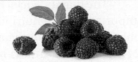

TABLE 1-4 Clinical Signs of Nutrient Deficiencies

CLINICAL SIGN	POSSIBLE DEFICIENCIES
Pallor; blue half circles beneath eyes	Iron, copper, zinc, B_{12}, B_6, biotin
Edema	Protein
Bumpy "gooseflesh"	Vitamin A
Lesions at corners of mouth	Riboflavin
Glossitis	Folic acid
Numerous "black-and-blue" spots and tiny, red "pinprick" hemorrhages under skin	Vitamin C
Emaciation	Carbohydrates, proteins; calories
Poorly shaped bones or teeth or delayed appearance of teeth in children	Vitamin D or calcium
Slow clotting time of blood	Vitamin K
Unusual nervousness, dermatitis, diarrhea in some client	Niacin
Tetany	Calcium, potassium, sodium
Goiter	Iodine
Eczema	Fat (linoleic acid)

© Cengage Learning 2014

The tests allow detection of malnutrition before signs appear. The following are some of the most commonly used tests for nutritional evaluation:

Serum albumin level measures the main protein in the blood and is used to determine protein status.

Serum transferrin level indicates iron-carrying protein in the blood. The level will be above normal if iron stores are low and below normal if the body lacks protein.

Blood urea nitrogen (BUN) may indicate renal failure, insufficient renal blood supply, or blockage of the urinary tract.

Creatinine excretion indicates the amount of creatinine excreted in the urine over a 24-hour period and can be used in estimating body muscle mass. If the muscle mass has been depleted, as in malnutrition, the level will be low.

Serum creatinine indicates the amount of creatinine in the blood and is used for evaluating renal function.

Examples of other blood tests are hemoglobin (Hgb), hematocrit (Hct), red blood cell (RBC), and white blood cell (WBC) tests. A low Hgb and Hct can indicate anemia. Not a routine test, but ordered on many clients with heart conditions, is the lipid profile, which includes total serum cholesterol, high-density lipoprotein (HDL), low-density lipoprotein (LDL), and serum triglycerides. Urinalysis also can detect protein and sugar in the urine, which can indicate kidney disease and diabetes.

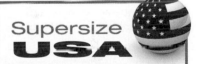

24-hour recall
listing the types, amounts, and preparation of all foods eaten in the past 24 hours

food diary
written record of all food and drink ingested in a specified period

EXPLORING
THE WEB

Search the Web for nutritional assessment tools. What resources are available for the health care professional in making nutritional assessments of clients? Assess the advantages and disadvantages of each tool you find.

The dietary-social history involves evaluation of food habits and is very important in the nutritional assessment of any client. It can be difficult to obtain an accurate dietary assessment. The most common method is the **24-hour recall**. In this method, the client is usually interviewed by the dietitian and is asked to give the types of, amounts of, and preparation used for all food eaten in the 24 hours prior to admission. Another method is the **food diary**. The client is asked to list all foods as they are eaten in a 3–4-day period. Neither method is totally accurate because clients forget or are not always truthful about their eating habits. They are sometimes inclined to say they have eaten certain foods because they know they should have done so. Computer analysis of the diet is the best way to determine if nutrient intake is appropriate. It will reveal any nutrient deficiencies or toxicities.

The dietary-social history is important to determine whether the client has the financial resources to obtain the needed food and the ability to properly store and cook food once home. After completing the dietary-social history, the dietitian can assess for risk of food–drug interactions that can lead to malnutrition (see Appendix E). Clients need to be instructed by a dietitian on possible interactions, if any.

When the preceding steps are evaluated together, and in the context of the client's medical condition, the dietitian has the best opportunity of making an accurate nutrition assessment of the client. This assessment can then be used by the entire health care team. The doctor will find it helpful in evaluating the client's condition and treatment. The dietitian can use the information to plan the client's dietary treatment and counseling, and other health care professionals will be able to use it in assisting and counseling the client.

HEALTH AND NUTRITION CONSIDERATIONS

The practice of good nutrition habits would help eliminate many health problems caused by malnutrition (Figure 1-4). The health professional is

FIGURE 1-4 Hands-on experiences foster the development of positive feelings about food.

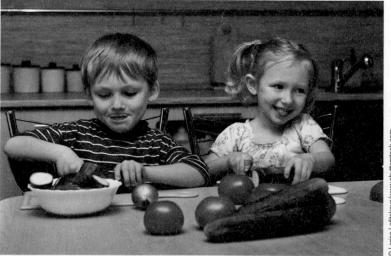

obligated to have a sound knowledge of nutrition. One's personal health, as well as that of one's family, depends on it. Parents must have a good, basic knowledge of nutrition for the sake of their personal health and that of their children. Children learn by imitating their parents. Family members and friends who know that the health professional has studied nutrition will ask questions. Anyone, in fact, who plans and prepares meals should value, have knowledge of, and be able to apply the principles of sound nutrition practice.

Clients will have questions and complaints about their diets. Their anxieties can be relieved by clear and simple explanations provided by the health professional. Sometimes clients must undergo diet therapy, prescribed by their physicians, which becomes part of their medical treatment in the hospital. The health professional must be able to check the client's tray quickly to see that it contains the correct foods for the diet prescribed. In many cases, diet therapy will have to be a lifelong practice for the client. In such cases, eating habits will have to be changed, and the client will need advice or instructions from a registered dietitian and support from other health professionals.

Nutrition is currently a popular subject. It is important to recognize that some books and articles concerning nutrition may not be scientifically correct. Also, food ads can be misleading. Nutrition information on websites may not always be accurate or even factual. People with knowledge of sound nutrition practices will be less likely to be misled. They will recognize fad and distinguish it from fact.

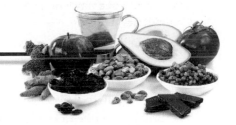

SUMMARY

Nutrition is directly related to health, and its effects are cumulative. Good nutrition is normally reflected by good health. Poor nutrition can result in poor health and even in disease. Poor nutrition habits contribute to atherosclerosis, osteoporosis, obesity, and some cancers.

To be well nourished, one must eat foods that contain the six essential nutrients: carbohydrates, fats, proteins, minerals, vitamins, and water. These nutrients provide the body with energy, build and repair body tissue, and regulate body processes. When there is a severe lack of specific nutrients, deficiency diseases may develop. The best way to determine deficiencies is to do a nutrition assessment.

With sound knowledge of nutrition, the health professional will be an effective health care provider and will also be helpful to family, friends, and self.

DISCUSSION TOPICS

1. Why is food commonly served at meetings and parties?

2. What relationship might nutrition and heredity have to each of the following?
   a. Development of physique
   b. Ability to resist disease
   c. Life span

3. What habits, in addition to good nutrition, contribute to making a person healthy?

4. What are the six classes of nutrients? What are their three basic functions?

5. Why are some foods called low-nutrient-density foods? Give some examples found in vending machines.

6. Ask anyone in the class who has been on a fad diet to discuss the diet's effects. Discuss possible reasons for those effects.

7. What is meant by the saying "You are what you eat"? Give specific examples of how the food we eat can affect our body and long-term consequences.

8. What is meant by the phrase "the cumulative effects of nutrition"? Describe some.

9. How could someone be overweight and at the same time suffer from malnutrition?

10. Discuss why health care professionals should be knowledgeable about nutrition.

SUGGESTED ACTIVITIES

1. List 10 signs of good nutrition and 10 signs of poor nutrition.

2. List the foods you have eaten in the past 24 hours. Underline those with low nutrient density.

3. Write a brief description of how you feel at the end of a day when you know you have not eaten wisely.

4. Name the laboratory tests used to determine nutritionally at-risk clients.

5. Write a brief paragraph discussing the nutrition assessment by a dietitian and its importance.

6. Briefly describe rickets, osteomalacia, and osteoporosis. Include their causes.

7. Ask a registered dietitian to speak to your class about nutrition problems commonly seen in your area.

REVIEW

Multiple choice. Select the *letter* that precedes the best answer.

1. The result of those processes whereby the body takes in and uses food for growth, development, and maintenance of health is
   a. respiration
   b. diet therapy
   c. nutrition
   d. digestion

2. Nutritional status is determined by
   a. heredity
   b. employment
   c. personality
   d. diet

3. To nourish the body adequately and to maintain health, one must
   a. avoid all low-nutrient-density foods
   b. eat foods containing the six classes of nutrients
   c. include fats at every meal
   d. restrict proteins at breakfast

4. Nutrients used primarily to provide energy to the body are
   a. vitamins, water, and minerals
   b. carbohydrates, proteins, and fats
   c. proteins, vitamins, and fats
   d. vitamins, minerals, and carbohydrates

5. Nutrients used mainly to build and repair body tissues are
   a. proteins, vitamins, and minerals
   b. carbohydrates, fats, and minerals
   c. fats, water, and minerals
   d. fats, vitamins, and minerals

6. Foods such as potato chips, cakes, sodas, and candy are
   a. high-nutrient-density foods
   b. essential nutrient foods
   c. low-nutrient-density foods
   d. nutritious foods

7. Overnutrition or undernutrition of the six classes of nutrients in the diet may result in
   a. increased energy
   b. malnutrition
   c. indigestion
   d. diabetes

8. The cumulative effect of a high-fat diet could be
   a. iron deficiency
   b. blindness
   c. heart disease
   d. diabetes mellitus

9. A cumulative condition is one that develops
   a. within a very short period of time
   b. over several years
   c. only in women under 52
   d. in premature infants

10. Malnutrition could be caused by
    a. poor posture
    b. constipation
    c. disease
    d. hypertension

11. Nutritional status
    a. is determined by heredity
    b. has no effect on mental health
    c. is not reflected in one's appearance
    d. can affect the body's ability to resist disease

12. Infants, young children, adolescents, pregnant adolescents, and the elderly
    a. are commonly overweight
    b. are among those prone to malnutrition
    c. all commonly suffer from osteomalacia
    d. never suffer from primary nutrient deficiencies

13. Organic nutrients are
    a. only found in products grown without pesticides
    b. only sold at health food stores
    c. substances that cannot be broken down
    d. substances containing a carbon atom

14. Which of the following would be an organic nutrient?
    a. fat
    b. folate
    c. calcium
    d. selenium

15. Anthropometric measures include measures of
    a. iron status
    b. fluid intake
    c. bone density
    d. weight

Case In Point

JAYDEN: COPING WITH MALNUTRITION

Jayden was living in an apartment with his mother Trina until recently when he was removed and placed in foster care. Jayden's aunt had contacted Child Protective Services because she was concerned about her sister's mental health and ability to care for Jayden. Jayden is only 5 years old and his mother Trina has multiple mental illnesses. Trina was diagnosed as a paranoid schizophrenic and has been on and off her medication depending on whether or not she can afford to purchase it. It was not uncommon for Trina to leave for extended periods of time without thought to Jayden's well-being. He often was without food, sufficient clothing, and clean surroundings. When Trina was home, she was often sleeping and Jayden was still left to fend for himself. When the social worker arrived at the home, she found it to be in disarray. There was very little food in the kitchen and trash and clutter was throughout the home. Jayden was found to be very thin, pale, and unclean. Jayden measured only 40 inches tall and weighed 30 pounds. The social worker noticed sores on his body, and his abdomen appeared to be very swollen. Jayden was complaining of pain in his legs and was having a difficult time walking. The social worker took Jayden to the emergency room for assessment and arranged for a foster family to be assigned to him.

ASSESSMENT

1. List five characteristics of poor nutritional status.
2. Identify characteristics of malnutrition that Jayden is experiencing.
3. Jayden needs to be provided with good nutrition and adequate calories. What would be important to consider in providing meals for Jayden?
4. Name five lab tests that the physician may order to help assess Jayden's nutrition and hydration status.

DIAGNOSIS

5. Write a nursing diagnosis for Jayden.

PLAN/GOAL

6. What two changes can you predict will occur with the introduction of a good, nutritionally sound diet?
7. Whom can you refer to for assistance?

IMPLEMENTATION

8. Name at least three nursing interventions that could be employed to improve Jayden's nutrition.
9. How might Jayden's dental status impact his nutrition?
10. Would a home visit be beneficial for Jayden and a caregiver?

EVALUATION/OUTCOME CRITERIA

11. What could the doctor assess at the next appointment to see if the plan is working?
12. What observations could the caregiver offer about the success of the plan?
13. What could be an important piece of information from Jayden?

THINKING FURTHER

14. How could the Internet be of benefit to the caregiver?

rate this **plate**

Jayden has been through a lot of heartache for a child his age. He is placed in a foster home, and his foster mother asks him what he would like to eat for his first dinner with them. He thought and thought and finally decided on the following plate. Rate this plate. Take into consideration that Jayden is malnourished, has not eaten much lately, and is lacking many nutrients.

Fried chicken thigh

½ cup mashed potatoes and 2 Tbsp gravy

½ cup corn with butter

Biscuit with butter

2% milk—8 oz.

Can Jayden eat all of this, and should he? Does this plate need to be changed, and how would you change it?

Case In Point

Asnaku lives in a small village in Ethiopia. Her family is not wealthy and is unable to travel to see a doctor. There is a nurse who visits the village a few times a year, but that is the extent of the medical care Asnaku's family receives. The last time the nurse visited she talked to Asnaku's mother about what her family typically eats. The nurse was a little concerned that Asnaku's family eats mostly grains. They rarely get meat, fruit, or vegetable sources. She spoke with Asnaku's mother about some of the signs and symptoms of vitamin deficiencies that could result from a diet with little access to a wider variety of foods. The nurse told her mother she would return in a few months and she would have a mission team with her. These nurses and doctors were coming to provide medical care and assistance to the entire village. She told Asnaku's mother they would be bringing vitamin supplements that would help prevent nutritional deficiencies as well as other medications. Asnaku's mother has been worried for a while that Asnaku may have a problem with her eyes. Asnaku is 7 years old now and has been fairly independent with her self-care. However, she has noticed that Asnaku has gotten lost in the night a couple of times trying to go to the bathroom. She also has had difficulty with tasks she has asked her to do after the sun goes down. She is worried that she is not able to see very well, yet during the day she seems fine. The mission team is to return in a couple of weeks and her mother has requested Asnaku be evaluated as to what could be wrong.

ASSESSMENT

1. What are the symptoms of vitamin A deficiency?
2. What is Asnaku experiencing that would suggest a vitamin A deficiency?
3. Make a list of foods that are high in vitamin A that should be incorporated in Asnaku's diet?
4. Think about Asnaku's grain-based diet. What other vitamin or mineral deficiencies could she have?

DIAGNOSIS

5. Write a nursing diagnosis for Asnaku.

PLAN/GOAL

6. What change can you predict will occur with the introduction of vitamin A?
7. What can be done to ensure that Asnaku is able to get the vitamin A her body needs?

IMPLEMENTATION

8. If Asnaku was hospitalized under your care, what interventions might you suggest for her care?
9. In the United States, vitamin A deficiency is nearly unheard of, when compared to Third World countries. There are children in the United States who have diets that do not meet their caloric needs and have little nutritional quality. Why is vitamin A deficiency in the United States so much lower than in other countries?
10. Can you think of other examples of food sources that have been fortified to avoid deficiencies in vitamins or minerals?

EVALUATION/OUTCOME CRITERIA

11. What could the nurse assess at her next visit to Asnaku's village to see if the plan is working?

THINKING FURTHER

12. Access the World Health Organization's web page and read about the programs in place to provide vitamin A supplements to countries worldwide. Briefly discuss this program and the severity of this problem.

rate this plate

Asnaku's night-blindness sounds like a vitamin A deficiency. As the family does not eat anything grown, such as vegetables and fruit, nutrient deficiencies can result. Having access to biofortified rice can provide Asnaku and her family with nutrients including vitamin A, iron, zinc, and iodine. Asnaku ate the following:

½ cup of fortified rice
¾ cup of vegetable stew
1 slice of flatbread

If Asnaku ate this meal three times a day, would the fortified rice be sufficient to provide her with 100% of her vitamin A and iron needs? What is the role of each nutrient within the biofortified rice?

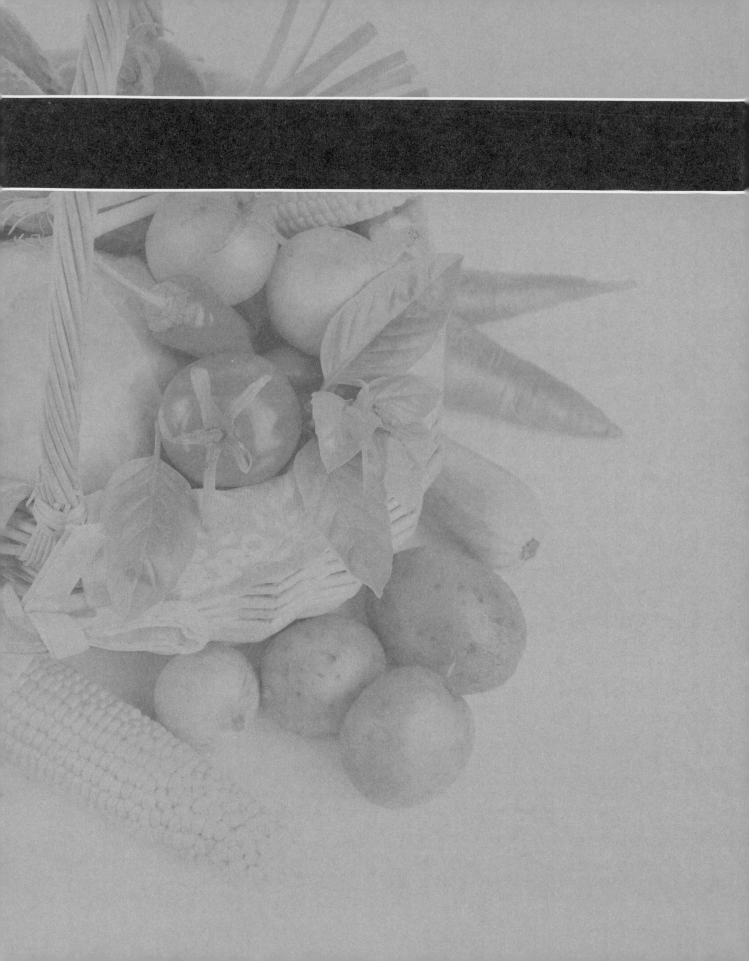

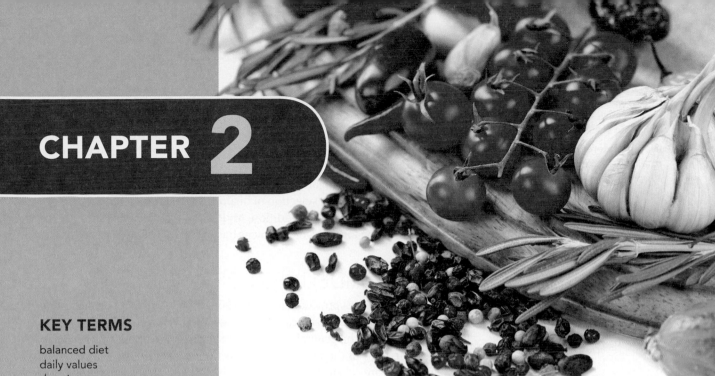

CHAPTER 2

KEY TERMS

balanced diet
daily values
descriptors
Dietary Guidelines for Americans
dietary laws
Dietary Reference Intakes (DRIs)
flavonoids
food customs
foodways
fusion
lacto-ovo vegetarians
lactose intolerance
lacto-vegetarians
legumes
masa harina
mirin
miso
MyPlate
vegans
wasabi

PLANNING
A HEALTHY DIET

OBJECTIVES

After studying this chapter, you should be able to:

- Define a balanced diet
- List the U.S. government's Dietary Guidelines for Americans and explain the reasons for each
- Identify the food groups and their placement on MyPlate
- Describe information commonly found on food labels
- List some food customs of various cultural groups
- Describe the development of food customs

The statement "eat a balanced diet" has been repeated so often that its importance may be overlooked. The value of this statement is so great, however, that it deserves serious consideration by people of all ages. A **balanced diet** includes all six classes of nutrients and calories in amounts that preserve and promote good health.

balanced diet
one that includes all the essential nutrients in appropriate amounts

Dietary Reference Intakes (DRIs)
combines the Recommended Dietary Allowances, Adequate Intake, Estimated Average Requirements, and the Tolerable Upper Intake Levels for individuals into one value representative of the average daily nutrient intake of individuals over time

Dietary Guidelines for Americans
general goals for optimal nutrient intake

MyPlate
outline for making selections based on *Dietary Guidelines for America, 2010*, from the U.S. Department of Agriculture

EXPLORING THE WEB

The *Dietary Guidelines for Americans 2010* (7th edition) offers science-based advice and suggestions for improving health through sound nutrition and physical activity. These guidelines serve as helpful reminders to many Americans, especially those who are overweight or obese, who eat too much fat, and who no longer think exercise is important. The Dietary Guidelines encourage a healthy diet, which means individuals should choose from the following:

- Fruits, vegetables, whole grains, and fat-free or low-fat milk and milk products
- Lean meats, poultry, fish, beans, eggs, and nuts
- Foods low in saturated fats, trans fats, cholesterol, salt (sodium), and added sugars

Visit http://www.choosemyplate.gov/dietary-guidelines.html to learn more about the *Dietary Guidelines for Americans, 2010*.

Daily review of the **Dietary Reference Intakes (DRIs)** and the Recommended Dietary Allowances (RDAs) would provide enough information to plan balanced diets. However, ordinary meal planning would be cumbersome and time consuming if that table had to be consulted each time a meal was planned. Fortunately, the U.S. Department of Agriculture (USDA) and the U.S. Department of Health and Human Services (USDHHS) developed a simple system to help with the selection of healthful diets. It is called the **Dietary Guidelines for Americans**. In addition, **MyPlate** was released in 2010 by the USDA as an outline for daily food choices based on the Dietary Guidelines.

DIETARY GUIDELINES FOR AMERICANS

The Dietary Guidelines provide science-based advice to promote health and to reduce the risk of chronic diseases through diet and physical activity. The guidelines are targeted to the general public over 2 years of age in the United States. Below are the titles of the topics for each section; all of the following key recommendations are taken from http://www.health.gov/dietaryguidelines. The Dietary Guidelines themselves form an integrated set of key recommendations in each of the topic areas and will be discussed under the respective topics.

- Adequate nutrients within calorie needs
- Weight management
- Physical activity
- Food groups to encourage
- Fats
- Carbohydrates
- Sodium and potassium
- Alcoholic beverages
- Food safety

Adequate Nutrients within Calorie Needs

A basic premise of the Dietary Guidelines is that recommended diets will provide all the nutrients needed for growth and health and that the nutrients consumed should come primarily from foods. Foods contain not only the vitamins and minerals found in supplements, but also hundreds of naturally occurring substances, including carotenoids, flavonoids and isoflavones, and protease inhibitors that may protect against chronic health conditions.

Key Recommendations

Maintain calorie balance over time to achieve and sustain a healthy weight. People who are most successful at achieving and maintaining a healthy weight do so through continued attention to consuming only enough calories from foods and beverages to meet their needs and by being physically active. To curb the obesity epidemic, many Americans must decrease the calories they consume and increase the calories they expend through physical activity. Focus on consuming nutrient-dense foods and beverages. Americans currently consume too much sodium and too many calories from solid fats, added sugars, and refined grains. These replace nutrient-dense foods and beverages and make it difficult for people to achieve recommended nutrient intake while controlling calorie and sodium intake. A healthy eating pattern limits the intake of sodium, solid fats, added sugars, and refined grains and emphasizes nutrient-dense foods and beverages—vegetables, fruits, whole grains, fat-free or low-fat milk and milk products, seafood, lean meats and poultry, eggs, beans and peas, and nuts and seeds.

Weight Management

Over the last 20 years, the prevalence of overweight in the general population, and especially among children and adolescents, has increased substantially. According to data from the 2007–2008 U.S. National Health and Nutrition Examination Survey program (NHANES), the prevalence of obesity reached 10% for children aged 2–5 years, 20% for children aged 6–11 years, and 18% for adolescents aged 12–19 years. Overweight and obesity of both adults and children are of great public health concern because excess body fat leads to a higher risk of premature death, type 2 diabetes, hypertension, dyslipidemia, cardiovascular disease, stroke, gallbladder disease, and other chronic diseases.

Key Recommendations

- Prevent and/or reduce overweight and obesity through improved eating and physical activity behaviors. Control total calorie intake to manage body weight. For people who are overweight or obese, this will mean consuming fewer calories from foods and beverages.

- Increase physical activity and reduce time spent in sedentary behaviors. Maintain appropriate calorie balance during each stage of life—childhood, adolescence, adulthood, pregnancy and breastfeeding, and older age.

Key Recommendations for Specific Population Groups

- *Women* are encouraged to achieve and maintain a healthy weight before becoming pregnant. This may reduce a woman's risk of complications during pregnancy, increase the chances of a healthy infant birth weight, and improve the long-term health of both mother and infant.

- *Pregnant women* are encouraged to gain weight within the 2009 Institute of Medicine (IOM) gestational weight gain guidelines. Maternal weight gain during pregnancy outside the recommended range is associated with increased risks for maternal and child health.

- *Adults ages 65 years and older* who are overweight are encouraged to not gain additional weight. Among older adults who are obese, particularly those with cardiovascular disease risk factors, intentional weight loss can be beneficial and result in improved quality of life and reduced risk of chronic diseases and associated disabilities.

- *Children and adolescents* are encouraged to maintain calorie balance to support normal growth and development without promoting excess weight gain. Children and adolescents who are overweight or obese should change their eating and physical activity behaviors so that their BMI-for-age percentile does not increase over time. Further more, a health care provider should be consulted to determine appropriate weight management for the child or adolescent.

Physical Activity

Americans are relatively inactive. Regular physical activity and physical fitness make important contributions to one's health, sense of well-being, and maintenance of a healthy body weight. Physical activity is defined as any bodily movement produced by skeletal muscles, resulting in energy expenditure. Regular physical activity has been shown to reduce the risk of certain chronic diseases, including high blood pressure, stroke, coronary artery disease, type 2 diabetes, colon cancer, and osteoporosis. Therefore, it is recommended that adults should participate in 150 minutes of moderate-intensity aerobic activity each week to maintain a healthy body weight. Regular physical activity is also a key factor in achieving and maintaining a healthy body weight for adults and children (Tables 2-1 and 2-2). It is recommended that males above age 40 and females above age 50 check with their health care provider before beginning aerobic activities.

Key Recommendations

- Engage in regular physical activity and reduce sedentary activities to promote health, psychological well-being, and healthy body weight.
  - To reduce the risk of chronic disease in adulthood, engage in at least 30 minutes of moderate-intensity physical activity, above usual activity, at work or home on most days of the week. For most people, greater health benefits can be obtained by engaging in physical activity of more vigorous intensity or longer duration.
- To help manage body weight and prevent gradual, unhealthy body weight gain in adulthood, engage in approximately 60 minutes of moderate- to vigorous-intensity activity on most days of the week while not exceeding caloric intake requirements.
- To sustain weight loss in adulthood, participate in at least 60 to 90 minutes of daily moderate-intensity physical activity while not exceeding caloric intake requirements. Some people may need to consult with a health care provider before participating in this level of activity.
- Achieve physical fitness by including cardiovascular conditioning, stretching exercises for flexibility, and resistance exercises or calisthenics for muscle strength and endurance.

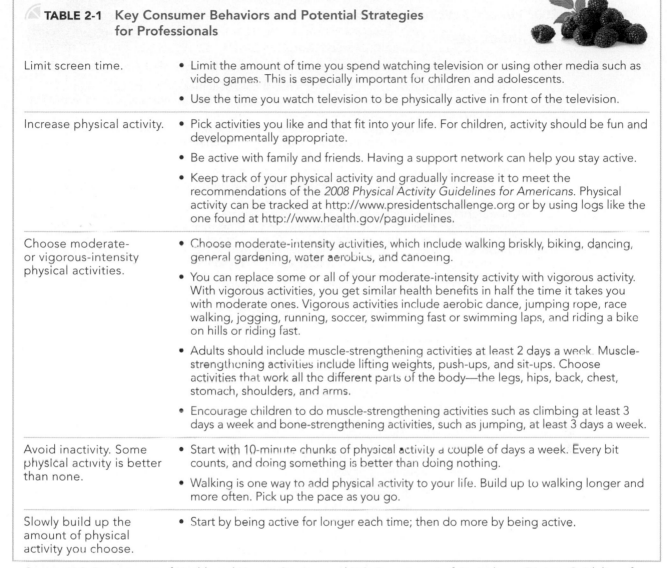

TABLE 2-1 Key Consumer Behaviors and Potential Strategies for Professionals

Limit screen time.	• Limit the amount of time you spend watching television or using other media such as video games. This is especially important for children and adolescents. • Use the time you watch television to be physically active in front of the television.
Increase physical activity.	• Pick activities you like and that fit into your life. For children, activity should be fun and developmentally appropriate. • Be active with family and friends. Having a support network can help you stay active. • Keep track of your physical activity and gradually increase it to meet the recommendations of the *2008 Physical Activity Guidelines for Americans*. Physical activity can be tracked at http://www.presidentschallenge.org or by using logs like the one found at http://www.health.gov/paguidelines.
Choose moderate- or vigorous-intensity physical activities.	• Choose moderate-intensity activities, which include walking briskly, biking, dancing, general gardening, water aerobics, and canoeing. • You can replace some or all of your moderate-intensity activity with vigorous activity. With vigorous activities, you get similar health benefits in half the time it takes you with moderate ones. Vigorous activities include aerobic dance, jumping rope, race walking, jogging, running, soccer, swimming fast or swimming laps, and riding a bike on hills or riding fast. • Adults should include muscle-strengthening activities at least 2 days a week. Muscle-strengthening activities include lifting weights, push-ups, and sit-ups. Choose activities that work all the different parts of the body—the legs, hips, back, chest, stomach, shoulders, and arms. • Encourage children to do muscle-strengthening activities such as climbing at least 3 days a week and bone-strengthening activities, such as jumping, at least 3 days a week.
Avoid inactivity. Some physical activity is better than none.	• Start with 10-minute chunks of physical activity a couple of days a week. Every bit counts, and doing something is better than doing nothing. • Walking is one way to add physical activity to your life. Build up to walking longer and more often. Pick up the pace as you go.
Slowly build up the amount of physical activity you choose.	• Start by being active for longer each time; then do more by being active.

Source: U.S. Department of Health and Human Services and U.S. Department of Agriculture. *Dietary Guidelines for Americans, 2010* (7th ed.). Accessed December 2011 from http://www.cnpp.usda.gov

Food Groups to Encourage

Increased intakes of fruits, vegetables, whole grains, and fat-free or low-fat milk products will have important health benefits. Those who eat more generous amounts of fruits and vegetables as part of a healthful diet may reduce the risk of chronic diseases, including stroke and other cardiovascular diseases, type 2 diabetes, and cancers in certain sites (oral cavity and pharynx, larynx, lung, esophagus, stomach, and colon-rectum). In addition to fruits and vegetables, whole grains are an important source of fiber and other nutrients. Consuming at least three or more ounce-equivalents of whole grains per day can reduce the risk of several chronic diseases and may help with weight maintenance. Table 2-3 can help one recognize the names of whole grains.

TABLE 2-2 2008 Physical Activity Guidelines

AGE GROUP	GUIDELINES
6 to 17 years	Children and adolescents should do 60 minutes (1 hour) or more of physical activity daily.

- Aerobic: Most of the 60 or more minutes a day should be either moderate (a) or vigorous (b) intensity aerobic physical activity, and should include vigorous-intensity physical activity at least 3 days a week.
- Muscle-strengthening (c): As part of their 60 or more minutes of daily physical activity, children and adolescents should include muscle-strengthening physical activity on at least 3 days of the week.
- Bone-strengthening (d): As part of their 60 or more minutes of daily physical activity, children and adolescents should include bone-strengthening physical activity on at least 3 days of the week.
- It is important to encourage young people to participate in physical activities that are appropriate for their age, that are enjoyable, and that offer variety.

AGE GROUP	GUIDELINES
18 to 64 years	All adults should avoid inactivity. Some physical activity is better than none, and adults who participate in any amount of physical activity gain some health benefits.

- For substantial health benefits, adults should do at least 150 minutes (2 hours and 30 minutes) a week of moderate-intensity, or 75 minutes (1 hour and 15 minutes) a week of vigorous-intensity aerobic physical activity, or an equivalent combination of moderate- and vigorous-intensity aerobic activity. Aerobic activity should be performed in episodes of at least 10 minutes, and preferably, it should be spread throughout the week.
- For additional and more extensive health benefits, adults should increase their aerobic physical activity to 300 minutes (5 hours) a week of moderate-intensity, or 150 minutes a week of vigorous-intensity aerobic physical activity, or an equivalent combination of moderate- and vigorous-intensity activity. Additional health benefits are gained by engaging in physical activity beyond this amount.
- Adults should also include muscle-strengthening activities that involve all major muscle groups on 2 or more days a week.

AGE GROUP	GUIDELINES
65 years and older	Older adults should follow the adult guidelines. When older adults cannot meet the adult guidelines, they should be as physically active as their abilities and conditions will allow.

- Older adults should do exercises that maintain or improve balance if they are at risk of falling.
- Older adults should determine their level of effort for physical activity relative to their level of fitness.
- Older adults with chronic conditions should understand whether and how their conditions affect their ability to do regular physical activity safely.

a. Moderate-intensity physical activity: Aerobic activity that increases a person's heart rate and breathing to some extent. On a scale relative to a person's capacity, moderate-intensity activity is usually a 5 or 6 on a 0 to 10 scale. Brisk walking, dancing, swimming, or bicycling on a level terrain are examples.

b. Vigorous-intensity physical activity: Aerobic activity that greatly increases a person's heart rate and breathing. On a scale relative to a person's capacity, vigorous-intensity activity is usually a 7 or 8 on a 0 to 10 scale. Jogging, singles tennis, swimming continuous laps, or bicycling uphill are examples.

c. Muscle-strengthening activity: Physical activity, including exercise, that increases skeletal muscle strength, power, endurance, and mass. It includes strength training, resistance training, and muscular strength and endurance exercises.

d. Bone-strengthening activity: Physical activity that produces an impact or tension force on bones, which promotes bone growth and strength. Running, jumping rope, and lifting weights are examples.

Source: U.S. Department of Health and Human Services. *2008 Physical Activity Guidelines for Americans.* Washington, DC: U.S. Department of Health and Human Services. 2008. ODPHP Publication No. U0036. Accessed December 2011 from http://www.health.gov/paguidelines

TABLE 2-3 Key Consumer Behaviors and Potential Strategies for Increasing Whole Grains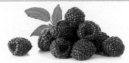

BEHAVIOR	STRATEGIES
Increase whole-grain intake. Consume at least half of all grains as whole grains.	• Substitute whole-grain choices for refined grains in breakfast cereals, breads, crackers, rice, and pasta. For example, choose 100% whole-grain breads; whole-grain cereals such as oatmeal; whole-grain crackers and pasta; and brown rice.
	• Check the ingredients list on product labels for the words "whole" or "whole grain" before the grain ingredient's name.
	• Note that foods labeled with the words "multi-grain," "stone-ground," "100% wheat," "cracked wheat," "seven-grain," or "bran" are usually not 100% whole-grain products, and may not contain any whole grains.
	• Use the Nutrition Facts label and the ingredients list to choose whole grains that are a good or excellent source of dietary fiber. Good sources of fiber contain 10 to 19 percent of the Daily Value per serving, and excellent sources of dietary fiber contain 20 percent or more.

Source: U.S. Department of Health and Human Services and U.S. Department of Agriculture. *Dietary Guidelines for Americans, 2010* (7th ed.). Accessed December 2011 from http://www.cnpp.usda.gov

SPOTLIGHT *on Life Cycle*

Adequate calcium intake and weight-bearing activity are important components in optimizing bone mass and decreasing the risk of osteoporosis. Calcium consumption is especially important during the preteen and teen years, when bones are growing at the fastest rate. By age 17 most teens have finished their growth spurts and have established 90% of their adult bone mass. Unfortunately, the majority of teens do not meet the recommended intake for calcium (1,300 mg/day). Rich sources of calcium include low-fat or fat-free milk, cheese, and yogurt; dark green leafy vegetables; calcium-fortified foods such as orange juice, cereal, bread, and tofu products; and nuts such as almonds. Adequate weight-bearing activity is also important in achieving and maintaining peak bone mass. Activities such as walking, playing tennis or basketball, jumping rope, dancing, and weightlifting can be incorporated into any exercise plan to keep bones healthy.

The most common nutrient deficiency in the world is lack of iron. This is particularly prevalent among infants, adolescents, and pregnant and menstruating women. It can result in iron-deficiency anemia. The health care provider can help by:

- Identifying those clients at risk (e.g., children under 2 years of age, adolescents, women with heavy menstrual flow, pregnant women, individuals with malabsorption syndromes, gastrointestinal bleedings, and gross dietary deficiencies).
- Performing complete nutritional assessments on high-risk clients.
- Encouraging clients to eat foods high in iron. These include lean meats, poultry, fish, enriched breads, legumes, leafy green vegetables, dried fruits, and nuts.

Key Recommendations

- Increase vegetable and fruit intake. Eat a variety of vegetables—especially dark green, red, and orange vegetables; beans and peas.

- Consume at least half of all grains as whole grains. Increase whole-grain intake by replacing refined grains with whole grains.

- Increase intake of fat-free or low-fat milk and milk products, such as milk, yogurt, cheese, or fortified soy beverages.
- Choose a variety of protein foods, which include seafood, lean meat and poultry, eggs, beans and peas, soy products, and unsalted seeds or nuts.
- Increase the amount and variety of seafood consumed by choosing seafood in place of some meat and poultry.
- Replace protein foods that are higher in solid fats with choices that are lower in solid fats and calories and/or are sources of oils.
- Use oils to replace solid fats where possible.
- Choose foods that provide more potassium, dietary fiber, calcium, and vitamin D, which are nutrients of concern in American diets. These foods include vegetables, fruits, whole grains, milk and milk products.

Key Recommendations for Specific Population Groups

- *Women capable of becoming pregnant.* Choose foods that supply heme iron, iron supplied through animal sources, which is more readily absorbed by the body, additional iron sources, and enhancers of iron absorption such as vitamin C-rich foods. Consume 400 micrograms (mcg) per day of synthetic folic acid (from fortified foods and/or supplements) in addition to food forms of folate from a varied diet.
- *Women who are pregnant or breastfeeding.* Consume 8–12 ounces of seafood per week from a variety of seafood types. Due to their methyl mercury content, limit white (albacore) tuna to 6 ounces per week and do not eat the following four types of fish: tilefish, shark, swordfish, and king mackerel. If pregnant, take an iron supplement as recommended by an obstetrician or other health care provider.
- *Individuals ages 50 years and older.* Consume foods fortified with vitamin B_{12}, such as fortified cereals, or dietary supplements.

Fats

Fats and oils are part of a healthful diet, but the type of fat makes a difference to heart health, and the total amount of fat consumed is also important. High intake of saturated fats, trans fats, and cholesterol increases the risk of coronary heart disease due to high blood lipid levels. Fats supply energy and essential fatty acids and serve as a carrier for the absorption of the fat-soluble vitamins A, D, E, and K and carotenoids.

Key Recommendations

- Consume less than 10% of calories from saturated fatty acids by replacing them with monounsaturated and polyunsaturated fatty acids.

- Consume less than 300 mg per day of dietary cholesterol. Keep trans fatty acid consumption as low as possible, especially by limiting foods that contain synthetic sources of trans fats, such as partially hydrogenated oils, and by limiting other solid fats. Focus on eating the most nutrient-dense forms of foods from all food groups. Limit the amount of solid fats and added sugars when cooking or eating (e.g., trimming fat from meat, using less butter and stick margarine, and using less table sugar).

Consume fewer and smaller portions of foods and beverages that contain solid fats and/or added sugars, such as grain-based desserts, sodas, and other sugar-sweetened beverages.

Carbohydrates

Carbohydrates are part of a healthful diet. Foods in the basic food groups that provide carbohydrates—fruits, vegetables, grains, and milk—are important sources of many nutrients. Dietary fiber is composed of nondigestible carbohydrates. Sugars and starches supply energy to the body in the form of glucose. Sugars can be naturally present in foods or added to the food. The greater the consumption of foods containing large amounts of added sugars, the more difficult it is to consume enough nutrients without gaining weight. See Table 2-4 to help identify the names of added sugar on labels.

Key Recommendations

At least half of recommended total grain intake should be whole grains. Americans should aim to replace many refined-grain foods with whole-grain foods that are in their nutrient-dense forms to keep total calorie intake within limits.

TABLE 2-4 Key Consumer Behaviors and Potential Strategies for Decreasing Added Sugar Consumption 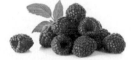	
BEHAVIOR	**STRATEGIES**
Cut back on foods and drinks with added sugars or caloric sweeteners (sugar-sweetened beverages).	• Drink few or no regular sodas, sports drinks, energy drinks, and fruit drinks. Eat less cake, cookies, ice cream, other desserts, and candy. If you do have these foods and drinks, have a small portion. These drinks and foods are the major sources of added sugars for Americans. • Choose water, fat-free milk, 100% fruit juice, or unsweetened tea or coffee as drinks rather than sugar-sweetened drinks. Select fruit for dessert. Eat less of high-calorie desserts. • Use the Nutrition Facts label to choose breakfast cereals and other packaged foods with less total sugars, and use the ingredients list to choose foods with little or no added sugars.

Source: U.S. Department of Health and Human Services and U.S. Department of Agriculture. *Dietary Guidelines for Americans, 2010* (7th ed.). Accessed December 2011 from http://www.cnpp.usda.gov

EXPLORING THE WEB

Explore the Web to learn how much sodium the average American is consuming on a daily basis and how this amount compares to the new recommendation set by the 2010 Dietary Guidelines for Americans. What foods are high in sodium? What are some strategies to help reduce the amount of sodium intake in the American diet? What are some health risks associated with increased sodium intake? Research the CDC and/or FDA for more information.

Sodium and Potassium

On average, the higher one's salt (sodium chloride) intake, the higher one's blood pressure. Keeping blood pressure in the normal range reduces one's risk of coronary heart disease, stroke, congestive heart failure, and kidney disease. When reading labels, look for the sodium content; foods that are low in sodium (less than 140 mg) are low in salt. Lifestyle changes including reducing salt intake, increasing potassium intake, losing excess body weight, increasing physical activity, and eating an overall healthful diet can prevent or delay the onset of high blood pressure and can lower elevated blood pressure.

Key Recommendations

Americans can reduce their consumption of sodium in a variety of ways:

- Consume less than 2,300 mg of sodium (approximately 1 teaspoon of salt) per day. Read the Nutrition Facts label for information on the sodium content of foods and purchase foods that are low in sodium.

- Consume more fresh foods and fewer processed foods that are high in sodium.

- Eat more home-prepared foods, where you have more control over sodium, and use little or no salt or salt-containing seasonings when cooking or eating foods.

    When eating at restaurants, ask that salt not be added to your food or order lower sodium options, if available.

Key Recommendations for Specific Population Groups

Americans should reduce their sodium intake to less than 2,300 mg or 1,500 mg per day depending on age and other individual characteristics (Table 2-5). African Americans, individuals with hypertension, diabetes, or chronic kidney disease, and individuals ages 51 and older comprise about half of the U.S. population ages 2 and older. While nearly everyone benefits from reducing their sodium intake, the blood pressure of these individuals tends to be even more responsive to the blood pressure–raising effects of sodium than others; therefore, they should reduce their sodium intake to 1,500 mg per day.

Alcoholic Beverages

Alcoholic beverages supply calories but few essential nutrients. As a result, excessive alcohol consumption makes it difficult to eat sufficient nutrients within one's daily calories and to maintain a healthy weight. Alcohol also interferes with nutritional processes, affecting digestion, storage, utilization, and excretion of nutrients. Alcoholic beverages are harmful when consumed in excess.

Key Recommendations

- Those who choose to drink alcoholic beverages should do so sensibly and in moderation—defined as the consumption of up to one drink per day for women and up to two drinks per day for men.

TABLE 2-5 Estimated Mean Daily Sodium Intake, by Age-Gender Group

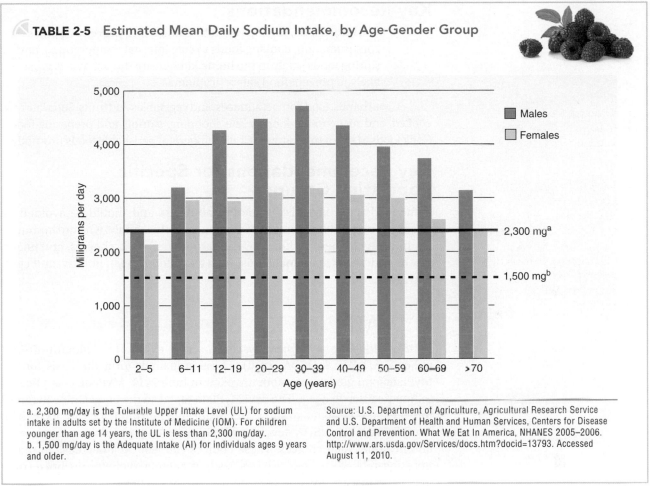

a. 2,300 mg/day is the Tolerable Upper Intake Level (UL) for sodium intake in adults set by the Institute of Medicine (IOM). For children younger than age 14 years, the UL is less than 2,300 mg/day.
b. 1,500 mg/day is the Adequate Intake (AI) for individuals ages 9 years and older.

Source: U.S. Department of Agriculture, Agricultural Research Service and U.S. Department of Health and Human Services, Centers for Disease Control and Prevention. What We Eat In America, NHANES 2005–2006. http://www.ars.usda.gov/Services/docs.htm?docid=13793. Accessed August 11, 2010.

Source: U.S. Department of Health and Human Services and U.S. Department of Agriculture. *Dietary Guidelines for Americans, 2010* (7th ed.). Accessed December 2011 from http://www.cnpp.usda.gov

- Alcoholic beverages should not be consumed by some individuals, including those who cannot restrict their alcohol intake, women of child-bearing age who may become pregnant, pregnant and lactating women, children and adolescents, individuals taking medications that can interact with alcohol, and those with specific medical conditions.
- Alcoholic beverages should be avoided by individuals engaging in activities that require attention, skill, or coordination, such as driving or operating machinery.

Food Safety

Avoiding foods that are contaminated with harmful bacteria, viruses, parasites, toxins, and chemical and physical contaminants is vital for healthful eating. It is estimated that every year about 76 million people in the United States become ill from pathogens in food. Chapter 10 discusses this further.

Key Recommendations

- Washing hands, rinsing vegetables and fruits, preventing cross-contamination, cooking foods to safe internal temperatures, and storing foods safely in the home kitchen are the behaviors most likely to prevent food safety problems.

Clean hands, food contact surfaces, and vegetables and fruits. Separate raw, cooked, and ready-to-eat foods while shopping, storing, and preparing foods. Cook foods to safe temperatures. Chill (refrigerate) perishable foods promptly.

Key Recommendations for Specific Population Groups

Some foods pose high risk of foodborne illness and should be avoided by infants, young children, pregnant women, and older adults who are immuno-compromised. These include raw (unpasteurized) milk, cheeses, and juices; raw or undercooked animal foods, such as seafood, meat, poultry, and eggs; and raw sprouts.

MYPLATE

Dietary Guidelines for Americans, 2010 serves as the U.S. federal nutrition policy (USDHHS & USDA, 2010). These guidelines form the basis for the MyPlate food guidance system unveiled in June 2011. MyPlate is applicable to Americans over age 2. The new MyPlate replaced the Food Guide Pyramid in 2011 and is designed to show Americans that nutrition does not have to be complicated. The USDA developed MyPlate to help people make informed and healthier food choices. These choices can lead to a decrease in major nutrition-related chronic diseases, such as anemia, diabetes mellitus, coronary heart disease, hypertension, and alcoholic cirrhosis.

MyPlate, by its divisions and colors, represents the types of foods that should be consumed. The size of the divisions within the plate denotes the approximate relative quantity of each food that should be consumed. MyPlate is based on a 9-inch plate, to encourage portion control. Personalization of one's diet is easier to accomplish by accessing the MyPlate website (http://www.choosemyplate.gov), where age and gender can be keyed in to customize guidelines. The exercise component for health and weight management can be accessed at this website as well. Clicking on MyPlate allows interaction and animation that can be used to explore additional information. By following the MyPlate method, an individual should be able to maintain a healthy body weight and decrease the risk of nutrition-related chronic diseases. Quantities are stated in household measures such as cups and ounces instead of servings that were used in the Food Guide Pyramid.

MyPlate Features

MyPlate has the following features:

- *Weight Management and Calories:* Provides detailed information about maintaining a healthy weight and making better food choices. The links provided on this site explain empty calories and how to manage calorie intake.

- *Physical Activity:* Defines physical activity, recommends how much physical activity is needed, and provides tips for physical activity. These features are important because being physically active can improve one's health.

- *SuperTracker:* Allows users to plan, analyze, and track their diet and physical activity. Using this resource, individuals can look up nutrition information for over 8,000 foods and compare foods side-by-side. Goals for weight management and healthy eating can be tracked using this feature.

- *Healthy Eating Tips:* Provides a wealth of information and suggestions that can help individuals get started toward a healthy diet. Sample menus and recipes, tips for vegetarians, tips for eating out, and food safety advice can be found within this feature.

MyPlate (Figure 2-1) has five colored portions representing five food groups. The divisions within the plate represent portions, but specifics about each group can be found on the website (http://www.choosemyplate.gov). The five food groups are the same as MyPyramid, but do not include fat. Fats and oils are listed on this website as well. The five groups are:

- Grains—bread, cereal, rice, and pasta group
- Vegetable group

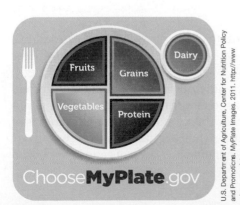

U.S. Department of Agriculture, Center for Nutrition Policy and Promotions. MyPlate Images. 2011. http://www .choosemyplate.gov

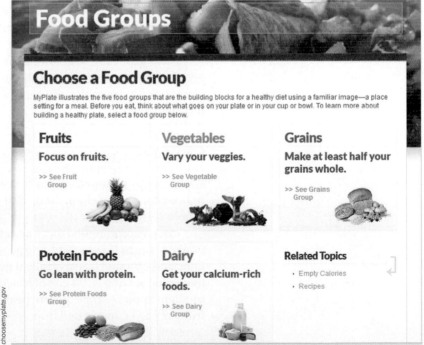

U.S. Department of Agriculture, Center for Nutrition Policy and Promotions. MyPlate Images. 2011. http://www.choosemyplate.gov

FIGURE 2-1 MyPlate guide for healthy eating.

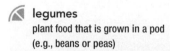

legumes
plant food that is grown in a pod
(e.g., beans or peas)

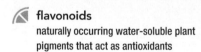

flavonoids
naturally occurring water-soluble plant
pigments that act as antioxidants

- Fruit group
- Dairy group
- Protein group

The emphasis of MyPlate, which takes its guidance from the *Dietary Guidelines for Americans, 2010*, is not based on a percentage of intake but on daily servings. Depending on the information one enters into MyPlate, a calorie level will be individually determined. See Table 2-6 for intake patterns for various caloric levels.

Grain Group

Any food made from wheat, rice, oats, cornmeal, barley, or another cereal grain is a grain product. Bread, pasta, oatmeal, breakfast cereals, tortillas, and grits are examples of grain products (Table 2-7). Intake of whole grains should be greater than refined grains (see Chapter 4 for more information). Whole grains provide dietary fiber, B vitamins, iron, and magnesium. Enriched products also contain B vitamins and iron, but if they are not made from whole grains, they contain little dietary fiber.

Vegetable Group

The food intake patterns have established the number of daily servings per calorie level of vegetable. All vegetables are included in the vegetable group: green and leafy, yellow, starchy, and **legumes** (Table 2-8). Vegetables provide carbohydrates; dietary fiber; vitamins A, B-complex, C, E, and K; and iron, calcium, phosphorus, potassium, magnesium, copper, manganese, and sometimes molybdenum.

This guideline, if followed, also guarantees that one will receive a variety of nutrients, phytochemicals, and **flavonoids**. One-half cup of cooked or chopped raw vegetables or 2 cups of uncooked, leafy vegetables is considered one serving.

Fruit Group

All fruits are included in the fruit group. They provide vitamins A and C, potassium, magnesium, iron, and carbohydrates, including dietary fiber (Table 2-9).

It is recommended that one eat a variety of fruit daily, following the food intake patterns for quantity, and go easy on the fruit juice. The calories in fruit juice add up quickly, especially if one is thirsty and drinks large amounts of juice. One serving is 3/4 cup of fruit juice; a half of a grapefruit; one whole raw medium apple, orange, peach, pear, or banana; 1/2 cup of canned or cooked fruit; and 1/4 cup of dried fruit.

TABLE 2-6 MyPlate Food Intake Patterns

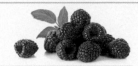

DAILY AMOUNT OF FOOD FROM EACH GROUP

The suggested amounts of food to consume from the basic food groups, subgroups, and oils to meet recommended nutrient intakes at 12 different calorie levels. Nutrient and energy contributions from each group are calculated according to the nutrient-dense forms of foods in each group (e.g., lean meats, fat-free milk). The table also shows the discretionary calorie allowance that can be accommodated within each calorie level, in addition to the suggested amounts of nutrient-dense forms of foods in each group.

CALORIE LEVEL[1]

	1,000	1,200	1,400	1,600	1,800	2,000	2,200	2,400	2,600	2,800	3,000	3,200
Fruits	1 cup	1 cup	1.5 cups	1.5 cups	1.5 cups	2 cups	2 cups	2 cups	2 cups	2.5 cups	2.5 cups	2.5 cups
Vegetables	1 cup	1.5 cups	1.5 cups	2 cups	2.5 cups	2.5 cups	3 cups	3 cups	3.5 cups	3.5 cups	4 cups	4 cups
Grains	3 oz–eq	4 oz–eq	5 oz–eq	5 oz–eq	6 oz–eq	6 oz–eq	7 oz–eq	8 oz–eq	9 oz–eq	10 oz–eq	10 oz–eq	10 oz–eq
Meat and beans	2 oz–eq	3 oz–eq	4 oz–eq	5 oz–eq	5 oz–eq	5 oz–eq	6 oz–eq	5 oz–eq	5 oz–eq	7 oz–eq	7 oz–eq	7 oz–eq
Milk	2 cups	2 cups	2 cups	3 cups	3 cups	3 cups	3 cups	3 cups	3 cups	3 cups	3 cups	3 cups
Oils	3 tsp	4 tsp	4 tsp	5 tsp	5 tsp	6 tsp	6 tsp	7 tsp	8 tsp	8 tsp	10 tsp	11 tsp
Discretionary calorie allowance	165	171	171	132	195	267	290	362	410	426	512	648

ESTIMATED DAILY CALORIE NEEDS

To determine which food intake pattern to use for an individual, the following chart gives an estimate of individual calorie needs. The calorie range for each age and gender is based on physical activity level, from sedentary to active. Sedentary means a lifestyle that includes only the light physical activity associated with typical day-to-day life. Active means a lifestyle that includes physical activity equivalent to walking more than 3 miles per day at 3 to 4 miles per hour, in addition to the light physical activity associated with typical day-to-day life.

	CALORIE RANGE				CALORIE RANGE		
	SEDENTARY	→	ACTIVE		SEDENTARY	→	ACTIVE
Children				**Males**			
2–3 years	1,000	→	1,400	4–8 years	1,400	→	2,000
Females				9–13	1,800	→	2,600
4–8 years	1,200	→	1,800	14–18	2,200	→	3,200
9–13	1,600	→	2,200	19–30	2,400	→	3,000
14–18	1,800	→	2,400	31–50	2,200	→	3,000
19–30	2,000	→	2,400	51+	2,000	→	2,800
31–50	1,800	→	2,200				
51+	1,600	→	2,200				

[1]Calorie levels are set across a wide range to accommodate the needs of different individuals

Source: U.S. Department of Agriculture, Center for Nutrition Policy and Promotions. *MyPlate Food Intake Patterns.* Accessed December 2011 from http://www.choosemyplate.gov

TABLE 2-7   Grain Group

BREADS

Whole wheat	Rolls or biscuits made with whole-wheat or enriched flour
Dark rye	
Enriched	Flour, enriched
Oatmeal bread	whole wheat, other whole-grain
Cornmeal, whole grain, or enriched	grits, enriched

CEREALS

Whole wheat	Other cereals, if whole grain or restored
Rolled oats	

RICE

Brown rice	Converted rice

PASTA

Noodles, spaghetti, macaroni

© Cengage Learning 2014

TABLE 2-8   Vegetable Subgroup Amounts

CALORIE LEVEL	1,000	1,200	1,400	1,600	1,800	2,000	2,200	2,400	2,600	2,800	3,000	3,200
Dark green veg.	1 c/wk	1.5 c/wk	1.5 c/wk	2 c/wk	3 c/wk	3 c/wk	3 c/wk	3 c/wk	3 c/wk	3 c/wk	3 c/wk	3 c/wk
Orange veg.	0.5 c/wk	1 c/wk	1 c/wk	1.5 c/wk	2 c/wk	2c/wk	2 c/wk	2 c/wk	2.5 c/wk	2.5 c/wk	2.5 c/wk	2.5 c/wk
Legumes	0.5 c/wk	1 c/wk	1 c/wk	2.5 c/wk	3 c/wk	3 c/wk	3 c/wk	3 c/wk	3.5 c/wk	3.5 c/wk	3.5 c/wk	3.5 c/wk
Starchy veg.	1.5 c/wk	2.5 c/wk	2.5 c/wk	2.5 c/wk	3 c/wk	3 c/wk	6 c/wk	6 c/wk	7 c/wk	7 c/wk	9 c/wk	9 c/wk
Other veg.	3.5 c/wk	4.5 c/wk	4.5 c/wk	5.5 c/wk	6.5 c/wk	6.5 c/wk	7 c/wk	7 c/wk	8.5 c/wk	8.5 c/wk	10 c/wk	10 c/wk

Source: U.S. Department of Agriculture, Center for Nutrition Policy and Promotions. *MyPlate Food Intake Patterns.* Accessed December 2011 from http://www.choosemyplate.gov

Dairy Group

Milk, yogurt, and cheese are excellent sources of carbohydrate (lactose); calcium, phosphorus, and magnesium; proteins; riboflavin, vitamins A, B_{12}, and, if the milk is fortified, vitamin D. Unfortunately, all contain sodium, and whole milk and whole-milk products also contain saturated fats and cholesterol. Fat-free milk has the fats removed.

TABLE 2-9   Fruit Group

SOURCES OF VITAMIN A	SOURCES OF VITAMIN C	
Bananas	Oranges	Cantaloupe
Cantaloupe	Lemons	Kiwi fruit
Avocados	Grapefruit	Honeydew melon
Apricots	Limes	Watermelon
Mangoes	Raspberries	Mangoes
	Strawberries	Papaya
	Pineapple	

© Cengage Learning 2014

It is recommended that two to three servings of these foods be included in one's daily diet. The serving size is one 8-ounce glass of milk or the equivalent in terms of calcium content.

Children	2 servings
Adolescents	3 servings
Adults	3 servings
Pregnant or lactating women	3 servings
Pregnant or lactating teens	4 servings

The following dairy foods contain calcium equal to that found in one 8-ounce cup of milk. The best choices would be low fat.

- 1½ ounces cheddar cheese
- 2 cups cottage cheese
- 1¾ cups of ice cream
- 1 cup yogurt

Milk used in making cream sauces, gravies, or baked products fulfills part of the calcium requirement. A cheese sandwich would fulfill one of the serving requirements, and a serving of ice cream could fulfill half of one of the serving requirements. Obviously, drinking milk is not the only way to fulfill the calcium requirement.

Some clients suffer from lactose intolerance and cannot digest milk or milk products. If they eat or drink foods containing untreated lactose, they experience abdominal cramps and diarrhea. This condition is caused by a deficiency of lactase (see Chapter 4). In such cases, milk that has been treated with lactase can be used, or commercial lactase can be added to the milk or taken in tablet form before drinking milk or eating dairy products.

Protein Group

All meats, poultry, fish, eggs, soybeans, dry beans and peas, lentils, nuts, and seeds are included in the protein group (Table 2-10). These foods provide

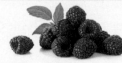

TABLE 2-10   Meats, Poultry, Fish, Dry Beans, Eggs, and Nuts

Beef	Dried beans
Lamb	Dried peas
Veal	Lentils
Pork, except bacon	Nuts
Organ meats, such as heart, liver, kidney, brain, tongue, sweetbread	Peanuts
	Peanut butter
Poultry, such as chicken, duck, goose, turkey	Soybean flour
	Soybeans
Fish, shellfish	

© Cengage Learning 2014

proteins, iron, copper, phosphorus, zinc, sodium, iodine, B vitamins, fats, and cholesterol.

Caution must be used so that the foods selected from this group are low in fat and cholesterol. Many meats contain large amounts of fat, and egg yolks and organ meats have very high cholesterol content.

Let the food intake patterns be the guide for the number of ounces one should eat daily. In general, 1 ounce of lean meat, poultry, or fish; 1 egg; 1 tablespoon of peanut butter; ¼ cup of cooked dry beans; or ½ ounce of nuts or seeds can be considered as a 1-ounce equivalent from the meat and beans group.

Fats

The fats group contains butter, margarine, cooking oils, mayonnaise and other salad dressings, sugar, syrup, honey, jam, jelly, and sodas. All of these foods have a low nutrient density, meaning they have few nutrients other than fats and carbohydrates and have a high calorie content. One's limit for fat will be figured and listed as oils in accordance with the food intake patterns shown in Table 2-6. It is recommended that the fat sources be from fish, nuts, and vegetable oils.

The Mediterranean diet has received attention because of the American Heart Association's recommendation to increase monounsaturated fats in the diet. The recommendations are outlined in Chapter 5. The following guidelines are recommended:

1. Eat the majority of food from plant sources, such as potatoes, grains and breads, beans, fruits, vegetables, nuts, and seeds.

2. Eat minimally processed foods, with an emphasis on fresh, locally grown foods.

3. Replace other fats and oils with olive oil.

4. Keep total fat in a range of less than 20–35% of energy. Saturated fat should be no more than 7–8% of energy.

5. Eat low to moderate amounts of cheese and yogurt (low-fat and fat-free types preferable).

6. Eat low to moderate amounts of fish and poultry and from zero to four eggs per week (those used in cooking need to be counted).

7. Eat fruit for dessert; desserts that contain a significant amount of sugar and saturated fat should be eaten only a few times per week.

8. Eat red meat a few times per month, not to exceed 12–16 ounces per month.

9. Engage in regular exercise to promote fitness, a healthy weight, and a feeling of physical well-being.

10. Drink wine in moderation (wine is optional). Wine with meals—one to two drinks per day for men and one drink per day for women.

FOOD LABELING

As a result of the passage by Congress of the Nutrition Labeling and Education Act (NLEA) in 1990, nutrition labeling regulations became mandatory in May 1994 for nearly all processed foods. The primary objective of the changes was to ensure that labels would be on most foods and would provide consistent nutrition information. The resulting food labels provide the consumer with more information on the nutrient contents of foods and how those nutrients affect health than former labels provided. Health claims allowed on labels are limited and set by the Food and Drug Administration (FDA). Serving sizes are determined by the FDA and not by the individual food processor. Descriptive terms used for foods are standardized. For example, "low fat" means that each serving contains 3 grams of fat or less.

Current Label

The nutrition label has a formatted space called Nutrition Facts (Figure 2-2) that includes required and optional information.

The items and amounts per serving that must be included on the food label are as follows:

- Total calories
- Calories from fat
- Total fat
- Saturated fat
- Trans fat
- Cholesterol
- Sodium
- Total carbohydrates
- Dietary fiber
- Sugars
- Protein
- Vitamin A
- Vitamin C

EXPLORING THE WEB

The website for the Center for Food Safety and Applied Nutrition, of the U.S. Food and Drug Administration (http://www.fda.gov), has an abundance of information on using the food label. Visit the website and create fact sheets on how to use the food label to lose weight, lower salt intake, control diabetes, and prevent heart disease. These sheets can also be used to aid in client teaching.

- Calcium
- Iron

The food processor can voluntarily include additional information on food products. If a health claim is made about the food or if the food is enriched or fortified with an optional nutrient, then nutrition information about that nutrient becomes required. The standardized serving size is based on amounts of the specific food commonly eaten, and it is given in both English and metric measurements (Table 2-11).

 daily values
represent percentage per serving of each nutritional item listed on food labels based on a daily intake of 2,000 calories

Daily values on the label give the consumer the percentage per serving of each nutritional item listed, based on a daily diet of 2,000 calories. For example, total fat in Figure 2-2 shows 3 grams, which represents 5% of the amount of fat someone on a 2,000-calorie diet should have. The label also shows the *maximum* amount of a nutrient that should be eaten (e.g., fat) or the *minimum* requirement for specified nutrients (e.g., carbohydrates) based on a daily diet of 2,000 calories and another based on 2,500 calories. The items included here are the amounts of total fat, saturated fat, cholesterol, sodium, total carbohydrate, and fiber. In addition, the label lists the calories per gram for fats, carbohydrates, and proteins.

Health Claims

Because diet has been implicated as a factor in heart disease, stroke, birth defects, and cancer, the following *health claims* linking a nutrient to a health-related condition are allowed on labels. They are intended to help consumers choose foods that are the most healthful for them and avoid being deceived by false advertisements on the label. The allowed claims are for the relationship between the following:

- Calcium and *osteoporosis*
- Sodium and *hypertension*
- Diets low in saturated fat and cholesterol and high in fruits, vegetables, and grains containing dietary fiber and *coronary heart disease*
- Diets low in fat and high in fruits and vegetables containing dietary fiber and the antioxidants, and vitamins A and C and *cancer*
- Diets low in fat and high in fiber-containing grains, fruits, and vegetables and *cancer*
- Folic acid and *neural tube defects*
- Soy protein and *coronary heart disease*

TABLE 2-11 Household and Metric Measures

- 1 teaspoon (tsp) = 5 milliliters (ml)
- 1 tablespoon (Tbsp) = 15 ml
- 1 cup (C) = 240 ml
- 1 fluid ounce (fl oz) = 30 ml
- 1 ounce (oz) = 28 grams (g)

© Cengage Learning 2014

U.S. Department of Agriculture and U.S. Department of Health and Human Services. *Dietary Guidelines for Americans, 2010 (7th ed.).* Washington, DC: U.S. Government Printing Office. December 2010

FIGURE 2-2 Food label.

Nutrition Facts

Serving Size 1 Bar (40g)

Amount Per Serving

Check Calories → **Calories** 170   Calories from Fat 60

	% Daily Value*
Total Fat 7g	**11%**
Saturated Fat 3g	**15%**
Trans Fat 0g	
Cholesterol 0mg	**0%**
Sodium 160mg	**7%**
Total Carbohydrate 24g	**8%**
Dietary Fiber 3g	**12%**
Sugars 10g	
Protein 5g	

Limit These Nutrients

Get Enough of These Nutrients →

Vitamin A 2%	•	Vitamin C 2%
Calcium 20%	•	Iron 8%

* Percent Daily Values are based on a 2,000 calorie diet. Your daily values may be higher or lower depending on your calorie needs:

Footnote →

	Calories	2,000	2,500
Total Fat	Less than	65g	80g
Sat Fat	Less than	20g	25g
Cholesterol	Less than	300mg	300mg
Sodium	Less than	2,400mg	2,400mg
Total Carbohydrate		300g	375g
Dietary Fiber		25g	30g

Calories per gram:
Fat 9 • Carbohydrate 4 • Protein 4

Ingredients

Granola Bar (Brown Rice Syrup, Granola [rolled oats, honey, canola oil], Dry Roasted Peanuts, Soy Crisps [soy protein isolate, rice flour, malt extract, calcium carbonate], Crisp Brown Rice [organic brown rice flour, evaporated cane juice, molasses, rice bran extract, sea salt], Glycerine, Peanut Butter [ground dry roasted peanuts], Inulin, Whey Protein Isolate, Gold Flax Seeds, Quinoa Flakes, Calcium Carbonate, Salt, Natural Flavors, Water, Soy Lecithin [an emulsifier]), Dark Compound Coating (evaporated cane juice, palm kernel oil, cocoa [processed with alkali], palm oil, soy lecithin [an emulsifier]).

Two additional criteria must also be met:

1. A food whose label makes a health claim must be a naturally good source (containing at least 10% of the daily value) of at least one of the following nutrients: protein, vitamin A, vitamin C, iron, calcium, or fiber.

2. Health claims cannot be made for a food if a standard serving contains more than 20% of the daily value for total fat, saturated fat, cholesterol, or sodium.

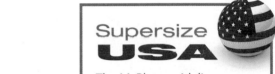

Supersize USA

The MyPlate guidelines were developed in the atmosphere of the growing obesity epidemic in this country. MyPlate is based on the 2010 Dietary Guidelines for Americans and helps consumers make better food choices. It illustrates the five food groups using a familiar mealtime visual—a place setting. The website features many practical tips and information to help Americans build healthier diets. Selected messages include:

- Enjoy your food, but eat less. Avoid oversized portions. Make half your plate fruits and vegetables. Switch to fat-free or low-fat (1%) milk.

- Make at least half your grains whole grains.

- Compare sodium in foods such as soup, bread, and frozen meals and choose foods with lower numbers.

- Drink water instead of sugary drinks.

Visit http://www.choosemyplate.gov for more information and ways you can take steps to a healthier you!

Terminology

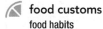

descriptors
terms used to describe something

The FDA has also standardized **descriptors** (terms used by manufacturers to describe products) on food labels to help the consumer select the most appropriate and healthful foods. The following are examples:

- *Low calorie* means 40 calories or less per serving.
- *Calorie free* means less than 5 calories per serving.
- *Low fat* means a food has no more than 3 grams of fat per serving or per 100 grams of the food.
- *Fat free* means a food contains less than 0.5 gram of fat per serving.
- *Low saturated fat* means 1 gram or less of saturated fat per serving.
- *Low cholesterol* means 20 mg or less of cholesterol per serving.
- *Cholesterol free* means less than 2 mg of cholesterol per serving.
- *No added sugar* means that no sugar or sweeteners of any kind have been added at any time during the preparation and packaging. When such a term is used, the package must also state that it is not low calorie or calorie reduced (unless it actually is).
- *Low sodium* means less than 140 mg of sodium per serving.
- *Very low sodium* means less than 35 mg of sodium per serving.

Obviously, the information on food labels is useful to all consumers and especially to those who must select foods for therapeutic diets. Health care professionals should become thoroughly knowledgeable about the labeling law. On request, many food manufacturers will provide the consumer with additional detailed information about their products.

FOOD CUSTOMS

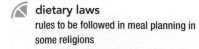

food customs
food habits

dietary laws
rules to be followed in meal planning in some religions

MyPlate and Nutrition Facts labels (if available) are useful in planning a nutritionally sound diet, but dietary and religious customs must also be taken into consideration. People from each country have favorite foods. Frequently, there are distinctive **food customs** originating in just a small section of a particular country. People of a particular area favor the foods that are produced in that area because they are available and economical. Some religions have **dietary laws** that require particular food practices. Because most people prefer the foods they were accustomed to while growing up, food habits are often based on nationality and religion.

One's economic status and social status also contribute to food habits. For example, the poor do not grow up with a taste for prime rib, whereas the wealthy may at least be accustomed to it—whether or not they like it. Those in a certain social class will be apt to consume the same foods as others in their class. And the foods they choose will probably depend on the work they do. For example, people doing hard, physical labor will require higher-calorie foods than will people in sedentary jobs.

When people move from one country to another or from one area to another, their economic status may change. They will be introduced to new foods and new food customs. Although their original food customs may have been nutritionally adequate, their new environment may cause them to change their eating habits. For example, if milk was a staple (basic) food in their diet before moving and is unusually expensive in the new environment, milk may be replaced by a cheaper, nutritionally inferior beverage such as soda, coffee, or tea. Candy, possibly a luxury in their former environment, may be inexpensive and popular in their new environment. As a result, a family might increase consumption of soda or candy and reduce purchases of more nutritious foods. Someone who is not familiar with the nutritive values of foods can easily make such mistakes in food selection.

The meal patterns of national and religious groups different from one's own may seem strange. However, the diet may well be nutritionally adequate. When a client's eating habits need to be corrected, such corrections are most easily made if the food customs of the client are known and understood. The health care professional can gain this knowledge by talking with the client and learning about her or his background. A dietitian can use that knowledge to plan nourishing menus consisting of foods that appeal to the client. The necessary adjustments in the diet can then be made gradually and effectively.

U.S. CULTURAL DIETARY INFLUENCES

American cuisine (cooking style) is a marvelous composite of countless national, regional, cultural, and religious food customs. Consequently, categorizing a client's food habits can be difficult. Nevertheless, it is sometimes helpful to be able to do so to a certain extent. People who are ill commonly have little interest in food. Sometimes comfort foods (foods that were familiar to them during their childhood) are more apt to tempt them than other types. The following section briefly discusses some food patterns typical of various cultures, regions, and countries. Of course, there can be and usually are enormous variations within any one classification.

Native American Influence

It is thought that approximately half of the edible plants commonly eaten in the United States today originated with the Native Americans. Examples are corn, potatoes, squash, cranberries, pumpkins, peppers, beans, wild rice, sunflower seeds, sweet potatoes, avocados, papayas, and cocoa beans (Figure 2-3). In addition, wild fruits, game, and fish are also popular. Foods are commonly prepared as soups and stews or are dried. The original Native American diets were probably more nutritionally adequate than are current diets, which frequently consist of too high a proportion of sweet and salty, snack-type low-nutrient-dense foods. Native American diets today may be deficient in calcium, vitamins A and C, and riboflavin.

U.S. Southern Influences

The foods of the South are as diverse as the people who settled the southern United States. Food influenced by the South is so much a part of our national food culture that you probably have eaten many of these foods without even realizing their origin.

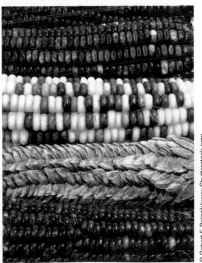

FIGURE 2-3 Corn is a major component in traditional Native American cooking.

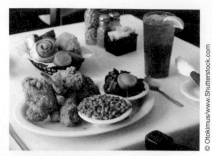

FIGURE 2-4 A traditional southern meal has foods like fried chicken, black-eyed peas, collard greens, cornbread and biscuits, and sweet tea.

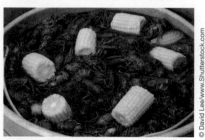

FIGURE 2-5 Crawfish are widely used in Cajun and Creole cooking.

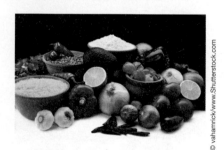

FIGURE 2-6 Ingredients used in Mexican cuisine include avocados, peppers, rice, and tomatoes.

 foodways
the food traditions or customs of a group of people

 fusion
a style of cooking that combines ingredients and techniques from different cultures or countries

masa harina
·ditional flour made from field corn

African American Influence

Down-home breads such as cornbread, biscuits, and cracklin' bread are served with most meals. Collard, turnip, and mustard greens are prepared with fatback (a cut along the back of pigs) for flavor. Black-eyed peas, okra, sweet potatoes, peanuts, corn, green beans, hot and sweet peppers, lima beans, and rice are an important part of African American heritage (Figure 2-4). Pork, chicken, and fried fish are served often. The term *soul food* was created in the 1960s to put emphasis on African American **foodways** (the food traditions or customs of a group of people) and preparation styles. Too much fat and sodium are consumed. This diet has too many carbohydrates but could be deficient in iron, calcium, fiber, potassium, and vitamin C.

French American Influence

Cajun and Creole cuisine is native to the "bayou" country in Louisiana and is a **fusion** of French and Spanish cooking. Cajuns lived off the land and waterways. Cajun cooks use wild game, seafood, vegetables, herbs, rice, tomatoes, sausage, hot peppers, and crawfish (resembling small lobsters) (Figure 2-5). Cajuns usually make their meals in one pot. Creole cooking uses many of the same foods but adds rich sauces that increase calories. Calcium and vitamins D, E, and C could be lacking in their diets, so the addition of fruit is needed.

Spanish Influences

The Spaniards were great seafaring explorers. They were responsible for finding and naming most of the islands in the Caribbean, along with Mexico and the west coast of South America. The Spanish and the natives who inhabited these countries have also greatly influenced our cuisine.

Mexican Influence

Mexican food is a combination of Spanish and Native American. Beans, rice, tomatoes, onions, jalapenos, other chilies, and **masa harina** (traditional flour made from field corn) are staples for Hispanics. Corn tortillas are made from masa harina and are used as bread as well as stuffed with cheese, beef, pork, and other ingredients to make enchiladas. Pork, goat, garlic, wheat and frijoles refritos (refried beans), avocados, and cheese are common foods (Figure 2-6). Flan, a custardlike pudding with caramel sauce, is a favorite dessert. The diet is lacking in vitamin C, and green and yellow vegetables and fruits. Cheese supplies some calcium in the diet, but calcium intake is low because of **lactose intolerance** (the body's inability to digest the lactose in milk and some milk products).

Puerto Rican Influence

Puerto Rican cuisine has been influenced by the Spanish, African, and Taino Indians (first inhabitants). Some of the foods in their diet are corn, wheat, seafood, beef, pork, rice, olive oil, chicken, pinto beans, and okra. Plantains, green bananas, white and yellow sweet potatoes, chayote squash, taro, and breadfruit are starchy vegetables and are eaten often. Tropical fruits such as pineapple, mango, papayas, guava, and coconut are used often in desserts (Figure 2-7). Traditional desserts includes flan, sweet potato balls with cinnamon, cloves and coconut, and guava jelly served with white cheese. From a nutrition standpoint, milk is not consumed often enough. Increased consumption of nonstarchy vegetables would add variety and eliminate some carbohydrates.

Mediterranean Influences

The Mediterranean diet is the healthiest in the world (Figure 2-8). The most important aspects of the Italian Mediterranean diet are the use of olive oil and the eating of small portions. The Italians on the Mediterranean have the lowest incidence of heart disease because of their eating habits.

lactose intolerance
inability to digest lactose because of a lack of the enzyme lactase; causes abdominal cramps and diarrhea

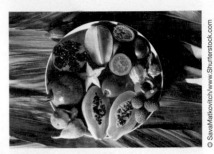

FIGURE 2-7 Tropical fruits like papaya are often used in Puerto Rican desserts.

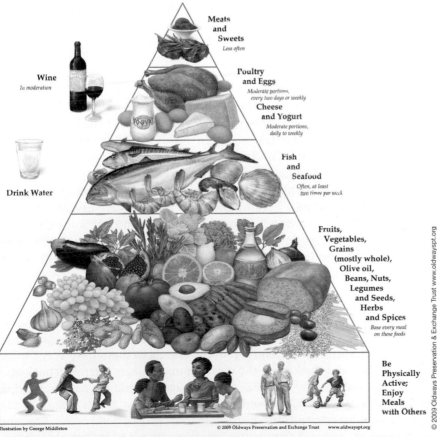

Mediterranean Diet Pyramid
A contemporary approach to delicious, healthy eating

Meats and Sweets *Less often*

Wine *In moderation*

Poultry and Eggs *Moderate portions, every two days or weekly*

Cheese and Yogurt *Moderate portions, daily to weekly*

Drink Water

Fish and Seafood *Often, at least two times per week*

Fruits, Vegetables, Grains (mostly whole), Olive oil, Beans, Nuts, Legumes and Seeds, Herbs and Spices *Base every meal on these foods*

Be Physically Active; Enjoy Meals with Others

Illustration by George Middleton

© 2009 Oldways Preservation and Exchange Trust   www.oldwayspt.org

© 2009 Oldways Preservation & Exchange Trust www.oldwayspt.org

FIGURE 2-8 Follow the Mediterranean Food Guide Pyramid, and you will be eating the healthiest diet in the world.

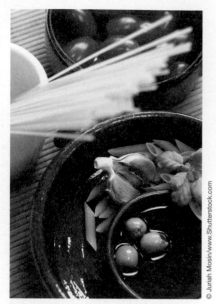

FIGURE 2-9 Olive oil, herbs, garlic, pasta, and tomatoes are ingredients commonly used in Italian cooking.

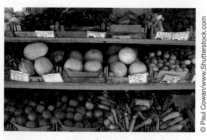

FIGURE 2-10 Fresh vegetables play a large role in Greek cooking and cuisine.

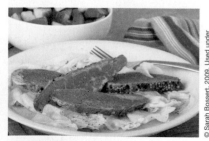

FIGURE 2-11 Countries in northern and western Europe have traditional "meat and potatoes" dishes like corned beef, cabbage, and potatoes.

Italian Influence

Italians consume a healthy mix of pasta, rice, beans, olives, fruits, vegetables, and seafood (Figure 2-9). Beef is seldom eaten on the Mediterranean side of Italy. Meats such as prosciutto salami, veal, and pork are favored. Cheese is important in Italian cooking but is often eaten by itself. Small portions are the norm. The primary fat used is olive oil. Dessert is usually fresh fruit. The Italians eat their main meal at lunch. Dinner is a light meal and could be pizza (not the Americanized version). Adding fat-free milk and low-fat meat would improve their already nutritious diet.

Greek Influence

In the past and even today in remote villages, the Greeks eat only what is in season at the time (Figure 2-10). Broccoli and cauliflower were first grown in Greece. Greeks eat salads of wild greens, artichokes, fava beans, green beans, eggplant, legumes, home-cured olives, yogurt, and feta cheese. Bread is the basis of a Greek meal, and fruity olive oil is the primary fat in the Greek diet. Fresh or cured fish and seafood are abundant and eaten regularly. Meats such as lamb, goat, and pork are also included in their diet. Dessert usually consists of fresh fruit. The Greeks have always eaten (and many continue to eat) a Mediterranean diet, but Western influence in the larger cities has changed the eating habits of younger generations.

Northern and Western European Influences

There are 20 countries in northern and western Europe that have influenced the foods we eat. These countries gave us our "meat and potato" mentality (Figure 2-11). The northern European diet consists of large servings of meat, poultry, or fish with small side dishes of vegetables and starch. Most countries use locally grown foods, such as greens, potatoes, beets, mushrooms, barley, plums, and rye. Sausages (including blood sausage), head cheese, dark breads, and dairy products are essential food in their diets. Pickled herring is favored in many countries. Some countries in northern and western Europe are extremely cold, limiting the growing season. The addition of fresh fruit and vegetables would add fiber and many vitamins and minerals.

Central European Influences

There are 16 countries in central Europe, and all of them have very similar cuisines. Pork and chicken are the most common meats eaten, but beef, sausages, fish, and game are popular too. Cabbage, sauerkraut, carrots, turnips, potatoes, beans, lentils, and onions appear in many meals (Figure 2-12). Spatzle, dark breads, and muesli are main sources of carbohydrates. Eggs and dairy products are used abundantly. Raw vegetables and fruit would increase vitamins, minerals, and fiber. Fewer eggs and the use of low-fat or fat-free dairy products would help to decrease fat in this diet.

Middle Eastern Influences

The foodways of the Middle East have intertwined and migrated to other countries. Lamb is the primary meat consumed. Pita and flat bread (unleavened) along with sourdough breads are eaten with meals (Figure 2-13). Legumes are an important part of the diet; these include chickpeas (garbanzo beans), which are used to make hummus. Dairy products in the form of yogurt and feta cheese are used extensively. Fortunately, fresh fruit is eaten for snacks and dessert. For centuries, dates and figs have been a staple in this diet. Pistachios are used to make baklava, a very sweet dessert. At the end of a meal, a dense, sweet coffee is served. The addition of fresh vegetables would be desirable to increase vitamins, minerals, and fiber.

Asian Influences

Each Asian country has its traditional foods. Most familiar is Chinese, but Japanese cuisine is becoming more available, as are the foods of Southeast Asia. Even though there may not be a wok in every kitchen, the art of stir-frying has become common practice. Cutting vegetables in small pieces and cooking them quickly preserves nutrients. Read the common foods consumed from each country and check how many you have eaten either at home or at a restaurant.

Chinese Influence

The Chinese believe that the five essential grains of life are rice, soybeans, barley, wheat, and millet. Their diet uses many vegetables, such as bean sprouts, shitake and other varieties of mushrooms, broccoli, peppers, snow peas, onions, green beans, bok choy, Napa cabbage, asparagus, chili peppers, seaweed, and cucumber (Figure 2-14). Protein is obtained from seafood, eggs, pork, chicken, beef, and tofu (soybean curd). Peanut oil for stir-frying and corn oil for deep frying are used extensively. Water chestnuts, walnuts, almonds, cashews, and sesame seeds are used in desserts and stir-fried dishes. Vegetarianism has expanded since the discovery of tofu. Some of the preferred seasonings are soy sauce, garlic, and fresh ginger along with various spices. The use of soy sauce and MSG (monosodium glutamate) may contribute to high blood pressure. Calcium sources are lacking in this diet, perhaps because of lactose intolerance in the Asian populations.

Japanese Influence

In ancient times, much of the traditional Japanese cuisine was influenced by the Chinese and Koreans. The medieval period triggered a gradual transformation with new tastes and flavors. The Japanese strive to use only the freshest ingredients. Essential ingredients include bamboo shoots, tofu, cucumbers, eggplant, enoki and other mushrooms, spinach, ginger, seaweed, rice, sesame, and green onions. Their protein is from seafood (both raw and cooked), eggs, and chicken. Seasonings used extensively are

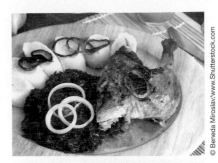

FIGURE 2-12 This Czechoslovakian dish of roast duck with dumplings and red cabbage is a traditional meal in many central European countries.

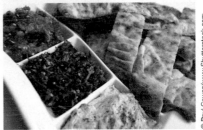

FIGURE 2-13 In Middle Eastern cuisine, flat bread is often eaten with hummus, tabouleh, or baba ganoush.

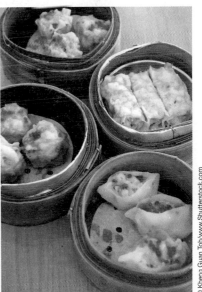

FIGURE 2-14 Steamed, baked, and fried dim sum is part of traditional Chinese cuisine.

◣ **mirin**
rice wine with 40–50% sugar

◣ **miso**
a thick fermented paste made from soybeans

◣ **wasabi**
Japanese horseradish

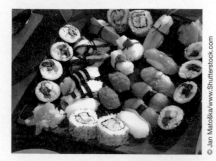

FIGURE 2-15 Sushi is a popular type of Japanese cuisine.

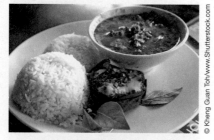

FIGURE 2-16 This Thai dish of spicy curry steamed fish pudding and rice is an example of traditional Southeast Asian cuisine.

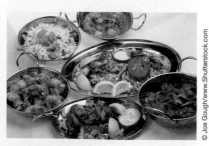

FIGURE 2-17 A sample of ʌditional Indian curry dishes.

mirin (rice wine with 40–50% sugar), soy sauce, **miso** (a thick fermented paste made from soybeans), and **wasabi** (Japanese horseradish). Sushi is a well-known food item (Figure 2-15). The Japanese drink green tea rather than milk. Lactose intolerance plays an important role in their choices. Fresh fruit is a needed addition.

Southeast Asian Influence

India and China have influenced much cooking. Many vegetables are eaten because 75% of the population is agriculture based. Rice is the staple food, but noodles are used often (Figure 2-16). Two times as much fish is consumed compared with other meats; pork, chicken, and beef are eaten less often. Southeast Asians prefer coconut milk to any dairy products. They, like other Asians, use soybean milk, soybean paste, and soy sauce. Fruits are part of the meals. The inhabitants of Southeast Asia, with the exception of Vietnam, eat with their fingers, but this is changing. The ginger plant was first grown here. High blood pressure caused by a high-sodium diet could be an issue. Cow's milk alternatives such as soy or rice milk are favored because of lactose intolerance.

Indian Influences

Religion and climate are two factors in the development of food habits in India. Vegetarianism is prevalent (over 80%) because of religious beliefs. Lentils, beans, and milk and milk products supply protein to their diet. The rest of the population eats small quantities of meat and fish for their protein. Vegetables grown locally are combined with rice in the south and wheat products in the north (Figure 2-17). Garlic and eggplants are native to India. Curry is a spice but also denotes Indian dishes. Eating with your fingers is acceptable. Oils used in cooking are sunflower, coconut, and mustard oils. A lack of calcium could be a problem if consumption of milk is inadequate.

New Immigrant Influences

The United States is made up of immigrants who bring with them wonderful foods that are native to their country. Immigrants will always prepare their native foods and, it is hoped, share them with others. Have you ever thought about what traditional foods your family eats and where they originated?

Somali Influence

No pork is eaten because of religious doctrine. Some foods in the diet are flat bread (Figure 2-18), millet, cornmeal, rice, noodles, bananas, mangoes, papayas, vegetables, liver, seafood, beans, eggs, pita bread, peanuts, bread, spiced tea with cardamom and cinnamon bark, chicken, lamb, goat, camel, sheep, and some beef. Frankincense is native to Somaliland. It is an aromatic gum resin obtained from various Arabian and East African trees and is chewed after a meal if desired. Lack of milk and milk products could lead to a calcium deficiency. Liver is an integral part of their diet but can lead to high cholesterol.

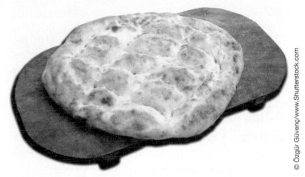

FIGURE 2-18 Flat bread is often part of traditional Somali meals.

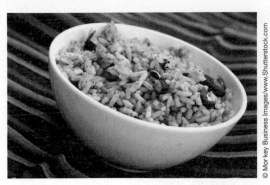

FIGURE 2-19 Haiti's national dish is beans and rice.

Haitian Influence

African, Spanish, and French culinary influences have shaped Haitian food-ways. The Haitian diet is based on starch staples, such as rice, corn, millet, yams, and beans. Only the wealthy can afford meat, lobster, shrimp, duck, and sweet desserts. The country's national dish is rice and beans (Figure 2-19). Haitians tend to fry their meals in pig fat (lard) for enhanced flavor. Tropical fruits, such as avocados, mangoes, pineapples, coconuts, and guava, grow abundantly in Haiti. Lack of milk and dairy products in the diet means that there will be a deficiency of calcium. If the poor eat only beans and rice with some fruits and vegetables, malnutrition is a real concern.

Korean Influence

In Korea, the growing of rice dates back to 2000 BC. Millet, soybeans, red beans, and other grains were also produced. Red meat is scarce, but chicken and sea-food are abundant. Rice is eaten with every meal, along with vegetables. The na-tional dish of Korea is kimchi, a fermented cabbage with spices, green onions, and radishes. Kimchi is native to Korea and is served with each meal. Korean food is very spicy with the use of red pepper paste, green onion, ginger, garlic, and bean paste (Figure 2-20). Soy sauce is used extensively. Fresh fruits, such as apples, pears, persimmons, and melons, or dried fruits, are eaten for snacks and dessert. Almost all (99%) of South Koreans receive adequate nutrition.

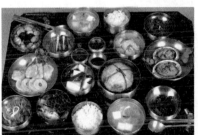

FIGURE 2-20 A traditional Korean meal, served with kimchi, rice, spicy pastes, and sauces.

Dominican Republic Influence

Dominican Republic cuisine is a mix of Spanish and Taino Indian. Goat and chicken are the meats eaten most often by local residents (Figure 2-21). Fresh seafood such as shrimp, mahi-mahi, rock lobster, and marlin are served of-ten in seaside towns. Tropical fruits such as bananas, papayas, pineapples, mangoes, and avocados are eaten often. Plantains, yuca (cassava), chayote, and rice are starchy foods in the diet. Salad is usually eaten with the midday meal. Enjoyed by many is a drink made by adding fruit juice to milk to make a smoothie. Spicy foods are normal in Caribbean countries but not in the Dominican Republic. A wide variety of foods are available, so choosing wisely will provide adequate nutrients.

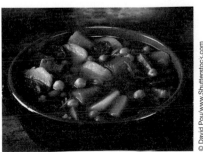

FIGURE 2-21 Cocido is a traditional Dominican Republican stew made with meat, vegetables, and garbanzo beans.

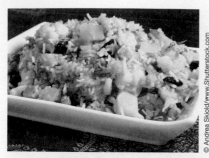

FIGURE 2-22 The Burmese version of biryani is often made with rice, chicken, cashew nuts, yogurt, raisins, peas, cloves, cinnamon, saffron, and bay leaves.

Burmese Influence

The Burmese people have many varieties of fruits and vegetables. Tropical fruits abound, such as pineapples, papayas, oranges, bananas, mangoes, melons, and coconuts. Cabbage, cucumbers, cauliflower, beets, carrots, bean sprouts, eggplant, kohlrabi, and tomatoes are just some of the vegetables eaten. Carbohydrate sources are rice, noodles, red lentils, and mung peas (Figure 2-22). Protein sources are pork, beef, lamb, chicken, duck, fish or prawns (large shrimp), tofu, and eggs. Vegetable and fruit salads are popular. Fresh fruits are served for dessert, but sweets are eaten as snacks or at breakfast. Choosing foods well will ensure good nutrition.

FOOD PATTERNS BASED ON RELIGION OR PHILOSOPHY
Jewish

Interpretations of the Jewish dietary laws vary. Persons who adhere to the Orthodox view consider tradition important and always observe the dietary laws. Foods prepared according to these laws are called *kosher* (Figure 2-23). Conservative Jews are inclined to observe the rules only at home. Reform Jews consider their dietary laws to be essentially ceremonial and so minimize their significance. Essentially the laws require the following:

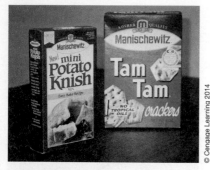

FIGURE 2-23 Kosher food label.

- Slaughtering must be done by a qualified person in a prescribed manner. The meat or poultry must be drained of blood, first by severing the jugular vein and carotid artery, then by soaking in brine before cooking.

- Meat and meat products may not be prepared with milk or milk products.

- The dishes used in the preparation and serving of meat products must be kept separate from those used for dairy foods.

- Dairy products and meat may not be eaten together. At least 6 hours must elapse after eating meat before eating dairy products, and 30 minutes to 1 hour must elapse after eating dairy products before eating meat.

- The mouth must be rinsed after eating fish and before eating meat.

- There are prescribed fast days: Passover Week, Yom Kippur, and the Feast of Purim.

- No cooking is done on the Sabbath, from sundown Friday to sundown Saturday.

Jewish dietary laws forbid the eating of the following:

- The flesh of animals without cloven (split) hooves or that do not chew their cud

- Hindquarters of any animal

- Shellfish or fish without scales or fins
- Birds of prey
- Creeping things and insects
- Leavened (contains ingredients that cause it to rise) bread during the Passover

In general, the food served is rich. Chicken and fresh-smoked and salted fish are popular, as are noodles, eggs, and flour dishes. These diets can be deficient in fresh vegetables and milk.

Although the dietary restrictions of the Roman Catholic religion have been liberalized, meat is not allowed on Ash Wednesday and Good Friday, but the Pope requests adherents to abstain on the other Fridays during Lent.

Eastern Orthodox

The Eastern Orthodox religion includes Christians from the Middle East, Russia, and Greece. Although interpretations of the dietary laws vary, meat, poultry, fish, and dairy products are restricted on Wednesdays and Fridays and during Lent and Advent.

Seventh-Day Adventist

In general, Seventh-Day Adventists are **lacto-ovo vegetarians**, which means they use milk products and eggs but no meat, fish, or poultry. They may also use nuts, legumes, and meat analogues (substitutes) and tofu. They consider coffee, tea, and alcohol to be harmful.

lacto-ovo vegetarians
vegetarians who will eat dairy products and eggs but no meat, poultry, or fish

Mormon (Latter-Day Saints)

The only dietary restriction observed by the Mormons is the prohibition of coffee, tea, and alcoholic beverages.

Islamic

Adherents of Islam are called Muslims. Their dietary laws prohibit the use of pork and alcohol, and other meats must be slaughtered according to specific laws. During the month of Ramadan, Muslims do not eat or drink during daylight hours.

Hindu

To the Hindus, all life is sacred, and animals contain the souls of ancestors. Consequently, most Hindus are vegetarians. They do not use eggs because eggs represent life.

> ## In The Media
>
> ### Vegetarian Meal Options at Colleges
>
> Pizza, hamburgers, and meat sub sandwiches are popular meals among college dining halls. For students who follow vegetarian, gluten-free, Kosher, or vegan diets, finding a wide selection can be difficult. According to a 2009-2010 Bon Appetit Mangement Company survey, 12% of college-aged vegetarians consider themselves part of the dietary description. Colleges across the country are developing different meals and programs to meet the needs of the growing meat-free population. Some schools, including St. Mary's College in Maryland, run campus farms where the produce is later served at the dining halls. Over 50 colleges have adopted a program called Meatless Mondays, to further promote vegetarian and vegan meals and make the public more aware of their food choices. Students today can make a difference at the universities by voicing their concerns to campus dining services and striving to encourage more nutritious alternatives.
>
> (Source: Adapted from Hopkins, Katy. Colleges that Offer Courses, Choices for Vegetarians. *U.S. News.* July 7, 2011. http://www.usnews.com)

OTHER FOOD PATTERNS
Vegetarians

There are several vegetarian diets. The common factor among them is that they do not include red meat. Some include eggs, some fish, some milk, and some even poultry. When carefully planned, these diets can be nutritious. They can even contribute to a reduction of obesity and a reduced risk of high blood pressure, heart disease, some cancers, and possibly diabetes. They must be carefully planned so that they include all the needed nutrients.

Lacto-ovo vegetarians use dairy products and eggs but no meat, poultry, or fish. **Lacto-vegetarians** use dairy products but no meat, poultry, or eggs. **Vegans** avoid all animal foods. They use soybeans, chickpeas, meat analogues, and tofu. It is important that their diets be carefully planned to include appropriate combinations of the essential amino acids. For example, beans served with corn or rice or peanuts eaten with wheat are better in such combinations than any of them would be if eaten alone. Vegans can show deficiencies of calcium; vitamins A, D, and B_{12}; and, of course, proteins.

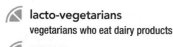

lacto-vegetarians
vegetarians who eat dairy products

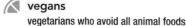

vegans
vegetarians who avoid all animal foods

Zen-Macrobiotic Diets

The macrobiotic diet is a system of 10 diet plans, developed from Zen Buddhism. Adherents progress from the lower number diet to the higher, gradually giving up foods in the following order: desserts, salads, fruits, animal foods, soups, and ultimately vegetables, until only cereals—usually brown rice—are consumed. Beverages are kept to a minimum, and only organically grown foods are used. Foods are grouped as yang (male) or yin (female). A ratio of 5:1 yang to yin is considered important. Most macrobiotic diets are nutritionally inadequate. As the adherents give up foods according to plans, their diets become increasingly inadequate. These diets can be especially dangerous because avid adherents promise medical cures from the diets that cannot be attained, and so medical treatment may be delayed when needed.

HEALTH AND NUTRITION CONSIDERATIONS

Learning and understanding the tools with which to plan a healthy diet are important for all health care professionals so that they can help their clients. All clients should be viewed as individuals whose food customs, which may be different from those of the health care professional, must be respected. A registered dietitian will help with a specific diet plan for a hospitalized client. The dietitian will take into account the client's likes, dislikes, and food customs.

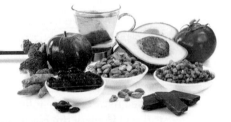

SUMMARY

MyPlate emphasizes grains, fruits, and vegetables—all plant foods. It also includes milk, yogurt, and cheese; meat, poultry, fish, dry beans, eggs, and nuts; and fats, oils, and sweets. Each group has a recommended number of portions based on specific calorie levels. The recommendations are useful in planning a nutritious diet. The Dietary Guidelines are important tools in the maintenance of good health through good nutrition. Their basic recommendation is to eat a balanced diet.

Food habits have many diverse origins. Nationality, religion, and economic and social status all affect their development. When food customs result in inadequate diets, corrections should be made gradually. Corrections are easier to make and are more effective when the reasons for the food habits are understood.

DISCUSSION TOPICS

1. Should health care professionals practice the rules of good nutrition themselves?

2. How do food habits originate?

3. What effects do environment have on particular food habits? When do the effects of a new environment improve diets, and when do they impair them?

4. From personal experience, explain why certain foods are enjoyed more than others that are commonly available in the local area.

5. Why might Scandinavians like fish more than Hungarians do?

6. Using your likes and dislikes, pick a cultural diet that reflects your likes and dislikes. If you were to move to this country, could you adapt to the food habits? Why or why not?

7. Discuss vegetarian diets. Are they safe? Explain.

8. Why is it difficult to convince someone to change her or his food habits? Discuss.

9. Define a balanced diet.

10. Describe MyPlate, including number of servings or portion size recommended for each group.

11. How might one include milk in the diet of a 4-year-old who refuses to drink it?

12. Why would yogurt be a good snack or dessert for a pregnant woman?

13. Alcohol is not considered a food, so why is a Dietary Guideline devoted to it?

14. Why should "crash" or "fad" diets be avoided? What is a better alternative? Why?

15. Discuss the sale of foods with low nutrient density in school cafeterias. Is it a good practice? If so, why? If not, why not? What would your position be on this subject if you were principal of an elementary school? Of a junior or senior high school?

SUGGESTED ACTIVITIES

1. Give a series of short reports on food customs. Each student should select a different country or area within a country for study. After the reports have been presented, hold a class discussion on whether climate, availability of food, or economic or other factors determine the food customs of the countries studied. Include answers to the following questions: What is the climate of the country? What types of crops are grown there? Are modern methods of agriculture used? Does the country depend on imports for much of its food supply? If so, what foods are imported? Are the majority of the citizens poor? What types of foods are popular? What types are expensive? Which of these foods are produced in the country? Which are imported? What is the prevalent religion?

2. Plan a diet for a client who adheres to no meat on Friday during Lent.

3. Role-play a situation in which a diet counselor tries to persuade a client to use more milk.

4. Buy some fruits and vegetables that are new to you. Bring them to class and sample them. Share ideas about their potential uses. Perhaps these might be added to family menus.

5. Using a restaurant menu, choose breakfast, lunch, and dinner. Check the selection of foods against MyPlate. Are they balanced meals?

Discuss the problems that people who eat all their meals in restaurants might have in maintaining a well-balanced diet.

6. Using the following table, fill in the "Menus" column with the foods eaten in the past 2 days. In the "Food Groups Used" column, list the group to which each food belongs. To evaluate personal dietary habits, fill in the "Food Groups Not Used" column. Compare the table with those of the rest of the class and discuss how your eating habits could be improved.

Menus	Food Groups Used	Food Groups Not Used
Breakfast		
Lunch		
Dinner		
Snacks		

7. Check labels on sour cream and yogurt containers. Which would be preferable for someone on a fat-restricted diet? Why? How does the calcium content compare?

8. Adapt the following menu for a person of the Orthodox Jewish faith.

Baked ham	Bread and butter
Scalloped potatoes	Fresh fruit
Buttered peas	Milk or coffee

9. Keep a food journal, writing down everything you eat for 3 days. Visit http://www.choosemyplate.gov and use the diet analysis to determine if your nutrient needs are met. For the nutrients that are deficient, what are you willing to add to your diet to improve your health?

REVIEW

Multiple choice. Select the *letter* that precedes the best answer.

1. Food customs mean one's
   a. food nutrients
   b. food habits
   c. food requirements
   d. all of the above

2. Food customs
   a. may be based on religion or nationality
   b. are always nutritious
   c. are easily changed
   d. are not affected by one's social status

3. Moving to a new environment or experiencing a change in salary
    a. rarely changes established food habits
    b. usually influences established food habits
    c. always reduces the amount of food eaten
    d. never reduces the quality of food eaten

4. Rice is a popular carbohydrate food in
    a. Puerto Rico
    b. central Europe
    c. northern Europe
    d. all of the above

5. In general, the diets of U.S. southerners, Mexicans, Puerto Ricans, and Italians would be improved by the addition of more
    a. rice   c. milk
    b. corn   d. pasta

6. A diet of dried beans, corn, and chili peppers would most likely be used by a(n)
    a. Mexican family
    b. Italian family
    c. Armenian family
    d. Orthodox Jewish family

7. A balanced diet is one that includes
    a. equal amounts of carbohydrates and fats
    b. has only corn, green beans, and potatoes as vegetables
    c. all six classes of nutrients
    d. more vegetables than fruits

8. Fruits and vegetables are rich sources of
    a. vitamins
    b. fats
    c. protein and fiber
    d. only B vitamins

9. Teenagers should have a serving of milk (or its substitute)
    a. not more than twice a day
    b. three times a day
    c. not more than four times a week
    d. not at all if they are overweight

10. Milk products are made from milk and include
    a. butter and margarine
    b. yogurt and cottage cheese
    c. bean curd and coconut milk
    d. all of the above

11. Milk and its products are the best dietary source of
    a. proteins and fats
    b. calcium and vitamin D
    c. carbohydrates
    d. all of the above

12. Breads, cereals, rice, and pasta are rich sources of
    a. vitamin D
    b. fats
    c. carbohydrates
    d. all of the above

13. Daily intake from the protein (meat) group for a 2,000-calorie diet should be
    a. 2 oz   c. 8 oz
    b. 5.5 oz   d. 11 oz

14. High-fat meats and egg yolks contain large amounts of
    a. sodium
    b. fiber
    c. fat and cholesterol
    d. carbohydrates and sodium

15. An example of a breakfast with high nutrient density is
    a. pancakes and cocoa
    b. melon, bran muffin, and cocoa made with fat-free milk
    c. fruit-flavored beverage, cinnamon bun, and coffee
    d. fried eggs, bacon, and coffee

16. Excessive amounts of salt in the diet
    a. raise cholesterol levels substantially
    b. are thought to contribute to hypertension
    c. cause cirrhosis of the liver
    d. have no relevance to one's nutritional status

17. MyPlate
    a. food groups are nutritionally interchangeable
    b. is an outline for meal planning for adults only
    c. advises that fruits and vegetables be eaten in moderation
    d. recommends portion ranges for the five food groups

18. The Nutrition Labeling and Education Act of 1990
    a. requires that descriptive words used for foods be standardized
    b. sets maximum amounts of cholesterol allowed for each food serving
    c. permits no health claims on food containers
    d. does not require the food manufacturer or processor to list the total amounts in each serving of calories, sodium, or dietary fiber

19. Foods rich in complex carbohydrates, such as whole-grain breads and cereals, are also excellent sources of
    a. calcium and phosphorus
    b. vitamins C and D
    c. dietary fiber and B vitamins
    d. proteins and fats

20. When choosing foods from the meats, poultry, and fish food group, one should be careful to select foods that
    a. are rich in calcium and phosphorus
    b. provide at least one-half of one's daily need for carbohydrates
    c. have limited amounts of protein and iron
    d. are low in saturated fats and cholesterol

21. The two vitamins that the Nutrition Labeling and Education Act of 1990 requires be included as amounts per serving on food labels are
    a. vitamin A and thiamine
    b. niacin and folic acid
    c. vitamins A and C
    d. vitamins D and K

22. Consuming alcoholic beverages
    a. by pregnant women can cause birth defects
    b. can cause cirrhosis of the liver only in men
    c. has little or no effect on one's nutritional status
    d. has no effect on one's appetite

23. People of the Jewish faith eat Kosher foods because
    a. they only like meat
    b. they believe it makes them live longer
    c. they adhere to strict dietary laws
    d. the diet contains more sodium

Case In Point

MARA: MAINTAINING A HEALTHY DIET WHILE GAINING INDEPENDENCE

Mara's parents immigrated to the United States from Mexico when she was young. She has lived with her parents who have worked for farmers since moving to the United States. They have been able to enjoy many of the fresh vegetables and fruits grown by the farmers. They also have access to a local farmer's market where her parents deliver produce from the farmers. They purchase fresh meats and seafood at the market as well. Her mother loves to cook and therefore they have rarely eaten at restaurants. Now that Mara has finished high school, she has received a scholarship to college. The college is nearby; however, Mara will be living on campus and not with her parents. Her mother is concerned about her health and nutrition as she goes away to college. She is concerned she will make poor nutritional choices if she is not educated on nutrition. She would like her to be aware of consequences of fast foods and alcohol consumption. Mara and her parents will be traveling to college to get her registered for classes soon. Mara's mother has made an appointment with a dietitian at the local hospital before they leave. She would like the dietitian to review healthy nutrition for Mara. She would like her to discuss with Mara how to incorporate American foods and eating out while still maintaining a healthy diet. Mara is currently 5 feet 4 inches and 119 pounds. She is happy with her current body weight and feels good about herself. She tells the dietitian she is interested in becoming more aware of what she is eating. She knows that in her new independence it will be easier to prepare healthy meals if she has the knowledge she needs to accomplish this task.

ASSESSMENT

1. What factors will be influencing Mara as she attends college?
2. List the subjective information that can be obtained from Mara and her mother about her eating habits
3. What can you caution Mara regarding her introduction into the college world of nutrition?
4. How significant are these problems?
5. Is Mara currently at a healthy weight for her height?

DIAGNOSIS

6. Write a nursing diagnosis for Mara.

PLAN/GOAL

7. What changes will Mara expect to see if she decides to eat less healthily?
8. What situations will be most stressful to Mara?
9. What could Mara do to help keep her nutrition and food consumption on track?
10. What goals could Mara set to also help maintain her weight and her health?

IMPLEMENTATION

11. List some strategies Mara can use to help keep healthy.
12. What substitutes could Mara make to be able to fit in with the crowd and still be eating well?

13. What would you caution Mara about in regard to stressful situations?

EVALUATION/OUTCOME CRITERIA

14. How will Mara be able to determine her success for healthy eating?
15. How well will Mara be able to associate body changes with poor food choices?
16. How could the dietitian evaluate Mara's progress?

THINKING FURTHER

17. Who else will benefit from Mara's food choices?
18. What resources could help Mara achieve her goals?

rate this plate

Analyze the meal that Mara has prepared for dinner. Are the portions the right size for Mara? How would you change the portion sizes you feel are not correct? Rework this plate.

2 chicken tacos with lettuce, tomato, cheese, and onion

1 cup rice

¾ cup refried beans made with lard

12 oz. regular soda

Case In Point

THOMAS: CONSIDERING A VEGAN LIFESTYLE

Thomas has always been an athlete. He played a wide variety of sports throughout his high school years. He continued to be very active even in college. He has done some bodybuilding and has always consumed a high percentage of his calories from protein and meat sources. Thomas is 26 years old and is Caucasian. He is currently 5 feet 9 inches tall and 215 pounds. Recently he has been dating a woman whom he is really in love with. His only concern is that she is of Indian decent and due to her cultural and religious beliefs, she is a vegan. She has not tried to persuade him into adapting the vegan lifestyle; however, he knows that meals at home with her would never contain animal proteins. He is not sure that he would ever be able to give up his meat sources for a different protein source. He is primarily concerned he would not get the adequate protein he needs for his weightlifting and bodybuilding activities. He has decided it may be in his best interest to discuss his concerns with his doctor. His doctor suggested meeting with a registered dietitian to review his calorie and protein needs and to discuss his options for alternative protein sources.

ASSESSMENT

1. Thomas is 5 feet 9 inches tall. What is the ideal body weight for him?
2. Is Thomas at a healthy body weight for his height?
3. Using Table 2-6, what would you expect an appropriate calorie range for Thomas to be?
4. What would be important to discuss with Thomas when considering a vegan diet plan?

DIAGNOSIS

5. Write a nursing diagnosis for Thomas.

PLAN/GOAL

6. What could Thomas do to help ensure he is receiving adequate nutrition and meeting his macro- and micronutrient needs?

IMPLEMENTATION

7. Name food sources Thomas could consume that are high in calcium.
8. Name food sources Thomas could consume that are high in vitamin B_{12}.
9. Name food sources Thomas could consume that are high in iron.
10. Name food sources that Thomas could consume that are high in omega-3 fatty acids.

EVALUATION/OUTCOME CRITERIA

11. How would you determine the success of Thomas's transition to his new vegan lifestyle?

THINKING FURTHER

12. What other types of vegetarian lifestyles are options for Thomas if he would like to incorporate some animal food sources?

rate this plate

Thomas is concerned about getting enough protein on a vegan diet. Will this meal provide Thomas with enough protein? What vegan protein sources could Thomas include in the meal or as a snack to meet his protein needs? Rate this plate.

Tofu stir-fry with broccoli, snow peas, carrots, and onion

½ cup brown rice

⅛ of a cantaloupe, sliced

Carbonated fruit beverage

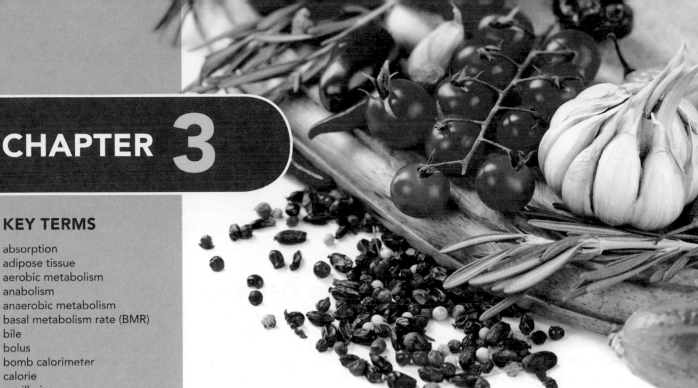

CHAPTER 3

KEY TERMS

absorption
adipose tissue
aerobic metabolism
anabolism
anaerobic metabolism
basal metabolism rate (BMR)
bile
bolus
bomb calorimeter
calorie
capillaries
cardiac sphincter
catabolism
catalyst
chemical digestion
cholecystokinin (CCK)
chyme
colon
digestion
duodenum
energy balance
energy requirement
enzymes
esophagus
feces
fundus (of stomach)
gastric juices
gastrin
gastrointestinal (GI) tract
hormones
hydrolysis
ileum
jejunum
kilocalorie (kcal)
Krebs cycle
lactase
lacteals
lean body mass
lymphatic system
maltase
mechanical digestion
metabolism
pancreas
pancreatic amylase
pancreatic lipase
pancreatic proteases
pepsin

DIGESTION, ABSORPTION, AND METABOLISM

OBJECTIVES

After studying this chapter, you should be able to:

- Describe the processes of digestion, absorption, and metabolism
- Name the organs in the digestive system and describe their functions
- Name the enzymes or digestive juices secreted by each organ and gland in the digestive system
- Calculate your basal metabolic rate

Although the body is infinitely more complex than the automobile engine, it may be compared to the engine because both require fuel to run. The body's fuel is, of course, food. For the body to use its fuel, it must first prepare the food and then distribute it appropriately. It does this through the processes of digestion and absorption. The actual use of the food as fuel, resulting in energy, is called **metabolism**.

57

KEY TERMS (continued)

peptidases
peristalsis
pylorus
resting energy expenditure (REE)
saliva
salivary amylase
secretin
sucrase
villi

 metabolism
the use of the food by the body after digestion which results in energy

 digestion
breakdown of food in the body in preparation for absorption

 gastrointestinal (GI) tract
pertaining to the digestive system

DIGESTION

Digestion is the process whereby food is broken down into smaller parts, chemically changed, and moved through the gastrointestinal system. The **gastrointestinal (GI) tract** consists of the body structures that participate in digestion. Digestion begins in the mouth and ends at the anus. Along the entire GI tract, secretions of mucus lubricate and protect the mucosal tissues. As the process of digestion is discussed, refer to Figure 3-1 and note the locations of the structures that perform the functions of digestion.

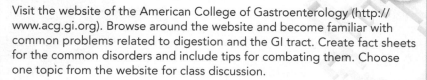

EXPLORING **THE WEB**

Visit the website of the American College of Gastroenterology (http://www.acg.gi.org). Browse around the website and become familiar with common problems related to digestion and the GI tract. Create fact sheets for the common disorders and include tips for combating them. Choose one topic from the website for class discussion.

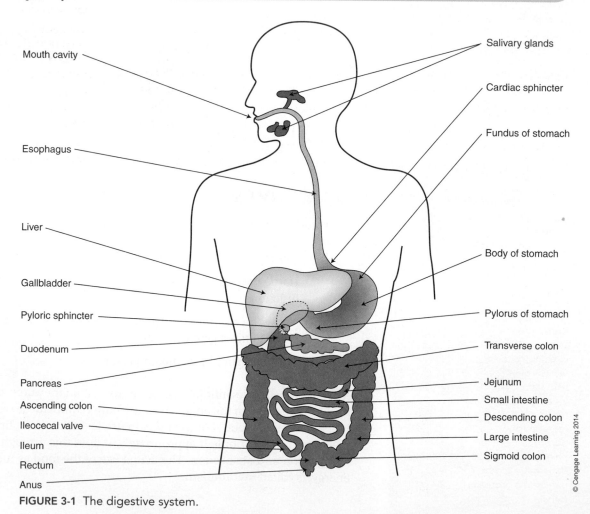

FIGURE 3-1 The digestive system.

© Cengage Learning 2014

Digestion occurs through two types of action—mechanical and chemical. During **mechanical digestion**, food is broken into smaller pieces by the teeth. It is then moved along the GI tract through the esophagus, stomach, and intestines. This movement is caused by a rhythmic contraction of the muscular walls of the tract called **peristalsis**. Mechanical digestion helps to prepare food for chemical digestion by breaking it into smaller pieces. Several small pieces collectively have more surface area than fewer large ones and thus are more readily broken down by digestive juices.

During **chemical digestion**, the composition of carbohydrates, proteins, and fats is changed. Chemical changes occur through the addition of water and the resulting splitting, or breaking down, of the food molecules. This process is called **hydrolysis**. Food is broken down into nutrients that the tissues can absorb and use. Hydrolysis also involves digestive **enzymes** that act on food substances, causing them to break down into simple compounds. An enzyme can also act as a **catalyst**, which speeds up the chemical reactions without itself being changed in the process. Digestive enzymes are secreted by the mouth, stomach, **pancreas**, and small intestine (Table 3-1). An enzyme is often named for the substance on which it acts. For example, the enzyme sucrase acts on sucrose, the enzyme maltase acts on maltose, and lactase acts on lactose.

Digestion in the Mouth

Digestion begins in the mouth, where the food is broken into smaller pieces by the teeth and mixed with saliva (Figure 3-2). At this point, each mouthful of food that is ready to be swallowed is called a **bolus**. **Saliva** is a secretion of

mechanical digestion
the part of digestion that requires certain mechanical movements such as chewing, swallowing, and peristalsis

peristalsis
rhythmical movement of the intestinal tract; moves the chyme along

chemical digestion
chemical changes in foods during digestion caused by hydrolysis

hydrolysis
the addition of water resulting in the breakdown of the molecule

enzymes
organic substances that cause changes in other substances

catalyst
a substance that causes another substance to react

pancreas
gland that secretes enzymes essential for digestion and insulin, which is essential for glucose metabolism

bolus
food in the mouth that is ready to be swallowed

saliva
secretion of the salivary glands

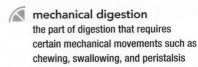

TABLE 3-1 Enzymes and Foods Acted Upon

SOURCE	ENZYME	FOOD ACTED UPON
Mouth	Salivary amylase	Starch
Stomach	Pepsin	Proteins
	Rennin	Proteins in milk
	Gastric lipase	Emulsified fat
Small intestine	Pancreatic amylase	Starch
	Pancreatic proteases (trypsin) (chymotrypsin) (carboxypeptidases)	Proteins
	Pancreatic lipase (steapsin)	Fats
	Lactase	Lactose
	Maltase	Maltose
	Sucrase	Sucrose
	Peptidases	Proteins

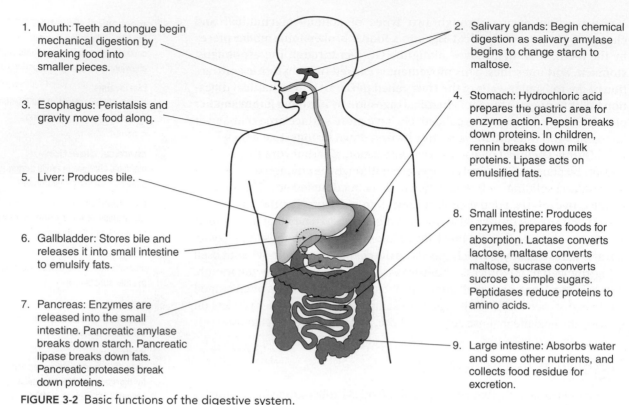

1. Mouth: Teeth and tongue begin mechanical digestion by breaking food into smaller pieces.

2. Salivary glands: Begin chemical digestion as salivary amylase begins to change starch to maltose.

3. Esophagus: Peristalsis and gravity move food along.

4. Stomach: Hydrochloric acid prepares the gastric area for enzyme action. Pepsin breaks down proteins. In children, rennin breaks down milk proteins. Lipase acts on emulsified fats.

5. Liver: Produces bile.

6. Gallbladder: Stores bile and releases it into small intestine to emulsify fats.

7. Pancreas: Enzymes are released into the small intestine. Pancreatic amylase breaks down starch. Pancreatic lipase breaks down fats. Pancreatic proteases break down proteins.

8. Small intestine: Produces enzymes, prepares foods for absorption. Lactase converts lactose, maltase converts maltose, sucrase converts sucrose to simple sugars. Peptidases reduce proteins to amino acids.

9. Large intestine: Absorbs water and some other nutrients, and collects food residue for excretion.

© Cengage Learning 2014

FIGURE 3-2 Basic functions of the digestive system.

salivary amylase
also called ptyalin; the enzyme secreted by the salivary glands to act on starch

the salivary glands that contains water, salts, and a digestive enzyme called **salivary amylase** (also called ptyalin), which acts on complex carbohydrates (starch). Food is normally held in the mouth for such a short time that only small amounts of carbohydrates are chemically changed there. The salivary glands also secrete a mucous material that lubricates and binds food particles to help in swallowing the bolus. The final chemical digestion of carbohydrates occurs in the small intestine.

The Esophagus

esophagus
tube leading from the mouth to the stomach; part of the gastrointestinal system

The **esophagus** is a 10-inch muscular tube through which food travels from the mouth to the stomach. When swallowed, the bolus of food is moved down the esophagus by peristalsis and gravity. At the lower end of the esophagus, the **cardiac sphincter** opens to allow passage of the bolus into the stomach. The cardiac sphincter prevents the acidic content of the stomach from flowing back into the esophagus. When this sphincter malfunctions, it causes acid reflux disease.

cardiac sphincter
the muscle at the base of the esophagus that prevents gastric reflux from moving into the esophagus

Digestion in the Stomach

fundus (of the stomach)
upper part of the stomach

pylorus
the end of the stomach nearest the intestine

The stomach consists of an upper portion known as the **fundus**, a middle area known as the body of the stomach, and the end nearest the small intestine called the **pylorus**. Food enters the fundus and moves to the body of the stomach, where the muscles in the stomach wall gradually knead the food, tear it, and mix it with gastric juices, and with the intrinsic factor necessary for the absorption of vitamin B_{12}, before it can be propelled forward in slow, controlled movements. The food becomes a semiliquid mass called **chyme** (pronounced "kime"). When the chyme enters the pylorus, it causes distention and the release of the hormone **gastrin**, which increases the release of gastric juices.

Gastric juices are digestive secretions of the stomach. They contain hydrochloric acid, **pepsin**, and mucus. Hydrochloric acid activates the enzyme pepsin, prepares protein molecules for partial digestion by pepsin, destroys most bacteria in the food ingested, and makes iron and calcium more soluble. As the hydrochloric acid is released, a thick mucus is also secreted to protect the stomach from this harsh acid. In children, there are two additional enzymes: rennin, which acts on milk protein and casein, and gastric lipase, which breaks the butterfat molecules of milk into smaller molecules.

In summary, the functions of the stomach include the following:

- Temporary storage of food
- Mixing of food with gastric juices
- Regulation of a slow, controlled emptying of food into the intestine
- Secretion of the intrinsic factor for vitamin B_{12} (to be discussed in Chapter 7)
- Destruction of most bacteria inadvertently consumed

Digestion in the Small Intestine

Chyme moves through the pyloric sphincter into the **duodenum**, the first section of the small intestine. It subsequently passes through the **jejunum**, the midsection of the small intestine, and the **ileum**, the last section of the small intestine.

When food reaches the small intestine, the hormone **secretin** causes the pancreas to release sodium bicarbonate to neutralize the acidity of the chyme. The gallbladder is triggered by the hormone **cholecystokinin (CCK)**, which is produced by intestinal mucosal glands when fat enters, to release **bile**. Bile is produced in the liver but stored in the gallbladder. Bile emulsifies fat after it is secreted into the small intestine. This action enables the enzymes to digest the fats more easily.

Chyme also triggers the pancreas to secrete its juice into the small intestine. Pancreatic juice contains the following enzymes:

- Trypsin, chymotrypsin, and carboxypeptidases split proteins into smaller substances. These are called **pancreatic proteases** because they are protein-splitting enzymes produced by the pancreas.
- **Pancreatic amylase** converts starches (polysaccharides) to simple sugars.
- **Pancreatic lipase** reduces fats to fatty acids and glycerol.

 chyme
the food mass as it has been mixed with gastric juices

 gastrin
hormone released by the stomach

 gastric juices
the digestive secretions of the stomach

 pepsin
an enzyme secreted by the stomach that is essential for the digestion of proteins

 duodenum
first (and smallest) section of the small intestine

 jejunum
middle section comprising about two fifths of the small intestine

 ileum
last part of the small intestine

 secretin
hormone causing the pancreas to release sodium bicarbonate to neutralize acidity of the chyme

 cholecystokinin (CCK)
hormone that triggers the gallbladder to release bile

 bile
secretion of the liver, stored in the gallbladder, essential for the digestion of fats

 pancreatic proteases
enzymes secreted by the pancreas that are essential for the digestion of proteins

 pancreatic amylase
the enzyme secreted by the pancreas that is essential for the digestion of starch

 pancreatic lipase
enzyme secreted by the pancreas that is essential for the digestion of fats

lactase
enzyme secreted by the small intestine for the digestion of lactose

maltase
enzyme secreted by the small intestine essential for the digestion of maltose

sucrase
enzyme secreted by the small intestine to aid in digestion of sucrose

peptidases
enzymes secreted by the small intestine that are essential for the digestion of proteins

colon
large intestine

absorption
passage of nutrients into the blood or lymphatic system

lymphatic system
transports fat-soluble substances from the small intestine to the vascular system

villi
tiny, hairlike structures in the small intestines through which nutrients are absorbed

capillaries
tiny blood vessels connecting veins and arteries

lacteals
lymphatic vessels in the small intestine that absorb fatty acids and glycerol

The small intestine itself produces an intestinal juice that contains the enzymes **lactase**, **maltase**, and **sucrase**. These enzymes split lactose, maltose, and sucrose, respectively, into simple sugars. The small intestine also produces enzymes called **peptidases** that break down proteins into amino acids.

The Large Intestine

The large intestine, or **colon**, consists of the cecum, colon, and rectum. The cecum is a blind, pouch-like beginning of the colon in the right lower quadrant of the abdomen. The appendix is a diverticulum that extends off the cecum. The cecum is separated from the ileum by the ileocecal valve and is considered to be the beginning of the large intestine (colon). Its primary function is to absorb water and salts from undigested food. It has a muscular wall that can knead the contents to enhance absorption. One of the end products of fermentation in the cecum is volatile fatty acids. The major volatile fatty acids are acetate, propionate, and butyrate. These are absorbed from the large intestine and used as sources of energy. The digested food then enters the ascending colon and moves through the transverse colon and on to the descending colon, the sigmoid colon, the rectum, and, finally, the anal canal.

ABSORPTION

After digestion, the next major step in the body's use of its food is absorption (Figure 3-3). **Absorption** is the passage of nutrients into the blood or **lymphatic system** (the lymphatic vessels carry fat-soluble particles and molecules that are too large to pass through the capillaries into the bloodstream).

To be absorbed, nutrients must be in their simplest forms. Carbohydrates must be broken down to the simple sugars (glucose, fructose, and galactose), proteins to amino acids, and fats to fatty acids and glycerol. Most absorption of nutrients occurs in the small intestine, although some occurs in the large intestine. Water is absorbed in the stomach, small intestine, and large intestine.

Absorption in the Small Intestine

The small intestine is approximately 22 feet long. Its inner surface has mucosal folds, villi, and microvilli to increase the surface area for maximum absorption. The fingerlike projections called **villi** have hundreds of microscopic, hairlike projections called microvilli. The microvilli are very sensitive to the nutrient needs of our bodies (Figure 3-4). Each villus contains numerous blood **capillaries** (tiny blood vessels) and **lacteals** (lymphatic vessels). The villi absorb nutrients from the chyme by way of these blood capillaries and lacteals, which eventually transfer them to the bloodstream. Glucose, fructose, galactose, amino acids, minerals, and water-soluble vitamins are absorbed by the capillaries. Fructose and galactose are subsequently carried to the liver, where they are converted to glucose. Lacteals absorb glycerol and fatty acids (end products of fat digestion) in addition to the fat-soluble vitamins.

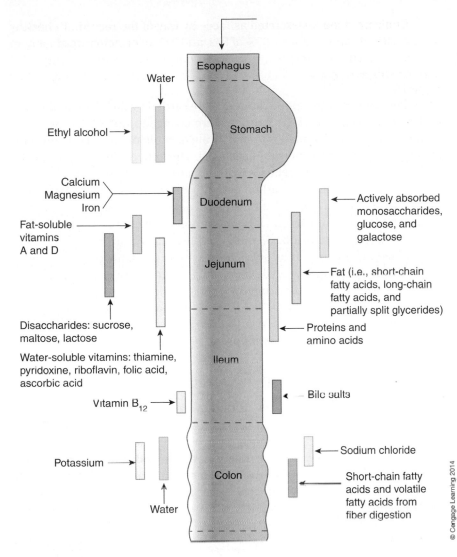

FIGURE 3-3 Absorption in the gastrointestinal tract.

Esophagus

Water

Stomach

Ethyl alcohol →

Calcium
Magnesium
Iron

Duodenum

Fat-soluble
vitamins
A and D

Jejunum

Disaccharides: sucrose,
maltose, lactose

Water-soluble vitamins: thiamine,
pyridoxine, riboflavin, folic acid,
ascorbic acid

Ileum

Vitamin B$_{12}$ →

Bile salts ◄

Potassium →

Sodium chloride

Colon

Short-chain fatty
acids and volatile
fatty acids from
fiber digestion

Water

→ Actively absorbed
monosaccharides,
glucose, and
galactose

← Fat (i.e., short-chain
fatty acids, long-chain
fatty acids, and
partially split glycerides)

← Proteins and
amino acids

Absorption in the Large Intestine

When the chyme reaches the large intestine, most digestion and absorption have already occurred. The colon walls secrete mucus as a protection from the acidic digestive juices in the chyme, which is coming from the small intestine through the ileocecal valve.

The major tasks of the large intestine are to absorb water, to synthesize some B vitamins and vitamin K (essential for blood clotting), and to collect food residue. Food residue is the part of food that the body's enzyme action cannot digest and consequently the body cannot absorb. Such residue is commonly called dietary fiber. Examples include the outer hulls of corn kernels and grains of wheat, celery strings, and apple skins. It is important that the diet contains adequate fiber because it promotes the health of the large intestine by helping to produce softer stools and more frequent bowel movements (see Chapter 4).

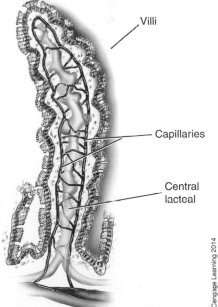

Villi

Capillaries

Central
lacteal

FIGURE 3-4 Wall of the small intestine.

EXPLORING THE WEB

For a fun animation showing the process of digestion and absorption, go to the National Geographic website (http://www.nationalgeographic.com), and search "digestive-system-article" to view an animation of the digestive system. Create a web link to this page to use as a teaching aid for your clients.

feces
solid waste from the large intestine

aerobic metabolism
combining nutrients with oxygen within the cell; also called oxidation

anaerobic metabolism
reduces fats without use of oxygen

Krebs cycle
a series of enzymatic reactions that serve as the main source of cellular energy

anabolism
the creation of new compounds during metabolism

catabolism
the breakdown of compounds during metabolism

hormones
chemical messengers secreted by a variety of glands

Undigested food is excreted as **feces** by way of the rectum. In healthy people, 99% of carbohydrates, 95% of fats, and 92% of proteins are absorbed.

METABOLISM

After digestion and absorption, nutrients are carried by the blood to the cells of the body. Within the cells, nutrients are changed into energy through a complex process called metabolism. During **aerobic metabolism**, nutrients are combined with oxygen within each cell. This process is known as oxidation. Oxidation ultimately reduces carbohydrates to carbon dioxide and water; Proteins are reduced to carbon dioxide, water, and nitrogen. **Anaerobic metabolism** reduces fats without the use of oxygen. The complete oxidation of carbohydrates, proteins, and fats is commonly called the **Krebs cycle**.

As nutrients are oxidized, energy is released. When this released energy is used to build new substances from simpler ones, the process is called **anabolism**. An example of anabolism is the formation of new body tissues. When released energy is used to reduce substances to simpler ones, the process is called **catabolism**. This building up (anabolism) and breaking down (catabolism) of substances is a continuous process (metabolism) within the body and requires a continuous supply of nutrients.

Metabolism and the Thyroid Gland

Metabolism is governed primarily by the **hormones** secreted by the thyroid gland. These secretions are *triiodothyronine* (T_3) and *thyroxine* (T_4). When the thyroid gland secretes too much of these hormones, a condition known as hyperthyroidism may result. In such a case, the body metabolizes its food too quickly, resulting in weight loss. When too little T_4 and T_3 are secreted, the condition called hypothyroidism may occur. In this case, the body metabolizes food too slowly, and the client tends to become sluggish and accumulates fat.

In The Media

Using Herbs to Aid the Digestive Process

The digestive system is a complex system that is involved with the feelings of fullness, gassiness, indigestion, constipation, and diarrhea. Herbalists have discovered that certain plants can aid in the digestive process, decreasing digestive discomfort. Plants that are bitter or aromatic have been proven safe and effective for aiding in digestion. The following plants or herbs have been known to assist in digestion: dandelion root and leaf, burdock root, orange peel, fennel seed, yellow dock root, gentian root, and ginger root. Some of their functions include relieving gas and cramps, laxative agents, decreasing motion sickness, and resolving heart burn. These bitters can be found year round and are available in Whole Food stores nationwide.

(Source: Kilham, Chris, *Herbs to Improve Digestion*. Fox News. December 21, 2011. http://www.foxnews.com)

ENERGY

Energy is constantly needed for the maintenance of body tissue and temperature and for growth (involuntary activity), as well as for voluntary activity. Examples of voluntary activity include walking, running, swimming, and gardening. The three groups of nutrients that provide energy to the body are carbohydrates, proteins, and fats. Carbohydrates are and should be the primary energy source (see Chapter 4).

Energy Measurement

The unit used to measure the energy value of foods is the **kilocalorie (kcal)**, commonly known as the large calorie, or **calorie**. In the metric system it is known as the kilojoule. One kilocalorie is equal to 4.184 kilojoules, but this may be rounded off to 4.2 kilojoules. One calorie is the amount of heat needed to raise the temperature of 1 kilogram of water by 1 degree Celsius (°C).

The number of calories in a food is its energy value, or caloric density. Energy values of foods vary a great deal because they are determined by the types and amounts of nutrients each food contains.

One gram of carbohydrate yields 4 calories; 1 gram of protein yields 4 calories; and 1 gram of fat yields 9 calories. One gram of alcohol yields 7 calories.

The energy values of foods are determined by a device known as a **bomb calorimeter**. The inner part of a calorimeter holds a measured amount of food, and the outer part holds water. The food is burned, and its caloric value is determined by the increase in the temperature of the surrounding water. The number of calories in average servings of common foods is listed in Appendix B.

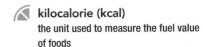
kilocalorie (kcal)
the unit used to measure the fuel value of foods

calorie
represents the amount of heat needed to raise the temperature of 1 kilogram of water by 1 degree Celsius (°C)

bomb calorimeter
device used to scientifically determine the kcal value of foods

Basal Metabolic Rate

One's basal metabolism is the energy necessary to carry on all involuntary vital processes while the body is at rest. These processes are respiration, circulation, regulation of body temperature, and cell activity and maintenance. The rate at which energy is needed only for body maintenance is called the **basal metabolism rate (BMR)**. The BMR may be referred to as the **resting energy expenditure (REE)**.

Medical tests can determine one's BMR (or REE). When such a test is given, the body is at rest and performing only the essential, involuntary functions. Voluntary activity is not measured in a BMR test. Factors that affect one's BMR are lean body mass, body size, sex, age, heredity, physical condition, and climate.

Lean body mass is muscle, as opposed to fat tissue. Because there is more metabolic activity in muscle tissue than in fat or bone tissue, muscle tissue requires more calories than does fat or bone tissue. People with large body frames require more calories than do people with small frames because the former have more body mass to maintain and move than do those with small frames.

Men usually require more energy than women. They tend to be larger and to have more lean body mass than women.

basal metabolism rate (BMR)
the rate at which energy is needed for body maintenance; also referred to as resting energy expenditure (REE)

resting energy expenditure (REE)
same as basal metabolism rate (BMR)

lean body mass
percentage of muscle tissue

Children require more calories per pound of body weight than adults because they are growing. As people age, the lean body mass declines, and the basal metabolic rate declines accordingly. Heredity is also a determining factor. Like appearance, one's BMR may resemble that of a parent. One's physical condition also affects the BMR. For example, women require more calories during pregnancy and lactation than at other times. The basal metabolic rate increases during fever and decreases during periods of starvation or severely reduced calorie intake. People living and working in extremely cold or warm climates require more calories to maintain normal body temperature than they would in a more temperate climate.

Thermic Effect of Food

The body requires energy to process food (digestion, absorption, transportation, metabolism, and storage); this requirement represents 10% of daily energy (calorie) intake. Multiply BMR by 0.10 and add to the BMR (REE) before an activity factor is calculated.

Estimating BMR

Dietitians commonly use the Harris-Benedict equation to determine the BMR (REE) of persons above the age of 18. This equation uses height, weight,

---

Supersize USA

When you drive through the fast-food restaurant, keep in mind the following worst fast-food choices:

Order	Calories	Fat	Carbs	Protein	Sodium
McDonald's Angus Chipotle BBQ Bacon Burger	800	39 g	66 g	45 g	2,202 mg
Burger King Tendercrisp Garden Salad with Ken's Ranch Dressing	600	42 g	30 g	27 g	1,610 mg
Denny's Country Fried Steak with gravy	1,170	74 g	74 g	55 g	2,920 mg
Burger King Sausage, Egg, & Cheese Croissan'wich	490	31 g	27 g	19 g	1,000 mg
Carl's Breakfast Burger	810	42 g	69 g	39 g	1,480 mg
Wendy's Caramel Frosty Shake, large	1,020	19 g	198 g	14 g	510 mg
Applebees Oriental Chicken Salad	1,340	98 g	85 g	37 g	1,200 mg
Pizza Hut Meat Lover's Pan Pizza (2 slices)	960	56 g	74 g	40 g	2,360 mg

Source: Data retrieved from website for each fast-food restaurant.

and age as factors and results in a more individualized estimate of the REE than some other methods (Figure 3-5).

Another method used to estimate one's BMR, or REE, is the following:

1. Convert body weight from pounds to kilograms (kg) by dividing pounds by 2.2 (2.2 pounds equal 1 kilogram).
2. Multiply the kilograms by 24 (hours per day).
3. Multiply the answer obtained in step 2 by 0.9 for a woman and by 1.0 for a man.

For example, assume that a woman weighs 110 pound. Divide 110 by 2.2 for an answer of 50 kg. Multiply 50 kg by 24 hours in a day for an answer of 1,200 calories. Then multiply 1,200 calories by 0.9 for an answer of 1,080 calories. This is the estimated basal metabolic energy requirement for that particular woman.

Female: **REE = 655 + (9.6 × weight in kg) + (1.8 × height in cm) − (4.7 × age)**

Male: **REE = 66 + (13.7 × weight in kg) + (5 × height in cm) − (6.8 × age)**

W = weight in kilograms (kg) (weight in pounds ÷ 2.2 = kg)
H = height in centimeters (cm) (height in inches × 2.54 = cm)
A = age in years

FIGURE 3-5 Harris-Benedict equation.

Harris & Benedict, 1919

Calculating Total Energy Requirements

An individual's average daily **energy requirement** is the total number of calories needed in a 24-hour period. Energy requirements of people differ, depending on BMR (REE) and activities. More energy is burned playing soccer than playing the piano. Refer to Table 3-2 for caloric guidelines according to MyPlate.

Table 3-3 shows suggested weights for adults according to height.

 energy requirement
number of calories required by the body each day

Energy Balance

A person who takes in fewer calories than she or he burns usually loses weight. If someone takes in more calories than she or he burns, the body stores them as **adipose tissue** (fat). Some adipose tissue is necessary to protect the body and support its organs. Adipose tissue also helps regulate body temperature, just as insulation helps regulate the temperature of a building. An excess of adipose tissue, however, leads to obesity, which can endanger health because it puts extra burdens on body organs and systems. For the healthy person, the goal is **energy balance**. This means that the number of calories consumed matches the number of calories required for one's BMR (REE) and activity.

adipose tissue
fatty tissue

 energy balance
occurs when the caloric value of food ingested equals the calories expended

TABLE 3-2   MyPlate Food Intake Patterns

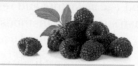

ESTIMATED DAILY CALORIE NEEDS

To determine which food intake pattern to use for an individual, the following chart gives an estimate of individual calorie needs. The calorie range for each age and gender is based on physical activity level, from sedentary to active. Sedentary means a lifestyle that includes only the light physical activity associated with typical day-to-day life. Active means a lifestyle that includes physical activity equivalent to walking more than 3 miles per day at 3–4 miles per hour, in addition to the light physical activity associated with typical day-to-day life.

| | CALORIE RANGE | | | | CALORIE RANGE | | |
	SEDENTARY	→	ACTIVE		SEDENTARY	→	ACTIVE
Children				**Males**			
2–3 years	1,000	→	1,400	4–8 years	1,400	→	2,000
Females				9–13	1,800	→	2,600
4–8 years	1,200	→	1,800	14–18	2,200	→	3,200
9–13	1,600	→	2,200	19–30	2,400	→	3,000
14–18	1,800	→	2,400	31–50	2,200	→	3,000
19–30	2,000	→	2,400	51+	2,000	→	2,800
31–50	1,800	→	2,200				
51+	1,600	→	2,200				

Source: U.S. Department of Agriculture, Center for Nutrition Policy and Promotions. *MyPlate Food Intake Patterns.* 2011. http://www.choosemyplate.gov

SPOTLIGHT *on Life Cycle*

Maintaining energy, or calorie, balance can be achieved by balancing "energy in" with "energy out." What you eat and drink is "energy in." Through daily activities and physical activity, energy is expended and can be considered as "energy out." When "energy in" equals "energy out" over time, body weight will stay the same. When there is more "in" than "out" over time, weight gain can result. When there is more "out" than "in" over time, weight loss can result. Eating an additional 150 calories per day for a year can result in a 10-pound weight gain. Reducing "energy in" or increasing "energy out" can help a person lose unwanted weight. Here are a few ways to cut 150 calories (energy in):

- Drink water instead of a 12-ounce regular soda.
- Order a small serving of French fries instead of a medium serving.
- Eat an egg-white omelet instead of whole eggs.
- Use tuna canned in water instead of oil.

Here are a few ways to burn 150 calories (energy out) in just 30 minutes (for a 150-pound person):

- Shoot hoops
- Walk 2 miles
- Do yard work
- Go for a bike ride
- Dance with family or friends

(Source: Adapted from the National Heart Lung and Blood Institute. *Balance Food and Activity.* Accessed February 13, 2012 from http://www.nhlbi .nih.gov)

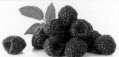

TABLE 3-3 Suggested Weights for Adults

| HEIGHT (WITHOUT SHOES) | WEIGHT IN POUNDS WITHOUT CLOTHES | |
	19–34 YEARS	35 YEARS AND OVER
5'0"	97–128	108–138
5'1"	101–132	111–143
5'2"	104–137	115–148
5'3"	107–141	119–152
5'4"	111–146	122–157
5'5"	114–150	126–162
5'6"	118–155	130–167
5'7"	121–160	134–172
5'8"	125–164	138–178
5'9"	129–169	142–183
5'10"	132–174	146–188
5'11"	136–179	151–194
6'0"	140–184	155–199
6'1"	144–189	159–205
6'2"	148–195	164–210
6'3"	152–200	168–216
6'4"	156–205	173–222
6'5"	160–211	177–228
6'6"	164–216	182–234

Note: The higher weights in the ranges generally apply to men, who tend to have more muscle and bone; the lower weights more often apply to women, who have less muscle and bone.

Source: U.S. Department of Health and Human Services and U.S. Department of Agriculture. *Dietary Guidelines for Americans* (3rd ed.). Accessed June 19, 2009 from http://www.cnpp.usda.gov

HEALTH AND NUTRITION CONSIDERATIONS

The health care professional will find that clients may make broad statements concerning the way their bodies work. An example would be: "Milk doesn't agree with me." This is when the appropriate questions need to be asked, such as "Does it cause flatulence (gas)?" or "Do you have to go to the bathroom immediately?" The first is a classic symptom of lactose intolerance, whereas the latter could indicate an allergy or other serious problems that would require further workup. Clients needing education about metabolism and energy requirements may tell you that they don't eat anything but keep gaining weight or that they exercise all the time but don't lose an ounce. Clients deserve current and correct health information; therefore, health care professionals must continually educate themselves in order to provide the most accurate information to their clients.

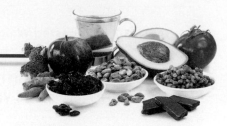

SUMMARY

The body is comparable to an automobile engine because both require fuel. Food acts as fuel, but to be usable, it must undergo a series of processes that include digestion, absorption, and metabolism. Digestion is the process whereby food is broken down into smaller parts, chemically changed, and moved along the gastrointestinal tract. Mechanical digestion refers to that part of the process performed by the teeth and muscles of the digestive system. Chemical digestion refers to that part of the process wherein food is broken down to molecules that the blood can absorb. Enzymes are essential for chemical digestion. After digestion, nutrients are transported by the blood and lymphatic system, primarily in the small intestine, and then carried to all body tissues. After absorption, food is metabolized. During metabolism, carbohydrates and proteins are combined with oxygen in a process called oxidation. Energy released during oxidation is measured by the calorie. Caloric values of foods vary, as do people's energy requirements. Requirements depend on age, body size, sex, lean body mass, physical condition, climate, and activity.

DISCUSSION TOPICS

1. Describe the process of digestion.
2. Of what value are enzymes to digestion? Name five enzymes and the nutrients on which they act.
3. Describe absorption of nutrients.
4. Describe metabolism.
5. Explain why the body requires fuel even during sleep.
6. Explain the differences between the terms *energy value* and *energy requirement.*

SUGGESTED ACTIVITIES

1. Using the method given in this chapter, calculate your total energy requirement.

2. Prepare a brief description of the processes of digestion and absorption that could be presented to a fourth-grade class.
3. Role-play a situation where the client asks the health care provider to explain *metabolism.*
4. Compare your total energy requirement with your intake from your 3-day food analysis in Chapter 2.

REVIEW

Multiple choice. Select the *letter* that precedes the best answer.

1. Digestion begins in the
   a. mouth   c. liver
   b. stomach   d. small intestine
2. Most of the digestive processes occur in the
   a. mouth
   b. stomach
   c. small intestine
   d. colon
3. The small intestine is divided into three segments. They are, in descending order,
   a. ileum, jejunum, duodenum
   b. jejunum, ileum, duodenum
   c. duodenum, ileum, jejunum
   d. duodenum, jejunum, ileum
4. The fluid mixture that moves from the stomach through the pyloric sphincter is called
   a. bolus
   b. chyme
   c. food
   d. gastrin
5. A muscular movement that moves food down the GI tract is called
   a. GI pump
   b. peristalsis
   c. lymphatic circulation
   d. circular propulsion

6. What body system transports fat throughout the body?
   a. lymphatic system
   b. circulatory system
   c. digestive system
   d. blood system

7. An organic substance that causes changes in other substances is a/an
   a. hormone
   b. bacterium
   c. enzyme
   d. acid

8. Maltase, sucrase, and lactase are produced in the
   a. stomach
   b. small intestine
   c. colon
   d. pancreas

9. Bile is needed to digest
   a. fats
   b. fiber
   c. proteins
   d. carbohydrates

10. When energy intake is greater than energy output, the body weight will
    a. remain the same
    b. decrease
    c. increase and then decrease
    d. increase

11. What is the BMR for a 170-pound male?
    a. 1,854
    b. 2,010
    c. 1,720
    d. 1,400

Case In Point

JANEESHA: WEIGHT MAINTENANCE AFTER SMOKING CESSATION

Janeesha has been smoking cigarettes for almost 10 years. Both of her parents were smokers, so she started smoking at about 15 years old. She began with just a few here and there, but gradually worked her way up to about a pack per day. When she first started smoking, she was not concerned about the health risks to her body. She thought it was cool, and many of her friends were also smoking. Now that she's older, she has seen first-hand what smoking can do. Her mother has been diagnosed with lung cancer and her father is now on oxygen to aid his breathing difficulties caused by his emphysema. In addition, Janeesha was married last year and her new husband is not a smoker. He has encouraged her to stop smoking. He is concerned for her health, and if they choose to have children, he would not want her to smoke during the pregnancy. Janeesha has decided she is ready to stop smoking. She has been attending a smoking cessation class. She has also discussed medication options for smoking cessation with her doctor. One of Janeesha's concerns about quitting is the weight gain that many people experience. Janeesha is African American, and she is currently 5 feet 2 inches tall and 140 pounds. She knows she is already slightly overweight, but likes her fuller figure. Her husband thinks she is beautiful at her current weight. However, she does not want to gain more weight and create additional health problems as she stops smoking. In discussing her concerns with her doctor, he suggests that Janeesha make an appointment with a dietitian to have some nutritional education as well as her calorie needs calculated. Janeesha is hopeful that the dietitian may also give her some suggestions for healthier meals and snacks.

ASSESSMENT

1. Identify the significant data in this case study.
2. Calculate Janeesha's REE using the Harris-Benedict equation, the thermic effect of food (TEF), and her calorie guidelines using Table 3-2.
3. What does Janeesha need to discuss with her doctor to assist with her smoking cessation?
4. What questions or concerns might Janeesha want to discuss with the dietitian?

DIAGNOSIS

5. Write a nursing diagnosis for Janeesha.

PLAN/GOAL

6. What changes can Janeesha implement to help prevent weight gain?
7. Set two measurable realistic goals for Janeesha during this process to prevent further weight gain.
8. How could information on exercise be helpful to Janeesha?

IMPLEMENTATION

9. What strategies can be used to help Janeesha become aware of her food consumption and the time it takes her to eat?
10. What actions would help Janeesha carry out these goals?
11. Who can help her?

EVALUATION/OUTCOME CRITERIA

12. What will Janeesha be able to identify if the plan is successful?

13. What will she be able to measure as evidence of her success?

THINKING FURTHER

14. Janeesha's husband is concerned about her smoking. He would like her to quit not only for her own health, but also his (exposure to secondhand smoke) and for their potential children if Janeesha were to become pregnant. What are some of the risks associated with smoking and some of the added benefits of quitting?

rate this **plate**

With smoking cessation, Janeesha needs to realize that her hands are going to miss the smoking since it's such a habit. Most people will eat something to fill the temptation. Rate this plate to see if Janeesha will be able to maintain her current weight.

Cheeseburger with lettuce, tomato, and onion

Medium French fries

Side salad with low-fat ranch dressing

32 oz. regular soda

Calculate the calories that are in this meal and determine if it's one-third of the calories she needs in a day. What can be eliminated from this meal to reduce fat and calories?

Case In Point

ED: CONTROLLING SYMPTOMS OF CROHN'S DISEASE

Ed was diagnosed with Crohn's disease when he was 16. Now that he is 28 years old, he is having increased difficulty controlling his symptoms. His disease is primarily affecting his large intestine. Ed is 6 feet 1 inch tall and weighs 223 pounds. He knows he is prone to flare-ups and must be careful about what he eats. His triggers can be malabsorption of any of the macronutrients: carbohydrate, protein, and fat. Ed and his wife recently took a trip to El Salvador to visit her family. He thoroughly enjoyed the food his mother-in-law prepared. She is a fabulous cook. During their visit, the symptoms began to flare up. He couldn't stop eating all the delicious foods. The cuisine was such a mix of spicy, salty, and sweet flavors, and he loved it all. For the last 2 weeks since returning home, he has been having mainly diarrhea and loose stools. He has lost 8 pounds. He has wanted to lose weight, however, he knows this is not the way to achieve weight loss. His wife feels terrible that the spicy foods may have caused his problem. She has encouraged Ed to go see his doctor. He makes an appointment with his physician. His physician orders a CBC, albumin, folic acid, and B_{12} levels to be drawn. She also would like Ed to see a dietitian. She would like for him to begin a low-lactose, low-fat, high-fiber, and high-protein diet.

ASSESSMENT

1. What are the pertinent objective and subjective data related to Ed's problem?
2. Calculate Ed's target caloric intake and weight range according to Tables 3-2 and 3-3.

DIAGNOSIS

3. Write a nursing diagnosis for Ed.
4. What is the cause of Ed's problem with elimination?

PLAN/GOAL

5. Write a measurable goal for controlling Ed's diarrhea.
6. Write a goal to help Ed adapt to his new diet. Incorporate Ed's desire to lose weight.
7. Where could the dietitian direct Ed to obtain information to increase his understanding of his disease and the related nutrition issues?

IMPLEMENTATION

8. List at least one action to help Ed meet each goal.
9. List two foods Carl should avoid.
10. List three things Ed needs to include in his diet.
11. How could the website http://www.ccfa.org for Crohn's and ulcerative colitis be helpful to Ed?

EVALUATION/OUTCOME CRITERIA

12. What will Ed report when your plan for his Crohn's disease is effective?
13. How will Ed know his new diet is successful?
14. What can the doctor measure when all the goals are successful?
15. If the plan were not successful, what would Ed be experiencing?
16. What could be an unplanned, undesirable outcome of this diet change?

THINKING FURTHER

17. What challenges does Ed face with chronic progressive disease?

rate this plate

Ed's doctor recommends a low-lactose, low-fat, high-fiber, and high-protein diet to begin treating his symptoms. Ed ate the following meal for dinner. Rate this plate.

10 oz. ribeye steak

Baked potato with sour cream, bacon bits, and butter

½ cup of lima beans

Whole wheat rolls with butter

10 oz. of whole milk

Whole wheat fruit crumble

What foods on this plate might give Ed continued symptoms of Crohn's disease? How might you adjust this meal to fit the diet prescribed by the physician?

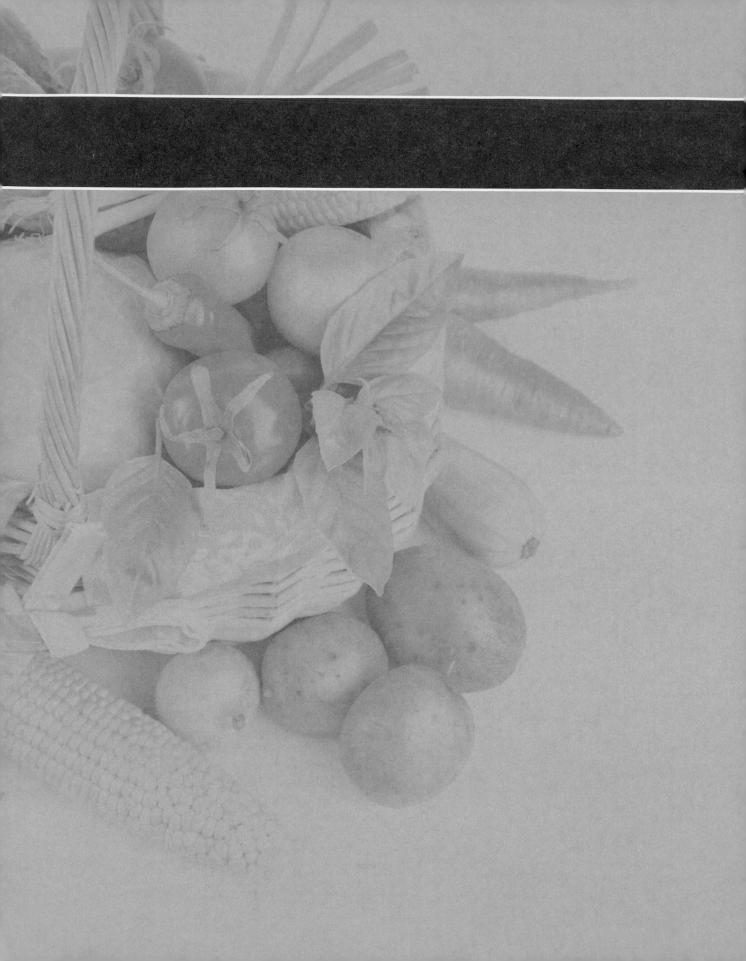

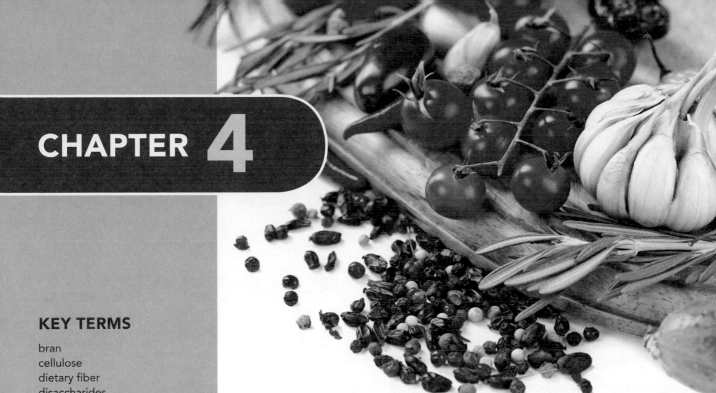

CHAPTER 4

CARBOHYDRATES

OBJECTIVES

After studying this chapter, you should be able to:

- Identify the functions of carbohydrates
- Name the primary sources of carbohydrates
- Describe the classification of carbohydrates

Carbohydrates are considered energy foods that can be rapidly oxidized by the body to release energy and its by-product, heat. Carbohydrates, fats, and proteins provide energy for the human body, but carbohydrates are the primary source. They are somewhat inexpensive compared to the other food groups and most abundant of the energy nutrients. Foods rich in carbohydrates grow easily in most climates. They keep well and are generally easy to digest.

Carbohydrates provide the major source of energy for people all over the world (Figure 4-1). They provide approximately half the calories for people living in the United States. In some areas of the world, where fats and proteins are scarce and expensive, carbohydrates provide as much as 80–100% of calories. Carbohydrates are named for the chemical elements they are composed of—carbon (C), hydrogen (H), and oxygen (O).

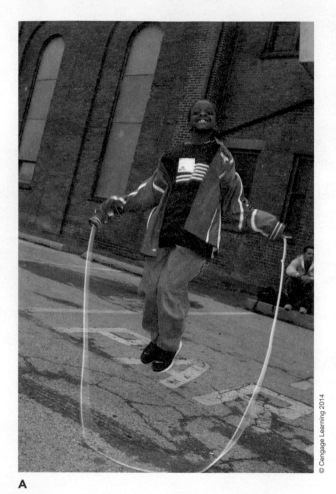

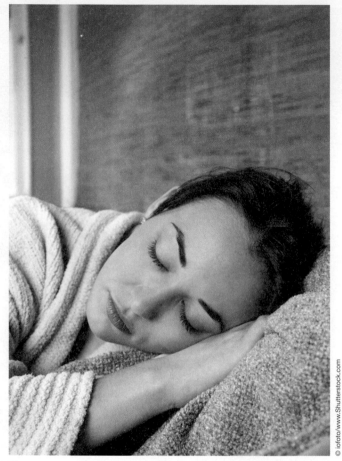

A   **B**

FIGURE 4-1 The need for carbohydrates is constant, whether you are active (A) or at rest (B).

FUNCTIONS

Providing energy is the major function of carbohydrates. Each gram of carbohydrate provides 4 calories. The body needs to maintain a constant supply of energy. Therefore, it stores approximately half a day's supply of carbohydrate in the liver and muscles for use as needed. In this form, it is called glycogen.

Protein-sparing action is also an important function of carbohydrates. When enough carbohydrates (at least 50–100 g/day) are ingested to supply a person's energy needs, they spare proteins for their primary function of building and repairing body tissues.

Normal fat metabolism requires an adequate supply of carbohydrates. If there are not enough carbohydrates to fulfill the energy requirement, an abnormally large amount of fat is metabolized to help meet it. During such an emergency need for energy, fat oxidization in the cells is not complete and substances called ketones are produced. **Ketones** are acids that accumulate in the blood and urine, upsetting the acid–base balance. Such a condition is called **ketoacidosis**. It can result from insulin-dependent diabetes mellitus

ketones
substances to which fatty acids are broken down in the liver

ketoacidosis
condition in which ketones collect in the blood; caused by insufficient glucose available for energy

(IDDM), also known as type 1 diabetes (see Chapter 17), from starvation, or from extreme low-carbohydrate diets. It can lead to coma and even death.

When sufficient carbohydrates are eaten, the body is protected against ketones. This is sometimes called the antiketogenic effect of carbohydrates.

Providing fiber in the diet is another important function of carbohydrates. Dietary fiber is found in grains, vegetables, and fruits. Fiber creates a soft, bulky stool that moves quickly through the large intestine.

FOOD SOURCES

The principal sources of carbohydrates are plant foods: cereal grains, vegetables, fruits, and sugars (Figure 4-2). The only substantial animal source of carbohydrates is milk.

Cereal grains and their products are dietary staples in nearly every part of the world. Rice is the basic food in Latin America, Africa, Asia, and many sections of the United States. Wheat and the various breads, pastas, and breakfast cereals made from it are basic to American and European diets. Rye and oats are commonly used in breads and cereals in the United States and Europe. Cereals also contain vitamins, minerals, and some proteins. During processing, some of these nutrients are lost. To compensate for this loss, food producers in the United States commonly add the B vitamins—thiamine, riboflavin, and niacin—plus the mineral iron to the final product. The product is then called *enriched*. When a nutrient that has never been part of a grain is added, the grain is said to be fortified. An example of fortification is the addition of folic acid to cereal grains to prevent neural tube defects (see Chapter 7).

Vegetables such as potatoes, beets, peas, lima beans, and corn provide substantial amounts of carbohydrates (in the form of starch). Green leafy vegetables provide dietary fiber. All of them also provide vitamins and minerals.

Fruits provide fruit sugar, fiber, vitamins, and minerals.

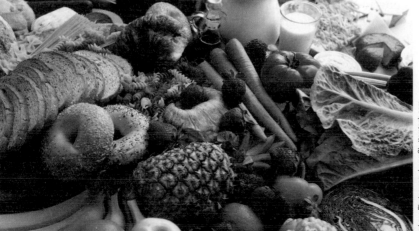

FIGURE 4-2 Fruits, vegetables, grains, and some dairy products are good sources of carbohydrates.

© Morgan Lane Photography/www.Shutterstock.com

Sugars such as table sugar, syrup, and honey and sugar-rich foods such as desserts and candy provide carbohydrates in the form of sugar with few other nutrients except for fats. Therefore, the foods in which they predominate are commonly called low-nutrient-dense foods.

CLASSIFICATION

Carbohydrates are divided into three groups: monosaccharides, disaccharides, and polysaccharides (Table 4-1).

Monosaccharides

Monosaccharides are the simplest form of carbohydrates. They are sweet, require no digestion, and can be absorbed directly into the bloodstream from the small intestine. They include glucose, fructose, and galactose.

Glucose, also called dextrose, is the form of carbohydrate to which all other forms are converted for eventual metabolism. It is found naturally in corn syrup and some fruits and vegetables. The central nervous system, the red blood cells, and the brain use only glucose as fuel; therefore, a continuous source is needed.

Fructose, also called levulose or fruit sugar, is found with glucose in many fruits and in honey. It is the sweetest of all the monosaccharides.

Galactose is a product of the digestion of milk. It is not found naturally.

Disaccharides

Disaccharides are pairs of the three sugars just discussed. They are sweet and must be changed to simple sugars by hydrolysis before they can be absorbed. Disaccharides include sucrose, maltose, and lactose.

Sucrose is composed of glucose and fructose. It is the form of carbohydrate present in granulated, powdered, and brown sugar and in molasses. It is one of the sweetest and least expensive sugars. Its sources are sugar cane, sugar beets, and the sap from maple trees.

Maltose is a disaccharide that is an intermediary product in the hydrolysis of starch. It is produced by enzyme action during the digestion of starch in the body. It is also created during the fermentation process that produces alcohol. It can be found in some infant formulas, malt beverage products, and beer. It is considerably less sweet than glucose or sucrose.

Lactose is the sugar found in milk. It is distinct from most other sugars because it is not found in plants. It helps the body absorb calcium. Lactose is less sweet than monosaccharides or other disaccharides.

Many adults are unable to digest lactose and suffer from bloating, abdominal cramps, and diarrhea after drinking milk or consuming a milk-based food such as processed cheese. This reaction is called lactose intolerance. It is caused by insufficient lactase, the enzyme required for digestion of lactose. There are special low-lactose milk products that can be used instead of regular milk. Lactase-containing products are also available.

monosaccharides
simplest carbohydrates; sugars that cannot be further reduced by hydrolysis; examples are glucose, fructose, and galactose

glucose
the simple sugar to which carbohydrate must be broken down for absorption; also known as *dextrose*

fructose
the simple sugar (monosaccharide) found in fruit and honey

galactose
the simple sugar (monosaccharide) to which lactose is broken down during digestion

disaccharides
double sugars that are reduced by hydrolysis to monosaccharides; examples are sucrose, maltose, and lactose

sucrose
a double sugar or disaccharide; examples are granulated, powdered, and brown sugar

maltose
the double sugar (disaccharide) occurring as a result of the digestion of grain

lactose
the sugar in milk; a disaccharide

TABLE 4-1 Carbohydrates

TYPE	SOURCE		FUNCTIONS	DEFICIENCY SYMPTOMS
Monosaccharides (Simple Sugars)				
Glucose	Berries	Grapes	Furnish energy	Fatigue
	Sweet corn	Corn syrup	Spare proteins	Weight loss
			Prevent ketoacidosis	
Fructose	Ripe fruits Honey	Soft drinks	Fruits and vegetables provide vitamins, minerals, and fiber	
Galactose	Lactose			
Disaccharides				
Sucrose	Sugar cane		Furnish energy	Fatigue
	Sugar beets		Spare proteins	Weight loss
	Granulated sugar		Prevent ketoacidosis	
	Confectioner's sugar			
	Brown sugar			
	Molasses			
	Maple syrup			
	Candy			
	Jams and jellies			
Maltose	Digestion of starch			
Lactose	Milk			
Polysaccharides (Complex Carbohydrates)				
Starch	Cereal grains and their products: cereals, breads, rice, flour, pasta, crackers		Furnish energy	Fatigue
			Prevent ketoacidosis	Weight loss
	Potatoes	Corn	Fruits and vegetables provide vitamins, minerals, and fiber	
	Lima beans	Yams		
	Navy beans	Green bananas		
	Sweet potatoes			
Dextrins	Starch hydrolysis			
Glycogen	Glucose stored in liver and muscles			
Cellulose	Wheat bran, whole grain cereals, green and leafy Vegetables, fruits, especially apples, pears, oranges, grapefruit, grapes		Provide fiber	Constipation Colon cancer Diverticulosis

During the process of making hard cheese, milk separates into curd (solid part from which hard cheese is made) and **whey** (liquid part). Lactose becomes part of the whey and not the curd. Therefore, lactose is not a component of natural cheese. However, manufacturers can add milk or milk solids

 whey
liquid part of milk that separates from the curd (solid part) during the making of hard cheese

to processed cheese, so it is important that persons who are lactose intolerant check the labels on cheese products.

There is no test for lactose intolerance. If eating dairy products consistently produces symptoms of flatulence, diarrhea, and abdominal pain, the doctor may recommend eliminating dairy products from the diet and adding them back after a period of time to ascertain the client's reaction. If the symptoms persist, the client is lactose intolerant.

Polysaccharides

Polysaccharides are commonly called *complex carbohydrates* because they are compounds of many monosaccharides (simple sugars). Three polysaccharides are important in nutrition: starch, glycogen, and fiber.

Starch is a polysaccharide found in grains and vegetables. It is the storage form of glucose in plants. Vegetables contain less starch than grains because vegetables have a higher moisture content. Legumes (dried beans and peas) are another important source of starch as well as of dietary fiber and protein. Starches are more complex than monosaccharides or disaccharides, and it takes the body longer to digest them. Thus, they supply energy over a longer period of time. The starch in grain is found mainly in the **endosperm** (center part of the grain). This is the part from which white flour is made. The tough outer covering of grain kernels is called the **bran** (Figure 4-3). The bran is used in coarse cereals and whole-wheat flour. The **germ** is the smallest part of the grain and is a rich source of B vitamins, vitamin E, minerals, and protein. Wheat germ is included in products made of whole wheat. It also can be purchased and used in baked products or as an addition to breakfast cereals.

polysaccharides
complex carbohydrates containing combinations of monosaccharides; examples include starch, dextrin, cellulose, and glycogen

starch
polysaccharide found in grains and vegetables

endosperm
the inner part of the kernel of grain; contains the carbohydrate

bran
outer covering of grain kernels

germ
embryo or tiny life center of each kernel of grain

FIGURE 4-3 A grain of wheat has three parts. All parts are used in whole-wheat flour; only the endosperm is used in white flour.

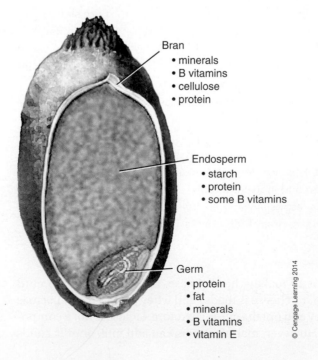

Bran
• minerals
• B vitamins
• cellulose
• protein

Endosperm
• starch
• protein
• some B vitamins

Germ
• protein
• fat
• minerals
• B vitamins
• vitamin E

© Cengage Learning 2014

Before the starch in grain can be used for food, the bran must be broken down. The heat and moisture of cooking break this outer covering, making the food more flavorful and more easily digested. Although bran itself is indigestible, it is important that some be included in the diet because of the fiber it provides.

Glycogen is sometimes called *animal starch* because it is the storage form of glucose in the body. In the healthy adult, approximately one-half day's supply of energy is stored as glycogen in the liver and muscles. The hormone **glucagon** helps the liver convert glycogen to glucose as needed for energy. (See Chapter 13 for information on glycogen loading.)

The Fibers

Dietary fiber, also called roughage, is indigestible because it cannot be broken down by digestive enzymes. Some fiber is insoluble (it does not readily dissolve in water), and some is soluble (it partially dissolves in water) (Figure 4-4). Insoluble fibers include cellulose, some hemicellulose, and lignins. Soluble fibers are gums, pectins, some hemicellulose, and mucilages. See Table 4-2 for food sources. **Cellulose** is a primary source of dietary fiber. It is found in the skins of fruits, the leaves and stems of vegetables, and legumes. Highly processed foods such as white bread, pasta (other than whole wheat), and pastries contain little if any cellulose because it is removed during processing. Because humans cannot digest cellulose, it has no energy value. It is useful because it provides bulk for the stool.

Hemicellulose is found mainly in whole-grain cereal. Some hemicellulose is soluble; some is not. **Lignins** are the woody part of vegetables such as carrots and asparagus or the small seeds of strawberries; they are not a carbohydrate.

Pectin, some hemicellulose, gums, and **mucilage** are soluble in water and form a gel that helps provide bulk for the intestines. They are useful also because they bind cholesterol, thus reducing the amount the blood can absorb.

Fiber is considered helpful to clients with diabetes mellitus because it lowers blood glucose levels. It may prevent some colon cancers by moving waste materials through the colon faster than would normally be the case, thereby reducing the colon's exposure time to potential carcinogens. Fiber helps prevent constipation, hemorrhoids, and diverticular disease by softening and increasing the size of the stool.

glycogen
glucose as stored in the liver and muscles

glucagon
hormone from alpha cells of the pancreas; helps cells release energy

dietary fiber
indigestible parts of plants; absorbs water in large intestine, helping to create soft, bulky stool; some is believed to bind cholesterol in the colon, helping to rid cholesterol from the body; some is believed to lower blood glucose levels

cellulose
indigestible carbohydrate; provides fiber in the diet

hemicellulose
dietary fiber found in whole grains

lignins
dietary fiber found in the woody parts of vegetables

pectin
edible thickening agent

mucilage
gel-forming dietary fiber

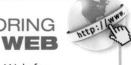

EXPLORING THE WEB

Search the Web for information on the role of carbohydrates and your health. What resources can you find? Has there been any new research in the area of carbohydrate metabolism? Create a report on new information you may have found. Create flash cards on the function and dietary recommendations of carbohydrates for self-review.

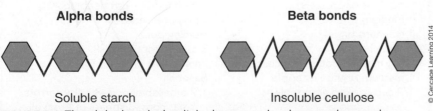

Alpha bonds　　　　　**Beta bonds**

Soluble starch　　　　Insoluble cellulose

© Cengage Learning 2014

FIGURE 4-4 The alpha bonds that link glucose molecules together can be broken down during digestion. The beta bonds in cellulose cannot be broken by digestive enzymes and are eliminated without being digested.

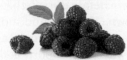

TABLE 4-2 Water-Soluble and Water-Insoluble Sources of Fiber

WATER-SOLUBLE FIBER		WATER-INSOLUBLE FIBER
Fruit (pectin)	**Grains**	All vegetables
Apples	Oats	Fruit
Peaches	Barley	Whole grains
Plums and prunes	**Legumes**	Brown rice
Bananas	Dried peas	Wild rice
	Beans	Wheat bran
	Lentils	Nuts
		Seeds

© Cengage Learning 2014

The optimal recommendation for fiber intake is 20–35 g/day. The normal U.S. diet is thought to contain approximately 11 grams. In general, Americans do not consume sufficient amounts of fruits and vegetables. They should eat no fewer than five servings of fruits and vegetables each day. Fiber intake should be increased gradually and should be accompanied by an

Supersize USA

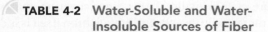

Portion distortion is an enormous contribution to overweight and obesity. Having a realistic visual image of portion size is helpful when preparing meals and choosing foods. Did you know . . .

Portion	Visualization of Size or Amount
3 oz meat, poultry, or fish	Deck of playing cards, cassette tape, or the palm of a woman's hand
1 oz meat, poultry, fish, or cheese	1-inch cube or rolling dice
1 pat butter or margarine (1 serving)	A scrabble tile
2 Tbsp peanut butter	Golf ball
1 oz salad dressing	1 small restaurant ladle
1 cup fresh greens	Tennis ball
1 lb uncooked spaghetti	Circle thumb and index finger
1 Tbsp mayonnaise	Woman's thumb
1 oz chips or pretzels	One handful—not heaping
1 medium potato	Computer mouse
1 standard bagel	Hockey puck
1 slice cheese	3.5-in. computer disk
1 cup mashed potatoes, rice, or pasta	Person's fist or tennis ball
1 medium orange or apple	Baseball
1/2 cup cooked vegetable	1/2 a baseball or 7–8 baby carrots, 1 ear corn, 3 spears of broccoli
1/2 cup frozen yogurt	Small fist
1 oz nuts, raisins, candy	Small handful, 2 Tbsp

increased intake of water. Eating too much fiber in a short time can produce discomfort, **flatulence** (abdominal gas), and diarrhea. It also could obstruct the GI tract if intake exceeds 50 grams. Insoluble fiber has binders (phytic acid or phytate), which are found in the outer covering of grains and vegetables. These can prevent the absorption of minerals such as calcium, iron, zinc, and magnesium, so excess intake should be avoided. The type of fiber consumed should be from natural food sources rather than from commercially prepared fiber products because the foods contain vitamins, minerals, and phytochemicals as well as fiber. Table 4-3 lists the dietary fiber content of selected foods.

DIGESTION AND ABSORPTION

Monosaccharides—glucose, fructose, and galactose—are simple sugars that may be absorbed from the intestine directly into the bloodstream. They are subsequently carried to the liver, where fructose and galactose are changed to glucose. The blood then carries glucose to the cells.

Disaccharides—sucrose, maltose, and lactose—require an additional step of digestion. They must be converted to the simple sugar glucose before they can be absorbed into the bloodstream. This conversion is accomplished by the enzymes sucrase, maltase, and lactase, which were discussed in Chapter 3 (see Table 3-1).

Polysaccharides are more complex, and their digestibility varies. After the cellulose wall is broken down, starch is changed to the intermediate product dextrin; it is then changed to maltose and finally to glucose. Cooking can change starch to dextrin. For example, when bread is toasted, it turns golden brown and tastes sweeter because the starch has been changed to dextrin.

The digestion of starch begins in the mouth, where the enzyme salivary amylase begins to change starch to dextrin. The second step occurs in the stomach, where the food is mixed with gastric juices. The final step occurs in the small intestine, where the digestible carbohydrates are changed to simple sugars by the enzyme action of pancreatic amylase and are subsequently absorbed into the blood.

METABOLISM AND ELIMINATION

All carbohydrates are changed to the simple sugar glucose before metabolism can take place in the cells. After glucose has been carried by the blood to the cells, it can be oxidized. Frequently, the volume of glucose that reaches the cells exceeds the amount the cells can use. In these cases, glucose is converted to glycogen and is stored in the liver and muscles. (Glycogen is subsequently broken down only from the liver and released as glucose when needed for energy.) When more glucose is ingested than the body can either use immediately or store in the form of glycogen, it is converted to fat and stored as adipose (fatty) tissue.

The process of glucose metabolism is controlled mainly by the hormone **insulin**, which is secreted by the **islets of Langerhans** in the pancreas and which maintains normal blood glucose at 70–110 mg/dl. When the secretion of insulin is impaired or absent, the glucose level in the blood becomes excessively high. This condition is called **hyperglycemia** (blood glucose more than 126 mg/dl) and is

 insulin
secretion of the islets of Langerhans in the pancreas gland; essential for the proper metabolism of glucose

 islets of Langerhans
part of the pancreas from which insulin is secreted

 hyperglycemia
excessive amounts of glucose in the blood

flatulence
gas in the intestinal tract

TABLE 4-3   Dietary Fiber Content of Selected Foods

GRAMS PER SERVING*	0.5 OR LESS	0.5–1.0	1.1–2.0	2.1–3.0	3.0 OR GREATER‡
Fruit[†]	Banana	Apricots (raw or dried)	Apple skin	Blackberries	Blackberries (4)
	Cherries	Apple (peeled or dried)	Cranberries, raw (1 cup)	Boysenberries	Elderberries (5)
	Coconut (shredded)	Applesauce	Figs	Gooseberries	Guava (5)
	Currants (dried)	Blueberries	Papaya	Kumquats	Raspberries (4)
	Dates	Cantaloupe		Pears	
	Fruit juice	Coconut, raw, 1/2 cup			
	Plums (cooked)	Cranberries, relish, 1/2 cup			
	Pomegranate	Honeydew			
	Prunes	Kiwifruit			
	Raisins	Mango			
	Rhubarb (raw)	Nectarine			
	Watermelon	Orange			
		Peach (raw or dried)			
		Pear (dried)			
		Pineapple			
		Plums (raw)			
		Prunes			
		Rhubarb, raw (1 cup) and cooked			
		Strawberries			
		Tangerine			
		Watermelon			
Vegetables[†]	Bamboo shoots	Artichoke hearts	Artichoke, Jerusalem		
	Bean sprouts (cooked or canned)	Asparagus	Broccoli (cooked)		
	Cabbage (cooked)	Bean sprouts (raw)	Brussels sprouts		
	Celery	Beans (string)	Chicory		
	Eggplant	Beets	Mushrooms		
	Endive	Broccoli (raw)	Pumpkin		
	Lettuce	Cabbage (raw)	Rutabagas		
	Onions	Carrots	Sauerkraut		
	Radishes	Cauliflower	Soybean sprouts (raw)		
	Summer squash	Cucumber	Spaghetti sauce		
	Vegetable juice	Green pepper	Tomato paste		

Vegetables	†Water chestnuts Watercress	Greens: Beet Collard Dandelion Kale Mustard Spinach Swiss chard Turnip Kohlrabi Mushrooms Okra Parsley Soybean sprouts (cooked) Summer squash (raw) Tomato puree Turnips (cooked)	Turnips (raw)		
Starches	Cornflakes Corn grits Cream of Wheat or Rice Farina Graham crackers Maltomeal Plantain Potato chips Potatoes Puffed cereals Rice, white Rice Krispies Saltines Spaghetti (refined)	Bread, white Cheerios Corn Flour, white Granola Oatmeal (cooked) Roll or bun, white Spaghetti and macaroni from whole wheat flour	Black-eyed peas Bread, whole wheat Flour, whole wheat Grapenuts Green peas Lima beans Popcorn Ralston (cooked cereal) Rice, brown or white Sesame seed kernels Soybeans Squash, winter Sweet potatoes	Beans (dried) 40% Branflakes Bulgur Lentils Parsnips Peas (dried) Pumpkin Raisin Bran Shredded Wheat Wheat germ	All-Bran (9) Bran Buds (8) 100% Bran (6) Bran muffin (3.5) Bulgur (3.5) RY KRISP Wheat bran (9)

Note: Based on the content of one diabetic exchange for each item listed.

* Serving sizes per the Dietary Guidelines for Americans.

† Includes all forms (raw, dried, cooked) for fruits and vegetables except where noted.

‡ Actual dietary fiber content listed in parentheses.

Reprinted with permission of the Mayo Clinic, Rochester, Minnesota.

hypoglycemia
subnormal levels of blood glucose

EXPLORING THE WEB

Search the Web for information on carbohydrate-reducing diets and products. Is the information provided at these sites accurate? If a client came to you with questions about a product such as these, how would you respond? Create a fact sheet that lists myths surrounding carbohydrates and the facts that dispel the myths. Visit the American Diabetes Association website for accurate information (http://www.diabetes.org).

usually a symptom of diabetes mellitus. If control by diet is ineffective, an oral hypoglycemic or insulin injections must be used to control blood sugar. When insulin is given, the diabetic client's intake of carbohydrates must be carefully controlled to balance the prescribed dosage of insulin (see Chapter 17). When blood glucose levels are unusually low, the condition is called **hypoglycemia** (blood glucose less than 70 mg/dl). A mild form of hypoglycemia may occur if one waits too long between meals or if the pancreas secretes too much insulin. Symptoms include fatigue, shaking, sweating, and headache.

Oxidation of glucose results in energy. With the exception of cellulose, the only waste products of carbohydrate metabolism are carbon dioxide and water. It is a very efficient nutrient.

DIETARY REQUIREMENTS

Although there is no specific daily dietary requirement for carbohydrates, the Food and Nutrition Board of the National Research Council recommends that half of one's energy requirement come from carbohydrates, preferably complex carbohydrates. (The recommendation is 10% of energy to come from simple carbohydrates.) For example, assume that one's total energy requirement is 2,000 calories. One half of this is 1,000. Divide 1,000 calories by 4 (the number of calories in each gram of carbohydrate) for an estimated carbohydrate requirement of 250 g/day.

A mild deficiency of carbohydrates can result in weight loss and fatigue. A diet seriously deficient in carbohydrates could cause ketoacidosis, a stage in metabolism occurring when the liver has been depleted of stored glycogen and switches to a fasting mode. At this point, energy from fat is mobilized to the liver and used to synthesize glucose. The by-products of fat breakdown are ketones that build up in the bloodstream and are then released through the kidneys. To prevent these effects, one needs a minimum of 50–120 grams of carbohydrates each day.

The overweight population constitutes a major health problem in the United States. Some believe eating excess carbohydrates to be the most common cause of obesity. Although surplus carbohydrates are changed to glycogen, the major part of any surplus becomes adipose tissue. Also, an excess of carbohydrate in the form of sugar can spoil an appetite for other nutrients that are more important. Too many carbohydrates may cause tooth decay, irritate the lining of the stomach, or cause flatulence.

HEALTH AND NUTRITION CONSIDERATIONS

The role of the health care professional in teaching about carbohydrates may be complicated. Some will have to be taught the nutritional differences between a baked potato and potato chips, between whole-wheat toast and Danish pastry, and between a fresh peach and canned fruit cocktail. Many will need to learn what dietary fiber is, where it can be found, and why it is needed. Some will need to learn that sugar should be used in moderation; others that it cannot be used in excess. All will require acceptance, understanding, and patience on the part of the health care professional.

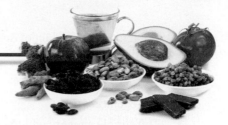

SUMMARY

Energy foods are those that can be rapidly oxidized by the body to release energy. Carbohydrates are and should be the major source of energy. They are composed of carbon, hydrogen, and oxygen. One gram of carbohydrate provides 4 calories. Carbohydrates are the least expensive and most abundant nutrient. The principal sources of carbohydrates are plant products such as grains and their products, vegetables, fruits, legumes, and sugars. In addition to providing energy, carbohydrates spare proteins, maintain normal fat metabolism, and provide fiber. Digestion of carbohydrates begins in the mouth, continues in the stomach, and is completed in the small intestine. Although they are obviously essential to the health and well-being of the body, eating an excess of carbohydrates can cause dental caries, digestive disturbances, and obesity.

DISCUSSION TOPICS

1. What are the three basic groups of carbohydrates? Name several foods in each group.

2. Discuss the effects of excessive intake of carbohydrates.

3. Why should one's diet contain dietary fiber? Name three sources of dietary fiber.

4. Describe the digestion and metabolism of carbohydrates.

5. Discuss the following menus. Which foods contain simple sugars and/or complex carbohydrates?

Orange juice	Baked chicken	Cheese sandwich
Cereal	Baked potato	on whole-wheat
Milk and sugar	Green beans	bread with
Toast	Coleslaw	lettuce and tomato
Butter and jelly	Bread and	Carrot and
Coffee	butter	celery sticks
	Raspberry	Fresh fruit
	sherbet	Cookies
	Milk	Milk

6. Why are complex carbohydrates preferable to simple sugars?

7. Discuss *enrichment*. What does it mean to enrich foods and what nutrients are returned? Why is it done? Which foods are typically enriched in the United States? Would you recommend that one purchase enriched foods? Why or why not?

8. Is it true, as many people say, that "carbs are fattening"? Explain your answer.

SUGGESTED ACTIVITIES

1. Hold a soda cracker in your mouth until you notice the change in flavor as the starch changes to dextrin. What causes this to happen?

2. Make a list of the foods you have eaten in the past 24 hours. Circle the carbohydrate-rich foods and underline the complex carbohydrates. Approximately what percentage of your calories were in the form of carbohydrates? In the form of complex carbs? Could your diet be improved? If so, how?

3. Role-play a situation between a diet counselor and a teenage girl who has placed herself on an extremely low–calorie diet. She refuses to eat anything that she thinks contains carbohydrates. Explain to her the functions of carbohydrates in the human body.

REVIEW

Multiple choice. Select the *letter* that precedes the best answer.

1. The three main groups of carbohydrates are
   a. fats, proteins, and minerals
   b. glucose, fructose, and galactose
   c. monosaccharides, disaccharides, and polysaccharides
   d. sucrose, cellulose, and glycogen

2. Galactose is a product of the digestion of
    a. milk
    b. fruit
    c. breads
    d. vegetables

3. The simple sugar to which all forms of carbohydrates are ultimately converted is
    a. sucrose   c. galactose
    b. glucose   d. maltose

4. A fibrous form of carbohydrate that cannot be digested is
    a. glucose   c. cellulose
    b. glycogen   d. fat

5. Glycogen is stored in the
    a. heart and lungs
    b. liver and muscles
    c. pancreas and gallbladder
    d. small and large intestines

6. Glucose, fructose, and galactose are
    a. polysaccharides
    b. disaccharides
    c. enzymes
    d. monosaccharides

7. How do we get lactose?
    a. bread   c. grains
    b. honey   d. yogurt

8. The only form of carbohydrate that the brain uses for energy is
    a. glycogen   c. glucose
    b. galactose   d. glucagon

9. When insufficient carbohydrates are eaten, the liver produces
    a. galactose   c. thyroxin
    b. estrogen   d. ketones

10. Starch is
    a. the form in which glucose is stored in plants
    b. a monosaccharide
    c. an insoluble form of dietary fiber
    d. found only in grains

11. Insoluble dietary fiber
    a. can increase blood glucose
    b. can decrease blood cholesterol
    c. commonly causes diverticular disease
    d. is preferably provided by commercially prepared fiber products

12. The enzyme in the mouth that begins the digestion of starch is
    a. salivary ptyalin
    b. salivary amylase
    c. sucrase
    d. lipase

13. Cellulose is
    a. not digestible by humans
    b. not to be included in the human diet
    c. a monosaccharide
    d. an excellent substitute for dextrose

14. Carbohydrates
    a. are rich in fat
    b. are generally expensive
    c. should provide approximately half of the calories in the U.S. diet
    d. frequently are an excellent substitute for proteins in the human diet

15. Glucose metabolism is
    a. controlled mainly by the hormone insulin
    b. not affected by any secretion of the islets of Langerhans in the pancreas
    c. managed entirely by glucagon
    d. not related to human energy levels

Case In Point

ANGELA: STEROIDS IMPACTING DIABETES CONTROL

Angela has been having problems for a couple of years with her left hip and has decided it is time to have it replaced. Her arthritis in combination with her lupus has made the pain in her hip intolerable. She is a 62-year-old Hispanic women who is 5 feet 6 inches tall and her current weight is 198 pounds. The day of her surgery she arrives at the hospital early. She has not taken anything by mouth, including her medications, in preparation for her surgery. Angela follows up with her surgeon 1 week after the surgery. He is concerned that the incision is not healing as well as it should. He decides since Angela takes prednisone routinely for her lupus that it would be wise to recheck her blood sugar levels. Her blood sugar in his office is 342 mg/dl. He diagnoses Angela with steroid-induced diabetes. He requests that she follows up with her family physician as soon as possible. He refers her to the local diabetes center to review meal planning for diabetes as well as other aspects of diabetes care.

ASSESSMENT

1. The dietitian can help Angela regulate her diet and in so doing lose weight. Calculate Angela's ideal caloric intake and weight using Tables 3-2 and 3-3, the Harris–Benedict equation, and thermic effect of food (TEF).
2. What does the dietitian need to know about Angela's meal choices?
3. What does the dietitian need to know about Angela's lifestyle?
4. What information will be helpful once Angela is discharged and at home?
5. What sources of carbohydrates would be most helpful in weight loss?

DIAGNOSIS

6. Write a nursing diagnosis for Angela.

PLAN/GOAL

7. Write a goal related to weight loss that Angela should achieve at the end of diabetic classes.
8. State two goals for Angela related to her diet and blood sugar.

IMPLEMENTATION

9. List the topics that you would teach Angela to achieve her goals.
10. What agencies or community resources can you provide to help Angela achieve her goals?

EVALUATION/OUTCOME CRITERIA

11. What can you expect from Angela to show she understands what you have taught?
12. What should Angela's fasting blood sugar read?
13. How long do you think it would take Angela to learn a new diet plan, check her blood sugar, learn a new exercise plan, and demonstrate integration into her everyday life?

THINKING FURTHER

14. What blood test could the doctor order to see if Angela had maintained her blood sugar at a normal level over the past few months?
15. What are some of the serious health consequences if Angela does not manage her diabetes well?

rate this **plate**

While at the diabetes center, Angela was educated about the diabetic meal plan. She continues to learn about how medications, along with her eating habits, can affect her blood sugar levels. Rate this plate to see how she has done with planning a 1,600–1,800 calorie meal plan.

2 pieces of French toast

2 strips of bacon

1 cup of mixed fruit

Coffee with cream and sugar

Case In Point

JEROME: COPING WITH GASTROPARESIS

Jerome has had type 1 diabetes since he was 6 years old. After being diagnosed at such a young age, his parents assisted with his insulin, blood sugar checks, and meal planning. Once he was grown and on his own, he began to slack off in caring for himself. He ate whatever he wanted, he rarely monitored his sugar, and he took his insulin only when he remembered. He has not seen his doctor in nearly 3 years, but now at age 41, he is starting to notice certain problems. Jerome is beginning to have difficulty with his vision. He has also had tingling and burning sensations in his feet and legs. Lately, he has even felt nauseated more often than not after he eats and has even vomited a few times after meals. He has decided it is time to see his doctor. His doctor is very concerned about his complications. He discusses with Jerome that it is extremely important he start caring for himself more aggressively. He tells Jerome that his nausea and vomiting are related to a diabetes complication known as gastroparesis. This is damage to the nerves surrounding the stomach. It causes paralysis of the stomach and delayed emptying of foods. It is going to require more focus on his meal planning to control the symptoms. He refers him to a registered dietitian for this instruction. The dietitian discusses with Jerome the key points to meal planning for gastroparesis. He is going to have to consume small but frequent (4–6) meals daily, and follow a low-fat, low-fiber diet. Jerome needs to chew his food thoroughly before swallowing and avoid foods that are difficult to digest, such as broccoli, corn, popcorn, nuts, and seeds.

ASSESSMENT

1. What has caused the gastroparesis that Jerome is now experiencing?
2. What symptoms did Jerome have?
3. How will the disease alter his life?
4. How significant is this disease?

DIAGNOSIS

5. Write a diagnostic statement for Jerome's potential alteration in nutrition.
6. Write a diagnosis for Jerome's deficient knowledge related to the new diet.

PLAN/GOAL

7. What dietary goals are measurable and appropriate for Jerome?
8. What education goals are specific and measurable for Jerome?

IMPLEMENTATION

9. What major topics about gastroparesis does Jerome need to understand to make necessary dietary changes?
10. What dietary changes does Jerome need to learn to control the symptoms?

EVALUATION/OUTCOME CRITERIA

11. At his follow-up doctor's appointment, what is his doctor likely to ask to determine if the plan was successful?

THINKING FURTHER

12. Can gastroparesis be cured?
13. What medications are typically used to help manage this disease?

rate this **plate**

Jerome has been instructed to consume a diet low in fat and fiber in order to make digestion easy and rest his gut. How did he do in planning the following meal according to the dietitian's recommendations? Rate his plate:

4 oz. beef roast with cooked potatoes, carrots, celery, and onions

¾ cup apple Waldorf salad

1 whole-wheat roll

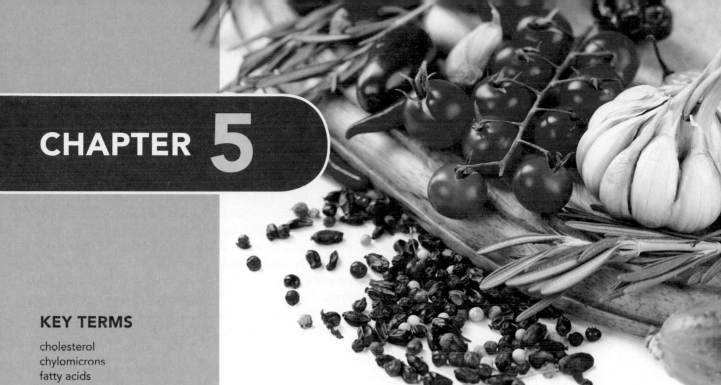

CHAPTER 5

KEY TERMS

LIPIDS (FATS)

OBJECTIVES

After studying this chapter, you should be able to:

- State the functions of fats in the body
- Identify sources of dietary fats
- Explain common classifications of fats
- Describe disease conditions with which excessive use of fats is associated

Fats belong to a group of organic compounds called **lipids**. The word *lipid* is derived from *lipos,* a Greek word for fat. Forms of this word are found in several fat-related health terms such as blood *lipids* (fats in the blood), hyper*lipid*emia (high levels of fat in the blood), and *lipo*proteins (carriers of fat in human blood).

Fats are greasy substances that are not soluble in water. They are soluble in some solvents such as ether, benzene, and chloroform. They provide a more concentrated source of energy than carbohydrates; each gram of fat contains 9 calories. This is slightly more than twice the calorie content of carbohydrates. Fat-rich foods are generally more expensive than

lipids
fats

carbohydrate-rich foods. Like carbohydrates, fats are composed of carbon, hydrogen, and oxygen but with a substantially lower proportion of oxygen.

FUNCTIONS

In addition to providing energy, fats are essential for the functioning and structure of body tissues (Table 5-1). Fats are a necessary part of cell membranes (cell walls). They contain essential fatty acids and act as carriers for fat-soluble vitamins A, D, E, and K. The fat stored in body tissues provides energy when one cannot eat, as may occur during some illness and after abdominal surgery. Adipose (fatty) tissue protects organs and bones from injury by serving as protective padding and support. Body fat also serves as insulation from cold. In addition, fats provide a feeling of **satiety** (satisfaction) after meals. This is due partly to the flavor fats give other foods and partly to their slow rate of digestion, which delays hunger.

satiety
feeling of satisfaction; fullness

FOOD SOURCES

Fats are present in both animal and plant foods. The animal foods that provide the richest sources of fats are meats, especially fatty meats such as bacon, sausage, and luncheon meats; whole, low-fat, and reduced-fat milk; cream; butter; cheeses made with cream; egg yolks (egg white contains no fat; it is almost entirely protein and water); and fatty fish such as tuna and salmon.

The plant foods containing the richest sources of fats are cooking oils made from olives, sunflower, safflower, or sesame seeds or from corn,

TABLE 5-1   Fats

FUNCTIONS	DEFICIENCY SIGNS	SOURCES
Provide energy	Eczema	Animal
Carry fat-soluble vitamins	Weight loss	Fatty meats
Supply essential fatty acids	Retarded growth	Lard
Protect and support organs and bones		Butter
		Cheese
Insulate from cold		Cream
Provide satiety after meals		Whole milk
		Egg yolk
		Plant
		Vegetable oils
		Nuts
		Chocolate
		Avocados
		Olives
		Margarine

peanuts, canola oil, or soybeans, margarine (which is made from vegetable oils), nuts, avocados, coconut, and cocoa butter.

Visible and Invisible Fats in Food

Sometimes fats are referred as visible or invisible, depending on their food sources. Fats that are purchased and used as fats such as butter, margarine, lard, and cooking oils are called **visible fats**. Hidden or **invisible fats** are those found in other foods such as meats, cream, whole milk, cheese, egg yolk, fried foods, pastries, avocados, and nuts.

It is often the invisible fats that can make it difficult for clients on limited-fat diets to regulate their fat intake. For example, one 3-inch doughnut may contain 12 grams of fat, whereas one 3-inch bagel contains only 2 grams of fat. One fried chicken drumstick may contain 11 grams of fat, whereas one roasted drumstick may contain only 2 grams of fat.

It is essential that the health care professional confirm that clients on limited-fat diets are carefully educated about sources of hidden fats.

CLASSIFICATION

Triglycerides, phospholipids, and *sterols* are all lipids found in food and the human body. Most lipids in the body (95%) are triglycerides. They are in body cells, and they circulate in the blood.

Triglycerides are composed of three (*tri*) fatty acids attached to a framework of **glycerol**, hence their name (Figure 5-1). Glycerol is derived from a water-soluble carbohydrate. **Fatty acids** are organic compounds of carbon atoms to which hydrogen atoms are attached. They are classified in two ways: essential or nonessential. *Essential fatty acids (EFAs)* are necessary fats that humans cannot synthesize; EFAs must be obtained through diet. EFAs are long-chain polyunsaturated fatty acids derived from **linoleic** and **linolenic** acids. There are two families of EFAs: omega-3 and omega-6. Necessary, but nonessential, are the omega-9 fatty acids because the body can manufacture a modest amount, provided EFAs are present. (Also see the later section on polyunsaturated fats.)

The other method of classification of fatty acids is by their degree of saturation with hydrogen atoms. In this method, they are described as *saturated, monounsaturated,* or *polyunsaturated,* depending on their hydrogen content (Figure 5-2).

Saturated Fats

When a fatty acid is **saturated**, each of its carbon atoms carries all the hydrogen atoms possible. In general, animal foods contain more saturated fatty acids than unsaturated. Examples include meat, poultry, egg yolks, whole milk, whole milk cheeses, cream, ice cream, and butter. Although plant foods generally contain more polyunsaturated fatty acids than saturated fatty acids, chocolate, coconut, palm oil, and palm kernel oils are exceptions. They contain substantial amounts of saturated fatty acids. Foods containing a high

visible fats
fats in foods that are purchased and used as fats, such as butter or margarine

invisible fats
fats that are not immediately noticeable such as those in egg yolk, cheese, cream, and salad dressings

triglycerides
three fatty acids attached to a framework of glycerol

glycerol
a component of fat; derived from a water-soluble carbohydrate

fatty acids
a component of fat that determines the classification of the fat

linoleic acid
fatty acid essential for humans; cannot be synthesized by the body

linolenic acid
fatty acid essential for humans; cannot be synthesized by the body

saturated fats
fats whose carbon atoms contain all of the hydrogen atoms they can; considered a contributory factor in atherosclerosis

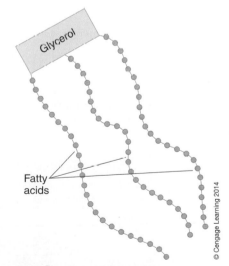

FIGURE 5-1 A triglyceride is composed of three fatty acids attached to a framework of glycerol.

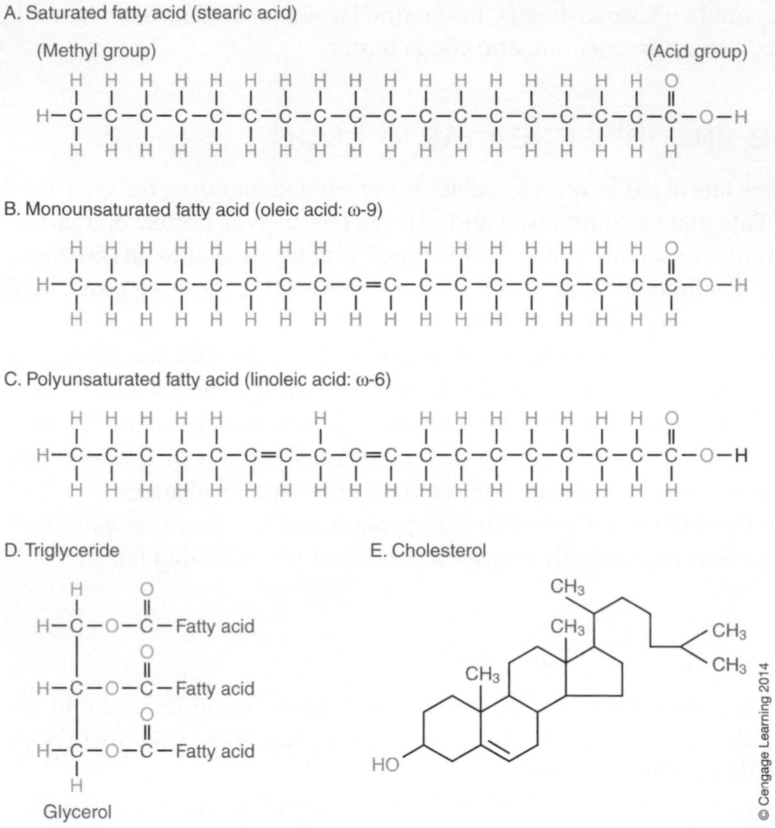

FIGURE 5-2 Chemical formula for (A) saturated fatty acid, (B) monounsaturated fatty acid, (C) polyunsaturated fatty acid, (D) triglyceride, and (E) cholesterol.

A. Saturated fatty acid (stearic acid)

B. Monounsaturated fatty acid (oleic acid: ω-9)

C. Polyunsaturated fatty acid (linoleic acid: ω-6)

D. Triglyceride   E. Cholesterol

© Cengage Learning 2014

proportion of saturated fats are usually solid at room temperature. It is recommended that one consume no more than 7% of total daily calories as saturated fats.

Monounsaturated Fats

monounsaturated fats
fats that are neither saturated nor polyunsaturated and are thought to play little part in atherosclerosis

If a fat is **monounsaturated**, there is one place among the carbon atoms of its fatty acids where there are fewer hydrogen atoms attached than in saturated fats. Examples of foods containing monounsaturated fats are olive oil, peanut oil, canola oil, avocados, and cashew nuts. Research indicates that monounsaturated fats lower the amount of low-density lipoprotein (LDL) ("bad cholesterol") in the blood, but only when they replace saturated fats in one's diet. They have no effect on high-density lipoproteins (HDLs) ("good cholesterol"). It is recommended that one consume 20% of total daily calories as monounsaturated fats (Table 5-2).

Polyunsaturated Fats

polyunsaturated fats
fats whose carbon atoms contain only limited amounts of hydrogen

If a fat is **polyunsaturated**, there are two or more places among the carbon atoms of its fatty acids where there are fewer hydrogen atoms attached than in saturated fats. The point at which carbon-carbon double bonds occur in a polyunsaturated fatty acid is the determining factor in how the body

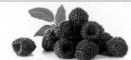

TABLE 5-2 Sources of Saturated, Monounsaturated, and Polyunsaturated Fatty Acids

SATURATED	MONOUNSATURATED	POLYUNSATURATED
Meats	Canola oil	Safflower oil
Coconut	Olive oil	Soybean oil
Palm oil, palm kernel oil	Peanut oil	Sunflower oil
Butter	Nuts	Soybeans
Egg yolks	Avocados	Tofu
Milk and milk products (except fat-free types)	Sardines	

metabolizes it. The two major fatty acids denoted by the placement of their double bonds are the omega-3 and omega-6 fatty acids. **Omega-3 fatty acids** have been reported to help lower the risk of heart disease. Because omega-3 fatty acids are found in fish oils, an increased intake of fatty fish is recommended. Omega-6 (linoleic acid) has a cholesterol-lowering effect. The use of supplements of either of these fatty acids is not recommended. Examples of foods containing polyunsaturated fats include cooking oils made from sunflower, safflower, or sesame seeds or from corn or soybeans; soft margarines whose major ingredient is *liquid* vegetable oil; and fish. Foods containing high proportions of polyunsaturated fats are usually soft or oily. Polyunsaturated fats should not exceed 10% of total daily calories.

 omega-3 fatty acids
help lower the risk of heart disease

Trans-Fatty Acid

Trans-fatty acids (TFAs) are produced when hydrogen atoms are added to monounsaturated or polyunsaturated fats to produce a semisolid product like margarine and shortening. A product is likely to contain a significant amount of TFAs if partially hydrogenated vegetable oil is listed in the first three ingredients on the label. The major source of TFAs in the diet is from baked goods and foods eaten in restaurants. TFAs raise LDLs and total cholesterol.

 trans-fatty acids (TFAs)
produced by adding hydrogen atoms to a liquid fat, making it solid

Hydrogenated Fats

Hydrogenated fats are polyunsaturated vegetable oils to which hydrogen has been added commercially to make them solid at room temperature. This process, called **hydrogenation**, turns polyunsaturated vegetable oils into saturated fats. Margarine is made in this way. (Soft margarine contains less saturated fat than firm margarine.)

 hydrogenation
the combining of fat with hydrogen, thereby making it a saturated fat and solid at room temperature

CHOLESTEROL

Cholesterol is a sterol (see Figure 5-2). It is not a true fat but a fatlike substance that exists in animal foods and body cells. It does not exist in plant foods. Cholesterol is essential for the synthesis of bile, sex hormones, cortisone, and vitamin D and is needed by every cell in the body. The body manufactures 800–1,000 mg of cholesterol a day in the liver.

 cholesterol
fatlike substance that is a constituent of body cells; is synthesized in the liver; also available in animal foods

hypercholesterolemia
unusually high levels of cholesterol in blood; also known as high serum cholesterol

plaque
fatty deposit on interior of artery walls

Cholesterol is a common constituent (part) of one's daily diet because it is found so abundantly in egg yolk, fatty meats, shellfish, butter, cream, cheese, whole milk, and organ meats (liver, kidneys, brains, sweetbreads) (Table 5-3).

Cholesterol is thought to be a contributing factor in heart disease because high serum cholesterol, also called **hypercholesterolemia**, is common in clients with atherosclerosis. Atherosclerosis is a cardiovascular disease in which **plaque** (fatty deposits containing cholesterol and other substances) forms on the inside of artery walls, reducing the space for blood flow. When the blood cannot flow through an artery near the heart, a heart attack occurs. When this is the case near the brain, a stroke occurs. (See Chapter 18.)

It is considered advisable that blood cholesterol levels not exceed 200 mg/dl (200 milligrams of cholesterol per 1 deciliter of blood). A reduction in the amount of total fat, saturated fats, and cholesterol and an increase in the amounts of monounsaturated fats in the diet, weight loss, and exercise all help to lower serum cholesterol levels. Soluble dietary fiber is also considered helpful in lowering blood cholesterol because the cholesterol binds to the fiber and is eliminated via the feces, thus preventing it from being absorbed in the small intestine. In some cases, medication may be prescribed if diet, weight loss, and exercise do not sufficiently lower serum cholesterol.

Because the development of plaque is cumulative, the preferred means of avoiding or at least limiting its development is to limit cholesterol and fat intake throughout life. If children are not fed high-cholesterol foods on a regular basis, their chances of overconsuming them as adults are reduced. Thus, their risk of heart attack and stroke is also reduced.

Supersize USA

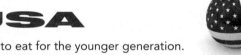

Taco Bell® is a favorite place to eat for the younger generation. My son would come home with three beef burritos, three tacos, nachos bellgrande, and a large cola. Let us look at the calories, fat, and sodium content of his meal.

Food Item	Calories	Fat/Sat Fat (g)	Sodium (mg)
Soft Beef Taco	210	9/4	530
Crunchy Beef Taco	170	10/3.5	290
Nachos BellGrande	770	42/7	1,020
Large Cola	200		13
Totals for son's meal:			
3 Soft Beef Tacos	630	27/12	1,590
3 Crunchy Beef Tacos	510	30/10.5	870
Nachos Bellgrande	770	42/7	1,020
Large Cola	200		40
Grand Total	**2,110**	**99/29.5**	**3,520**

What a tasty meal! Because it is his favorite place to eat and it fits within his budget, should he continue to eat there? As a mother and dietitian I tried to tell him the cons for his body, but like all kids he knows everything. He doesn't exercise much and worries about his weight. He should—he is on the way to supersizing himself.

Source: Retrieved October 2011 from http://www.tacobell.com/nutrition/information.

EXPLORING THE WEB

Search the Web for cholesterol-lowering products. What claims do these products make? Are food–drug interactions mentioned? Are the claims based on scientific research and facts? What advice would you give a client who is inquiring about such products? Create a fact sheet that lists the myths regarding fats and cholesterol and present the facts that dispel these myths.

TABLE 5-3 Fat and Cholesterol Content of Some Common Foods

FOOD	AMOUNT	SATURATED FAT (g)	CHOLESTEROL (mg)	TOTAL FAT (g)	TOTAL KCAL
Dairy					
Creamed cottage cheese (4% fat)	1 cup	6.4	34	10	235
Uncreamed cottage cheese (0.5% fat)	1 cup	0.4	10	1	125
Cream cheese	1 oz	6.2	31	10	100
Swiss cheese	1 oz	5.0	24	8	105
American processed cheese	1 oz	5.6	27	9	105
Half and half	1 Tbsp	1.1	6	2	20
Heavy cream	1 Tbsp	3.5	21	6	54
Nondairy creamer	1 Tbsp	1.4	0	1	20
Whole milk	1 cup	5.1	33	8	150
Reduced-fat milk	1 cup	2.9	18	5	120
Low-fat milk	1 cup	1.6	10	3	100
Fat-free milk	1 cup	0	4	0	90
Chocolate milk shake	10 oz	4.8	30	8	335
Ice cream (11% fat)	½ cup	8.9	59	14	270
Egg (large)	1	1.6	213	5	75
Oils					
Butter	1 Tbsp	7.1	31	11	100
Margarine	1 Tbsp	2.2	0	11	100
Corn oil	1 Tbsp	1.8	0	14	125
Seafood					
Crabmeat (canned)	1 cup	0.5	135	3	135
Salmon (canned)	3 oz	0.9	34	5	120
Shrimp (canned)	3 oz	0.2	128	1	100
Tuna					
Water-packed	3 oz	0.3	48	1	135
Oil-packed	3 oz	1.4	55	7	165
Vegetable					
Avocado	½	2.2	0	15	150
Bread					
Bagel	1	0.3	0	2	200
Doughnut	1	2.8	20	12	210
English muffin	1	0.3	0	1	140
Nuts					
Peanuts (dry roasted)	1 oz	2.0	0	15	170
Meat					
Ground beef (lean)	3 oz	6.2	74	16	230
Roast beef (lean)	4.4 oz	7.2	100	18	300
Leg lamb (lean)	5.2 oz	4.8	130	12	280
Leg lamb (lean and fat)	6 oz	11.2	156	26	410
Bacon	3 slices	3.3	16	9	110
Pork chop (lean)	5 oz	5.2	142	16	330
Frankfurter	1.5 oz	4.8	23	13	145
Chicken leg, fried (meat and skin)	5 oz	6.0	124	22	390
Chicken leg, roasted (meat only)	3.2 oz	1.4	82	4	150

Source: U.S. Department of Agriculture. *Nutritive Values of Foods.* Home and Garden Bulletin, No. 72. 2002 (rev. ed.). Revised 2011

DIGESTION AND ABSORPTION

Although 95% of ingested fats are digested, it is a complex process. The chemical digestion of fats occurs mainly in the small intestine. Fats are not digested in the mouth. They are digested only slightly in the stomach, where gastric lipase acts on emulsified fats such as those found in cream and egg yolk. Fats must be mixed well with the gastric juices before entering the small intestine. In the small intestine, bile emulsifies the fats, and the enzyme pancreatic lipase reduces them to fatty acids and glycerol, which the body subsequently absorbs through villi (Figure 5-3).

Lipoproteins

Fats are insoluble in water, which is the main component of blood. Therefore, special carriers must be provided for the fats to be absorbed and transported by the blood to body cells. In the initial stages of absorption, bile joins with the products of fat digestion to carry fat. Later, protein combines with the final products of fat digestion to form special carriers called **lipoproteins**. The lipoproteins subsequently carry the fats to the body cells by way of the blood.

Lipoproteins are classified as **chylomicrons**, **very-low-density lipoproteins (VLDLs)**, **low-density lipoproteins (LDLs)**, and **high-density lipoproteins (HDLs)**, according to their mobility and density. Chylomicrons are the first lipoprotein identified after eating. They are the largest lipoproteins and the lightest in weight. They are composed of 80–90% triglycerides. Lipoprotein lipase acts to break down the triglycerides into free fatty acids and glycerol. Without this enzyme, fat could not get into the cells.

Very-low-density lipoproteins are made primarily by the liver cells and are composed of 55–65% triglycerides. They carry triglycerides and other lipids to all cells. As the VLDLs lose triglycerides, they pick up cholesterol from other lipoproteins in the blood, and they then become LDLs. Low-density lipoproteins are approximately 45% cholesterol with few triglycerides. They carry most of the blood cholesterol from the liver to the cells. Elevated blood levels greater than 130 mg/dl of LDL are thought to be contributing factors in atherosclerosis. LDL is sometimes termed *bad cholesterol.*

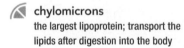 **lipoproteins**
carriers of fat in the blood

chylomicrons
the largest lipoprotein; transport the lipids after digestion into the body

very-low-density lipoproteins (VLDLs)
lipoproteins made by the liver to transport lipids throughout the body

low-density lipoproteins (LDLs)
carry blood cholesterol to the cells

high-density lipoproteins (HDLs)
lipoproteins that carry cholesterol from cells to the liver for eventual excretion

FIGURE 5-3 The body absorbs fatty acids and glycerol through the villi of the small intestine.

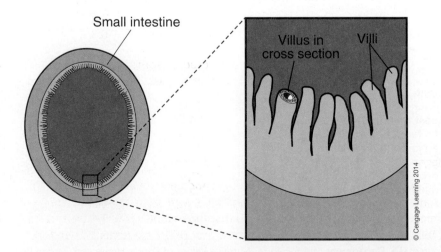

Small intestine

Villus in cross section   Villi

© Cengage Learning 2014

High-density lipoproteins carry cholesterol from the cells to the liver for eventual excretion. The level at which low HDL becomes a major risk factor for heart disease has been set at 40 mg/dl. Research indicates that an HDL level of 60 mg/dl or more is considered protective against heart disease. High-density lipoproteins are sometimes called *good cholesterol*. Exercising, maintaining a desirable weight, and giving up smoking are all ways to increase one's HDL.

METABOLISM AND ELIMINATION

The liver controls fat metabolism. It hydrolyzes triglycerides and forms new ones from this hydrolysis as needed. Ultimately, the metabolism of fats occurs in the cells, where fatty acids are broken down to carbon dioxide and water, releasing energy. The portion of fat that is not needed for immediate use is stored as adipose tissue. Carbon dioxide and water are by-products that are used or removed from the body by the circulatory, respiratory, and excretory systems.

FATS AND THE CONSUMER

Fats continue to be of particular interest to the consumer. Most people know that fats are high-calorie foods and that they are related to heart disease. But people who are not in the health field may not know *how* fats affect health. Consequently, they may be easily duped by clever ads or salespersons marketing nutritional supplements or new "health food" products.

It is important that the health care professional carefully evaluate any new dietary "supplement" for which a nutrition claim is made. For example, supplements for omega-3 fatty acids, fish oil, and vitamin E should be approved by your physician before taking. If the item is not included in the RDA, DRI, or AI, it is safe to assume that medical research has not determined that it is essential. Ingestion of dietary supplements of unknown value could, ironically, be damaging to one's health.

Lecithin

Lecithin is a fatty substance classified as a phospholipid. It is found in both plant and animal foods and is synthesized in the liver. It is a natural emulsifier that helps transport fat in the bloodstream. It is used commercially to make food products smooth.

Lecithin supplements have been promoted by some health food salespersons as being able to prevent cardiovascular disease. To date, this has not been scientifically proven.

lecithin
fatty substance found in plant and animal foods; a natural emulsifier that helps transport fats in the bloodstream; used commercially to make food products smooth

Fat Alternatives

Research into fat alternatives has been in progress for decades. Olestra is an example of a fat alternative made from sugar and fatty acids. The FDA has approved olestra for use only in snack foods such as potato chips, tortilla chips, and crackers. The government requires that food labels indicate that olestra "inhibits the absorption of some vitamins and other nutrients." Therefore, the fat-soluble vitamins A, D, E, and K have been added to foods containing olestra. Olestra contains no calories, but it can cause cramps and diarrhea. The products manufactured with olestra should be used in moderation.

Simplesse is made from either egg white or milk protein and contains 1.3 kcal/g. It can be used only in cold foods such as ice cream because it becomes thick or gels when heated. It is not available for home use.

Oatrim is carbohydrate-based and is derived from oat fiber. Oatrim is heat-stable and can be used in baking but not in frying. Manufacturers have used carbohydrate-based compounds for years as thickeners. Oatrim does provide calories, but significantly less fat.

The long-term effects these products may have on human health and nutrition are unknown. If they are used in the way the U.S. population uses artificial sweeteners, they probably will not reduce the actual fat content in the diet. They may simply be additions to it. One concern among nutritionists is that they will be used in place of nutritious food that, in addition to fat, also provides vitamins, minerals, proteins, and carbohydrates.

DIETARY REQUIREMENTS

Although no specific dietary requirement for fats is included in the RDA and DRIs, deficiency symptoms do occur when fats provide less than 10% of the total daily calorie requirement. When gross deficiency occurs, eczema (inflamed and scaly skin condition) can develop. This has been observed in infants who were fed formulas lacking the essential fatty acid linoleic acid and in clients maintained for long periods on intravenous feedings that lack linoleic acid. Also, growth may be retarded, and weight loss can occur when diets are seriously deficient in fats.

In The Media

Fat Tax

Denmark became the first country to tax saturated fats. The tax applies to all foods with a saturated fat content above 2.3 percent, which calculates to about $6.27 per pound. The tax was implemented to encourage the Danes to get healthier and improve their life expectancy. Research conducted by directors at the Centers of Disease Control (CDC) found it takes a 1 cent-per-ounce tax on unhealthy foods to change consumer behavior. The Denmark government is unsure how the tax will affect the people, but they hope the Danes will begin to consume healthier items.

(Source: Adapted from Kliff, Sarah. Will a Fat Tax Make Denmark Healthier? *The Washington Post.* October 4, 2011. http://www .washingtonpost.com)

SPOTLIGHT *on Life Cycle*

When we think about exercise activities for adults, we think of running on a treadmill or joining a gym, but for children exercise consists of playing with friends, being physically active in school, and participating in extracurricular activities. Sadly, studies have shown that children are becoming more sedentary, with the average child spending 3 hours a day watching television. Television, video games, and computer time has replaced the time that children should be spending riding their bikes, playing outside, and being physically active. The American Academy of Pediatrics recommends that children under the age of 2 years watch no TV at all and that quality programming should be limited to 1–2 hours for children 2 years and older. Parents need to ensure that their child is getting enough exercise in order to positively influence bone and muscle growth and prevent childhood overweight or obesity. Keeping physical activity fun and embracing a healthier lifestyle will encourage children, as well as their families, to participate in regular exercise.

(Source: Adapted from KidsHealth. *Kids and Exercise.* Retrieved February 13, 2012 from http://www.kidshealth.org)

On the other hand, excessive fat in the diet can lead to obesity or heart disease. In addition, studies point to an association between high-fat diets and cancers of the colon, breast, uterus, and prostate.

The Food and Nutrition Board's Committee on Diet and Health recommends that people reduce their fat intake to 30% of total calories. The American Heart Association's newest recommendation is to consume less or no more than 7% of saturated fats, 10% polyunsaturated fats, and 20% monounsaturated fats. According to the Mayo Clinic, currently 35% of calories in U.S. diets are derived from solid fats and sugar.

HEALTH AND NUTRITION CONSIDERATIONS

To accomplish dietary change, the health care professional should review clients' usual diets *with* them. Changes then can be introduced clearly and sensitively and with the clients' active participation. Unless clients understand *why* dietary changes are needed and want to make them, they are unlikely to change their diets.

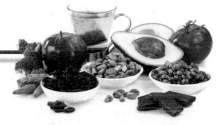

SUMMARY

In addition to providing an important source of energy, fats carry essential fatty acids and fat-soluble vitamins, protect organs and bones, insulate from cold, and provide satiety to meals. They are composed of carbon, hydrogen, and oxygen and are found in both animal and plant foods. Each gram of fat provides 9 calories. Digestion of fats occurs mainly in the small intestine, where they are reduced to fatty acids and glycerol. An excess of fat in the diet can result in obesity and possibly heart disease or cancer.

DISCUSSION TOPICS

1. Why are fats considered a more concentrated source of energy than carbohydrates?

2. Of what value are fats to the body? List some foods rich in fats.

3. Discuss adipose tissue. Is it good? Is it bad? Explain.

4. Describe atherosclerosis. It is said that its effects are cumulative. Explain.

5. Describe the digestion and metabolism of fats. What are the end products of fat digestion?

6. Why might a client on a low-fat diet complain? How might the health care professional be helpful in such a case?

7. What are hydrogenated fats? Are they polyunsaturated? Explain.

8. Why is there a greater danger of excess fat in the U.S. diet than a deficiency of fat?

9. Discuss invisible fats and their potential impact on low-fat diets.

10. What are the probable reasons that omega-3 fatty acid capsules and lecithin have become so popular with the general public?

SUGGESTED ACTIVITIES

1. List the foods you ate yesterday. Circle those containing visible fats. Underline those containing invisible fats. Explain why some foods are both circled and underlined. Revise your list, making it appropriate for someone on a limited-fat diet.

2. Using a cookbook, review recipes for baked products and answer the following questions about them.
   a. Why do bagels contain no cholesterol?
   b. Why does angel food cake contain no cholesterol?
   c. Why does a doughnut contain cholesterol when an English muffin does not?
   d. Why does French toast contain cholesterol when the white bread it is made from may not?
   e. Why does lemon meringue pie filling contain cholesterol when apple pie filling does not?
   f. Why does a cheeseburger contain more cholesterol than a hamburger?

3. Write down five typical meals in your family's diet—one breakfast, one lunch, one dinner, and two snacks. How could you modify them to reduce the fat content?

4. Visit a fast-food restaurant and review the menu. How many items are high in fat? How many are not? Is there any invisible fat in the more "healthy" items? Share your findings with the class.

REVIEW

Multiple choice. Select the *letter* that precedes the best answer.

1. Fats provide the most concentrated form of
   a. carbon
   b. oxygen
   c. lipase
   d. energy

2. Adipose tissue is useful because it
   a. protects and insulates
   b. prevents eczema
   c. provides satiety
   d. can synthesize triglycerides

3. Atherosclerosis is thought to increase the risk of
   a. cancer
   b. plaque
   c. heart attacks
   d. hypercholesterolemia

4. A diet grossly deficient in fats may be deficient in
   a. lipase
   b. linoleic acid
   c. cholesterol
   d. triglycerides

5. Invisible fats can be found in
   a. cake and cookies
   b. orange and tomato juice
   c. egg white and skim milk
   d. lettuce and tomatoes

6. Plant foods that contain saturated fats are
   a. olives and avocados
   b. coconut and chocolate
   c. corn and soybeans
   d. cashew nuts and canola oil

7. When a polyunsaturated vegetable oil is changed to a saturated fat, the process is called
   a. hydrolysis
   b. hypercholesterolemia
   c. hydrogenation
   d. hyperlipidemia

8. Linoleic acid is one of the fatty acids that is known to be
   a. a triglyceride
   b. saturated
   c. monounsaturated
   d. essential to the human diet

9. Cholesterol is
   a. not essential to the human diet
   b. thought to contribute to atherosclerosis
   c. not found in animal foods
   d. classified as a mineral

10. I work at an ice cream factory and am responsible for choosing a fat alternative for the ice cream. Which product should I use?
    a. oatrim   c. simplesse
    b. truvia   d. olestra

11. Three groups of lipids found naturally in the human body and in food are triglycerides, phospholipids, and
    a. cortisone
    b. steroids
    c. sterols
    d. hydrogenated fats

12. Fatty acids are organic compounds of carbon atoms and
    a. hydrogen atoms
    b. arachidonic acids
    c. triglycerides
    d. glycerol

13. Cholesterol
    a. is found in both plants and animals
    b. is found only in plants
    c. does not contribute in any way to heart disease
    d. is a sterol

14. HDL (high-density lipoprotein)
    a. is sometimes called good cholesterol
    b. carries lipids to the cells
    c. is the same as lipase
    d. levels should be less than 40 mg/dl of human blood

15. For digestion, fats require the help of gastric lipase,
    a. bile, and fatty acids
    b. bile, and pancreatic lipase
    c. pancreatic lipase, and glycerol
    d. cholesterol, and bile

16. How many calories are in 13 grams of fat?
    a. 117
    b. 130
    c. 210
    d. 155

17. Which would be the healthiest fat to use when frying a chicken?
    a. lard
    b. olive oil
    c. solid shortening
    d. canola oil

Case In Point

MURALI: FAMILY HISTORY AND ELEVATED CHOLESTEROL

Murali is from Sri Lanka. He moved to the United States when he was 19 years old. His family has a history of heart disease and high cholesterol. Murali's father and brother both died of heart attacks in their 40s. Murali is now 52 years old. His wife Annika is worried about his health. Annika has tried to be careful in preparing his meals. For many years, Murali's cholesterol has been in the high-normal range and he has not needed medication. He has recently landed a new contract with a Fortune 500 company at work. He has been very busy with luncheons and dinner meetings. He has been taking clients to many of the classy restaurants in town for four-course meals that always include dessert. He has been working on this contract for several months. Due to the added stress of this new lifestyle, he is rarely taking time to eat healthy. He also has resumed his old habit of smoking. He is so busy, he rarely has time for any exercise. Annika is worried and convinces Murali to see his physician. His physician orders blood work that reveals a total cholesterol of 428 mg/dl, an LDL of 263 mg/dl, and an HDL of 28 mg/dl. Due to his family history his physician orders a cholesterol-lowering medication. However, he stresses to Murali that this is no replacement for good nutrition and exercise. He refers Murali to a cardiac education class for both nutrition and fitness information. He also refers Murali to a smoking-cessation program.

ASSESSMENT

1. What data do you have about Murali?
2. As a nurse, what conclusion can you draw from Murali's lab results?
3. What do you need to know about his current eating habits? Could foods with unknown fat content have a bearing on his current diet? How could a 24-hour food diary help?
4. What about his health habits, like smoking and alcohol use?
5. What is Murali doing that is healthy for his heart?

DIAGNOSIS

6. What is the cause of Murali's imbalanced nutrition, more than body requirements?
7. Complete this statement: Murali's change of lifestyle is related to _____.

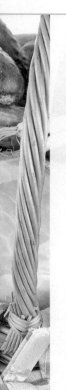

PLAN/GOAL

8. What two goals do you have for Murali?

IMPLEMENTATION

9. What topics do you need to cover related to dietary fats?
10. Name three things Murali can do to help him recognize hidden fats in fast-food restaurants.
11. Who else should be in class with Murali?
12. What agencies or resources could you provide to support Murali at home?
13. How could the information on the American Heart Association website (http://www.americanheart.org) be helpful to Murali?

EVALUATION/OUTCOME CRITERIA

14. What can the physician measure to determine the effectiveness of the plan?
15. What can Murali provide to demonstrate his compliance with the plan?

THINKING FURTHER

16. What is the worst consequence if Murali does not reduce his cholesterol?
17. What does family history have to do with Murali's results?
18. What are the challenges of maintaining a diet and exercise plan for life?

rate this plate

Murali attended the nutrition class to learn how to choose healthy foods while eating out. He attended a dinner meeting with his clients and ordered the following meal. Rate this plate for foods that contain large amounts of cholesterol and fat.

4 oz. shrimp cocktail appetizer

2 cups chicken Caesar salad with 2 Tbsp light vinaigrette dressing

2 hot dinner rolls with creamy butter

1 slice of cheesecake with strawberries

20 oz. iced tea

Case In Point

CECELIA: ELEVATED CHOLESTEROL AND TRANS FATS

Cecelia moved to New York City from Italy with her mother and father when she was a young girl. Her parents opened an Italian bakery and Cecelia spent much of her time there growing up. Her parents are now ready to hand the bakery over to Cecelia so they can retire. At 42 years old, she is very excited about taking charge of the bakery. She has always enjoyed baking and has learned so much through the years about running a business. Her parents recently had physicals and they both had elevated cholesterol. They were concerned for Cecelia and asked her to see her doctor and have her cholesterol tested as well. Cecelia has always been in pretty good health, but decides this wouldn't be a bad idea. When Cecelia sees her doctor, he informs her that she, too, has elevated cholesterol. Her total cholesterol is 282. Her LDL is 186 and her HDL is 27. He discusses with her the importance of weight loss. She is currently 5 feet 4 inches tall and 173 pounds. He also refers her to a dietitian for an assessment of her diet. The dietitian discusses with her the foods that can affect her cholesterol level. In addition to saturated fats, she mentions trans fats. Cecelia has heard this term before, but never understood its meaning. The dietitian explains that trans fats are created from hydrogenating (solidifying) vegetable oils. The dietitian tells Cecelia that trans fats are usually present in baked goods. She also discusses with Cecelia that New York City passed a law banning trans fats in restaurants. She educates Cecelia on the importance of not just eliminating the trans fats from her diet, but making sure that her parents adjusted the recipes for their bakery items to remove all trans fats as well.

ASSESSMENT

1. Why were Cecelia's parents concerned about her cholesterol levels?
2. Cecelia's doctor shares with her the results of her lipid panel. What are the recommendations for total cholesterol, LDL, and HDL levels for Cecelia?
3. What is Cecelia's ideal body weight range? Is her current weight within her ideal body weight range?
4. What is trans fat and what are the impacts of trans fats on the body?

DIAGNOSIS

5. Write a nursing diagnosis for Cecelia.

PLAN/GOAL

6. Cecelia should be educated on what foods will elevate her cholesterol. What are some of these foods?
7. Cecelia should understand that cholesterol comes not only from foods, but also from what other source?
8. What goals would you set for Cecelia?

IMPLEMENTATION

9. What is important for Cecelia to understand about trans fats?
10. How often should Cecelia have her cholesterol assessed?

EVALUATION/OUTCOME CRITERIA

11. How will Cecelia and her doctor know if she has been successful with her goals?

THINKING FURTHER

12. Search guidelines on the National Cholesterol Education Program website (http://www.nhlbi.nih.gov) for cholesterol levels and take the 10-year risk assessment at the bottom of the page. Are you at risk for a cardiac event in the next 10 years? Are there changes in your diet that could help to decrease your risk?

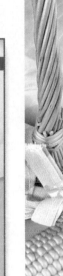

rate this **plate**

Cecelia would like to modify the following recipe for dark chocolate cake in order to make it healthier for her family and customers. What ingredient(s) needs to be eliminated and replaced with a trans-fat-free option? What can you substitute to eliminate trans fat?

- 2 cups boiling water
- 1 cup unsweetened cocoa powder
- 2¾ cups all-purpose flour
- 2 teaspoons baking soda
- ½ teaspoon baking powder
- ½ teaspoon salt
- 1 cup butter, softened
- 2¼ cups white sugar
- 4 eggs
- 1½ teaspoons vanilla extract

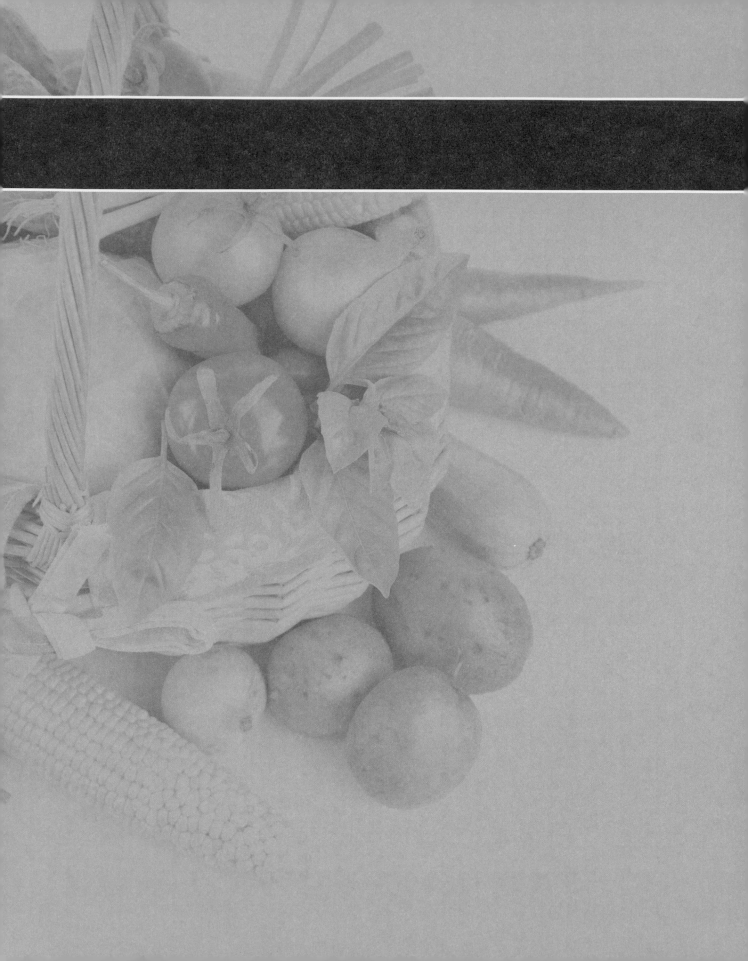

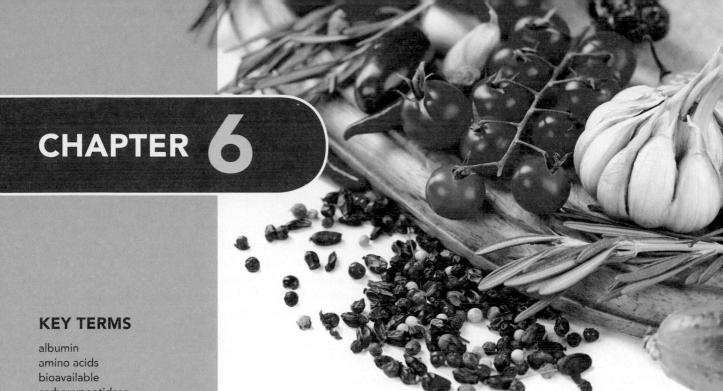

CHAPTER 6

PROTEINS

OBJECTIVES

After studying this chapter, you should be able to:

- State the functions of proteins in the body
- Identify the elements of which proteins are composed
- Describe the effects of protein deficiency
- State the energy yield of proteins
- Identify at least six food sources of complete proteins and six food sources of incomplete proteins

Proteins are the basic material of every body cell. By the age of 4, body protein content reaches the adult level of about 18% of body weight. An adequate supply of proteins in the daily diet is essential for normal growth and development and for the maintenance of health. Proteins are appropriately named. The word *protein* is of Greek derivation and means "of first importance."

FUNCTIONS

Proteins build and repair body tissue, play major roles in regulating various body functions, and provide energy if there is insufficient carbohydrate and fat in the diet.

Building and Repairing Body Tissue

The primary function of proteins is to build and repair body tissues. This is made possible by the provision of the correct type and number of amino acids in the diet. Also, as cells are broken down during metabolism (catabolism), some amino acids released into the blood are recycled to build new and repair other tissue (anabolism). The body uses the recycled amino acids as efficiently as those obtained from the diet.

Regulating Body Functions

Proteins are important components of hormones and enzymes that are essential for the regulation of metabolism and digestion. Proteins help maintain fluid and electrolyte balances in the body and thus prevent edema (abnormal retention of body fluids). Proteins are also essential for the development of antibodies and, consequently, for a healthy immune system.

Providing Energy

Proteins can provide energy if and when the supply of carbohydrates and fats in the diet is insufficient. Each gram of protein provides 4 calories. This is not a good use of proteins, however. In general, they are more expensive than carbohydrates, and most of the complete proteins also contain saturated fats and cholesterol.

FOOD SOURCES

Proteins are found in both animal and plant foods (Table 6-1). The animal food sources provide the highest quality of complete proteins. They include meats, fish, poultry, eggs, milk, and cheese.

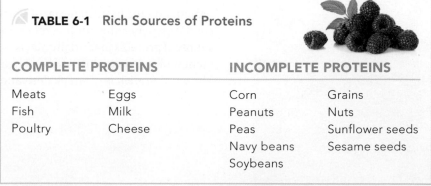

TABLE 6-1 Rich Sources of Proteins

COMPLETE PROTEINS		INCOMPLETE PROTEINS	
Meats	Eggs	Corn	Grains
Fish	Milk	Peanuts	Nuts
Poultry	Cheese	Peas	Sunflower seeds
		Navy beans	Sesame seeds
		Soybeans	

Despite the high biologic value of proteins from animal food sources, they also provide saturated fats and cholesterol. Consequently, complete proteins should be carefully selected from low-fat animal foods such as fish, lean meats, and low-fat dairy products. Whole eggs should be limited to two or three a week if hyperlipidemia is a problem.

Proteins found in plant foods are incomplete proteins and are of a lower biologic quality than those found in animal foods. Even so, plant foods are important sources of protein. Examples of plant foods containing protein are corn, grains, nuts, sunflower seeds, sesame seeds, and legumes such as soybeans, navy beans, pinto beans, split peas, chickpeas, and peanuts.

Plant proteins can be used to produce textured soy protein and tofu, also called analogues. Meat alternatives (analogues) made from soybeans contain soy protein and other ingredients mixed together to simulate various kinds of meat. Meat alternatives may be canned, dried, or frozen. Analogues are excellent sources of protein, iron, and B vitamins.

Tofu is a soft cheese-like food made from soy milk. Tofu is a bland product that easily absorbs the flavors of other ingredients with which it is cooked. Tofu is rich in high-quality proteins and B vitamins, and it is low in sodium. Textured soy protein and tofu are both economical and nutritious meat replacements.

Because of their inclusion of either dairy products and eggs or dairy products alone, most individuals who follow lacto-ovo vegetarian or lacto-vegetarian diets will be able to meet their protein requirements through a balanced diet that includes milk and milk products, enriched grains, nuts, and legumes. Strict vegetarians who consume no animal products will need to be more careful to include other protein-rich food sources such as soybeans, soy milk, and tofu.

CLASSIFICATION

The classification and quality of a protein depends on the number and types of amino acids it contains. There are 20 amino acids, but only 10 are considered essential to humans (Table 6-2). Two additional amino acids are sometimes incorporated into proteins during translation: selenocyteine and pyrrolysine.

TABLE 6-2 Amino Acids

ESSENTIAL		NONESSENTIAL	
Arginine*	Phenylalanine	Alanine	Glutamine
Histidine*	Threonine	Arginine*	Glycine
Isoleucine	Tryptophan	Asparagine	Histidine*
Leucine	Valine	Aspartic acid	Proline
Lysine		Cysteine	Serine
Methionine		Glutamic acid	Tyrosine

*Essential during childhood only.

© Cengage Learning 2014

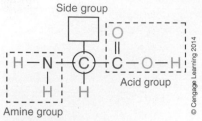

FIGURE 6-1 Two different foods (e.g., grains and dairy products) alone may not provide all the essential amino acids. Combined, however, they form a complete protein and therefore are considered complementary.

complete proteins
proteins that contain all the essential amino acids

bioavailable
ability of a nutrient to be readily absorbed and used by the body

incomplete proteins
proteins that do not contain all of the essential amino acids

complementary proteins
incomplete proteins that when combined provide all 10 essential amino acids

nitrogen
chemical element found in protein; essential to life

amino acids
nitrogen-containing chemical compounds of which protein is composed

TABLE 6-3 Examples of Complementary Protein Foods

Corn	and	Beans
Rice	and	Beans
Bread	and	Peanut butter
Bread	and	Split pea soup
Bread	and	Cheese
Bread	and	Baked beans
Macaroni	and	Cheese
Cereal	and	Milk

© Cengage Learning 2014

Essential amino acids are necessary for normal growth and development and must be provided in the diet. Proteins containing all the essential amino acids are of high biologic value; these proteins are called **complete proteins** and are extremely **bioavailable**. The nonessential amino acids can be produced in the body from the essential amino acids, vitamins, and minerals.

Incomplete proteins are those that lack one or more of the essential amino acids. Consequently, incomplete proteins cannot build tissue without the help of other proteins. The value of each is increased when it is eaten in combination with another incomplete protein, not necessarily at the same meal but during the same day. In this way, one incomplete protein food can provide the essential amino acids the other lacks. The combination may thereby provide all the essential amino acids (Figure 6-1). When this occurs, the proteins are called **complementary proteins** (Table 6-3). Gelatin is the only protein from an animal source that is an incomplete protein.

COMPOSITION

Like carbohydrates and fats, proteins contain carbon, hydrogen, and oxygen, but in different proportions. In addition, and most important, they are the only nutrient group that contains **nitrogen**, and some contain sulfur. Figure 6-1 is an example of an amino acid with a nitrogen (N) molecule.

Proteins are composed of chemical compounds called **amino acids** (Figure 6-2). Amino acids are sometimes called the building blocks of protein because they are combined to form the thousands of proteins in the human body. Heredity determines the specific types of proteins within each person.

DIGESTION AND ABSORPTION

The mechanical digestion of protein begins in the mouth, where the teeth grind the food into small pieces. Chemical digestion begins in the stomach. Hydrochloric acid prepares the stomach so that the enzyme pepsin can begin its task of reducing proteins to **polypeptides**.

After the polypeptides reach the small intestine, three pancreatic enzymes (**trypsin**, **chymotrypsin**, and **carboxypeptidase**) continue chemical digestion. Intestinal peptidases finally reduce the proteins to amino acids.

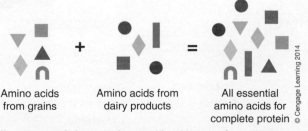

Amino acids from grains + Amino acids from dairy products = All essential amino acids for complete protein

FIGURE 6-2 All amino acids have a chemical backbone of a carbon atom; an amine group, which contains nitrogen; an acid group; and a side group. It is the chemical structure of the side group that gives each amino acid its unique identity.

After digestion, the amino acids in the small intestine are absorbed by the villi and are carried by the blood to all body tissues. There, they are used to form needed proteins.

METABOLISM AND ELIMINATION

All essential amino acids must be present to build and repair the cells as needed. When amino acids are broken down, the nitrogen-containing amine group is stripped off. This process is called deamination. Deamination produces ammonia, which is released into the bloodstream by the cells. The liver picks up the ammonia, converts it to urea, and returns it to the bloodstream for the kidneys to filter out and excrete. The remaining parts are used for energy or are converted to carbohydrate or fat and stored as glycogen or adipose tissue.

DIETARY REQUIREMENTS

One's protein requirement is determined by size, age, sex, and physical and emotional conditions. A large person has more body cells to maintain than a small person. A growing child, a pregnant woman, or a woman who is breast-feeding needs more protein for each pound of body weight than the average adult. When digestion is inefficient, fewer amino acids are absorbed by the body; consequently the protein requirement is higher. This is sometimes thought to be the case with the elderly. Extra proteins are usually required after surgery, severe burns, or during infections in order to replace lost tissue and to manufacture antibodies. In addition, emotional trauma can cause the body to excrete more nitrogen than it normally does, thus increasing the need for protein foods.

The National Research Council of the National Academy of Sciences considers the average adult's daily requirement to be 0.8 gram of protein for each kilogram of body weight. To determine your requirement, do the following:

1. Divide body weight by 2.2 (the number of pounds per kilogram).
2. Multiply the answer obtained in step 1 by 0.8 (gram of protein per kilogram of body weight).

polypeptides
ten or more amino acids bonded together

trypsin
pancreatic enzyme; helps digest proteins

chymotrypsin
pancreatic enzyme necessary for the digestion of proteins

carboxypeptidase
pancreatic enzyme necessary for protein digestion

Supersize USA

Are you aware that increasing your protein intake by 50% can lead to a 1% bone loss each year? High protein diets are becoming more popular with adults wanting to limit calorie intake through carbohydrates and build muscle. However, too much protein can lead to heart disease, kidney damage, constipation, tumors and growths, arthritis, and bone loss. "Stacking" your protein, such as eating a sausage, cheese, and egg breakfast muffin, can yield additional calories and fat. As explained above, it is easy to consume an excess amount of protein as well as additional calories, fat, and cholesterol in a breakfast meal. Ordering your burgers without the added bacon and eating breakfast sandwiches with no added cheese will save you hundreds of calories in the long run.

(Source: Adapted from *Lesson 85: The Dangers of a High Protein Diet. The Problems with Protein. Raw Food Explained.* Accessed November 15, 2011 from www.rawfoodexplained.com)

In 2002, the Dietary Reference Intakes (DRIs) for protein were published by the National Academy of Sciences (see Table 6-4). An Adequate Intake (AI) was established for infants 0–6 months, with all other recommendations based on 0.8 g/kg of body weight. Table 6-5 provides an idea of the amount of protein in an average day's diet. (For specific amounts of protein in other foods, refer to Appendix D.)

TABLE 6-4 Recommended Dietary Allowances for Protein

LIFE STAGE GROUP	AGE	PROTEIN (GRAMS/DAY)
Infants	0–6 mo	9.1*
	7–12 mo	11*
Children	1–3 y	13
	4–8 y	19
Males	9–13 y	34
	14–18 y	52
	19–30 y	56
	31–50 y	56
	51–70 y	56
	>70 y	56
Females	9–13 y	34
	14–18 y	46
	19–30 y	46
	31–50 y	46
	51–70 y	46
	>70 y	46
Pregnancy	14–18 y	71
	19–30 y	71
	31–50 y	71
Lactation	14–18 y	71
	19–30 y	71
	31–50 y	71

* Infant values are Adequate Intakes (AI); all other values are Recommended Dietary Allowances (RDA).

Source: Reprinted with permission from the National Academies Press, Copyright © 2006, National Academy of Sciences. *Dietary Reference Intakes: The Essential Guide to Nutrient Requirements.*

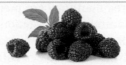

TABLE 6-5 Protein in an Average Diet for 1 Day	SERVING SIZE	PROTEIN (g)	CALORIE
Breakfast			
Orange juice	1/2 cup	1	45
Cornflakes	3/4 cup	1	75
with sugar	2 tsp		30
Toast	2 slices	4	140
Butter	1 Tbsp		65
Jelly	1 Tbsp		60
Fat-free milk	1/2 cup	4	50
Lunch			
Grapefruit juice	1/2 cup	1	50
Tuna salad sandwich	2/3 cup tuna salad	20	220
on bread with	2 slices bread	4	140
lettuce			
Carrot sticks	1 carrot	1	25
Canned pears	1/2 cup	1	100
Oatmeal cookies	2	1	160
Fat-free milk	1 cup	8	100
Dinner			
Chicken breast	3 oz	26	160
Baked potato	1	4	145
Asparagus	1/2 cup		25
Sliced tomato salad	1 tomato	1	25
Roll	1	2	100
with butter	1 Tbsp		65
Ice cream	2/3 cup	3	200
Fat-free milk	1 cup	8	100
		90	2,080

© Cengage Learning 2014

In The Media

Weight Loss: Calories versus Protein

Some dieters think that manipulating the amount of protein in their diet can cause weight loss. A new study published in the *Journal of the American Medical Association* discovered that the amount of protein in a diet had no effect on weight gain when 1,000 additional calories were added to the diet. Eating less protein can lead to a reduction in lean body mass and a higher percentage of calories stored as fat. Those overeating protein gained more lean body mass and stored fewer calories as fat. Research concluded that overeating, regardless of protein amount, can cause weight gain. Practicing mindful eating will manage calorie intake and prevent weight gain.

Source: Adapted from Jaslow, Ryan. *Calories Count More Than Protein for Weight Loss.* CBS News. Accessed January 5, 2012 from CBSNews.com

Protein Excess

It is easy for people living in the developed parts of the world to ingest more protein than the body requires. There are a number of reasons why this should be avoided. The saturated fats and cholesterol common to complete protein foods may contribute to heart disease and provide more calories than desirable. Some studies seem to indicate a connection between long-term high-protein diets and colon cancer and high calcium excretion, which depletes the bones of calcium and may contribute to osteoporosis. People who eat excessive amounts of protein-rich foods may ignore the also essential fruits and vegetables, and excess protein intake may put more demands on the liver (which converts nitrogen to urea) and the kidneys to excrete excess urea than they are prepared to handle. Therefore, the Centers for Disease Control and Prevention recommends that protein intake represent no more than 10–35% of one's daily calorie intake and not exceed double the amount given in the table of DRIs (see Table 6-4).

Protein and Amino Acid Supplements

Protein and amino acid supplements are taken for a number of reasons. Information in the media may lead consumers to think that protein and amino acid supplements should be taken for the following: "bulking up" for athletes, sparing body protein in weight loss, and maintaining health. In reality, it is weightlifting, not protein bars or supplements, that build muscle. To determine how much protein is needed in maintaining a healthy weight, dieters need a balanced diet using the guidelines of MyPlate.

High-quality protein foods are more bioavailable than expensive supplements. Single amino acids can be harmful to the body and never occur naturally in food. The body was designed to handle food, not supplements. If a single amino acid has been recommended, it is very important that a physician be consulted before the amino acid is used.

Nitrogen Balance

nitrogen balance
when nitrogen intake equals nitrogen excreted

positive nitrogen balance
nitrogen intake exceeds outgo

physical trauma
extreme physical stress

negative nitrogen balance
more nitrogen lost than taken in

Protein requirements may be discussed in terms of **nitrogen balance**. This occurs when nitrogen intake equals the amount of nitrogen excreted. **Positive nitrogen balance** exists when nitrogen intake exceeds the amount excreted. This indicates that new tissue is being formed, and it occurs during pregnancy, during children's growing years, when athletes develop additional muscle tissue, and when tissues are rebuilt after **physical trauma** such as illness or injury. **Negative nitrogen balance** indicates that protein is being lost. It may be caused by fevers, injury, surgery, burns, starvation, or immobilization.

Protein Deficiency

albumin
protein that occurs in blood plasma

When people are unable to obtain an adequate supply of protein for an extended period, muscle wasting will occur, and arms and legs become very thin. At the same time, **albumin** (protein in blood plasma) deficiency will cause edema, resulting in an extremely swollen appearance. The water is excreted when sufficient protein is eaten. People may lose appetite, strength, and weight, and wounds may heal very slowly. Clients suffering from edema become lethargic and depressed. These signs are seen in grossly neglected children or in the elderly, poor, or incapacitated. It is essential that people following vegetarian diets, especially vegans, carefully calculate the types and amount of protein in their diets so as to avoid protein deficiency.

Protein Energy Malnutrition

　protein energy malnutrition (PEM)
malnutrition resulting from inadequate intake of protein and energy-rich foods; marasmus and kwashiorkor

People suffering from **protein energy malnutrition (PEM)** lack both protein and energy-rich foods. Such a condition is not uncommon in developing countries where there are long-term shortages of both protein and energy

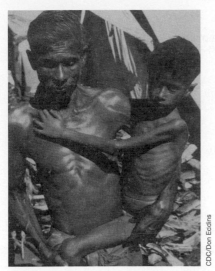

CDC/Don Eddins

FIGURE 6-3 Visible signs of marasmus include extreme wasting, wrinkled skin, and irritability.

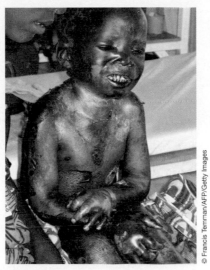

© Francis Temman/AFP/Getty Images

FIGURE 6-4 Edema, skin lesions, and hair changes are common signs of kwashiorkor.

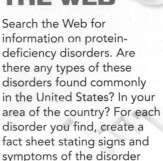

EXPLORING THE WEB

Search the Web for information on protein-deficiency disorders. Are there any types of these disorders found commonly in the United States? In your area of the country? For each disorder you find, create a fact sheet stating signs and symptoms of the disorder and dietary changes that can be made to correct the deficiency.

foods. Children who lack sufficient protein do not grow to their potential size. Infants born to mothers eating insufficient protein during pregnancy can have permanently impaired mental capacities.

Two deficiency diseases that affect children are caused by a grossly inadequate supply of protein or energy, or both. **Marasmus**, a condition resulting from severe malnutrition, afflicts young children and adults who lack both energy and protein foods as well as vitamins and minerals. The infant with marasmus appears emaciated but does not have edema. Hair is dull and dry, and the skin is thin and wrinkled (Figure 6-3). The other protein-deficiency disease that affects children as well as adults is kwashiorkor (Figure 6-4). **Kwashiorkor** appears when there is a sudden or recent lack of protein-containing food (such as during a famine). This disease causes fat to accumulate in the liver, and the lack of protein and hormones results in edema, painful skin lesions, and changes in the pigmentation of skin and hair. The mortality rate for kwashiorkor clients is high.

Those who survive these deficiency diseases may suffer from permanent **mental retardation**. The ultimate cost of food deprivation among young children is high, indeed. Table 6-6 lists some signs that help distinguish marasmus from kwashiorkor.

 marasmus
severe wasting caused by lack of protein and all nutrients or faulty absorption; PFM

 kwashiorkor
deficiency disease caused by extreme lack of protein

 mental retardation
below-normal intellectual capacity

HEALTH AND NUTRITION CONSIDERATIONS

Proteins have acquired an unfairly high value among the general public in the United States. Also, many people think that proteins are found only in animal food sources. As a result, complete proteins tend to be overused in most diets.

Research about the cumulative effects of the overuse of proteins in the diet is beginning to suggest that excessive use of protein could damage

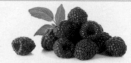

TABLE 6-6 Differentiating Marasmus and Kwashiorkor	
MARASMUS	**KWASHIORKOR**
Total surface fat (TSF)* and mid-arm circumference (MAC) decreased	TSF and MAC within normal limits
Weight decreased	Weight possibly within normal limits
Visceral proteins (albumin) within normal limits or decreased	Visceral proteins decreased
Immune function within normal limits	Immune function decreased
Dull, dry hair	Reddish-color hair
Emaciated, wrinkled appearance	Puffy appearance
Lack of protein and total energy	Edema

*TSF and MAC can be determined by anthropometric measurements (see Chapter 1), which are done by a dietitian. The results are then compared with standard values obtained from measurement of a large number of people.

© Cengage Learning 2014

kidneys, possibly contribute to osteoporosis and cancer, and cause over-weight and heart disease.

The health care professional may find that reeducating clients about the need to reduce their protein intake to 10–35% of total calories is a challenging task.

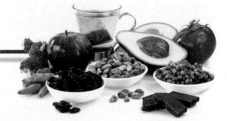

SUMMARY

Proteins contain nitrogen, an element that is necessary for growth and the maintenance of health. In addition to building and repairing body tissues, proteins regulate body processes and can supply energy. Each gram of protein provides 4 calories. Proteins are composed of amino acids, 10 of which are essential for growth and repair of body tissues.

Complete proteins contain all of the essential amino acids and can build tissues. The best sources of complete proteins are animal foods such as meat, fish, poultry, eggs, milk, and cheese. Incomplete proteins do not contain all of the essential amino acids, and two or more of these proteins must be combined in order to build tissues. The best sources of incomplete proteins are legumes, corn, grains, and nuts. The nutritional value of incomplete protein foods can be increased by eating two or more incomplete protein foods during the day. Chemical digestion of proteins occurs in the stomach and small intestine. Proteins are reduced to amino acids and ultimately are absorbed into the blood through the villi in the small intestine.

A severe deficiency of protein in the diet can cause kwashiorkor and can contribute to marasmus in children and adults. Both conditions can result in impaired physical and mental development.

DISCUSSION TOPICS

1. Why are proteins especially important to children, pregnant women, and people who are ill?

2. Of which elements are proteins composed?

3. What functions do proteins perform in the body?

4. Discuss why it may be unwise to use protein foods as energy foods.

5. Discuss the effects of protein deficiency in both children and adults.

6. Describe the digestion of proteins.

7. Describe the metabolism of proteins.

8. Tell what amino acids are and explain their importance. Tell where they are found.

9. Describe complete and incomplete protein foods and name several of each type.

10. How does one determine protein requirements? Calculate your mother's or father's protein requirements.

11. Why might someone with a broken hip develop negative nitrogen balance in the hospital?

SUGGESTED ACTIVITIES

1. Keep a record of the foods you eat in a 24-hour period. Using Appendix D or the diet analysis software at MyPlate, compute the grams of protein consumed. Did your diet provide the recommended amount of protein as indicated in Table 6-4?

2. Plan a day's menu for yourself. Include foods especially rich in complete proteins.

   a. Alter your planned menu by replacing some of the complete protein foods with those containing incomplete proteins.

   b. Visit a local supermarket and compute the cost of the menu that contains complete proteins. Compute the cost of the menu that contains incomplete proteins. Which is less expensive? Why?

REVIEW

Multiple choice. Select the *letter* that precedes the best answer.

1. The building blocks of proteins are
   a. ascorbic acids
   b. amino acids
   c. nitrogen and sulfur only
   d. meat and fish

2. Proteins are essential because they are the only nutrient that contains
   a. nitrogen
   b. niacin
   c. hydrochloric acid
   d. carbon

3. Corn, peas, and beans
   a. are complete protein foods
   b. are incomplete protein foods
   c. contain no protein
   d. lose proteins during cooking

4. Protein deficiency may result in
   a. beriberi
   b. goiter
   c. edema
   d. leukemia

5. Good sources of complete protein foods are
   a. eggs and ground beef
   b. breads and cereals
   c. butter and margarine
   d. legumes and nuts

6. One gram of protein provides
   a. 4 calories
   b. 9 calories
   c. 7 calories
   d. 19 calories

7. Proteins are broken down in the body to
   a. peptides
   b. ascorbic acids
   c. amino acids
   d. calories

8. The *primary* function of protein is to
   a. build and repair body cells
   b. provide energy
   c. digest minerals and vitamins
   d. none of the above

9. Once proteins reach the small intestine, chemical digestion continues through the action of
    a. rennin
    b. pancreatic enzymes
    c. bile
    d. hydrochloric acid

10. It is unwise to regularly ingest excessive amounts of protein because
    a. it can cause positive nitrogen balance
    b. it may reduce the work of the kidneys
    c. it can contribute to the heart disease
    d. it may cause uremic poisoning

11. The following symptoms describe Marasmus except for
    a. protein deficient
    b. edema
    c. calorie malnutrition
    d. emaciated appearance

12. Arrange the following foods into two lists, one containing those that are the best sources of complete proteins and one containing those that are the best sources of incomplete proteins.

Scrambled eggs	Refried beans
Corn on the cob	Hot chocolate milk
Chickpeas and rice	Fat-free milk
Beef burgers	Baked navy beans
Filet of sole	Fried chicken
Peanuts	Swiss cheese

Case In Point

Anneliese is a college exchange student from Germany. While attending college, she noticed she had gained some weight. She is 5 feet 6 inches tall and is now 163 pounds. Some of her friends were using the Atkins diet in an attempt to lose weight. They discussed how to follow the diet with her. She has been trying it out for the past 2 months and has seen some weight loss. However, she is finding it increasingly difficult to adhere to. She grew up in Germany eating many fruits and vegetables daily. She has been trying to find a new diet that will allow her to consume a larger variety of foods. In researching further, she discovers many diets that all promise the weight loss she desires. She decides a different diet might be the answer to her dilemma. She would definitely prefer one that will incorporate more fruits and vegetables in with the high-protein foods. She believes this may help with the constipation she has been experiencing as well. One of her friends is studying nutrition and suggests Anneliese meet with a dietitian to help her choose a diet that is healthy. Anneliese hopes meeting with a dietitian will be the best way for her to lose weight, keep it off, and enjoy the foods she loves.

ASSESSMENT

1. What data do you have about Anneliese's eating habits?
2. What do you know about her ability to develop habits?
3. What is the cause of the current problem?

DIAGNOSIS

4. Complete the following diagnostic statement: Imbalanced nutrition, more than body requirements, as evidenced by _____.
5. Complete the following diagnostic statement: Deficient knowledge related to a lack of information about _____.

PLAN/GOAL

6. What are two measurable, reasonable goals for Anneliese?

IMPLEMENTATION

7. What foods need to be altered in Anneliese's diet?
8. What does Anneliese need to add to her diet?
9. Using preferences, suggest some alternative menus that would help Anneliese lose weight.

EVALUATION/OUTCOME CRITERIA

10. What criterion would a dietitian use to measure Anneliese's success?

11. What diseases would Anneliese avoid by reducing her high-fat protein intake?

THINKING FURTHER

12. Which protein sources are most economical and are low in calories?
13. How could this information be useful in other situations?

rate this **plate**

Anneliese does not need a high amount of protein in order to lose weight. She only needs 5½ oz of protein per day. By lowering the amount of protein in the diet, calories will decrease and weight will be lost. Rate what she ate on the Atkins diet before seeing the dietitian.

7 oz. deep fried chicken breast

Spinach salad with tomatoes, onions, egg, dried cranberries, and croutons

Vinaigrette dressing

¾ cup of broccoli

What changes can be made to this plate to encourage healthy choices and continued weight loss without the Atkins diet plan?

Case In Point

TALIL: PROTEIN ENERGY MALNUTRITION

Erin is a registered dietitian who is currently traveling with a medical missionary team of nurses and physicians throughout southern Asia. Their team's goal is to reach many of the people in that area who have never received any kind of medical attention. Talil lives in southern Asia with his family. Their primary source of food is the rice they grow and the fruits and berries they find on trees and bushes nearby. His mother is concerned about 2-year-old Talil. After giving birth to her second child 8 months ago, she weaned Talil so she could feed the new baby. Since that time, Talil has become extremely thin, yet his belly is distended and his face is puffy. She doesn't understand why he is only gaining weight in his belly and his face. She has also noticed recently that some areas of his skin are lighter in pigment and others are more reddened and rashlike. He seems lethargic and irritable and has even had several bouts of diarrhea. His mother brings him to the clinic where the mission team is working. The doctor diagnoses Talil with kwashiorkor. He asks Erin to meet with his mother and explain what kwashiorkor is and what needs to be done to improve the health and well-being of Talil. Erin explains to Talil's mother that he is not getting adequate protein. She discusses the need for either meat or dairy sources in his diet. If meat and dairy are not available then lentil beans need to be incorporated with the rice in his diet. She gives Talil's mom a case of lentils. The team brought several cases knowing the high incidence of kwashiorkor in this area of the world. She discussed with Talil's mom the importance of finding an additional source of protein for him before the lentils run out. Talil's mom asks Erin if consuming fish from the nearby lake would be a good protein source. Erin assures her that this would be an excellent way to start incorporating protein.

ASSESSMENT

1. What is deficient in Talil's diet?
2. What causes kwashiorkor?
3. What caused Talil to develop kwashiorkor?
4. If Talil's kwashiorkor continues, what consequence could follow as a result?

DIAGNOSIS

5. Write a nursing diagnosis for Talil.

PLAN/GOAL

6. What can Erin do as a dietitian to help Talil's mother correct his kwashiorkor?

IMPLEMENTATION

7. What could Talil's mom do to help prevent further kwashiorkor in her children or other children in their village?
8. Explain what happens in kwashiorkor that causes edema, skin lesions, and changes in pigment of the skin?

EVALUATION/OUTCOME CRITERIA

9. How will Talil's mom know that the strategies she has implemented have resolved the kwashiorkor?

THINKING FURTHER

10. Shown in Table 6-6, what are the key differences between kwashiorkor and marasmus?

rate this plate

Talil was diagnosed with kwashiorkor due to inadequate protein intake. His mother has asked the dietitian for good sources of protein and milk she would have in her area. Talil's mother prepared the following meal. Rate this plate on protein content:

1 oz. cooked fish

⅓ cup rice

¼ cup of vegetables

4 oz. soy milk

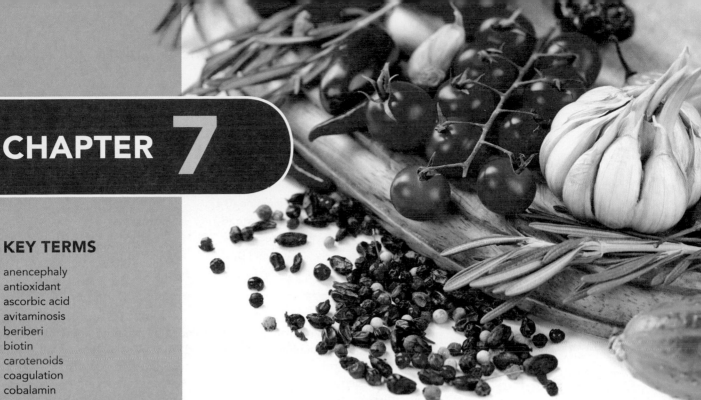

VITAMINS

OBJECTIVES

After studying this chapter, you should be able to:

- State one or more functions of each of the 13 vitamins discussed
- Identify at least two food sources of each of the vitamins discussed
- Identify some symptoms of, or diseases caused by, deficiencies of the vitamins discussed

Vitamins are organic (carbon-containing) compounds that are essential in small amounts for body processes. Vitamins themselves do not provide energy. They enable the body to use the energy provided by carbohydrates, fats, and proteins. The name vitamin implies their importance, as in Latin *vita* means "life." They do not, however, represent a panacea (universal remedy) for physical or mental illness or a way to alleviate the stressors in life. They should not be overused—more is not necessarily better. In fact, **megadoses** can be toxic (poisonous). In the past, it was believed that a healthy person eating a balanced diet would obtain all the nutrients—including vitamins— needed. That was in the past. Today's reality is such that with after-school sports, dance lessons, band practice or lessons, both parents working, and more, people are in a time and energy crunch. So in many homes,

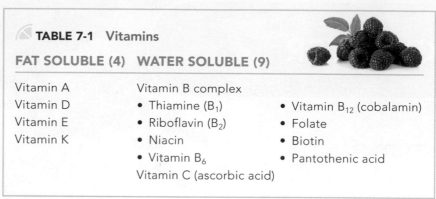

TABLE 7-1 Vitamins	
FAT SOLUBLE (4)	**WATER SOLUBLE (9)**
Vitamin A	Vitamin B complex
Vitamin D	• Thiamine (B$_1$) • Vitamin B$_{12}$ (cobalamin)
Vitamin E	• Riboflavin (B$_2$) • Folate
Vitamin K	• Niacin • Biotin
	• Vitamin B$_6$ • Pantothenic acid
	Vitamin C (ascorbic acid)

© Cengage Learning 2014

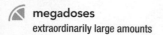

megadoses
extraordinarily large amounts

home-cooked family meals have been replaced by fast food, home delivery, carry-out, vending machines, and processed foods. Most of these choices are not found in the fruit and vegetable recommendation from MyPlate.

The existence of vitamins has been known since early in the 20th century. It was discovered that animals fed diets of pure proteins, carbohydrates, fats, and minerals did not thrive as did those fed normal diets that included vitamins.

Vitamins were originally named by letter. Subsequent research has shown that many of the vitamins that were originally thought to be a single substance are actually groups of substances doing similar work in the body. Vitamin B proved to be more than one compound—B$_1$, B$_6$, B$_{12}$, and so on—and consequently is now known as B complex. Many of the 13 known vitamins are currently named according to their chemical composition or function in the body (Table 7-1).

Vitamins are found in minute amounts in foods. The specific amounts and types of vitamins in foods vary.

DIETARY REQUIREMENTS

Since 1997, the Food and Nutrition Board of the Institute of Medicine has been establishing Dietary Reference Intakes (DRIs) to replace the Recommended Dietary Allowances (RDAs) as outlined in Table 7-2. Tolerable Upper Limits (ULs) have also been set for some vitamins and minerals. The UL is the maximum level of daily intake unlikely to cause adverse effects and is not a recommended level of intake. Vitamin allowances are given by weight—milligrams (mg) or micrograms (µg or mcg).

Vitamin deficiencies can occur and can result in disease. Persons inclined to vitamin deficiencies because they do not eat balanced diets include alcoholics, the poor and incapacitated elderly, clients with serious diseases that affect appetite, intellectually disabled persons, and young children who receive inadequate care. Also, deficiencies of fat-soluble vitamins occur in clients with chronic malabsorption diseases such as cystic fibrosis, celiac disease, and Crohn's disease.

The term **avitaminosis** means "without vitamins," whereas hypervitaminosis is the excess of one or more vitamins. Either term followed by the

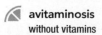

avitaminosis
without vitamins

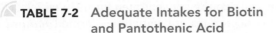
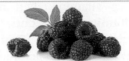

CATEGORY	AGE	BIOTIN (mg)	PANTOTHENIC ACID (mg)
Infants	0–6 mo	5	1.7
	7–12 mo	6	1.8
Children and adolescents	1–3 y	8	2
	4–8 y	12	3
	9–13 y	20	4
	14–18 y	25	5
Adults	19–70 y	30	5
Pregnancy		30	6
Lactation		35	6

TABLE 7-2 Adequate Intakes for Biotin and Pantothenic Acid

Source: Reprinted with permission from the National Academies Press, Copyright © 2006, National Academy of Sciences. *Dietary Reference Intakes: The Essential Guide to Nutrient Requirements.*

SPOTLIGHT *on Life Cycle*

Hypervitaminosis can be very dangerous. Several years ago, I received a letter from my sister informing me that she had been diagnosed with Alzheimer's and she had approximately 3 years until she would no longer recognize me. I was devastated. My sister is a very intelligent person who keeps up with the latest nutrition information about diabetes (she has type 2), nutrition in general, and supplements. Over the years, we had many discussions about what supplements would be beneficial for her age, which is currently 84.

What I didn't know was that she and my brother-in-law, who live in Florida, had been going to a health food store and had been talked into taking a multitude, I mean handfuls, of vitamins, minerals, and herbal supplements. During my next visit, I discovered one entire dresser drawer full of bottles of vitamins, minerals, and herbal supplements that they had been taking for about 2 years. My brother, who visited more often than I, knew that there had been a change in my sister's cognition. She would stop talking in midsentence, lose her train of thought, and even slur her speech. That explained why, when I would call, she would not want to talk very long. My brother and I found it hard to believe she really had Alzheimer's, given her symptoms.

During my next visit, my brother and I got rid of all the supplements, and we helped my sister apply and thankfully be accepted into the assisted-living section of a retirement community. We did this so that my sister's medication and approved supplements would be given at designated times. Since then, 2 years have gone by, and my sister does not have Alzheimer's. Her cognition is fine, no more slurred speech or low blood pressure (caused by excessive potassium), and just a little forgetfulness. I almost lost my sister because of overconsumption of vitamins, minerals, and herbal supplements, and now I have her back. I am so grateful!

name of a specific vitamin is used to indicate a serious lack thereof or excess of that particular vitamin. Either a lack or excess of vitamins can be detrimental to a person's health. This word followed by the name of a specific vitamin is used to indicate a serious lack of that particular vitamin. **Hypervitaminosis** is the excess of one or more vitamins. Either a lack or excess of vitamins can be detrimental to a person's health.

hypervitaminosis
condition caused by excessive ingestion of one or more vitamins

vitamin supplements
concentrated forms of vitamins; may be in tablet or liquid form

Vitamins taken in addition to those received in the diet are called **vitamin supplements**. One can acquire concentrated forms in tablets, capsules, and drops. Vitamin concentrates are sometimes termed *natural* or *synthetic* (manufactured). Some people believe that a meaningful difference exists between the two types and that the natural are far superior in quality to the synthetic. However, according to the U.S. Food and Drug Administration (FDA), the body cannot distinguish between a vitamin of plant or animal origin and one manufactured in a laboratory because once they have been dismantled by the digestive system, the two types of the same vitamin are chemically identical.

Synthetic vitamins are frequently added to foods during processing. When this is done, the foods are described as enriched or fortified. Examples of these foods are enriched breads and cereals to which thiamine, niacin, riboflavin, folate, and the mineral iron have been added. Vitamins A and D are added to milk and fortified margarine.

Preserving Vitamin Content in Food

Occasionally, vitamins are lost during food processing. In most cases, food producers can replace these vitamins with synthetic vitamins, making the processed food nutritionally equal to the unprocessed food. Foods in which vitamins have been replaced are called enriched foods.

Because some vitamins are easily destroyed by light, air, heat, and water, it is important to know how to preserve the vitamin content of food during its preparation and cooking. Vitamin loss can be avoided by the following:

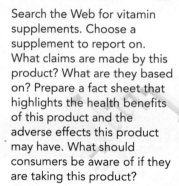

EXPLORING THE WEB

Search the Web for vitamin supplements. Choose a supplement to report on. What claims are made by this product? What are they based on? Prepare a fact sheet that highlights the health benefits of this product and the adverse effects this product may have. What should consumers be aware of if they are taking this product?

- Buying the freshest, unbruised vegetables and fruits locally and using them within a day's time
- Preparing fresh vegetables and fruits just before serving
- Heating canned vegetables quickly and in their own liquid
- Following package directions when using frozen vegetables or fruit
- Using as little water as possible when cooking and having it boiling before adding vegetables, or preferably steaming them
- Covering the pan, cooking vegetables until bright in color and crisp tender
- Saving any cooking liquid for later use in soups, stews, and gravies
- Storing fresh vegetables and most fruits in a cool, dark place
- Microwaving fruits and vegetables in 1–2 tablespoons of water
- Cooking corn on the cob in a microwave by wrapping in a paper towel
- Roasting vegetables to retain nutrients rather than boiling them

CLASSIFICATION

 fat soluble
can be dissolved in fat

 water soluble
can be dissolved in water

Vitamins are commonly grouped according to solubility. Vitamins A, D, E, and K are **fat soluble**, and B complex and C are **water soluble** (Table 7-3). In addition, vitamin D is sometimes classified as a hormone, and the

TABLE 7-3 Fat-Soluble and Water-Soluble Vitamins

NAME	FOOD SOURCES	FUNCTIONS	DEFICIENCY/TOXICITY
Fat-Soluble Vitamins			
Vitamin A (retinol)	Animal • Liver • Whole milk • Butter • Cream • Cod liver oil Plants • Dark green leafy vegetables • Deep yellow or orange fruit • Fortified margarine	• Maintenance of vision in dim light • Maintenance of mucous membranes and healthy skin • Growth and development of bones • Reproduction • Healthy immune system • Antioxidant	Deficiency • Night blindness • Xerophthalmia • Respiratory infections • Bone growth ceases Toxicity • Birth defects • Bone pain • Anorexiant • Enlargement of liver
Vitamin D (calciferol)	Animal • Eggs • Liver • Fortified milk • Fortified margarine • Oily fish Plants • None Other sources • Sunlight	• Regulation of absorption of calcium and phosphorus • Building and maintenance of normal bones and teeth • Prevention of tetany	Deficiency • Rickets • Osteomalacia • Osteoporosis • Poorly developed teeth and bones • Muscle spasms Toxicity • Kidney stones • Calcification of soft tissues
Vitamin E (tocopherol)	Animal • None Plants • Green and leafy vegetables • Margarine • Salad dressing • Wheat germ • Vegetable oils • Nuts	• Antioxidant • Considered essential for protection of cell structure, especially of red blood cells	Deficiency • Destruction of red blood cells Toxicity
Vitamin K	Animal • Liver • Milk Plants • Green leafy vegetables • Cabbage, broccoli • Brussels sprouts	• Blood clotting	Deficiency • Prolonged blood clotting or hemorrhaging Toxicity • Hemolytic anemia • Interferes with anticlotting medications

(continues)

TABLE 7-3 (*continued*)

NAME	FOOD SOURCES	FUNCTIONS	DEFICIENCY/TOXICITY
Water-Soluble Vitamins			
Thiamine (vitamin B_1)	Animal • Lean pork • Beef • Liver • Eggs • Fish Plants • Whole and enriched grains • Legumes • Brewer's yeast	• Metabolism of carbohydrates and some amino acids • Maintains normal appetite and functioning of nervous system	Deficiency • Gastrointestinal tract, nervous system, and cardiovascular system problems • Beriberi Toxicity • None
Riboflavin (vitamin B_2)	Animal • Liver, kidney, heart • Milk • Cheese Plants • Green, leafy vegetables • Cereals • Enriched bread	• Aids release of energy from food • Health of the mouth tissue • Healthy eyes	Deficiency • Cheilosis • Eye sensitivity • Dermatitis • Glossitis • Photophobia Toxicity • None
Niacin (nicotinic acid)	Animal • Milk • Eggs • Fish • Poultry Plants • Enriched breads and cereals	• Energy metabolism • Healthy skin and nervous and digestive systems	Deficiency • Pellagra—dermatitis, dementia, diarrhea Toxicity • Vasodilation of blood vessels
Pyridoxine (vitamin B_6)	Animal • Pork • Fish • Poultry • Liver, kidney • Milk • Eggs Plants • Whole-grain cereals • Legumes	• Conversion of tryptophan to niacin • Release of glucose from glycogen • Protein metabolism and synthesis of nonessential amino acids	Deficiency • Cheilosis • Glossitis • Dermatitis • Confusion • Depression • Irritability Toxicity • Depression • Nerve damage

(*continues*)

TABLE 7-3 *(continued)*

NAME	FOOD SOURCES	FUNCTIONS	DEFICIENCY/TOXICITY
Vitamin B_{12} (cobalamin)	Animal • Seafood • Poultry • Liver, kidney • Muscle meats • Eggs • Milk • Cheese Plants • None	• Synthesis of red blood cells • Maintenance of myelin sheaths • Treatment of pernicious anemia • Folate metabolism	Deficiency • Degeneration of myelin sheaths • Pernicious anemia • Sore mouth and tongue • Anorexia • Neurological disorders Toxicity • None
Folate (folic acid)	Animal • Liver Plants • Leafy green vegetables • Spinach • Legumes • Seeds • Broccoli • Cereal and flour fortified with folate • Fruit	• Synthesis of RBCs • Synthesis of DNA	Deficiency • Anemia • Glossitis • Neural tube defects such as anencephaly and spina bifida Toxicity • Could mask a B_{12} deficiency
Biotin	Animal • Milk • Liver and kidney • Egg yolks Plants • Legumes • Brewer's yeast • Soy flour • Cereals • Fruit	• Coenzyme in carbohydrate and amino acid metabolism • Niacin synthesis from tryptophan	Deficiency • Dermatitis • Nausea • Anorexia • Depression • Hair loss Toxicity • None
Pantothenic acid	Animal • Eggs • Liver • Salmon • Poultry Plants • Mushrooms • Cauliflower • Peanuts • Brewer's yeast	• Metabolism of carbohydrates, lipids, and proteins • Synthesis of fatty acids, cholesterol, steroid hormones	Deficiency • Rare: burning feet syndrome; vomiting; fatigue Toxicity • None

(continues)

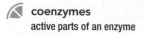

TABLE 7-3 *(continued)*

NAME	FOOD SOURCES	FUNCTIONS	DEFICIENCY/TOXICITY
Vitamin C (ascorbic acid)	Animal • None Plants • All citrus fruits • Broccoli • Melons • Strawberries • Tomatoes • Brussels sprouts • Potatoes • Cabbage • Green peppers	• Prevention of scurvy • Formation of collagen • Healing of wounds • Release of stress hormones • Absorption of iron • Antioxidant • Resistance to infection	Deficiency • Scurvy • Muscle cramps • Ulcerated gums • Tendency to bruise easily Toxicity • Raised uric acid level • Hemolytic anemia • Kidney stones • Rebound scurvy

© Cengage Learning 2014

 coenzymes
active parts of an enzyme

 precursor
something that comes before something else; in vitamins it is also called a provitamin, something from which the body can synthesize the specific vitamin

 provitamin
a precursor of a vitamin

 carotenoids
plant pigments, some of which yield vitamin A

B-complex group may be classified as catalysts or **coenzymes**. When a vitamin has different chemical forms but serves the same purpose in the body, these forms are sometimes called vitamers. Vitamin E is an example. Sometimes a **precursor**, or **provitamin**, is found in foods. This is a substance from which the body can synthesize (manufacture) a specific vitamin. **Carotenoids** are examples of precursors of vitamin A and are referred to as provitamin A.

FAT-SOLUBLE VITAMINS

The fat-soluble vitamins A, D, E, and K are chemically similar. They are not lost easily in cooking but are lost when mineral oil is ingested. Mineral oil is not absorbed by humans. After absorption, fat-soluble vitamins are transported through the blood by lipoproteins because they are not soluble in water. Excess amounts can be stored in the liver. Therefore, deficiencies of fat-soluble vitamins are slower to appear than are those caused by a lack of water-soluble vitamins. Because of the body's ability to store them, megadoses of fat-soluble vitamins should be avoided, as they can reach toxic levels.

Vitamin A

 retinol
the preformed vitamin A

Vitamin A consists of two basic dietary forms: preformed vitamin A, also called **retinol**, which is the active form of vitamin A; and carotenoids, the inactive form of vitamin A, which are found in plants.

Functions

Vitamin A is a family of fat-soluble compounds that play an important role in vision, bone growth, reproduction, and cell division. It helps regulate the immune system, which helps fight infections. Vitamin A has been labeled as an **antioxidant** when, in fact, provitamin A (carotenoids) is the part of the family that functions as an antioxidant. Antioxidants protect cells from **free radicals**. Free radicals are atoms or groups of atoms with an odd (unpaired) number of electrons and can be formed when oxygen interacts with certain molecules. Once formed, these highly reactive radicals can start a chain reaction. When they react with important cellular components such as DNA or cell membranes, the most damage occurs. Antioxidants have the capability of safely interacting with free radicals and stopping the chain reaction before vital cells are damaged.

The first organic free radical was discovered in 1900 by Moses Gomberg. In the 1950s, Dr. Denman Harman was the first to propose the free radical theory of aging.

Sources

There are two forms of vitamin A: preformed vitamin A and provitamin A. Retinol is a preformed vitamin A and is one of the most active and usable forms of vitamin A. Retinol can be converted to retinal and retinoic acid, other active forms of vitamin A.

Provitamin A carotenoids can be converted to vitamin A from darkly colored pigments, both green and orange, in fruits and vegetables. Common carotenoids are beta-carotene, lutein, lycopene, and zeaxanthin. Beta-carotene is most efficiently converted to retinol. Eating "five-a-day" of fruits and vegetables is highly recommended. The best sources of beta-carotene are carrots, sweet potatoes, spinach, broccoli, pumpkin, squash (butternut), mango, and cantaloupe.

Research has shown that regular consumption of foods rich in carotenoids decreases the risk of some cancers because of its antioxidant effect. Taking a beta-carotene supplement has not shown the same results.

Preformed vitamin A (retinol) is found in fat-containing animal foods such as liver, butter, cream, whole milk, whole-milk cheeses, and egg yolk. It is also found in low-fat milk products and in cereals that have been fortified with vitamin A, but these are not the best sources.

Requirements

A well-balanced diet is the preferred way to obtain the required amounts of vitamin A. Vitamin A values are commonly listed as a **retinol equivalent (RE)**. A retinol equivalent is 1 mcg retinol or 6 mcg beta-carotene.

Hypervitaminosis

The use of a single vitamin supplement should be discouraged because an excess of vitamin A can have serious consequences. Signs of hypervitaminosis A may include birth defects, hair loss, dry skin, headaches, nausea, dryness of mucous membranes, liver damage, and bone and joint pain. In general, these symptoms tend to disappear when excessive intake is discontinued.

 antioxidant
a substance preventing damage from oxygen

 free radicals
atoms or groups of atoms with an odd (unpaired) number of electrons and can be formed when oxygen interacts with certain molecules

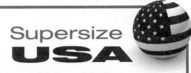

Nutrients are found in all foods. Explore the MyPlate food model to learn how to meet your individual food needs through the various food groups. When grocery shopping make sure to check that the products you are buying are enriched or fortified for optimal health. Go to *The Journal of Nutrition*'s website (http://www.jn.nutrition.org) to check the vitamins and minerals found in enriched and fortified products.

(Source: Adapted from Fulgoni, V.L., Keast, D.R., Bailey, R.L., and Dwyer, J. (October 2011). Foods, Fortificants, and Supplements: Where Do Americans Get Their Nutrients? *The Journal of Nutrition* 141:1847–1854.)

 retinol equivalent (RE)
the equivalent of 3.33 IUs of vitamin A

Deficiency

Signs of a deficiency of vitamin A include night blindness; dry, rough skin; and increased susceptibility to infections. Vitaminosis A can result in blindness or **xerophthalmia**, a condition characterized by dry, lusterless, mucous membranes of the eye. Lack of vitamin A is the leading cause of blindness in the world (discounting accidents).

xerophthalmia
serious eye disease characterized by dry mucous membranes of the eye, caused by a deficiency of vitamin A

Vitamin D

Vitamin D exists in two forms—D_2 (ergocalciferol) and D_3 (cholecalciferol). Each is formed from a provitamin when irradiated with (exposed to) ultraviolet light. They are equally effective in human nutrition, but D_3 is the one that is formed in humans from cholesterol in the skin. D_2 is formed in plants. Vitamin D is considered a **prohormone** because it is converted to a hormone in the human body.

Vitamin D is heat-stable and not easily oxidized, so it is not harmed by storage, food processing, or cooking.

prohormone
substance that precedes the hormone and from which the body can synthesize the hormone

Functions

The major function of vitamin D is the promotion of calcium and phosphorus absorption in the body. By contributing to the absorption of these minerals, it helps to raise their concentration in the blood so that normal bone and tooth mineralization can occur and tetany (involuntary muscle movement) can be prevented. (Tetany can occur when there is too little calcium in the blood. This condition is called hypocalcemia.)

Vitamin D is absorbed in the intestines and is chemically changed in the liver and kidneys. Excess amounts of vitamin D are stored in the liver and in adipose tissue.

Sources

The best source of vitamin D is sunlight, which changes a provitamin to vitamin D_3 in humans. It is sometimes referred to as the sunshine vitamin. The amount of vitamin D that is formed depends on the individual's pigmentation (coloring matter in the skin) and the amount of sunlight available. The best food sources of vitamin D are milk, fish liver oils, egg yolk, butter, and fortified margarine. Because of the rather limited number of food sources of vitamin D and the unpredictability of sunshine, health authorities decided that the vitamin should be added to a common food. Since 1930, cow's milk has been fortified with 100 IU of vitamin D per cup.

Requirements

In late 2010, the Institute of Medicine (IOM) recommended an increase in vitamin D intake to 600 **international units (IUs)**—that is, 15 mcg for men and women aged 1–70 years old. To meet the vitamin D requirements through diet, one would have to consume 3 cups of milk, 1 egg, 6 oz. of fortified yogurt, and 1 cup of fortified orange juice. Additional sources of vitamin D are

international units (IUs)
a unit of measurement of some vitamins; 5 mcg = 200 IUs

listed in Table 7-4. Often it is difficult for consumers to fulfill their vitamin D requirement through diet, therefore a vitamin D supplement may be necessary. Many general multivitamins contain 400 IUs of vitamin D_3. Calcium supplements contain varying amounts of vitamin D as well.

Vitamin D, or specifically cholecalciferol values, are given in micrograms on the DRI chart (Table 7-5); however, most supplements will state the IUs as 5 mcg = 200 IUs.

Hypervitaminosis

Hypervitaminosis D must be avoided because it can cause deposits of calcium and phosphorus in soft tissues, kidney and heart damage, and bone fragility. Based on new research, the IOM has increased the tolerable upper limit that is safe to consume daily to 4,000 IUs for adults.

TABLE 7-4 Selected Food Sources of Vitamin D

Salmon (sockeye), cooked, 3 oz	447 IU
Tuna, water packed, drained, 3 oz	154 IU
Milk, fortified (nonfat, reduced fat, whole), 1 cup	115–124 IU
Yogurt, 6 oz fortified with 20% daily value of vitamin D	88 IU
Egg, 1 large	41 IU
Fortified margarine, 1 Tbsp	60 IU
Ready-to-eat cereal, fortified with 10% of daily value of vitamin D, ¾–1 cup	40 IU
Orange juice fortified with vitamin D, 1 cup	137 IU

Source: U.S. Department of Agriculture, Agricultural Research Service. 2011. USDA National Nutrient Database for Standard Reference, Release 24. Nutrient Data Laboratory Home Page, http://www.ars.usda.gov/ba/bhnrc/ndl

TABLE 7-5 Recommended Dietary Allowances (RDAs) for Vitamin D

AGE	MALE	FEMALE	PREGNANCY	LACTATION
0–12 months*	400 IU (10 mcg)	400 IU (10 mcg)		
1–13 years	600 IU (15 mcg)	600 IU (15 mcg)		
14–18 years	600 IU (15 mcg)	600 IU (15 mcg)	600 IU (15 mcg)	600 IU (15 mcg)
19–50 years	600 IU (15 mcg)	600 IU (15 mcg)	600 IU (15 mcg)	600 IU (15 mcg)
51–70 years	600 IU (15 mcg)	600 IU (15 mcg)	600 IU (15 mcg)	600 IU (15 mcg)
>70 years	800 IU (20 mcg)	800 IU (20 mcg)		

*Adequate Intake (AI)

Source: Reprinted with permission from the National Academies Press, Copyright © 2011, National Academy of Sciences. *Dietary Reference Intakes for Calcium and Vitamin D.*

Deficiency

The deficiency of vitamin D inhibits the absorption of calcium and phosphorus in the small intestine and results in poor bone and tooth formation. Vitamin D deficiency in children may lead to rickets, which causes malformed bones, pain, and poorly formed teeth. Adults lacking sufficient vitamin D may develop osteomalacia, which is softening of the bones. Deficiency contributes to osteoporosis (brittle, porous bones).

People who are seldom outdoors, those who use sunscreens, and those who live in areas where there is little sunlight for 3–4 months a year should be especially careful that they attain the RDA for vitamin D. Other groups at risk for vitamin D deficiency include breast-fed infants, older adults, people with dark skin, those who have fat malabsorption, and those who are obese or who have undergone gastric bypass surgery. Vitamin D deficiency has been found to be widespread in the normal population with some estimating deficiency as high as 40–75% of individuals. Recent research has shown that optimal blood levels are much higher than previously thought (>30 ng/ml versus >20 ng/ml). Emerging science is linking higher levels of vitamin D with reduced incidence of numerous diseases. Researchers document that vitamin D influences the expression of 229 genes in our bodies. If the current studies are confirmed, vitamin D status will play a central role in cancer protection, immunity, neuromuscular function, cardiovascular health, autoimmune disease protection, glucose tolerance, and diabetes.

Vitamin E

Vitamin E consists of two groups of chemical compounds. They are the **tocopherols** and the **tocotrienols**. There are four types of tocopherols: alpha, beta, delta, and gamma. The most biologically active of these is alpha-tocopherol.

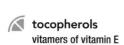

tocopherols
vitamers of vitamin E

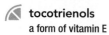

tocotrienols
a form of vitamin E

Functions

Vitamin E is an antioxidant. It is aided in this process by vitamin C and the mineral selenium. It is carried in the blood by lipoproteins. When the amount of vitamin E in the blood is low, the red blood cells become vulnerable to a higher-than-normal rate of **hemolysis**. Vitamin E has been found helpful in the prevention of hemolytic anemia among premature infants. It may also enhance the immune system. Because of its antioxidant properties, it is commonly used in commercial food products to retard spoilage.

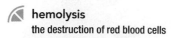

hemolysis
the destruction of red blood cells

Sources

Vegetable oils made from corn, soybean, safflower, and cottonseed and products made from them, such as margarine, are the best sources of vitamin E. Wheat germ, nuts, green leafy vegetables, peanut butter, broccoli, and kiwi are also good sources. Animal foods, fruits, and most vegetables are poor sources.

Requirements

Research indicates that the vitamin E requirement increases if the amount of polyunsaturated fatty acids in the diet increases. In general, however, the U.S. diet is thought to contain sufficient vitamin E.

Hypervitaminosis

Although vitamin E appears to be relatively nontoxic, it is a fat-soluble vitamin, and the excess is stored in adipose tissue. Consequently, it would seem advisable to avoid long-term megadoses of vitamin E.

Deficiency

A deficiency of vitamin E has been detected in premature, low-birthweight infants and in clients who are unable to absorb fat normally. Malabsorption can cause serious neurological defects in children, but in adults, it takes 5–10 years before deficiency symptoms occur.

Vitamin K

Vitamin K is made up of several compounds that are essential to blood clotting. Vitamin K_1, commonly called phylloquinone, is found in dietary sources, especially green leafy vegetables such as spinach and in animal tissue. Vitamin K_2, called menaquinone, is synthesized in the intestine by bacteria and is also found in animal tissue. In addition, there is a synthetic vitamin K, called menadione. Vitamin K is destroyed by light and alkalies.

Vitamin K is absorbed like fats, mainly from the small intestine and slightly from the colon. Its absorption requires a normal flow of bile from the liver, and it is improved when there is fat in the diet.

Functions

Vitamin K is essential for the formation of prothrombin, which permits the proper clotting of the blood. It may be given to newborns immediately after birth because human milk contains little vitamin K and the intestines of newborns contain few bacteria. With insufficient vitamin K, newborns may be in danger of intracranial hemorrhage (bleeding within the head).

Vitamin K may be given to clients who suffer from faulty fat absorption; to clients after extensive antibiotic therapy (ingestion of antibiotic drugs to combat infection) because these drugs destroy the bacteria in the intestines; as an antidote for an overdose of anticoagulant (blood thinner such as warfarin—sometimes sold as Coumadin or warnerin); or to treat cases of **hemorrhage**.

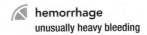
hemorrhage
unusually heavy bleeding

Sources

The best dietary sources of vitamin K are green leafy vegetables such as broccoli, cabbage, spinach, and kale. Dairy products, eggs, meats, fruits, and cereals also contain some vitamin K. Cow's milk is a much better source of vitamin K than human milk. The synthesis of vitamin K by bacteria in the small intestine does not provide a sufficient supply by itself. It must be supplemented by dietary sources.

Requirements

Vitamin K is measured in micrograms. The AI for vitamin K is 120 mcg for men and 90 mcg for women. This is not increased during pregnancy or lactation. Infants up to 6 months should have 2.0 mcg a day. Those between 6 months and 1 year should receive 2.5 mcg a day. Vitamin K must be ingested daily. What is absorbed today will be utilized immediately with very little storage in the liver.

Hypervitaminosis

Ingestion of excessive amounts of synthetic vitamin K can be toxic and can cause a form of anemia.

Deficiency

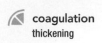
coagulation
thickening

The only major sign of a deficiency of vitamin K is defective blood **coagulation**. This increases clotting time, making the client more prone to hemorrhage. Human deficiency may be caused by faulty fat metabolism, antacids, antibiotic therapy, inadequate diet, or anticoagulants.

WATER-SOLUBLE VITAMINS

Water-soluble vitamins include B complex and C. These vitamins dissolve in water and are easily destroyed by air, light, and cooking. They are not stored in the body to the extent that fat-soluble vitamins are stored.

Vitamin B Complex

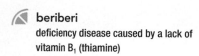
beriberi
deficiency disease caused by a lack of
vitamin B₁ (thiamine)

Beriberi is a disease that affects the nervous, cardiovascular, and gastrointestinal systems. The legs feel heavy, the feet burn, and the muscles degenerate. The client is irritable and suffers from headaches, depression, anorexia, constipation, tachycardia (rapid heart rate), edema, and heart failure.

Toward the end of the 19th century, a doctor in Indonesia discovered that chickens that were fed table scraps of polished rice developed symptoms much like those of his clients suffering from beriberi. When these same chickens were later fed brown (unpolished) rice, they recovered.

Some years later, this mysterious component of unpolished rice was recognized as an essential food substance and was named vitamin B. Subsequently, it was named vitamin *B complex* because the vitamin was found to be composed of several compounds. The B-complex vitamins are listed in Table 7-1.

Thiamine

thiamine
vitamin B₁

Thiamine, a coenzyme, was originally named vitamin B_1. It is partially destroyed by heat and alkalies, and it is lost in cooking water.

Functions

Thiamine is essential for the metabolism of carbohydrates and some amino acids. It is also essential to nerve and muscle action. It is absorbed in the small intestine.

Sources

Thiamine is found in many foods, but generally in small quantities. (See Appendix D.) Some of the best natural food sources of thiamine are unrefined and enriched cereals, whole grains, lean pork, liver, seeds, nuts, and legumes.

Requirements

Thiamine is measured in milligrams. The daily thiamine requirement for the average adult female is 1.1 mg a day, and for the average adult male it is 1.2 mg a day. The requirement is not thought to increase with age. In general, however, an increase in calories increases the need for thiamine.

Most breads and cereals in the United States are enriched with thiamine, so that the majority of people can and do easily fulfill their recommended intake.

Deficiency

Symptoms of thiamine deficiency include loss of appetite, fatigue, nervous irritability, and constipation. An extreme deficiency causes beriberi. Its deficiency is rare, however, occurring mainly among alcoholics whose diets include reduced amounts of thiamine while their requirements are increased and their absorption is decreased. Others at risk include renal clients undergoing long-term dialysis, clients undergoing bypass surgery for weight loss, and those who eat primarily rice.

Because some raw fish contain thiaminase, an enzyme that inhibits the normal action of thiamine, frequent consumption of large amounts of raw fish could cause thiamine deficiency. Eating raw fish is not recommended. Cooking inactivates this enzyme.

There are no known ill effects from excessive oral intake of thiamine, but it may be toxic if excessive amounts are given intravenously.

Riboflavin

Riboflavin is sometimes called B_2. It is destroyed by light and irradiation and is unstable in alkalies.

 riboflavin
vitamin B_2

Functions

Riboflavin is essential for carbohydrate, fat, and protein metabolism. It is also necessary for tissue maintenance, especially the skin around the mouth, and for healthy eyes. Riboflavin is absorbed in the small intestine.

Sources

Riboflavin is widely distributed in animal and plant foods but in small amounts. Milk, meats, poultry, fish, and enriched breads and cereals are some of its richest sources. Some green vegetables such as broccoli, spinach, and asparagus are also good sources.

Requirement

Riboflavin is measured in milligrams. The average adult female daily requirement is thought to be 1.1 mg, and the adult male requirement is 1.3 mg. The riboflavin requirement appears to increase with increased energy expenditure. The requirement does not diminish with age.

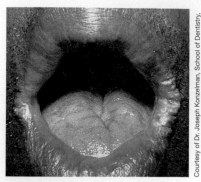

Courtesy of Dr. Joseph Konzelman, School of Dentistry, Medical College of Georgia

FIGURE 7-1 Cheilosis at the corners of the mouth is an indication of a riboflavin deficiency.

niacin
B vitamin

pellagra
deficiency disease caused by a lack of niacin

niacin equivalent (NE)
unit of measuring niacin; 1 NE equals 1 mg niacin or 60 mg tryptophan

Deficiency

Because of the small quantities of riboflavin in foods and its limited storage in the body, deficiencies of riboflavin can develop. The generous use of fat-free milk in the diet is a good way to prevent deficiency of this vitamin. It is important, however, that milk be stored in opaque containers because riboflavin can be destroyed by light. It appears that fiber laxatives can reduce riboflavin absorption, and their use over long periods should be discouraged.

A deficiency of riboflavin can result in cheilosis, a condition characterized by sores on the lips and cracks at the corners of the mouth (Figure 7-1), glossitis (inflammation of the tongue), dermatitis, and eye strain in the form of itching, burning, and eye fatigue. Its toxicity is unknown.

Niacin

Niacin is the generic name for nicotinic acid and nicotinamide. Niacin is fairly stable in foods. It can withstand reasonable amounts of heat and acid and is not destroyed during food storage.

Functions

Niacin serves as a coenzyme in energy metabolism and consequently is essential to every body cell. In addition, niacin is essential for the prevention of **pellagra**. Pellagra is a disease characterized by sores on the skin and by diarrhea, anxiety, confusion, irritability, poor memory, dizziness, and untimely death if left untreated. Niacin, when used as a cholesterol-lowering agent, must be closely supervised by a physician because of possible adverse side effects such as liver damage and peptic ulcers.

Sources

The best sources of niacin are meats, poultry, and fish. Peanuts and other legumes are also good sources. Enriched breads and cereals also contain some. Milk and eggs do not provide niacin per se, but they are good sources of its precursor, tryptophan (an amino acid). Vegetables and fruits contain little niacin.

Requirements

Niacin is measured in as a **niacin equivalent (NE)**. One NE equals 1 mg of niacin or 60 mg of tryptophan. The general recommendation is a daily intake of 14 mg/NE for adult women and 16 mg/NE for adult men. Because excessive amounts of niacin have caused flushing due to vascular dilation (expansion of blood vessels), self-prescribed doses of niacin concentrate should be discouraged. Other symptoms include gastrointestinal problems and itching. If excessive amounts of niacin are ingested, liver damage may result.

Deficiency

A deficiency of niacin is apt to appear if there is a deficiency of riboflavin. Symptoms of niacin deficiency include weakness, anorexia, indigestion, anxiety, and irritability. In extreme cases, pellagra may occur.

Vitamin B$_6$

Vitamin B$_6$ is composed of three related forms: pyridoxine, pyridoxal, and pyridoxamine. It is stable to heat but sensitive to light and alkalies.

Functions

Vitamin B$_6$ is essential for protein metabolism and absorption, and it aids in the release of glucose from glycogen. With the help of vitamin B$_6$, amino acids present in excessive amounts can be converted to those in which the body is temporarily deficient. It also serves as a catalyst in the conversion of tryptophan to niacin, and it is helpful in the formation of other substances from amino acids. An example is the synthesis of neurotransmitters such as serotonin and dopamine.

Sources

Some of the nutrient-dense sources of vitamin B$_6$ are poultry, fish, liver, kidney, potatoes, bananas, and spinach. Whole grains, especially oats and wheat, are good sources of vitamin B$_6$, but because this vitamin is lost during milling and is not replaced during the enrichment process, refined grains are not a good source.

Requirements

Vitamin B$_6$ is measured in milligrams, and the need increases as the protein intake increases. For adult females, the daily requirement is 1.3–1.5 mg and for males, 1.3–1.7 mg. Vitamin B$_6$ is required for the body to manufacture the nonessential amino acids from the essential amino acids. Oral contraceptives interfere with the metabolism of vitamin B$_6$ and can result in a deficiency.

Deficiency

A deficiency of vitamin B$_6$ is usually found in combination with deficiencies of other B vitamins. Symptoms include irritability, depression, and dermatitis. In infants, its deficiency can cause various neurological symptoms and abdominal problems. Although its toxicity is rare, it can cause temporary neurological problems.

Vitamin B$_{12}$

Vitamin B$_{12}$ (**cobalamin**) is a compound that contains the mineral cobalt. It is slightly soluble in water and fairly stable to heat, but it is damaged by strong acids or alkalies and by light. It can be stored in the human body for 3–5 years.

cobalamin
organic compound known as vitamin B$_{12}$

Functions

Vitamin B$_{12}$ is involved in folate metabolism, maintenance of the **myelin** sheath, and healthy red blood cells. In order for vitamin B$_{12}$ to be absorbed, it must bind with a glycoprotein (**intrinsic factor**) present in gastric secretions in the stomach and travel to the small intestine, where it combines with pancreatic proteases, then travels to the ileum, where it attaches to special receptor cells to complete the absorption process. A client who has lost

myelin
lipoprotein essential for the protection of nerves

intrinsic factor
secretion of stomach mucosa essential for B$_{12}$ absorption

pernicious anemia
severe, chronic anemia caused by a deficiency of vitamin B_{12}; usually due to the body's inability to absorb B_{12}

the ability to produce the gastric secretions, pancreatic proteases, intrinsic factor, or the special receptor cells because of disease or surgery will develop **pernicious anemia**.

Sources

The best food sources of B_{12} are animal foods, especially organ meats, lean meat, seafood, eggs, and dairy products.

Requirements

Vitamin B_{12} is measured in micrograms. The DRI for adults is 2–4 mcg a day, but it increases during pregnancy and lactation. The amount absorbed will depend on current needs.

Deficiency

Fortunately, a vitamin B_{12} deficiency is rare and is thought to be caused by congenital problems of absorption, which inhibit the body's ability to absorb or synthesize sufficient amounts of vitamin B_{12}. Vegan-vegetarians must choose their food wisely to avoid a B_{12} deficiency.

When the amount of B_{12} is insufficient, megaloblastic anemia may result. If the intrinsic factor is missing, pernicious anemia develops. Intrinsic factor could be missing because of surgical removal of the stomach, or a large portion of it, or because of disease or surgery affecting the ileum. Dietary treatment will be ineffective; the client must be given intramuscular injections of B_{12}, usually on a monthly basis.

Vitamin B_{12} deficiency may also result in inadequate myelin synthesis. This deficiency causes damage to the nervous system. Signs of vitamin B_{12} deficiency include anorexia, glossitis, sore mouth and tongue, pallor, neurological upsets such as depression and dizziness, and weight loss.

In The Media

Fat-Soluble Versus Water-Soluble Nutrients

It is important to know the differences and recommendations for both fat- and water-soluble vitamins. Getting too many of either one can be dangerous. Taking vitamins and minerals above the upper limit of the DRI may harm tissues where vitamins are commonly stored. When the body takes in more water-soluble nutrients than it needs, the excess is excreted in the urine. However, research has shown that some water-soluble vitamins are handled differently by the body than others. It is important to include vitamins and nutrients from food sources as well as those you may drink or receive through supplements. Excess of fat-soluble vitamins can interfere with kidney function and the absorption of other essential nutrients. When taking supplements it is important to know the upper limit values and to include the vitamins and minerals found in enriched foods as part of your intake.

(Source: Adapted from Zelman, Kathleen. Know the Difference Between Fat- and Water-Soluble Nutrients. Accessed December 13, 2011 from http://www.webmd.com)

Folate

Folate, folacin, and **folic acid** are chemically similar compounds. Their names are often used interchangeably.

Functions

Folate is needed for DNA synthesis, protein metabolism, and the formation of hemoglobin. Researchers have concluded that folic acid helps to prevent colon, cervical, esophageal, stomach, and pancreatic cancers. Folic acid also increases homocysteine levels that help prevent strokes, blood vessel disease, macular degeneration, and Alzheimer's disease.

Sources

Folate is found in many foods, but the best sources are cereals fortified with folate, green leafy vegetables, legumes, sunflower seeds, and fruits such as orange juice and strawberries. Heat, oxidation, and ultraviolet light all destroy folate, and it is estimated that 50–90% of folate may be destroyed during food processing and preparation. Consequently, it is advisable that fruits and vegetables be eaten uncooked or lightly cooked when possible.

Requirements

Folate is measured in micrograms. The average daily requirement for all adults, both female and male, is 400 mcg. There is an increased need for folate during pregnancy and periods of growth because of the increased rate of cell division and the DNA synthesis in the body of the mother and of the fetus. Consequently, it is extremely important that women of child-bearing age maintain good folate intake. The recommended amount for a woman 1 month before conception and through the first 6 weeks of pregnancy is 600 mcg a day.

Deficiency

Folate deficiency has been linked to **neural tube defects (NTDs)** in the fetus, such as **spina bifida** (spinal cord or spinal fluid bulge through the back) and **anencephaly** (absence of a brain). Other signs of deficiency are inflammation of the mouth and tongue, poor growth, depression and mental confusion, problems with nerve functions, and **megaloblastic anemia**, a condition in which red blood cells are large and immature and cannot carry oxygen properly.

Hypervitaminosis

The FDA limits the amount of folate in over-the-counter (OTC) supplements to 100 mcg for infants, 300 mcg for children, and 400 mcg for adults because consuming excessive amounts of folate can mask a vitamin B_{12} deficiency and inactivate phenytoin, an anticonvulsant drug used by epileptics.

Biotin

Function and Sources

Biotin participates as a coenzyme in the synthesis of fatty acids and amino acids. Some of its best dietary sources are egg yolks, milk, poultry, fish, broccoli,

 folate/folic acid
a form of vitamin B, also called folacin; essential for metabolism

 neural tube defects (NTDs)
congenital malformation of brain and/or spinal column due to failure of neural tube to close during embryonic development

 spina bifida
spinal cord or spinal fluid bulge through the back

 anencephaly
absence of brain

 megaloblastic anemia
anemia in which the red blood cells are unusually large and are not completely mature

 biotin
a B vitamin; necessary for metabolism

spinach, and cauliflower. Biotin is also synthesized in the large intestine by microorganisms, but the amount that is available for absorption is unknown.

Requirements

Biotin is measured in micrograms. The Food and Nutrition Board of the Institute of Medicine has established an AI of 30 mcg for adults (see Table 7-2).

Deficiency

Deficiency symptoms include nausea, anorexia, depression, pallor (paleness of complexion), dermatitis (inflammation of skin), and an increase in serum cholesterol. Toxicity from excessive intake is unknown.

Pantothenic Acid

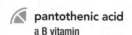
pantothenic acid
a B vitamin

Pantothenic acid is appropriately named because the Greek word *pantothen* means "from many places." It is fairly stable, but it can be damaged by acids and alkalies.

Functions

Pantothenic acid is involved in metabolism of carbohydrates, fats, and proteins. It is also essential for the synthesis of the neurotransmitter acetylcholine and of steroid hormones.

Sources

Pantothenic acid is found extensively in foods, especially animal foods such as meats, poultry, fish, and eggs. It is also found in whole-grain cereals and legumes. In addition, it is thought to be synthesized by the body.

Requirements

There is no DRI for pantothenic acid, but the Food and Nutrition Board has provided an estimated intake of 4–7 mg a day for normal adults (see Table 7-2).

Deficiency

Natural deficiencies are unknown. However, deficiencies have been produced experimentally. Signs include weakness, fatigue, and a burning sensation in the feet. Toxicity from excessive intake has not been confirmed.

Vitamin C

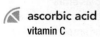
ascorbic acid
vitamin C

Vitamin C is also known as **ascorbic acid**. It has antioxidant properties and protects foods from oxidation, and it is required for all cell metabolism. It is readily destroyed by heat, air, and alkalies, and it is easily lost in cooking water.

Functions

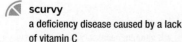
scurvy
a deficiency disease caused by a lack of vitamin C

Vitamin C is known to prevent **scurvy**. This is a disease characterized by gingivitis (soft, bleeding gums, and loose teeth); flesh that is easily bruised; tiny, pinpoint hemorrhages of the skin; poor wound healing; sore joints and muscles; and weight loss. In extreme cases, scurvy can result in death. Scurvy used to be common among sailors, who lived for months on bread, fish, and salted meat, with no fresh fruits or vegetables. During the mid-18th century, it was discovered that the addition of limes or lemons to their diets prevented this disease.

Vitamin C also has an important role in the formation of **collagen**, a protein substance that holds body cells together, making it necessary for wound healing. Therefore, the requirement for vitamin C is increased during trauma, fever, and periods of growth. Tiny, pinpoint hemorrhages are symptoms of the breakdown of collagen.

Vitamin C aids in the absorption of **nonheme iron** (from plant and animal sources and less easily absorbed than **heme iron**—see Chapter 8) in the small intestine when both nutrients are ingested at the same time. Because of this, it is called an iron enhancer.

Vitamin C also appears to have several other functions in the human body that are not well understood. For example, it may be involved with the formation or functioning of norepinephrine (a neurotransmitter and vasoconstrictor that helps the body cope with stressful conditions), some amino acids, folate, leukocytes (white blood cells), the immune system, and allergic reactions.

It is believed to reduce the severity of colds because it is a natural antihistamine, and it can reduce cancer risk in some cases by reducing nitrites in foods. Vitamin C is absorbed in the small intestine.

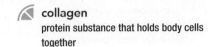

collagen
protein substance that holds body cells together

nonheme iron
iron from animal foods that is not part of the hemoglobin molecule, and all iron from plant foods

heme iron
part of the hemoglobin molecule in animal foods

Sources

The best sources of vitamin C are citrus fruits, melon, strawberries, tomatoes, potatoes, red and green peppers, cabbage, and broccoli.

Requirements

Vitamin C is measured in milligrams. Under normal circumstances, an average female adult in the United States requires 75 mg a day and an average male 90 mg. In times of stress, the need is increased. Regular cigarette smokers are advised to ingest 125 mg or more a day.

It is generally considered nontoxic, but this has not been confirmed. An excess can cause diarrhea, nausea, cramps, an excessive absorption of food iron, rebound scurvy (when megadoses are stopped abruptly), and possibly oxalate kidney stones.

Deficiency

Deficiencies of vitamin C are indicated by bleeding gums, loose teeth, tendency to bruise easily, poor wound healing, and, ultimately, scurvy.

SUPPLEMENTS

Healthy people who eat a variety of foods using the guidelines of MyPlate should be able to obtain all the vitamins needed to maintain good health. However, some people take supplements because they believe that food no longer contains the right nutrients in adequate quantities; supplements can "bulk up" muscles and enhance athletic performance; vitamins provide

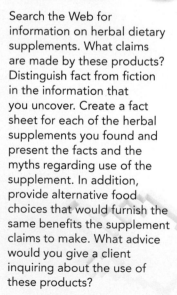

EXPLORING THE WEB

Search the Web for information on vitamin deficiency disorders. Choose a disorder and research the signs and symptoms related to it. Prepare a diet for a client suffering from the disorder that would provide the vitamin content that is lacking in the client's current diet. What other factors do you need to consider in regard to planning a therapeutic diet?

EXPLORING THE WEB

Search the Web for information on herbal dietary supplements. What claims are made by these products? Distinguish fact from fiction in the information that you uncover. Create a fact sheet for each of the herbal supplements you found and present the facts and the myths regarding use of the supplement. In addition, provide alternative food choices that would furnish the same benefits the supplement claims to make. What advice would you give a client inquiring about the use of these products?

needed energy; and vitamins and minerals can cure anything, including heart trouble, the common cold, and cancer.

The facts are as follows: (1) A balanced diet would provide for the nutritional needs of healthy people, but many do not follow a healthy eating plan, they rely on fast food; processed foods; and heat, eat, and go foods. Therefore, the American Medical Association has recommended that everyone take one multivitamin a day. (2) No amount of vitamins will build muscles; only weightlifting will do that. (3) Vitamins do not provide energy themselves. They help to release the energy within the carbohydrates, proteins, and fats that people ingest. (4) Only certain diseases caused by vitamin deficiencies (such as beriberi, scurvy, and rickets) can be cured with the help of vitamin supplements. Heart disease, cancer, and the common cold cannot.

Almost everyone can take a daily multivitamin and mineral supplement without fear of toxicity, but a megadose (10 times the RDA/DRI) to correct a deficiency or to help prevent disease should be prescribed by a physician. If a multivitamin-mineral is taken as a supplement, it is best not to exceed 100% of the RDA/DRI for each vitamin and mineral. An excess of one vitamin or one mineral can negatively affect the absorption or utilization of other vitamins and minerals. If vitamin supplements are thought to be necessary, it is best to consult a physician or registered dietitian.

Herbal products are also included under the heading "dietary supplements." Some people are interested in herbs because they believe certain ones can improve their health, they require no prescription, and they are often less expensive than prescription drugs.

The U.S. Food and Drug Administration (FDA) requires that manufacturers of prescription and over-the-counter drugs run, monitor, and report results of clinical trials of their products before selling them. Doses are established, and side effects and adverse reactions are reported in scientific journals. Also the FDA can inspect drug manufacturing facilities to confirm the purity of ingredients.

The Dietary Supplement Health and Education Act of 1994 exempts dietary supplements from FDA evaluation unless the FDA has evidence that a product is harmful. But before a suspect product can be removed from store shelves, the FDA must prove it is not safe. Manufacturers of supplements cannot claim their products can treat or prevent diseases, but they can make "structure-function" claims. For example, they cannot say vitamin A prevents cancer, but they can say vitamin A has antioxidant properties and antioxidants have been linked to reduced rates of cancer.

Misinformation concerning supplements is widely available. Health care professionals must stay well informed concerning supplements, provide accurate information to their clients, and urge clients to consult with their physicians or registered dietitians before using any supplement. Some herbal products may indeed be helpful, but some may be harmful.

HEALTH AND NUTRITION CONSIDERATIONS

Vitamins are a popular subject about which many people have strong beliefs. Some beliefs are based on fact; many are incorrect. Today's magazines, the

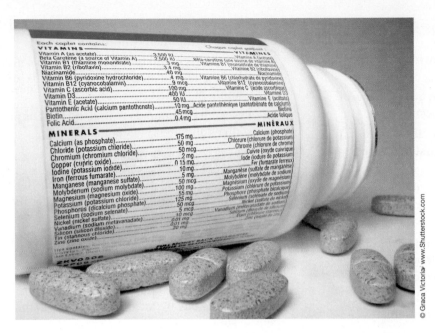

FIGURE 7-2 Client education about vitamins is important.

Internet, and newspapers frequently contain articles about vitamins, but they are not always factual. Clients who have no other source of nutrition information tend to believe the statements in those articles. It is important that the client have correct information about vitamins (Figure 7-2). Continuation of a poor diet or continued abuse of vitamin supplements is potentially dangerous to the client.

Health care professionals will need a solid knowledge of vitamins, a convincing manner, and enormous patience to reeducate clients as may be needed. Some will believe that vitamin E will prevent heart attack, that the only source of vitamin C is orange juice, or that megadoses of vitamin A will prevent cancer. Others will confuse milligrams with grams.

Client education about vitamins may be difficult until the health care professional gains the confidence of the client. Simple and clear written materials to reinforce the information will be helpful to the client.

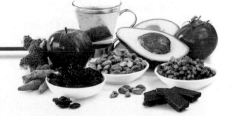

SUMMARY

Vitamins are organic compounds that regulate body functions and promote growth. Each vitamin has a specific function or functions within the body. Food sources of vitamins vary, but generally a well-balanced diet provides sufficient vitamins to fulfill body requirements. Vitamin deficiencies can result from inadequate diets or from the body's inability to utilize vitamins. Vitamins are available in concentrated forms, but their use should be carefully monitored because overdoses can be detrimental to health. Vitamins A, D, E, and K are fat soluble. Vitamin B complex and vitamin C are water soluble. Water-soluble vitamins can be destroyed during food preparation. It is important that care is taken during the preparation of food to preserve its vitamin content.

DISCUSSION TOPICS

1. How do vitamins help to provide energy to the body?

2. Discuss possible times when avitaminosis of one or more vitamins may occur.

3. Discuss any vitamin deficiencies that class members have observed. What treatments were prescribed?

4. Discuss why it may be unwise for anyone but a physician or dietitian to prescribe vitamin supplements.

5. Discuss the terms *enriched* and *fortified*. What do they mean in relation to food products? Name foods that are enriched or fortified.

6. Discuss the proper storage and cooking of foods to retain their vitamin content.

7. If any member of the class has experienced night blindness, ask her or him to describe it. Discuss how this condition occurs and how it can be prevented.

8. Why is it advisable to use liquids left over from vegetable cooking? How might these be used?

9. Explain the role of vitamin C in collagen formation and wound healing.

10. If anyone in the class has taken concentrated vitamin C, ask why. If it was useful, ask how it helped.

11. Why are some vitamins called prohormones? Coenzymes? Give examples.

12. What is a precursor? Give an example.

13. Discuss appropriate nutritional advice for a young mother who is giving her 4-year-old 50 mcg of vitamin D each day.

14. What is beriberi, and how can it be prevented?

15. Why should milk be sold in opaque containers?

SUGGESTED ACTIVITIES

1. Write a menu for 1 day that is especially rich in the B-complex vitamins. Underline the foods that are the best sources of these vitamins.

2. List the foods you have eaten in the past 24 hours. Write the names of the vitamins supplied by each food. What percentage of your day's food did *not* contain vitamins? Could this diet be nutritionally improved? How?

3. Plan a day's menu for a person who has been instructed to eat an abundance of foods rich in vitamin A.

4. Research carotenoids to find the various food sources and their benefit to the body.

REVIEW

Multiple choice. Select the *letter* that precedes the best answer.

1. The daily vitamin requirement is best supplied by
   a. eating a well-balanced diet
   b. eating one serving of citrus fruit for breakfast
   c. taking one of the many forms of vitamin supplements
   d. eating at least one serving of meat each day

2. All of the following measures preserve the vitamin content of food except
   a. using raw vegetables and fruits
   b. preparing fresh vegetables and fruits just before serving
   c. adding raw, fresh vegetables to a small amount of cold water and heating to boiling
   d. storing fresh vegetables in a cool place

3. Fat-soluble vitamins
   a. cannot be stored in the body
   b. are lost easily during cooking
   c. are dissolved by water
   d. are slower than water-soluble vitamins to exhibit deficiencies

4. Night blindness is caused by a deficiency of
   a. vitamin A   c. niacin
   b. thiamine   d. vitamin C

5. Good sources of thiamine include
   a. citrus fruits and tomatoes
   b. wheat germ and liver
   c. carotene and fish liver oils
   d. nuts and milk

6. Water-soluble vitamins include
   a. A, D, E, and K
   b. A, B_6, and C
   c. thiamine, niacin, and retinol
   d. thiamine, riboflavin, niacin, B_6, and B_{12}

7. Blindness can result from a severe lack of
   a. vitamin K
   b. vitamin A
   c. thiamine
   d. vitamin E

8. Organ meats are good sources of the vitamins
   a. thiamine, riboflavin, and B_{12}
   b. biotin and vitamin C
   c. vitamins E and K
   d. all of the above

9. Fortified milk is a good source of
   a. vitamin E
   b. vitamin D
   c. vitamin K
   d. vitamin C

10. Good sources of vitamin C are
    a. meats
    b. milk and milk products
    c. breads and cereals
    d. citrus fruits

11. The vitamin that aids in the prevention of rickets is
    a. vitamin A
    b. thiamine
    c. vitamin C
    d. vitamin D

12. The vitamin that is necessary for the proper clotting of the blood is
    a. vitamin A
    b. vitamin K
    c. vitamin D
    d. niacin

13. Vitamins commonly added to breads and cereals are
    a. vitamins A, D, and K
    b. thiamine, riboflavin, niacin, and folate
    c. vitamins E, B_6, and B_{12}
    d. ascorbic acid, pantothenic acid, and folate

14. The vitamin known to prevent scurvy is
    a. vitamin A
    b. vitamin B complex
    c. vitamin C
    d. vitamin D

15. The vitamin deficiency linked to neural tube defects such as spina bifida is
    a. vitamin K
    b. folate
    c. biotin
    d. vitamin E

16. Pernicious anemia is caused by a deficiency of
    a. vitamin B_6
    b. folate
    c. vitamin B_{12}
    d. vitamins A, C, and E

Case In Point

KRYSTYNA: DEEP VEIN THROMBOSIS

Krystyna recently gave birth to her first child. She had lots of trouble with premature labor and had to be on bed rest the last month of her pregnancy. She has been so relieved to be out of the house and enjoying her new baby and the sunshine. This morning she awoke and as she was getting out of bed she noticed quite a bit of pain in her left leg and calf. As she was getting dressed she noticed that her left leg was very swollen and even looked reddened. She was used to her legs being swollen during her pregnancy, but that had resolved since she gave birth. In addition, the leg swelling typically involved both legs, so Krystyna was concerned that it was just the left one.

She decided she was in enough pain that she would call the doctor. After examining Krystyna, the doctor told her that she had developed what is called a deep vein thrombosis. She told Krystyna that it was a blood clot that can sometimes occur after giving birth. Krystyna's doctor told her she needed to admit her to the hospital for treatment. She would run some additional tests and give Krystyna some blood thinning medications. In addition, she told Krystyna she would need to be cautious in consuming foods that had high levels of vitamin K in them, such as green leafy vegetables among other things. The vitamin K in these foods could increase the chance of further clotting. Krystyna's doctor requested the hospital dietitian come and speak to her about these food sources.

ASSESSMENT

1. What data do you have about Krystyna?
2. What factors put Krystyna at risk for developing a deep vein thrombosis?
3. As the dietitian, what would you find helpful in Krystyna's history?

DIAGNOSIS

4. Write a nursing diagnosis for Krystyna.

PLAN/GOAL

5. What is a specific measurable goal for Krystyna in regard to her diet?

IMPLEMENTATION

6. What food sources are high in vitamin K and should be avoided by Krystyna?

EVALUATION/OUTCOME CRITERIA

7. What criteria should Krystyna use to evaluate the success of her actions?

THINKING FURTHER

8. Who else needs to be aware of Krystyna's vitamin K restriction?

rate this **plate**

The dietitian educated Krystyna on high vitamin K vegetables to avoid until her thrombosis had healed. Rate the plate that Krystyna ordered for lunch.

13 × 3 slice of spinach lasagna

1 garlic breadstick

½ cup steamed broccoli

⅙ slice of apple pie

12 oz. ice tea

List the foods that are high in vitamin K and replace them with low sources of vitamin K.

Case In Point

Tina began drinking at a very young age. She can remember her parents drinking heavily at times as well. She was caught a few times in her early days, but Tina thought nothing of it. She had lots of friends who had experimented with alcohol. It was no big deal. When Tina went to college, she had a great time. There were bars and fraternities and all kinds of parties. Alcohol was everywhere. She would typically go out with a group of girls to the bar or a party, but often would find they were ready to go home long before she was. She would often tell her friends to go ahead and leave. She knew she could always find a ride home. One night, Tina's friends were really worried about her. By morning, she hadn't returned home and she hadn't called any of them. Finally, about noon she made it home. She had no shoes and her clothes were filthy with stains. She had walked home more than 2 miles from the party where they had been the night before. Tina assured her friends that she was fine. Over the course of time, this began happening again and again.

Tina would often arrive home in the morning with little memory of what happened the night before. Finally, one night the police arrested Tina for public intoxication. Prior to transporting her to jail, she was taken to a local hospital for medical clearance. The emergency room doctor discovered that Tina had a blood alcohol level of 0.25. Tina's roommate arrived at the hospital and let the staff know that Tina had blacked out several times recently from alcohol abuse. She and her other friends were worried that Tina was an alcoholic. She would rarely eat, she had lost quite a bit of weight, and she could be found anytime day or night with a drink in hand.

At the hospital, Tina's doctor assesses her thiamin status. Knowing that many heavy abusers of alcohol are unable to absorb and utilize thiamin, this is one of the most common deficiencies among alcoholics. Indeed Tina's thiamin levels are very low. He prescribes a thiamin replacement regimen and admits Tina to a rehabilitation facility.

ASSESSMENT

1. What are some of the red flags that may indicate that Tina is an alcoholic?
2. If Tina's body cannot absorb thiamin as a result of excessive alcohol consumption, what are the consequences of this?
3. Tina was arrested with a blood alcohol level of 0.24. How does her level compare to the legal blood alcohol limit in most states?

DIAGNOSIS

4. Write a nursing diagnosis for Tina related to her nutritional intake.
5. Write a nursing diagnosis for her alcohol abuse and rehabilitation.

PLAN/GOAL

6. Tina needs to begin reintroducing foods into her body. What would be the best way to go about this?

IMPLEMENTATION

7. What must Tina understand about her nutrition and her recovery?

EVALUATION/OUTCOME CRITERIA

8. What would you expect from Tina in 6 months if her recovery plan is successful?

THINKING FURTHER

9. Look at the web page for Alcoholics Anonymous. Read about this organization's programs and what it offers clients. Note the historical timeline of AA at http://www.aa.org/aatimeline/.

rate this plate

Rate this plate that the dietitian at the rehabilitation facility ordered for Tina.

3 oz. pulled pork on a whole-wheat bun

2 oz. potato chips

1 medium orange

1–2 × 2 walnut brownie

8 oz. milk

Did the dietitian do a good job at planning at meal rich in thiamin for Tina? Where could improvements be made in this meal?

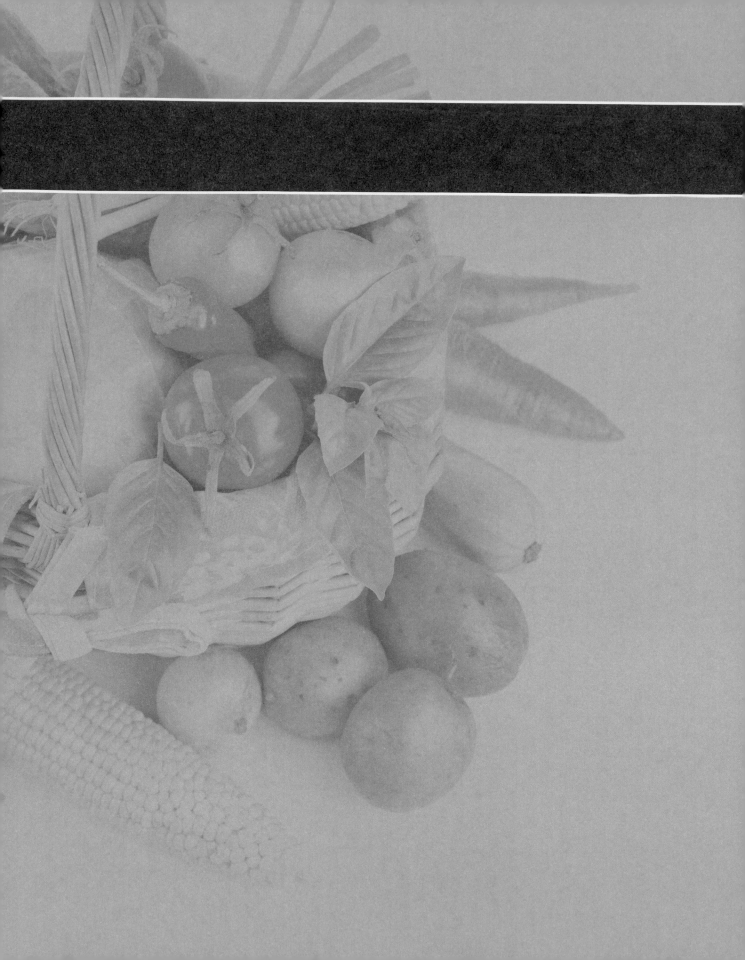

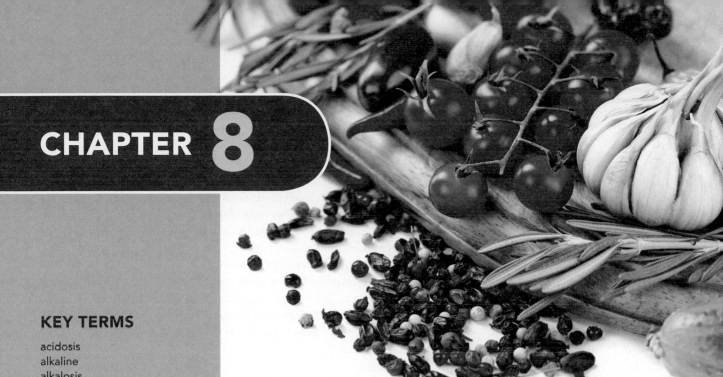

CHAPTER 8

MINERALS

OBJECTIVES

After studying this chapter, you should be able to:

- List at least two food sources of given minerals
- List one or more functions of given minerals
- Describe the recommended method of avoiding mineral deficiencies

Chemical analysis shows that the human body is made up of specific chemical elements. Four of these elements—oxygen, carbon, hydrogen, and nitrogen—make up 96% of body weight. All the remaining elements are *minerals*, which represent only 4% of body weight. Nevertheless, these minerals are essential for good health.

A mineral is an inorganic (noncarbon-containing) element that is necessary for the body to build tissues, regulate body fluids, or assist in various body functions. Minerals are found in all body tissues. Any abnormal concentration of minerals in the blood can help diagnose different disorders. Minerals cannot provide energy by themselves, but in their role as body regulators, they contribute to the production of energy within the body.

Minerals are found in water and in natural (unprocessed) foods, together with proteins, carbohydrates, fats, and vitamins. Minerals in the soil are absorbed by growing plants. Humans obtain minerals by eating plants grown in mineral-rich soil or by eating animals that have eaten such plants. The specific mineral content of food is determined by burning the food and then chemically analyzing the remaining ash.

Highly processed or refined foods such as sugar and white flour contain almost no minerals. Iron, together with the vitamins thiamine, riboflavin, niacin, and folate, are commonly added to white flour and cereals, which are then labeled **enriched foods**.

Most minerals in food occur as salts, which are soluble in water. Therefore, the minerals leave the food and remain in the cooking water. Foods should be cooked in as little water as possible or, preferably, steamed, and any cooking liquid should be saved to be used in soups, gravies, and white sauces. Using this liquid improves the flavor as well as the nutrient content of foods to which it is added.

CLASSIFICATION

Minerals are divided into two groups. First are the major minerals, so named because each is required in amounts greater than 100 mg a day. Second, the trace minerals are needed in amounts smaller than 100 mg a day (Tables 8-1 and 8-2).

As mineral salts dissolve in water, they break into separate, electrically charged particles called **ions**. Ions, if positively charged, are called cations. When negatively charged, they are anions. The cations and anions must be balanced within the body fluids to maintain electroneutrality. For example, if body fluid contains 200 positive (+) charges, it must also contain 200 negative (−) charges. These ions are known as **electrolytes**.

Electrolytes are essential in maintaining the body's fluid balance, and they contribute to its electrical balance, assist in its transmission of nerve impulses and contraction of muscles, and help regulate its acid-base balance (see Chapter 9).

Normally, a balanced diet will maintain electrolyte balance. However, in cases of severe diarrhea, vomiting, high fever, or burns, electrolytes are lost, and the electrolyte balance can be upset. Medical intervention will be necessary to replace the lost electrolytes.

Scientists lack exact information on some of the trace elements, although they do know that trace elements are essential to good health. The study of these elements continues to reveal their specific relationships to human nutrition. A balanced diet is the only safe way of including minerals in the amounts necessary to maintain health.

The Food and Nutrition Board of the National Academy of Sciences, National Research Council (NRC) has recommended dietary allowances for minerals where research indicates knowledge is adequate to do so.

For those minerals where there remains some uncertainty as to amounts of specific human requirements, the NRC has provided a table of Adequate Intakes of selected minerals (Table 8-3). The NRC recommends that the upper levels of listed amounts not be habitually exceeded. (Tables 8-1 and 8-2 list the best sources, functions, and deficiency symptoms of minerals.)

---

enriched foods
foods to which nutrients, usually B vitamins and iron, have been added to improve their nutritional value

ions
electrically charged atoms resulting from chemical reactions

electrolytes
chemical compounds that dissolve in water break up into electrically charged atoms called ions

EXPLORING THE WEB

Search the Web for information on sports drinks, drinks containing electrolytes, and energy drinks. What are the claims made by the makers of these drinks? What are the benefits, if any, that these drinks provide? Who is the target market for these drinks? What are some other dietary alternatives to these drinks? Are any warnings included for giving these drinks to babies?

TABLE 8-1 **Major Minerals**

NAME	FOOD SOURCES	FUNCTIONS	DEFICIENCY/TOXICITY
Calcium (Ca^{++})	• Milk, cheese • Sardines • Salmon • Some dark green leafy vegetables • Yogurt	• Development of bones and teeth • Transmission of nerve impulses • Blood clotting • Normal heart action • Normal muscle activity	Deficiency • Osteoporosis • Osteomalacia • Rickets • Tetany • Retarded growth • Poor teeth and bone formation
Phosphorus (P)	• Milk, cheese • Lean meat • Poultry • Fish • Whole-grain cereals • Legumes • Nuts	• Development of bones and teeth • Maintenance of normal acid-base balance of the blood • Constituent of all body cells • Necessary for effectiveness of some vitamins • Metabolism of carbohydrates, fats, and proteins	Deficiency • Poor teeth and bone formation • Weakness • Anorexia • General malaise
Potassium (K$^+$)	• Oranges, bananas • Dried fruits • Vegetables • Legumes • Milk • Cereals • Meat	• Contraction of muscles • Maintenance of fluid balance • Transmission of nerve impulses • Osmosis • Regular heart rhythm • Cell metabolism	Deficiency • Hypokalemia • Muscle weakness • Confusion • Abnormal heartbeat Toxicity • Hyperkalemia • Potentially life-threatening irregular heartbeats
Sodium (Na$^+$)	• Table salt • Beef, eggs • Poultry • Milk, cheese	• Maintenance of fluid balance • Transmission of nerve impulses • Osmosis • Acid-base balance • Regulation of muscle and nerve irritability	Deficiency • Nausea • Exhaustion • Muscle cramps Toxicity • Increase in blood pressure • Edema
Chloride (Cl$^-$)	• Table salt • Eggs • Seafood • Milk	• Gastric acidity • Regulation of osmotic pressure • Osmosis • Fluid balance • Acid-base balance • Formation of hydrochloric acid	Deficiency • Imbalance in gastric acidity • Imbalance in blood pH • Nausea • Exhaustion

(continues)

TABLE 8-1 (*continued*)

NAME	FOOD SOURCES	FUNCTIONS	DEFICIENCY/TOXICITY
Magnesium (Mg^{++})	• Green leafy vegetables • Whole grains • Avocados • Nuts • Milk • Legumes • Bananas	• Synthesis of ATP • Transmission of nerve impulses • Activation of metabolic enzymes • Constituent of bones, muscles, and red blood cells • Necessary for healthy muscles and nerves	Deficiency • Normally unknown • Mental, emotional, and muscle disorders
Sulfur (S)	• Eggs • Poultry • Fish	• Maintenance of protein structure • For building hair, nails, and all body tissues • Constituent of all body cells	Unknown

© Cengage Learning 2014

TABLE 8-2   Trace Minerals

NAME	FOOD SOURCES	FUNCTIONS	DEFICIENCY/TOXICITY
Iron (Fe^+)	• Muscle meats • Poultry • Shellfish • Liver • Legumes • Dried fruits • Whole-grain or enriched breads and cereals • Dark green and leafy vegetables • Molasses	• Transports oxygen and carbon dioxide • Component of hemoglobin and myoglobin • Component of cellular enzymes essential for energy production	Deficiency • Iron deficiency anemia characterized by weak ness, dizziness, loss of weight, and pallor Toxicity • Hemochromatosis (genetic) • Can be fatal to children • May contribute to heart disease • Injure liver
Iodine (I^-)	• Iodized salt • Seafood	• Regulation of basal metabolic rate	Deficiency • Goiter • Cretinism • Myxedema
Zinc (Zn^+)	• Seafood, especially oysters • Liver • Eggs • Milk • Wheat bran • Legumes	• Formation of collagen • Component of insulin • Component of many vital enzymes • Wound healing • Taste acuity • Essential for growth • Immune reactions	Deficiency • Dwarfism, hypogo-nadism, anemia • Loss of appetite • Skin changes • Impaired wound healing • Decreased taste acuity

(*continues*)

TABLE 8-2 (*continued*)

NAME	FOOD SOURCES	FUNCTIONS	DEFICIENCY/TOXICITY
Selenium (Se⁻)	• Seafood • Kidney • Liver • Muscle meats • Grains	• Constituent of most body tissue • Needed for fat metabolism • Antioxidant functions	Deficiency • Unclear, but related to Keshan disease • Muscle weakness Toxicity • Vomiting • Loss of hair and nails • Skin lesions
Copper (Cu⁺)	• Liver • Shellfish, oysters • Legumes • Nuts • Whole grains	• Essential for formation of hemoglobin and red blood cells • Component of enzymes • Wound healing • Needed metabolically for the release of energy	Deficiency • Anemia • Bone disease • Disturbed growth and metabolism Toxicity • Vomiting; diarrhea • Wilson's disease (genetic)
Manganese (Mn⁺)	• Whole grains • Nuts • Fruits • Tea	• Component of enzymes • Bone formation • Metabolic processes	Deficiency • Unknown Toxicity • Possible brain disease
Fluoride (F⁻)	• Fluoridated water • Seafood	• Increases resistance to tooth decay • Component of bones and teeth	Deficiency • Tooth decay • Possibly osteoporosis Toxicity • Discoloration of teeth (mottling)
Chromium (Cr)	• Meat • Vegetable oil • Whole-grain cereal and nuts • Yeast	• Associated with glucose and lipid metabolism	Deficiency • Possibly disturbances of glucose metabolism
Molybdenum (Mo)	• Dark green leafy vegetables • Liver • Cereal • Legumes	• Enzyme functioning • Metabolism	Deficiency • Unknown Toxicity • Inhibition of copper absorption

© Cengage Learning 2014

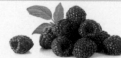

TABLE 8-3 Recommended Dietary Allowances (RDA) and Adequate Intakes (AI) for Selected Trace Minerals

CATEGORY	AGE	COPPER (mcg)	MANGANESE (mg)	CHROMIUM (mcg)	MOLYBDENUM (mcg)
Infants	0–6 mo	200*	0.003*	0.2*	2*
	6–12 mo	220*	0.6*	5.5*	3*
Children and adolescents	1–3 y	340	1.2*	11*	17
	4–8 y	440	1.5*	15*	22
	9–13 y	700	1.9 males* 1.6 females*	25 males* 21 females*	34
	14–18 y	890	2.2 males* 1.6 females*	35 males* 24 females*	43
Adults	19–50 y	900	2.3 males* 1.8 females*	35 males* 25 females*	45
Adults	51–70		2.3 males* 1.8 females*	30 males* 20 females*	45
Pregnancy	14–18 y	1,000	2.0*	29*	50
	19–50	1,000	2.0*	30*	50
Lactation	14–18	1,300	2.6*	44*	50
	19–50	1,300	2.6*	45*	50

Adequate Intake (AI)

Reprinted with permission from the National Academies Press, Copyright © 2006, National Academy of Sciences. *Dietary Reference Intakes: The Essential Guide to Nutrient Requirements.*

In addition, the Institute of Medicine has developed Daily Reference Intakes (DRIs) for calcium, fluoride, phosphorus, and magnesium. The DRI incorporates Estimated Average Requirements (EAR), the RDA, and Tolerable Upper Intake Levels.

TOXICITY

Because it is known that minerals are essential to good health, some would-be nutritionists will make claims that "more is better." Ironically, more can be hazardous to one's health when it comes to minerals. In a healthy individual who is eating a balanced diet, there will be some normal mineral loss through perspiration and saliva, and amounts in excess of body needs will be excreted in urine and feces. However, when concentrated forms of minerals are taken on a regular basis, over a period of time, they become more than the body can handle, and **toxicity** develops. An excessive amount of one mineral can sometimes cause a deficiency of another mineral. In addition, excessive amounts of minerals can cause hair loss and changes in the blood, hormones, bones, muscles, blood vessels, and nearly all tissues. Concentrated forms of minerals should be used only on the advice of a physician.

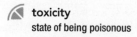
toxicity
state of being poisonous

MAJOR MINERALS
Calcium

The human body contains more calcium (Ca) than any other mineral. The body of a 154-pound person contains approximately 4 pounds of calcium. Of that calcium, 99% is found in the skeleton and teeth. The remaining 1% is found in the blood.

Functions

Calcium, in combination with phosphorus, is a component of bones and teeth, giving them strength and hardness. Bones, in turn, provide storage for calcium. Calcium is needed for normal nerve and muscle action, blood clotting, heart function, and cell metabolism.

Regulation of Blood Calcium

Each cell requires calcium. It is carried throughout the body by the blood, and its delivery to the cells is regulated by the hormonal system. Normal blood calcium levels are maintained even if intake is poor.

When blood calcium levels are low, the parathyroid glands release a hormone that tells the kidneys to retrieve calcium before it is excreted. In addition, this hormone, working with calcitriol (the active hormone form of vitamin D), causes increased release of calcium from the bones by stimulating the activity of the osteoclasts (cells that break down bones). Both of these actions increase blood calcium levels. If calcium intake is low for a period of years, the amount withdrawn from the bones will cause them to become increasingly fragile. Osteoporosis may result.

If the blood calcium level is high, osteoblasts (cells that make bones) will increase bone mass. During growth, osteoblasts will make more bone mass than will be broken down. Bone mass is acquired until one is approximately 30 years old. With adequate consumption of calcium, phosphorus, and vitamin D, bone mass will remain stable in women until menopause. After menopause, bones will begin to weaken owing to the lack of the hormone estrogen. A special x-ray, a DEXA scan, can be taken to determine bone density. If a person is at risk for injury due to decreased bone density, the physician will decide the best course of action. Drugs that help prevent further loss of bone mass are available.

Sources

The best sources of calcium are milk and milk products. They provide large quantities of calcium in small servings. For example, 1 cup of milk provides 300 mg of calcium (Figure 8-1). One ounce of cheddar cheese provides 250 mg of calcium.

Calcium is also found in some dark green leafy vegetables. However, when the vegetable contains oxalic acid, as spinach and Swiss chard do, the calcium remains unavailable because the oxalic acid binds it and prevents it from being absorbed. When the intake of fiber exceeds 35 g a day, calcium will also bind with phytates (phosphorus compounds found in some high-fiber cereal), which also limits its absorption.

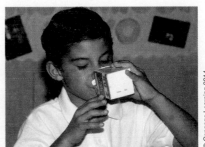

© Cengage Learning 2014

FIGURE 8-1 Milk is an important source of calcium and phosphorus. These minerals are essential for the normal growth and development of bones and teeth.

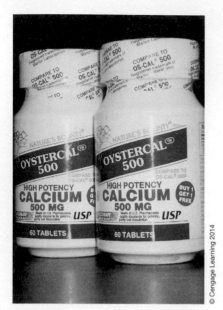

FIGURE 8-2 Always look for the USP seal of approval when purchasing supplements.

TABLE 8-4	Recommended Dietary Intakes for Calcium (mg/day)
0–6 mo*	200 mg
6–12 mo*	260 mg
1–3 y	700 mg
4–8 y	1,000 mg
9–18 y	1,300 mg
19–50 y	1,000 mg
51–70 y	1,000 mg males
	1,200 mg females
70+	1,200
Pregnant women, 14–18 y	1,300 mg
Pregnant women, 19–50 y	1,000 mg
Lactating women	Same as for nonlactating women of same age

*Adequate Intake (AI)

Reprinted with permission from the National Academies Press, Copyright © 2011, National Academy of Sciences. *Dietary Reference Intakes: Calcium and Vitamin D.*

Factors that are believed to enhance the absorption of calcium include adequate vitamin D, a calcium-to-phosphorus ratio that includes no more phosphorus than calcium, and the presence of lactose. A lack of weight-bearing exercise reduces the amount of calcium absorbed.

Requirements

The estimated requirement for calcium is now given as an Adequate Intake (AI) level. Calcium is measured in milligrams (mg). The AIs for calcium at different ages and conditions are shown in Table 8-4. The recommendations were made to achieve optimal bone health and to reduce the probability of fractures in later life.

Calcium supplements are recommended for persons who are lactose intolerant, those who dislike milk, and those who are unable to consume enough dairy products to meet their needs. Calcium carbonate, the form found in calcium-based antacid tablets, has the highest concentration of bioavailable calcium. Calcium supplements appear to be absorbed most efficiently when consumed in doses of 500 mg.

When purchasing calcium supplements, check for the USP (United States Pharmacopeia) seal of approval on the product you select (Figure 8-2). USP-approved products are unlikely to contain lead or other toxins. Avoid bone meal products because they may contain lead.

Deficiency

Calcium deficiency may result in rickets. This is a disease that occurs in early childhood and results in poorly formed bone structure. It causes bowed legs, "pigeon chest," and enlarged wrists or ankles. Severe cases can result in

TABLE 8-5 Adequate Intakes and Recommended Dietary Allowances for Phosphorus	
AI FOR PHOSPHORUS	
0–6 mo	100 mg*
7–12 mo	275 mg*
RDA FOR PHOSPHORUS	
1–3 y	460 mg
4–8 y	500 mg
9–18 y	1,250 mg
19–70 y	700 mg
Pregnant and lactating women	Same as for nonpregnant and nonlactating women of same age

*Adequate Intake (AI)

Reprinted with permission from the National Academies Press, Copyright © 2006, National Academy of Sciences. *Dietary Reference Intakes: The Essential Guide to Nutrient Requirements.*

stunted growth. Insufficient calcium can also cause "adult rickets" (osteomalacia), a condition in which bones become soft. And although the precise **etiology** of osteoporosis is unknown, it is thought that long-term calcium deficiency is a contributing factor. Other factors contributing to osteoporosis include deficiency of vitamin D and certain hormones.

Insufficient calcium in the blood can cause a condition characterized by involuntary muscle movement, known as **tetany**. Excessive intake may cause constipation, or it may inhibit the absorption of iron and zinc.

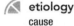
etiology
cause

tetany
involuntary muscle movement

Phosphorus

Phosphorus (P), together with calcium, is necessary for the formation of strong, rigid bones and teeth. Phosphorus is also important in the metabolism of carbohydrates, fats, and proteins. Phosphorus is a constituent of all body cells. It is necessary for a proper acid-base balance of the blood and is essential for the effective action of several B vitamins. Like calcium, phosphorus is stored in bones, and its absorption is increased in the presence of vitamin D.

Sources

Although phosphorus is widely distributed in foods, its best sources are protein-rich foods such as milk, cheese, meats, poultry, and fish. Cereals, legumes, nuts, and soft drinks also contain substantial amounts of this mineral.

Requirements

The requirement for phosphorus is provided as AI for the first 12 months and as EAR (Estimated Average Requirements) after that (Table 8-5). Phosphorus is measured in milligrams.

Deficiency

Because phosphorus is found in so many foods, its deficiency is rare. Excessive use of antacids can cause it, because they affect its absorption. Symptoms of phosphorus deficiency include bone **demineralization** (loss of minerals), fatigue, and anorexia.

demineralization
loss of mineral or minerals

Potassium

intracellular
within the cell

osmosis
movement of a substance through a semipermeable membrane

Potassium (K) is an electrolyte found primarily in **intracellular** fluid. Like sodium, it is essential for fluid balance and osmosis. Potassium maintains the fluid level *within* the cell, and sodium maintains the fluid level *outside* the cell. **Osmosis** moves the fluid into and out of cells as needed to maintain electrolyte (and fluid) balance. There is normally more potassium than sodium inside the cell and more sodium than potassium outside the cell. If this balance is upset and the sodium inside the cell increases, the fluid within the cell also increases, swelling it and causing edema. If the sodium level outside the cell drops, fluid enters the cell to dilute the potassium level, thereby causing a reduction in **extracellular** fluid. With the loss of sodium and reduction of extracellular fluid, a decrease in blood pressure and dehydration can result.

extracellular
outside the cell

Potassium is also necessary for transmission of nerve impulses and for muscle contractions.

Sources

Potassium is found in many foods. Fruits—especially melons, oranges, bananas, and peaches—and vegetables—notably mushrooms, Brussels sprouts, potatoes, tomatoes, winter squash, lima beans, and carrots—are particularly rich sources of it.

Deficiency or Excess

hypokalemia
low level of potassium in the blood

diuretics
substances used to increase the amount of urine excreted

hyperkalemia
excessive amounts of potassium in the blood

Potassium deficiency (**hypokalemia**) can be caused by diarrhea, vomiting, diabetic acidosis, severe malnutrition, or excessive use of laxatives or **diuretics**. Nausea, anorexia, fatigue, muscle weakness, and heart abnormalities (tachycardia) are symptoms of its deficiency. **Hyperkalemia** (high blood levels of potassium) can be caused by dehydration, renal failure, or excessive intake. Cardiac failure can result.

Sodium

Sodium (Na) is an electrolyte whose primary function is the control of fluid balance in the body. It controls the extracellular fluid and is essential for osmosis. Sodium is also necessary to maintain the acid-base balance in the body. In addition, it participates in the transmission of nerve impulses essential for normal muscle function.

Sources

The primary dietary source of sodium is table salt (sodium chloride), which is 40% sodium. One teaspoon of table salt contains 2,000 mg sodium. It is also naturally available in animal foods. Salt is typically added to commercially prepared foods because it enhances flavor and helps to preserve

Supersize USA

Two-for-One Portion Is Double Trouble

Consumers must totally rethink the way they eat. With obesity or overweight now affecting at least one out of three adult Americans, it is time to look at our portion distortion. We look at a meal and think that more is better, and it doesn't help that fast-food companies will offer double portions of French fries or soft drinks for less money than a normal size. Even dinner plates and serving bowls have gotten larger. With larger portions creating obesity, there are more incidences of children and teenagers with diabetes, heart and kidney disease, and other potentially fatal illnesses as well as menstruation problems. Obesity also significantly cuts life expectancy. A well-balanced diet can result in adequate vitamin and mineral intake; however, consuming large amounts of foods not recommended in the MyPlate program may result in an inadequate balance of vitamins and minerals, in addition to obesity.

(Source: Adapted from Centers for Disease Control and Prevention, Overweight and Obesity. Adult Obesity Facts. July 2011. http://www.cdc.gov)

some foods by controlling growth of microorganisms. Fruits and vegetables contain little or no sodium. Drinking water contains sodium but in varying amounts. "Softened" water has a much higher sodium content than "hard," or unsoftened, water.

Requirements

The DRI for sodium has been established at 1,500 mg, or 3,800 mg of salt. The UL for salt is 5,800 mg, with the majority of men and women exceeding that limit.

Deficiency or Excess

Either deficiency or excess of sodium can cause upsets in the body's fluid balance. Although rare, a deficiency of sodium can occur after severe vomiting, diarrhea, or heavy perspiration. In such cases, **dehydration** can result. A sodium deficiency also can upset the acid-base balance in the body. Cells function best in a neutral or slightly **alkaline** medium. If too much acid is lost (which can happen during severe vomiting), tetany due to **alkalosis** may develop. If the alkaline reserve is deficient as a result of starvation or faulty metabolism, as in the case of diabetes, **acidosis** (too much acid) may develop.

An excess of sodium is a more common problem and may cause **edema**. This edema adds pressure to artery walls that can cause **hypertension**. Thus, an excess of sodium is frequently associated with **cardiovascular** conditions such as hypertension and congestive heart failure. Certain groups have greater (or lesser) reduction in blood pressure in response to reduced sodium intake. Those with the greatest reductions in blood pressure have been termed *salt sensitive*, whereas those with little or no reduction in blood pressure have been termed *salt resistant*. Working with your cardiologist is the best way to determine which you are—sensitive or resistant. Depending on the diagnosis, the diet order may be either a 3–4 g (also called no-added salt or NAS) or a 1–2 g sodium-restricted diet. A physician rarely prescribes a diet of 1 g of sodium because compliance is difficult.

 dehydration
loss of water

 alkaline
base; capable of neutralizing acids

 alkalosis
condition in which excess base accumulates in, or acids are lost from, the body

 acidosis
condition in which excess acids accumulate or there is a loss of base in the body

 edema
abnormal retention of fluid by the body

 hypertension
higher than normal blood pressure

 cardiovascular
pertaining to the heart and entire circulatory system

Chloride

Chloride (Cl) is an electrolyte that is essential for maintenance of fluid, electrolyte, and acid-base balance in the body. Like sodium, it is a constituent of extracellular fluid. It is also a component of gastric juices, where, in combination with hydrogen, it is found in hydrochloric acid, cerebrospinal fluid (of the brain and spinal cord), and muscle and nerve tissue. It helps the blood carry carbon dioxide to the lungs and is necessary during immune responses when white blood cells attack foreign cells.

Sources

Chloride is found almost exclusively in table salt (sodium chloride) or in foods containing sodium chloride.

Requirements

The DRI for chloride for normal adults is 2,300 mg a day.

Deficiency

Because chloride is found in salt, deficiency is rare. It can occur, however, with severe vomiting, diarrhea, or excessive use of diuretics, and alkalosis can result. Also, it could occur in clients who follow long-term sodium-restricted diets. In such cases, clients can be provided with an alternative source of chloride.

Magnesium

Magnesium (Mg) is vital to both hard and soft body tissues. It is essential for metabolism and regulates nerve and muscle function, including the heart, and plays a role in the blood-clotting process.

Sources

Like phosphorus, magnesium is widely distributed in foods, but it is found primarily in plant foods. The nutrient-dense foods are green leafy vegetables, legumes, nuts, whole grains, and some fruits such as avocados and bananas. Milk is also a good source if taken in sufficient quantity. For example, 2 cups of fat-free milk provide about 60 mg of magnesium.

Magnesium is lost during commercial food processing and in cooking water, so it is preferable to eat vegetables and fruits raw rather than cooked.

Requirements

The requirement for magnesium is provided as AIs (Table 8-6). Magnesium is measured in milligrams.

TABLE 8-6 Adequate Intakes (AIs) for Potassium, Sodium, Chloride, and Recommended Dietary Allowances for Magnesium

	POTASSIUM (g/d)	SODIUM (g/d)	CHLORIDE (g/d)	MAGNESIUM (mg/d)
LIFE STAGE GROUP				
Infants				
0–6 mo	0.4	0.12	0.18	30*
6–12 mo	0.7	0.37	0.57	75*
Children				
1–3 y	3.0	1.0	1.5	80
4–8 y	3.8	1.2	1.9	130
Males				
9–13 y	4.5	1.5	2.3	240
14–18 y	4.7	1.5	2.3	410
19–30 y	4.7	1.5	2.3	400
31–50 y	4.7	1.5	2.3	420
51–70 y	4.7	1.3	2.0	420
>70 y	4.7	1.2	1.8	420
Females				
9–13 y	4.5	1.5	2.3	240
14–18 y	4.7	1.5	2.3	360
19–30 y	4.7	1.5	2.3	310
31–50 y	4.7	1.5	2.3	320
51–70 y	4.7	1.3	2.0	320
>70 y	4.7	1.2	1.8	320
Pregnancy				
14–18 y	4.7	1.5	2.3	400
19–30 y	4.7	1.5	2.3	350
31–50 y	4.7	1.5	2.3	360
Lactation				
14–18 y	5.1	1.5	2.3	360
19–30 y	5.1	1.5	2.3	310
31–50 y	5.1	1.5	2.3	320

*Values are Adequate Intakes (AI) for Magnesium for Infants

Reprinted with permission from the National Academies Press, Copyright © 2006, National Academy of Sciences. Dietary Reference Intakes: The Essential Guide to Nutrient Requirements.

Deficiency

Because of the wide availability of magnesium, its deficiency among people on normal diets is unknown. When deficiency was experimentally induced, the symptoms included nausea and mental, emotional, and muscular disorders.

Sulfur

Sulfur (S) is necessary to all body tissues and is found in all body cells. It contributes to the characteristic odor of burning hair and tissue. It is necessary for metabolism.

Sources

Sulfur is a component of some amino acids and is consequently found in protein-rich foods.

Requirements or Deficiency

Neither the amount of sulfur required by the human body nor its deficiency is known.

TRACE MINERALS

Iron

The principal role of iron (Fe) is to deliver oxygen to body tissues. It is a component of hemoglobin, the coloring matter of red blood cells (erythrocytes). Hemoglobin allows red blood cells to combine with oxygen in the lungs and carry it to body tissues.

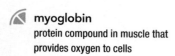

myoglobin
protein compound in muscle that
provides oxygen to cells

Iron is also a component of **myoglobin**, a protein compound in muscles that provides oxygen to cells, and it is a constituent of other body compounds involved in oxygen transport. Iron is utilized by enzymes that are involved in the making of amino acids, hormones, and neurotransmitters.

Sources

Meat, poultry, and fish are the best sources of iron because only the flesh of animals contains heme iron. Heme iron is absorbed more than twice as efficiently as nonheme iron. Nonheme iron is found in whole-grain cereals, enriched grain products, vegetables, fruit, eggs, meat, fish, and poultry. The rate of absorption of nonheme iron is strongly influenced by dietary factors and the body's iron stores. Factors affecting the absorption of both heme and nonheme iron are listed in Table 8-7.

For iron to be absorbed, it must be chemically changed from ferric to ferrous iron. This change is accomplished by the hydrochloric acid in the stomach. Absorption of nonheme iron can be enhanced by consuming a vitamin C–rich food and a nonheme iron–rich food at the same meal. Vitamin C holds onto and keeps the iron in its ferrous form, which facilitates absorption. Meat protein factor (MPF) is a substance in meat, poultry, and fish that aids in the absorption of nonheme iron.

Phytic acid and oxalic acid can bind iron and reduce the body's absorption of it. Polyphenols, such as tannins in tea and related substances in coffee,

TABLE 8-7 Factors That Affect Iron Absorption

INCREASE	DECREASE
Acid in the stomach	Phytic acid (in fiber)
Heme iron	Oxalic acid
High body demand for red blood cells (blood loss, pregnancy)	Polyphenols in tea and coffee
Low body stores of iron	Full body stores of iron
Meat protein factor (MPF)	Excess of other minerals (Zn, Mn, Ca) (especially when taken as supplements)
Vitamin C	Some antacids

© Cengage Learning 2014

also reduce the absorption of iron. Antacids containing calcium and calcium supplements should be taken several hours before or after a meal high in iron because calcium also interferes with iron absorption.

Requirements

The NRC has determined that men lose approximately 1 mg of iron a day and that women lose 1.5 mg a day. On the assumption that only 10% of ingested iron is absorbed, the DRI for men has been set at 10 mg and for women from the age of 11 through the child-bearing years at 15 mg. This is doubled during pregnancy and is difficult to meet by diet alone. Consequently, an iron supplement is commonly prescribed during pregnancy. Women should make a special effort to include iron-rich foods in their diets at all times. The rapid growth periods of infancy and adolescence also produce a heavy need for iron.

Deficiency or Toxicity

Iron deficiency continues to be a problem, especially for women. Iron deficiency can be caused by insufficient intake, malabsorption, lack of sufficient stomach acid, or excessive blood loss, any or all of which can deplete iron stores in the body. Decreased stores of iron prevent hemoglobin synthesis. The result is an insufficient number of red blood cells to carry needed oxygen. What begins as iron deficiency can become **iron deficiency anemia**. Iron deficiency anemia takes a long time to develop, but it is the most common nutrient deficiency worldwide. Symptoms include fatigue, weakness, irritability, and shortness of breath. Clinical signs include pale skin and spoon-shaped fingernails.

Some people suffer from *hemochromatosis*. This is a condition due to an inborn error of metabolism and causes excessive absorption of iron. The onset of this disorder can happen at any age. Unless treated, this condition can damage the liver, spleen, and heart. To control the buildup of iron, clients with this condition must give blood on a regular basis.

iron deficiency anemia
condition resulting from inadequate amount of iron in the diet, reducing the amount of oxygen carried by the blood to the cells

Iodine

Iodine (I) is a component of the thyroid hormones, thyroxine (T_4) and triiodo-thyronine (T_3). It is necessary for the normal functioning of the thyroid gland, which determines the rate of metabolism.

Sources

The primary sources of iodine are **iodized salt**, seafood, and some plant foods grown in soil bordering the sea. Iodized salt is common table salt to which iodine has been added in an amount that, if used in normal cooking, provides sufficient iodine.

Requirements

The DRI for adults is 150 mg a day. Additional amounts are needed during pregnancy and lactation.

Deficiency

When the thyroid gland lacks sufficient iodine, the manufacture of thyroxine and triiodothyronine is retarded. In its attempt to take up more iodine, the gland grows, forming a lump on the neck called a goiter (Figure 8-3). Goiter appears to be more common among women than among men. A thyroid gland that doesn't function properly causes myxedema (hypothyroidism) in adults. The children of mothers lacking sufficient iodine may suffer from cretinism (retarded physical and mental development).

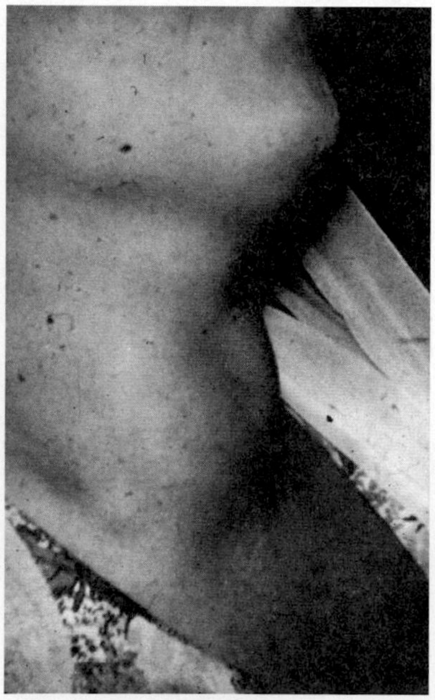

Zinc

Zinc (Zn) is a cofactor for more than 300 enzymes. Consequently, it affects many body tissues. It appears to be essential for growth, wound healing, taste acuity, glucose tolerance, and the mobilization of vitamin A within the body.

Sources

The best sources of zinc are protein foods, especially meat, fish, eggs, dairy products, wheat germ, and legumes.

Requirements

The DRI for zinc is 11 mg in normal adult males and 8 mg in adult females, with increased requirements during pregnancy and further increases during lactation.

Deficiency

Decreased appetite and taste acuity, delayed growth, dwarfism, hypogonadism (subnormal development of male sex organs), poor wound healing, anemia, acne-like rash, and impaired immune response are all symptoms of zinc deficiency.

Selenium

Selenium (Se) is a constituent of most body tissues, but the heaviest concentration of the mineral is in the liver, kidneys, and heart.

iodized salt
salt that has the mineral iodine added for the prevention of goiter

Centers for Disease Control and Prevention, Public Health Image Library

FIGURE 8-3 A goiter on the neck, which results primarily from iodine deficiency, is an enlargement of the thyroid gland.

In The Media

Safe Use of Dietary Supplements

The use of dietary supplements is increasing worldwide with 17.7% of Americans using natural products in the year 2007. Many believe that supplements providing daily vitamins and minerals will enhance overall health, but there are a few safety considerations when choosing to take dietary supplements. Safety and effectiveness of a product does not have to be proven or stated on the label before being marketed to the public. Manufacturers are, however, required to follow specific standards to developing supplements. It is important to keep in mind that certain medications may interact with dietary supplements. Reading the label and talking to a health care professional before deciding to take a supplement is highly recommended.

(Source: Adapted from U.S. Department of Health and Human Services, National Institutes of Health, National Center for Complementary and Alternative Medicine. *Get the Facts: Using Dietary Supplements Wisely.* March 2010.)

Functions

Selenium is a component of an enzyme that acts as an antioxidant. In this way, it protects cells against oxidation and spares vitamin E.

Sources

The best sources of selenium are seafood, kidney, liver, and muscle meats.

Requirements

The DRI for selenium for an adult male and female is 70 mcg.

Deficiency or Toxicity

Symptoms of selenium deficiency are unclear, but selenium supplements appear to be effective in treating **Keshan disease**. High doses (1 mg or more daily) are toxic and can cause vomiting, loss of hair and nails, and skin lesions.

 Keshan disease
condition causing abnormalities in the heart muscle

Copper

Copper (Cu) is found in all tissues, but its heaviest concentration is in the liver, kidneys, muscles, and brain. As an essential component of several enzymes, it helps in the formation of hemoglobin, aids in the transport of iron to bone marrow (soft tissue in bone center) for the formation of red blood cells, and participates in energy production.

Sources

Copper is available in many foods, but its best sources include organ meats, shellfish, legumes, nuts, cocoa, and whole-grain cereals. Human milk is a good source of copper, but cow's milk is not.

Requirements

The DRI for copper is 900 mg for adults.

Deficiency or Toxicity

Copper deficiency is extremely rare among adults, occurring only in people with malabsorption conditions and in cases of gross protein deficiency, such as kwashiorkor. It is apparent sometimes in premature infants and in people on long-term parenteral nutrition (feeding via a vein) programs lacking copper. A copper deficiency can be caused by taking excess zinc supplements. Anemia, bone demineralization, and impaired growth may result.

Excess copper can be highly toxic. A single dose of 10–15 mg can cause vomiting. Wilson's disease is an inherited condition, resulting in accumulation of copper in the liver, brain, kidneys, and cornea. It can cause damage to liver cells and neurons. If the excess is detected early, copper-binding agents can be used to bind copper in the bloodstream and increase excretion.

Manganese

Manganese (Mn) is a constituent of several enzymes involved in metabolism. It is also important in bone formation.

Sources

The best sources of manganese are whole grains and tea. Vegetables and fruits also contain moderate amounts.

Requirements

The AI for adults is 2.3 mg for men and 1.8 mg for women.

Deficiency and Toxicity

Its deficiency has not been documented. Toxicity from excessive ingestion of manganese is unknown. However, people who have inhaled high concentrations of manganese dust have developed neurological problems.

Fluoride

Fluoride (F) increases one's resistance to dental caries. It appears to strengthen bones and teeth by making the bone mineral less soluble and thus less inclined to being reabsorbed.

Sources

The principal source of fluoride is fluoridated water (water to which fluoride has been added). In addition, fish and tea contain fluoride. Commercially prepared foods in which fluoridated water has been used during the preparation process also contain fluoride.

Requirements

The requirement for fluoride is given as AI levels (Table 8-8). Fluoride is measured in milligrams.

TABLE 8-8	Adequate Intakes for Fluoride	
Boys and girls	0–6 mo	0.01 mg
	6–12 mo	0.5 mg
	1–3 y	0.7 mg
	4–8 y	1 mg
	9–13 y	2 mg
Boys	14–18 y	3 mg
Girls	14–18 y	3 mg
Males	19+ y	4 mg
Females	19+ y	3 mg
Pregnant and lactating women	Same as for nonpregnant and nonlactating women of same age	

Reprinted with permission from the National Academies Press, Copyright © 2006, National Academy of Sciences. *Dietary Reference Intakes: The Essential Guide to Nutrient Requirements.*

Deficiency or Toxicity

The deficiency of fluoride can result in increased tooth decay. Excessive amounts of fluoride in drinking water have been known to cause permanent discoloration or mottling of children's teeth.

Chromium

Chromium (Cr) is associated with glucose and lipid metabolism. Chromium levels decrease with age except in the lungs, where chromium accumulates.

Sources

The best sources of chromium include meat, mushrooms, nuts, organ meats, and wheat germ.

Requirements

Although there is no DRI for chromium, there is AI for adults, which is 35 mg for men and 25 mg for women. There appears to be no difficulty fulfilling this requirement when one has a balanced diet.

Deficiency

Chromium deficiency appears to be related to disturbances in glucose metabolism.

Molybdenum

Molybdenum (Mo) is a constituent of enzymes and is thought to play a role in metabolism.

Sources

The best sources of molybdenum include milk, liver, legumes, and cereals.

Requirements

The estimated safe and adequate daily intake for adults is 45 mcg. This is normally fulfilled with a balanced diet.

Deficiency or Toxicity

No deficiencies have been noted in people who consume a normal diet. Excessive intake can inhibit copper absorption.

HEALTH AND NUTRITION CONSIDERATIONS

Second to vitamins, minerals are of great interest to the general public. They often are given mythic powers in current articles. It is imperative that the health care professional be aware of the dangers of even small doses of minerals and be able to transmit this information in a meaningful way to the clients.

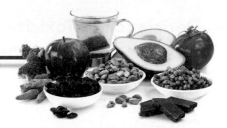

SUMMARY

Minerals are necessary to promote growth and regulate body processes. They originate in soil and water and are ingested via food and drink. Deficiencies can result in conditions such as anemia, rickets, and goiter. A well-balanced diet can prevent mineral deficiencies. Concentrated forms of minerals should be taken only on the advice of a physician. Excessive amounts of minerals can be toxic, causing hair loss and changes in nearly all body tissues.

DISCUSSION TOPICS

1. Discuss the special importance of calcium and phosphorus to children and to pregnant women.

2. List ways of supplying an adequate amount of calcium in the diet of an adult who dislikes milk. Plan a day's menu for this adult.

3. Ask if any member of the class has suffered from anemia. If anyone has, ask the class member to describe the symptoms and treatment. What kind of anemia was it? If it's preventable, what measures are being taken to prevent a recurrence of the condition?

4. If a person is to decrease sodium in her or his diet, should animal foods be increased or decreased? Why?

5. Why does the FNB/NAS recommend that the upper limits of DRIs for minerals not be habitually exceeded?

6. If anyone in class knows someone with osteoporosis, ask for a description of the client, including sex, age, physical appearance, physical complaints, lifelong dietary habits, and medical treatment.

7. Explain the relationship of sodium and edema.

8. Why is it recommended that clients on sodium-restricted diets have the mineral content of their local water supply evaluated?

9. Explain the relationship of sodium and potassium.

10. Why would a doctor prescribe potassium at the same time a diuretic is prescribed?

11. Although rare, why does chloride deficiency sometimes occur in clients on long-term sodium-restricted diets?

12. Discuss the differences between heme and nonheme iron.

13. Why is iron commonly prescribed for pregnant women?

14. Why is selenium said to spare vitamin E?

SUGGESTED ACTIVITIES

1. Using outside sources, prepare a report on how sodium and potassium regulate the body's fluid balance.

2. Using other sources, write a report on at least one of the following:

   Rickets
   Goiter
   Hypothyroidism and hyperthyroidism
   Edema
   Osteoporosis
   Osteomalacia

3. Check four or five varieties of bread at the local supermarket. Using the labels on the breads, evaluate their mineral content.

4. List five good sources of heme iron and five sources of nonheme iron.

5. Spend 5–10 minutes observing customers at a drugstore display of various vitamin and mineral compounds. Write a short report on which minerals were most frequently purchased. Include your opinion about why this was the case.

6. Write a short essay on why iodized salt is a better choice than plain salt.

REVIEW

Multiple choice. Select the *letter* that precedes the best answer.

1. Minerals are inorganic elements that
   a. help to build and repair tissues
   b. are found only in bones
   c. provide energy when carbohydrates are lacking
   d. can substitute for proteins

2. The trace minerals in the human body are defined as
   a. those minerals that cannot be detected in laboratory tests
   b. those essential minerals found in very small amounts
   c. those minerals that are not essential to health
   d. only those minerals that are found in the blood

3. What mineral works with calcium to strengthen and maintain healthy bones and teeth?
   a. iron   c. phosphorus
   b. sulfur   d. molybdenum

4. Phosphorus is found in
   a. poultry
   b. common table salt
   c. vegetable oils
   d. leafy vegetables

5. The coloring matter of the blood is
   a. marrow   c. hemoglobin
   b. lymph   d. plasma

6. The main causes of iron deficiency are
   a. malabsorption
   b. lack of stomach acid
   c. insufficient intake
   d. all of the above

7. Some of the common signs of iron deficiency anemia are
   a. muscle spasms and pain in the liver
   b. bowed legs and an enlarged thyroid gland
   c. edema and loss of vision
   d. fatigue and weakness

8. Iodine is essential to health because it
   a. is necessary for red blood cells
   b. strengthens bones and teeth
   c. helps the blood to carry oxygen to the cells
   d. affects the rate of metabolism

9. Sodium is often restricted in cardiovascular conditions because it
   a. causes the heart to beat slowly
   b. encourages the growth of the heart
   c. contributes to edema
   d. raises the blood sugar

10. Iron is known to be a necessary component of
    a. adipose tissue   c. thyroxine
    b. hemoglobin   d. amino acids

11. Liquid from cooking vegetables should be used in preparing other dishes because
    a. mineral salts are soluble in water
    b. the hydrogen and oxygen in water aid the digestion of minerals
    c. the amino acids are soluble in water
    d. none of the above

12. Goiter can result from a deficiency of
    a. manganese
    b. magnesium
    c. copper
    d. iodine

13. A deficiency of calcium can cause
    a. lactose intolerance   c. tetany
    b. severe nausea   d. hypertension

14. Sodium is especially important in
    a. the blood-clotting process
    b. curing osteoporosis
    c. the prevention of osteomalacia
    d. osmosis

15. Sulfur
    a. is found only in bones and teeth
    b. is richly supplied in carbohydrates
    c. is found in all body cells
    d. deficiency is very common

16. Hypokalemia is
    a. caused by an abnormal heartbeat
    b. caused by potassium deficiency
    c. often a precursor of hyperkalemia
    d. a common result of chronic overeating

17. Delayed growth and hypogonadism are symptoms of what mineral deficiency?
    a. arsenic   c. selenium
    b. zinc   d. copper

18. What type of milk is a good source of copper?
    a. soy milk   c. goat's milk
    b. cow's milk   d. human milk

Case In Point

LIAN: BALANCING EDEMA AND POTASSIUM LEVELS

Lian currently works as a secretary at a law firm. At work, she is primarily sitting at a desk during the day. She has never been particularly active, other than her household work and an occasional walk with her husband. She does try and take the stairs instead of the elevator while she is working to incorporate some activity throughout her day. Lian is 56 years old and is from China. She is small in stature with a height of only 4 feet 10 inches. She weighs 170 pounds. She is currently 80 pounds above her ideal body weight. She has noticed that she is increasingly out of breath when she does take the stairs. She rarely can climb more than one flight before needing to rest. Until recently, she has assumed her shortness of breath was related to her inactivity. Lately though, she has noticed her ankles are swelling. She has been trying to keep her feet elevated after work to decrease the swelling. Finally, she has decided that she needs to see her doctor. At her appointment the nurse finds her blood pressure to be 192/98 and her heart rate is 96 bpm. Her doctor orders an EKG and the results are within normal limits. Lian's doctor suggests that she decrease the sodium in her diet to no more than 2,400 mg daily. He also tells Lian that she needs to work on losing weight and increasing her activity. The doctor explains that both of these will improve her stamina. In addition, her doctor prescribes a diuretic to help with both the swelling and the blood pressure. He explains that the diuretic could deplete her body of potassium so he also prescribes a potassium supplement. He asks her to return in 3 months for blood work. In an effort to cut back on her sodium intake, Lian begins replacing the salt in her diet with a salt substitute. She is unaware that the salt substitute contains potassium instead of sodium. When Lian returns in 3 months for her blood work, her doctor is really concerned. Her potassium level is very high. He explains that this can be a very dangerous problem and he will have to admit her to the hospital so she can be treated for hyperkalemia.

ASSESSMENT

1. How would you identify hidden sources of sodium in Lian's diet?
2. What contributing factors would cause her to have swelling?
3. What questions about thirst would be helpful to pinpoint?
4. What information from a 24-hour food diary could the doctor obtain?
5. What information about no added salt could be causing stress for Lian?
6. What information about Lian's lack of physical activity could benefit her in the future?

DIAGNOSIS

7. Write a nursing diagnosis for Lian.

PLAN/GOAL

8. What prepared foods can Lian have when starting to diet that would not interfere with her sodium restriction?
9. What foods are high in potassium that Lian may want to watch her consumption of?
10. What two goals would you set for Lian?

IMPLEMENTATION

11. What are the main topics you would have Lian understand about a no-added-salt, low-fat diet?

12. Explain the importance of drinking lots of water, even with edema.

EVALUATION/OUTCOME CRITERIA

13. How will Lian know if she is successful?

THINKING FURTHER

14. Look ahead to Chapter 18. What other factors could be influencing Lian's hypertension?
15. Why is it important for Lian to control her hypertension and what are some of the consequences if she does not?

rate this plate

During her admission to the hospital, a registered dietitian educated Lian on a low-potassium, low-sodium diet. The dietitian regularly checked on the foods Lian ordered. Rate this plate.

Spaghetti and meatballs

1 breadstick

Side salad with Italian dressing

Are these food items permitted on a low-potassium, low-sodium diet? List some vegetables and fruits that are high in potassium.

Case In Point

Aisha first started her periods when she was 13 years old. She always had a great deal of difficulty with them each month. It was not uncommon for them to be 7–8 days in length, with 5 days of heavy bleeding. Her pediatrician told her that she would eventually outgrow this problem. Through the years, Aisha has learned to just live with her symptoms. She often had to stay home from school or work the first couple of days of her period. She usually was so fatigued she would have to nap throughout the day.

Aisha is now a 32-year-old woman. She is married and has a 2-year-old daughter. It took 3 years for her to conceive and give birth to her daughter. Since her daughter's birth, things have not improved for Aisha. She is increasingly more tired and short-tempered with her husband and family. She and her husband would like to have a second child, but Aisha feels too exhausted to even consider the idea. Aisha makes an appointment to see her OB/GYN. Results of her blood work reveal that Aisha has low iron stores and a low iron count. Her doctor diagnoses Aisha with iron deficiency anemia. He prescribes a medication to help regulate her periods. He also recommends an iron supplement as well as a stool softener. Her physician asks her to meet with a dietitian to help her better understand her nutritional needs. The dietitian discusses foods high in iron with Aisha. She also recommends Aisha take her iron tablet with vitamin C. She tells Aisha that this will help her body absorb the iron better.

ASSESSMENT

1. Would a 48-hour diet diary be helpful to you as a nurse?
2. What would you look for in the diet diary that would indicate a low iron store for Aisha?
3. What blood tests do you expect to see the doctor order for Aisha?
4. How much iron is lost by women, per day, according to the NRC?
5. What is the daily requirement for iron for women?

DIAGNOSIS

6. Complete the following diagnostic statement: Activity intolerance related to impaired oxygen transport secondary to diminished red blood cell count related to _____.

7. Complete the following diagnostic statement: Health-seeking behaviors related to lack of understanding of _____.

PLAN/GOAL

8. Name two reasonable goals for Aisha.

IMPLEMENTATION

9. Which food categories are priorities to include in Aisha's diet?
10. What can Aisha include as part of daily living to assist in absorption of iron?
11. Would Aisha benefit from taking an iron supplement?

EVALUATION/OUTCOME CRITERIA

12. In 4 months, when Aisha sees her doctor again, what could the doctor measure to evaluate the effectiveness of Aisha's compliance?

THINKING FURTHER

13. What changes could Aisha expect to see if she complies with her program?

rate this plate

No wonder Aisha is tired. She does not have enough iron to keep her going. The dietitian helped her realize that she could eventually keep her iron levels up by taking an iron supplement and eating a healthy diet. Rate this plate for iron intake.

10 oz. medium-rare ribeye steak
¾ cup rice pilaf
Vegetable medley with cauliflower and broccoli
Whole-wheat dinner roll with butter
Slice of chocolate cream pie
Lemonade

What on this plate is high in iron?

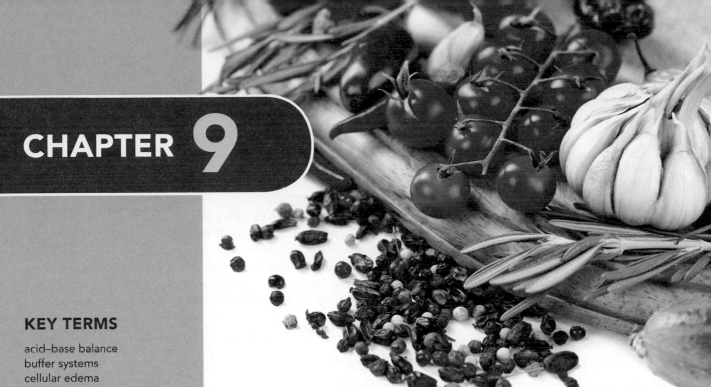

CHAPTER 9

WATER

OBJECTIVES

After studying this chapter, you should be able to:

- Describe the functions of water in the body
- Explain fluid balance and its maintenance
- Name causes and consequences of water depletion
- Give causes and consequences of positive fluid balance
- Describe the acid-base balance of the human body

Although humans can live about 30–45 days without food, it is possible to live only 10–14 days without water. Water is a component of all body cells and constitutes 50–60% of normal adult body weight. The percentage is higher in males than females because men usually have more muscle tissue than women. The water content of muscle tissue is higher than that of fat tissue. The percentage of water content is highest in newborns (75%) and decreases with age.

Body water is divided into two basic compartments: intracellular and extracellular. **Intracellular fluid (ICF)** is water within the cells and accounts for about 65% of total body fluid (Figure 9-1). **Extracellular fluid (ECF)** is water outside the cells and accounts for about 35% of total body fluid. Extracellular fluid is made up of intravascular and **interstitial fluids**.

intracellular fluid (ICF)
water within cells; approximately 65% of total body fluid

extracellular fluid (ECF)
water outside the cells; approximately 35% of total body fluid

interstitial fluid
fluid between cells

solvent
liquid part of a solution

Although it is a component of all body tissues, water is the major component of blood plasma. It is a **solvent** for nutrients and waste products and helps transport both to and from body cells through blood. It is necessary for the hydrolysis of nutrients in the cells, making it essential for metabolism. It functions as a lubricant in joints and in digestion. In addition, it cools the body through perspiration and may, depending on its source, provide some mineral elements (Table 9-1).

The best source of water is drinking water. Table 9-2 lists the Dietary Reference Intake for water. Beverages of all types are the second-best source. A considerable amount is also found in foods, especially fruits, vegetables, soups, milk, and gelatin desserts. In addition, energy metabolism produces water. When carbohydrates, fats, and proteins are metabolized, their end products include carbon dioxide and water (Table 9-3). See Appendix D for water content of foods.

FLUID AND ELECTROLYTE BALANCE

homeostasis
state of physical balance; stable condition

milliequivalents
the concentrations of electrolytes in a solution

solute
the substance dissolved in a solution

osmolality
number of particles per kilogram of solution; solutions with high osmolality exert more pressure than do those with fewer particles

For optimum health there must be **homeostasis**. For this to exist, the body must be in *fluid and electrolyte balance.* This means the water lost by healthy individuals through urination, feces, perspiration, and the respiratory tract must be replaced in terms of both volume and electrolyte content. Electrolytes are measured in **milliequivalents**/liter (mEq/L). An illness causing vomiting and diarrhea can result in large losses of water and electrolytes and must be addressed quickly. Water lost through urine is known as sensible (noticeable) water loss. Insensible (unnoticed) water loss is in feces, perspiration, and respiration. The body must excrete 500 ml of water as urine each day in order to get rid of the waste products of metabolism (Table 9-4).

Water moves through cell walls by osmosis (Figure 9-2). Water flows from the side with the lesser amount of **solute** to the side with the greater solute concentration. The electrolytes sodium, chloride, and potassium are the solutes that maintain the balance between intracellular and extracellular fluids. Potassium is the principal electrolyte in intracellular fluid. Sodium is the principal electrolyte in extracellular fluid. **Osmolality** is the measure of particles in a solution.

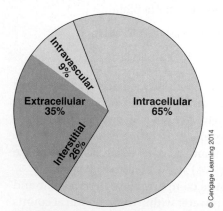

FIGURE 9-1 Body fluid compartments as percentage of total body fluid. All fluid in the body can be classified as either intracellular or extracellular.

© Cengage Learning 2014

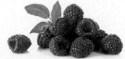

TABLE 9-1   **Functions of Water**

- Component of all body tissues providing structure and form
- Solvent for nutrients and body wastes and chemical reactions
- Provides transport for nutrients and wastes via the blood and lymphatic system
- Essential for hydrolysis and thus metabolism
- Lubricant in joints and in digestion
- Helps regulate body temperature by evaporation of perspiration
- Serves as a shock absorber

© Cengage Learning 2014

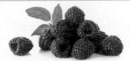

TABLE 9-2 Dietary Reference Intake (Adequate Intake) for Water*

LIFE STAGE GROUP	ADEQUATE INTAKE (L/DAY)
Infants	
0–6 mo	0.7
6–12 mo	0.8
Children	
1–3 y	1.3
4–8 y	1.7
Males	
9–13 y	2.4
14–18 y	3.3
19–30 y	3.7
31–50 y	3.7
51–70 y	3.7
>70 y	3.7
Females	
9–13 y	2.1
14–18 y	2.3
19–30 y	2.7
31–50 y	2.7
51–70 y	2.7
>70 y	2.7
Pregnancy	3.0
Lactation	3.8

*Total water includes all water contained in food, beverages, and drinking water.

Source: Reprinted with permission from the National Academies Press, Copyright © 2006, National Academy of Sciences. *Dietary Reference Intakes: The Essential Guide to Nutrient Requirements.*

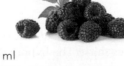

TABLE 9-3 Estimated Daily Fluid Intake for an Adult

Ingested liquids	1,500 ml
Water in foods	700 ml
Water from oxidation	200 ml
Total	2,400 ml

© Cengage Learning 2014

In The Media

Sports Drinks, Vitamin Waters, and Water

We all know it is important to stay hydrated while participating in physical activity, but which type of beverage, whether sports drink or water, provides the most benefit? Sports drinks have the greatest benefit when continuous activity is occurring longer than 60 minutes, based on *Exercise Physiology: Basis of Human Movement in Health and Disease.* Participating in strenuous activity for longer than 60 minutes causes the body to deplete carbohydrate and electrolyte stores. While drinking water is encouraged for shorter durations of exercise, sports drinks will provide the calories and energy needed for longer, more strenuous exercises. Although your body needs essential vitamins and minerals to perform daily functions, drinking vitamin water is not needed unless there is a deficiency. Adequate amounts of vitamins and minerals can be provided through a healthy diet containing all five food groups.

(Source: Adapted from Jason Machowsky, MS, RD, ACSM-cPT. *Sports Drinks and Vitamin Waters: Are They Right for Me?* 2010. http://www.rd411.com)

When the electrolytes in the extracellular fluid are *increased,* ICF moves to the ECF in an attempt to equalize the concentration of electrolytes on both sides of the membrane. This movement reduces the amount of water in the cells. The cells of the **hypothalamus** (regulates appetite and thirst) then become

 hypothalamus
area at base of brain that regulates appetite and thirst

TABLE 9-4 Factors That Lead to Fluid Imbalances

FACTORS	FLUID DEFICIT	FLUID EXCESS
Environmental factors	• Exposure to sun or high atmospheric temperatures	
Personal behaviors	• Fasting • Fad diets • Exercise without adequate fluid replacement	• Excessive sodium or water intake • Venous compression due to pregnancy
Psychological influences	Decreased motivation to drink due to • Fatigue • Depression Excessive use of • Laxatives • Enemas • Alcohol • Caffeine	• Low protein intake due to anorexia
Consequences of diseases	Fluid losses due to • Fever • Wound drainage • Vomiting • Diarrhea • Heavy menstrual flow • Burns Difficulty swallowing due to • Oral pain • Fatigue • Neuromuscular weakness Excessive urinary output due to uncontrolled • Diabetes mellitus • Diabetes insipidus	Fluid retention due to • Renal failure • Cardiac conditions • Congestive heart failure • Valvular diseases • Left ventricular failure • Cirrhosis • Cancer • Impaired venous return

© Cengage Learning 2014

dehydrated
having lost large amounts of water

vascular osmotic pressure
high concentration of electrolytes in the blood; low blood volume or blood pressure

cellular edema
swelling of body cells caused by inadequate amount of sodium in extracellular fluid

dehydrated, as do those in the mouth and tongue, and the body experiences thirst. The hypothalamus stimulates the pituitary gland to excrete ADH (antidiuretic hormone) whenever the electrolytes become too concentrated in the blood or whenever blood volume or blood pressure is too low. This measurement is called **vascular osmotic pressure**. The ADH causes the kidneys to reabsorb water rather than excrete it. At such times, thirst causes the healthy person to drink fluids, which provide the water and electrolytes needed by the cells.

When the sodium in the ECF is reduced, water flows from the ECF into the cells, causing **cellular edema**. When this occurs, the adrenal glands secrete aldosterone, which triggers the kidneys to increase the amount of sodium reabsorbed. When the missing sodium is replaced in the ECF, the excess water that has been drawn from the ECF into the cells moves back to the ECF, and the edema is relieved.

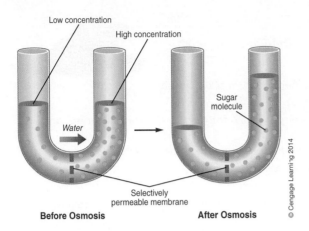

Low concentration

High concentration

Water

Sugar molecule

Selectively permeable membrane

Before Osmosis

After Osmosis

© Cengage Learning 2014

FIGURE 9-2 In osmosis, water passes through the selectively permeable cell membrane from an area of low-solute concentration to an area of high-solute concentration.

The amount of water used and thus needed each day varies, depending on age, size, activity, environmental temperature, and physical condition. The average adult water requirement is 1 ml (milliliter) for every calorie in food consumed. For example, for every 1,800 kcal in food consumed, one needs to drink 7.5 glasses of fluid. The Institute of Medicine determined that the AI for men is roughly 3 liters or about 13 cups of total fluid per day. The AI for women is 2.2 liters or about 9 cups of total fluid per day. Youth, fever, diarrhea, unusual perspiration, and hyperthyroidism increase the requirement.

Dehydration

When the amount of water in the body is inadequate, dehydration can occur. It can be caused by inadequate intake or abnormal loss. Such loss can occur from severe diarrhea, vomiting, hemorrhage, burns, diabetes mellitus, excessive perspiration, excessive urination, or the use of certain medications such as diuretics. Symptoms of dehydration include low blood pressure, thirst, dry skin, fever, and mental disorientation.

As water is lost, electrolytes are also lost. Thus, treatment includes replacement of electrolytes and fluids. Electrolyte content must be checked and corrections made if necessary. A loss of 10% of body water can cause serious problems. Blood volume and nutrient absorption are reduced, and kidney function is upset. A loss of 20% of body water can cause circulatory failure and death. Infants, for example, are at high risk of dehydration when fever, vomiting, and diarrhea occur. Intravenous fluids are often necessary if sufficient fluids cannot be consumed by mouth.

The thirst sensation often lags behind the body's need for water, especially in the elderly, children, athletes, and the ill. Feeling thirsty is not a reliable indicator of when the body needs water. Fluids should be drunk throughout the day to prevent dehydration (Figure 9-3 and Table 9-5).

Dehydration can occur in hot weather when one perspires excessively but fails to drink sufficient water to replace the amount lost through perspiration. Failure to replace water lost through perspiration could lead to progression through the four stages of heat illness: (1) *Heat fatigue* causes thirst, feelings of weakness, or fatigue. To combat this, one should go to a cool place, rest, and drink fluids. (2) *Heat cramp,* due to the loss of sodium and potassium, causes leg cramps and thirst. One should go to a cool place, rest, and

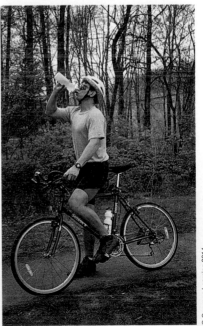

© Cengage Learning 2014

FIGURE 9-3 Preventing dehydration is an important element of proper nutrition.

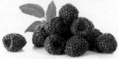

> **TABLE 9-5**   Signs of Dehydration
>
> - Health history reveals inadequate intake of fluids.
> - Decrease in urine output.
> - Weight loss (% body weight): 3–5% for mild, 6–9% for moderate, and 10–15% for severe dehydration.
> - Eyes appear sunken; tongue has increased furrows and fissures.
> - Oral mucous membranes are dry.
> - Decreased skin turgor (normal skin resiliency).
> - Changes in neurological status may occur with moderate to severe dehydration.

© Cengage Learning 2014

drink fluids. (3) *Heat exhaustion* causes thirst, dizziness, nausea, headache, and profuse sweating. Treatment includes sponge baths with cool water, a 2- to 3-day rest, and the ingestion of a great deal of water. (4) *Heat stroke* involves fever and could produce brain and kidney damage. Emergency medical service (911) should be called, and the client should be put in chilled water and transported to the hospital. People can die from heat stroke. Those who are unable to perspire are at high risk for any of the stages of heat illness.

Excess Water Accumulation

Some conditions cause an excessive accumulation of fluid in the body. This condition is called positive water balance. It occurs when more water is taken in than is used and excreted, and edema results. Hypothyroidism, congestive heart failure, hypoproteinemia (low amounts of protein), some infections, some cancers, and some renal conditions can cause such water retention because sodium is not being excreted normally. Fluids and sodium may then be restricted. Those without a medical or psychological condition are not prone to excess water intake.

Supersize USA

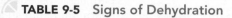

Cycling is my passion. I love cycling and have competed in some short races. Now I am ready for my first long race that will take at least 5 hours to complete. The day of the race is hot and humid, but I have my water, and there will be stations for water along the way. I am racing well and have downed my first bottle of water (480 ml) and have been riding for about 1 hour. I am drinking my second bottle of water (480 ml) and am into my second hour of racing. The hot and humid weather is taking its toll on me, and I am feeling dehydrated, so I start my third bottle (480 ml) and a fourth bottle (480 ml)—I have been riding for 3 hours. I continue to drink, and after two more bottles of water I begin to feel nauseated and really tired; I feel like I can't remember how much water I have had or how much more I need—I'm confused. I have to stop racing. I learn from the physician that I have hyponatremia (low sodium concentrations) caused by overhydration. How did I end up drinking too much water? I thought I needed a lot of water because I was perspiring so much.

The physician recognized my symptoms. After he obtained my weight and discovered I had gained weight, he knew definitively that I was suffering from overhydration. I was told that fluid intake of 500 ml/hr would have been sufficient for this 5-hour race. I also learned that I should not limit my sodium intake before the race. I will be better prepared for the next race.

ACID–BASE BALANCE

In addition to maintaining fluid and electrolyte balance, the body must also maintain **acid–base balance**. This is the regulation of hydrogen ions in body fluids (**pH** balance).

In a water solution, an acid gives off hydrogen ions and a base picks them up. Hydrochloric acid is an example of an acid found in the body. It is secreted by the stomach and is necessary for the digestion of proteins. Ammonia is a base produced in the kidneys from amino acids.

Acidic substances run from pH 1 to 7, with the lowest numbers representing the most acidic (which contain the most hydrogen ions). Alkaline substances run from pH 7 to 14, with the alkalinity increasing with the number (as the number of hydrogen ions decreases). A pH of 7 is considered neutral. Blood plasma runs from pH 7.35 to 7.45. Intracellular fluid has a pH of 6.8. The kidneys play the primary role in maintaining the acid–base balance by selecting which ions to retain and which to excrete. For the most part, what a person eats affects the acidity not of the body but of the urine.

Buffer Systems

The body has **buffer systems** that regulate hydrogen ion content in body fluids. Such a system is a mixture of a weak acid and a strong base that reacts to protect the nature of the solution in which it exists. In a normal buffer system, the ratio of base to acid is 20:1. For example, when a strong acid is added to a buffered solution, the base takes up the hydrogen ions of the strong acid, thereby weakening it. When a strong base is added to a solution, the acid of the buffer system combines with this base and weakens it.

A mixture of carbonic acid and sodium bicarbonate forms the body's main buffer system. Carbonic acid moves easily to buffer a strong alkali, and sodium bicarbonate moves easily to buffer a strong acid. Amounts are easily adjusted by the lungs and kidneys to suit needs. For example, the end products of metabolism are carbon dioxide and water, and together they can form carbonic acid. The hemoglobin in the blood carries carbon dioxide to the lungs, where the excess is excreted. If the amount of carbon dioxide is more concentrated than it should be, the medulla oblongata in the brain causes the breathing rate to increase. This increase, in turn, increases the rate at which the body rids itself of carbon dioxide. Excess sodium bicarbonate is excreted via the kidneys. The kidneys can excrete urine from pH 4.5–8. The pH of average urine is 6.

Acidosis and Alkalosis

The healthy person eating a balanced diet does not normally have to think about acid–base balance. Upsets can occur in some disease conditions, however. Renal failure, uncontrolled diabetes mellitus, starvation, or severe diarrhea can cause acidosis. This is a condition in which the body is unable to balance the need for bases with the amount of acids it is retaining. Alkalosis can occur when the body has suffered a loss of hydrochloric acid from severe vomiting or has ingested too much alkali, such as too many antacid tablets.

EXPLORING THE WEB

Search the Web for information related to the water needs of elderly and pediatric clients. How do the water needs differ in these two client populations? Why is there a difference? Why are these two populations at increased risk for dehydration? What tips can you provide to clients to maintain adequate water intake in these two client groups?

 acid–base balance
the regulation of hydrogen ions in body fluids

 pH
symbol for the degree of acidity or alkalinity of a solution

buffer systems
protective systems regulating amounts of hydrogen ions in body fluids

HEALTH AND NUTRITION CONSIDERATIONS

Clients who are required to limit both their salt and liquid intake will probably be unhappy with their diets. In such cases, it is helpful when the dietitian can discuss realistic ways of planning menus for them and *with* them. These menus should be based, of course, on good nutrition, but they also must be based on the client's normal habits and desires as much as possible. The client's former diet should be reviewed with the client. The high-salt and high-liquid foods should be pointed out and alternative foods presented in a positive manner.

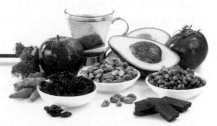

SUMMARY

Water is a component of all tissues. It is a solvent for nutrients and body wastes and provides transport for both. It is essential for hydrolysis, lubrication, and maintenance of normal temperature. Its best sources are water, beverages, fruits, vegetables, soups, and water-based desserts.

Fluid balance and electrolyte balance are dependent upon one another. An upset in one can cause an upset in the other. An inadequate supply of water can result in dehydration, which can be caused by severe diarrhea, vomiting, hemorrhage, burns, or excessive perspiration or urination. Symptoms include thirst, dry skin, fever, lowered blood pressure, and mental disorientation. Dehydration can result in death. Positive water balance is an excess accumulation of water in the body. It causes edema.

Acid–base balance is the regulation of hydrogen ions in the body. Excessive acids or inadequate amounts of base can cause acidosis. Excessive base or inadequate amounts of acids can cause alkalosis.

Healthy people eating a balanced diet need not be concerned about fluid, electrolyte, or acid–base balance, as the body has intricate maintenance systems for all.

DISCUSSION TOPICS

1. Why can people live longer without food than without water?
2. Why does water constitute a larger proportion of a man's body weight than of a woman's?
3. Describe homeostasis.
4. How do the lungs help to prevent excess acid from developing in the body?
5. What happens to the skin when it touches a red-hot pan? How might such developments on a large scale upset the body's fluid and electrolyte balance?
6. What is alkalosis? What causes it?
7. Explain how dehydration is dangerous in adults and in infants and children.
8. What does pH mean? How is it related to the homeostasis of the body?

SUGGESTED ACTIVITIES

1. Ask a nurse to describe what happens to body tissue when it is badly burned. Also ask about the treatment of burn clients, including diet.
2. Ask a nurse to describe a diabetic coma, explaining what causes it, why it can be life threatening, and how it can be treated.

REVIEW

Multiple choice. Select the *letter* that precedes the best answer.

1. Fluid within the cells is called
   a. interstitial fluid
   b. extracellular fluid
   c. intracellular fluid
   d. none of the above

2. Intravascular fluid contains
   a. interstitial fluid
   b. extracellular fluid
   c. intracellular fluid
   d. none of the above

3. In a mixture of sugar and water, water is the
   a. solute
   b. solvent
   c. solution
   d. none of the above

4. Water
   a. is essential for hydrolysis
   b. causes hydrogenation
   c. reduces hypoproteinemia
   d. is produced by hypothyroidism

5. Good sources of water include
   a. oranges and melon
   b. seafood and meats
   c. baked desserts and rice
   d. all of the above

6. The solute in the extracellular fluid principally responsible for maintaining fluid balance is
   a. potassium
   b. phosphorus
   c. calcium
   d. sodium

7. The solute in the intracellular fluid principally responsible for maintaining fluid balance is
   a. calcium
   b. phosphorus
   c. potassium
   d. sodium

8. ADH causes the kidneys to
   a. reabsorb water
   b. conserve fluid
   c. release additional sodium
   d. excrete increased amounts of urine

9. The amount of water needed by individuals
   a. varies from day to day
   b. is not affected by one's activities
   c. decreases with fever
   d. all of the above

10. Thirst is a symptom of
    a. osmosis
    b. hydrolysis
    c. cellular edema
    d. dehydration

11. What system in the body regulates acid–base balance?
    a. circulatory system
    b. buffer system
    c. respiratory system
    d. GI system

12. What are the three electrolytes that maintain the balance between intracellular and extracellular fluids?
    a. sodium, magnesium, and phosphorus
    b. sodium, chloride, and phosphorus
    c. sodium, chloride, and potassium
    d. sodium, potassium, and magnesium

Case In Point

ESHE: COPING WITH DEHYDRATION

Eshe is very excited to have gotten a job working in a steel factory that makes parts for large machines. She was told when she was hired that the factory floor could often reach temperatures of 105°F. She was told that the shifts were 12 hours in length with periodic breaks in accordance with law. Her employer encouraged Eshe to take advantage of the breaks and to drink plenty of fluids. Eshe is a 52-year-old woman from South Africa. She has recently migrated to the United States. She is overwhelmed by the new lifestyle and culture that surrounds her. She is eager to please her boss and is a very hard worker.

Eshe had been working at the plant for 2 weeks. The factory is very warm and she finds herself sweating much more than she ever has. All aspects of her job are new to her so she has been working really hard to learn the tasks she is required to do. She has been taking her routine breaks, but has spent much of her break time asking questions and learning tips from other employees. She has not been able to drink as much water as she would like to at her breaks because of this. By the time she gets home she is so exhausted she will often go right to bed. The past two nights she was so tired after work, she even skipped dinner. Last night she was awakened with excruciating cramps in her calf and ankles.

ASSESSMENT

1. How can you explain to Eshe what is happening to her?
2. What data support your conclusion?
3. What does Eshe's increasing her physical exertion at work have to do with her condition?
4. What can be expected to occur if Eshe ignores the leg cramps?

DIAGNOSIS

5. Write a nursing diagnosis for Eshe.

PLAN/GOAL

6. What would be your immediate concern for Eshe?
7. What is your concern for her nursing shift?

IMPLEMENTATION

8. What fluid is most helpful to Eshe? Why?
9. How much fluid does she need to drink?
10. What else should Eshe's nurse be aware of during her nursing shift?

EVALUATION/OUTCOME CRITERIA

11. What should Eshe look for when her plan is effective?
12. Who else could benefit from this information?

THINKING FURTHER

13. At what point could Eshe have avoided her cramping problem?

rate this plate

Eshe is becoming dehydrated due to not drinking enough fluids to replace the water lost through perspiration. How could Eshe's food intake improve her hydration status? Rate the plate.

Ham sandwich on whole-wheat bun

(the sandwich contains 3 oz. lean ham, tomato, and lettuce)

2 oz. corn chips

1 cup apple slices

8 oz. milk

Use Appendix D to look up the percentage of water in these foods. Which food ranked the highest in percent water and which one was the lowest? Would you change anything in this meal, and if so, what?

Case In Point

BRANDON: CHRONIC RENAL FAILURE

Brandon is a 49-year-old African American male. He has a strong positive family history for hypertension. Brandon was diagnosed with hypertension in his early 20s. His doctor prescribed an antihypertensive medication, but Brandon felt fine and decided not to take it. He figured if there were truly something wrong with him he would have symptoms. Several years later he had a physical for work and was again told his blood pressure was elevated. The doctor again prescribed a medication to lower his blood pressure. Brandon did take the medication this time, but only for a while. His position was eliminated about a year later and Brandon lost his insurance. Frustrated, he quit taking the medication because now he was unable to afford it. In fact, he avoided seeing a doctor for several years so he didn't have to worry about his lack of insurance. Finally, after several months of not feeling well he began to worry about his health. He was having difficulty breathing and his legs had been swollen for months. He often felt disoriented and confused. Finally, his symptoms are severe enough that Brandon decides to go to emergency room. Upon admission, Brandon's blood pressure is 232/108 with a heart rate of 112. The doctor orders several blood tests to further assess Brandon's problems. It is discovered that Brandon's BUN is 176 and his creatinine is 6.3. The doctor decides that Brandon needs immediate dialysis. A Quentin catheter is placed in Brandon's jugular vein as soon as possible and dialysis is initiated.

ASSESSMENT

1. What do you know about Brandon that puts him at risk for this problem?
2. How significant is his health problem?
3. How will dialysis alter his life?

DIAGNOSIS

4. Write a diagnostic statement about what Brandon needs to know about high blood pressure and renal failure.
5. Write a statement about the risk of excess fluid in the body.
6. Write a statement about the risk of noncompliance for renal clients.

PLAN/GOAL

7. Brandon's new renal diet is 3 grams of sodium, 3 grams of potassium, and 80 grams of protein. How could you as a nurse help improve Brandon's knowledge of his new diet and encourage compliance?
8. What goals are important for Brandon?

IMPLEMENTATION

9. What major topics would be important for the dietitian to discuss with Brandon?
10. Create a day's menu for Brandon using the dietitian's new diet. Spread the protein intake throughout the day.
11. What teaching aids could the dietitian give Brandon to help him remember his new diet?
12. How could the website http://www.choosemyplate.gov help with meal planning?
13. What impact will his CRF have on his ability to be employed? What impact will it have on his physical and psychological status?

EVALUATION/OUTCOME CRITERIA

14. After discharge from the hospital, how will the physician know that Brandon has been compliant with his diet and medications?
15. During the dialysis treatment, what is important for Brandon to do in order to have the appropriate clearances of his blood and ultrafiltration of his fluids?

THINKING FURTHER

16. Why is it important for clients with hypertension to control it?
17. Why is it important for clients with diabetes to control it?

rate this **plate**

Now that Brandon is receiving dialysis, his protein, sodium, and potassium intake will have to be closely monitored. Before experiencing complications with his health, Brandon liked to prepare and eat the following meal. Rate the plate.

5 oz. fried catfish filet

1 cup sweet potato fries

¾ cup collard greens made with fatback

1 slice cornbread with butter

½ cup watermelon and cantaloupe

20 oz. sweet iced tea

In order to prevent further health complications, should Brandon continue to prepare this type of meal? How could this meal be changed to comply with his new meal plan?

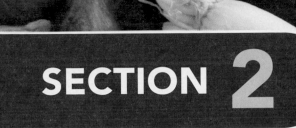

ACHIEVING HEALTH THROUGH GOOD NUTRITION

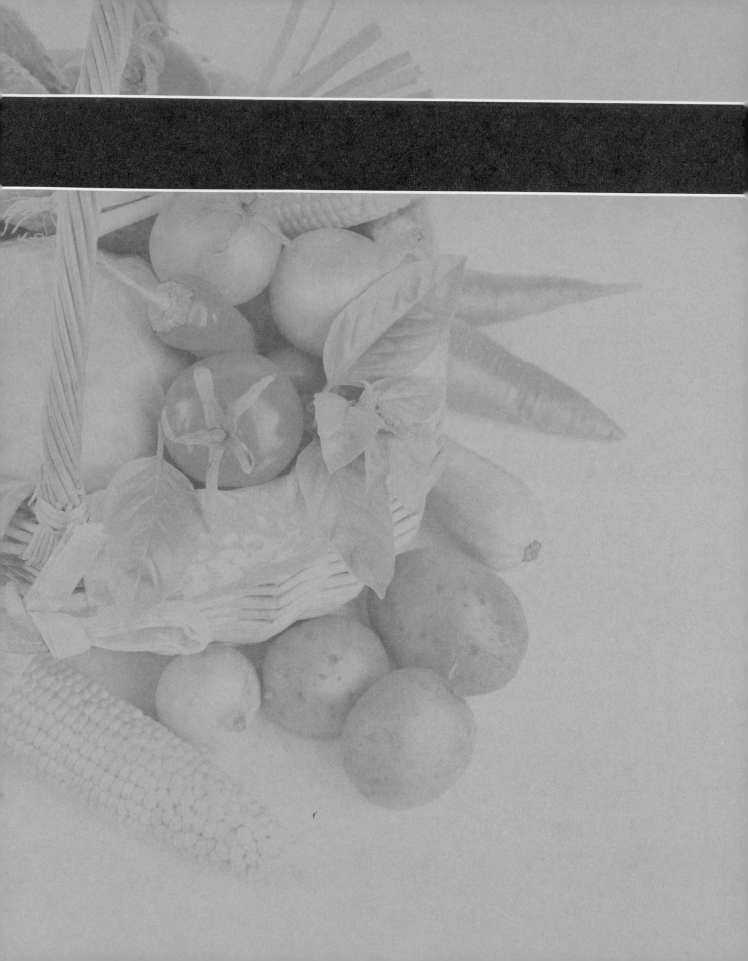

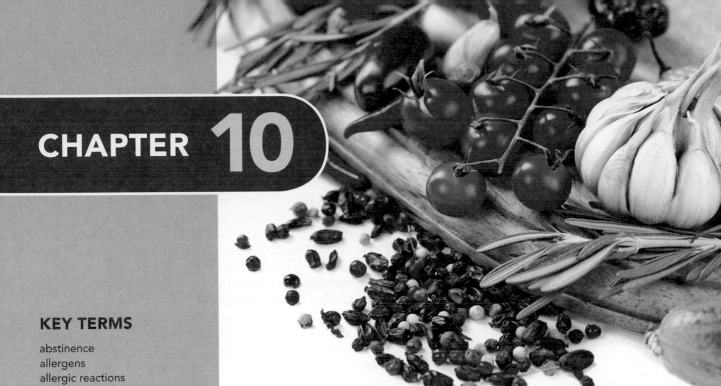

CHAPTER 10

FOODBORNE ILLNESSES AND ALLERGIES

OBJECTIVES

After studying this chapter, you should be able to:

- Identify diseases caused by contaminated food, their signs, and the means by which they are spread
- List signs of food contamination
- State precautions for protecting food from contamination
- Describe allergies and elimination diets and their uses

The most nutritious food can cause illness if it is contaminated with **pathogens** (disease-causing agents) or certain chemicals. Some of the pathogens that can cause foodborne illness include certain bacteria, viruses, molds, worms, and protozoa. The chemicals may be a natural component of specific foods, intentionally added during production or processing or accidentally added through carelessness or pollution.

There are always microorganisms in the environment. Some are useful, such as the bacteria used to make yogurt and certain cheeses. Others are

pathogens
disease-causing agents

food poisoning
foodborne illness

enterotoxins
toxins affecting mucous membranes

neurotoxins
toxins affecting the nervous system

pathogens. Pathogens may be in the air, on equipment, in food, on the skin, or in mucus and feces. Food is a particularly good breeding place for them because it provides nutrients, moisture, and often warmth. Although pathogens can be found in all food groups, they are most commonly found in foods from animal sources. Contaminated food seldom smells, looks, or tastes different from noncontaminated food.

Food poisoning is a general term for foodborne illness. When food poisoning develops as a result of a pathogen's infecting someone, it is a *foodborne infection*. When it is caused by toxins produced by the pathogen, it is called *food intoxication* and, in the case of botulism, can kill. Toxins can be produced by bacteria during food preparation or storage or by bacteria in one's digestive tract. **Enterotoxins** affect mucous membranes in the digestive tract, and **neurotoxins** affect the nervous system.

It is thought that as many as one in six Americans may experience food poisoning each year. Its typical symptoms include vomiting, diarrhea, headache, and abdominal cramps. Many never know they are suffering from food poisoning and assume they have the flu. Others, especially young children, the elderly, pregnant women, or those with compromised immune systems (such as people who are HIV positive) may become very ill, and some may die.

BACTERIA THAT CAUSE FOODBORNE ILLNESS

Campylobacter jejuni, Clostridium botulinum, Clostridium perfringens, Cyclospora Cayetanensis, Escherichia coli 0157:H7, Listeria monocytogenes, Salmonella, Shigella, and *Staphylococcus aureus* are examples of bacteria that can cause foodborne illness. Refer to Table 10-1.

Campylobacter jejuni

Campylobacter jejuni is believed to be one of the most prevalent causes of diarrhea. It is commonly found in the intestinal tracts of cattle, pigs, sheep, chickens, turkeys, dogs, and cats and can contaminate meat during slaughter. It is caused by the ingestion of live bacteria.

It can take 2–5 (or more) days to develop after infection and may last up to 7 days. Symptoms include diarrhea (sometimes bloody), fever, headache, and muscle and abdominal pain. It can be transmitted to humans via unpasteurized milk; contaminated water; and raw or undercooked meats, poultry, and shellfish.

Clostridium botulinum

Clostridium botulinum is found in soil and water, on plants, and in the intestinal tracts of animals and fish. The spores of these bacteria can divide and produce toxin in the absence of oxygen. (Spores are single cells that are produced asexually, each of which is able to develop into a new organism. They have thick, protective walls that allow them to survive unfavorable conditions.) This means that the toxin can be produced in sealed containers such as cans, jars, and vacuum-packaged foods.

TABLE 10-1 Foodborne Illnesses

BACTERIA	ASSOCIATED FOODS	SYMPTOMS AND POTENTIAL IMPACT	PREVENTION
Campylobacter jejuni	Contaminated water, raw or unpasteurized milk, and raw or undercooked meat, poultry, or shellfish.	Diarrhea (sometimes bloody), cramping, abdominal pain, and fever that appear 2–5 days after eating; may last 7 days. May spread to bloodstream and cause a life-threatening infection.	Cook meat and poultry to a safe minimum internal temperature; do not drink or consume unpasteurized milk or milk products; wash your hands after coming in contact with feces.
Clostridium botulinum	Improperly canned foods, garlic in oil, vacuum-packed and tightly wrapped food.	Bacteria produce a nerve toxin that causes illness, affecting the nervous system. Toxin affects the nervous system. Symptoms usually appear 18–36 hours, but can sometimes appear as few as 6 hours or as many as 10 days after eating; double vision, blurred vision, drooping eyelids, slurred speech, difficulty swallowing, dry mouth, and muscle weakness. If untreated, these symptoms may progress causing muscle paralysis and even death.	Do not use damaged canned foods or canned foods showing signs of swelling, leakage, punctures, holes, fractures, extensive deep rusting, or crushing/denting severe enough to prevent normal stacking. Follow safety guidelines when home canning food. Boil home canned foods for 10 minutes before eating to ensure safety. (Note: Safe home canning guidelines may be obtained from State University or County Extension Office).
Clostridium perfringens	Meats, meat products and gravy called "the cafeteria germ" because many outbreaks result from food left for long periods in steam tables or at room temperature.	Intense abdominal cramps, nausea, and diarrhea may appear 6–24 hours after eating; usually last about 1 day, but for immune-comprised individuals, symptoms may last 1–2 weeks. Complications and/or death can occur only very rarely.	Keep hot foods hot and cold foods cold! Once food is cooked, it should be held hot, at an internal temperature of 140°F or above. Use a food thermometer to make sure. Discard all perishable foods left at room temperature longer than 2 hours; 1 hour in temperatures above 90°F.
Cryptosporidium	Soil, food, water, contaminated surfaces. Swallowing contaminated water, including that from recreational sources, (e.g., a swimming pool or lake); eating uncooked or contaminated food; placing a contaminated object in the mouth.	Dehydration, weight loss, stomach cramps or pain, fever, nausea, and vomiting; respiratory symptoms may also be present. Symptoms begin 2–10 days after becoming infected, and may last 1–2 weeks. Immune-comprised individuals may experience a more serious illness.	Wash your hands before and after handling raw meat products, and after changing diapers, going to the bathroom, or touching animals. Avoid water that might be contaminated. (Do not drink untreated water from shallow wells, lakes, rivers, springs, ponds, and streams.)

(continues)

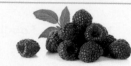

TABLE 10-1 (continued)

BACTERIA	ASSOCIATED FOODS	SYMPTOMS AND POTENTIAL IMPACT	PREVENTION
Escherichia coli O157:H7	Uncooked beef (especially ground beef), unpasteurized milk and juices (e.g., "fresh" apple cider); contaminated raw fruits and vegetables, or water. Person-to-person contamination can also occur.	Severe diarrhea (often bloody diarrhea), abdominal cramps, and vomiting. Usually little or no fever. Can begin 2–8 days, but usually 3–4 days after consumption of contaminated food or water and last about 5–7 days, depending on severity. Children under 5 are at greater risk of developing hemolytic uremic syndrome (HUS), which causes acute kidney failure.	Cook hamburgers and ground beef to a safe minimum internal temperature of 160°F. Drink only pasteurized milk, juice, or cider. Rinse fruits and vegetables under running tap water, especially those that will not be cooked. Wash your hands with warm water and soap after changing diapers, using the bathroom, handling pets, or having any contact with feces.
Listeria monocytogenes	Ready-to-eat foods such as hot dogs, luncheon meats, cold cuts, fermented or dry sausage, and other deli-style meat and poultry. Also, soft cheeses made with unpasteurized milk. Smoked seafood and salads made in the store such as ham salad, chicken salad, or seafood salad.	Fever, muscle aches, and sometimes gastrointestinal symptoms such as nausea or diarrhea. If infection spreads to the nervous system, symptoms such as headache, stiff neck, confusion, loss of balance, or convulsions can occur. Those at risk (including pregnant women and newborns, older adults, and people with weakened immune systems) may later develop more serious illness; death can result from Listeria. Can cause severe problems with pregnancy, including miscarriage or death in newborns.	Cook raw meat, poultry, and seafood to a safe minimum internal temperature; prevent cross-contamination, separating ready-to-eat foods from raw eggs, and raw meat, poultry, seafood, and their juices; wash your hands before and after handling raw meat, poultry, seafood, and egg products. Those with a weakened immune system should avoid eating hot dogs and deli meats, unless they are reheated to 165°F or steaming hot. Do not drink raw (unpasteurized) milk or foods that have unpasteurized milk in them (e.g., soft cheeses). Do not eat deli salads made in store, such as ham, egg, tuna, or seafood salad.
Salmonella (over 2,300 types)	Raw or undercooked eggs, poultry, and meat; unpasteurized milk and juice; cheese and seafood; and contaminated fresh fruits and vegetables.	Diarrhea, fever, and abdominal cramps usually appear 12–72 hours after eating; may last 4–7 days. In people with weakened immune system, the infection may be more severe and lead to serious complications, including death.	Cook raw meat, poultry, and egg products to a safe temperature. Do not eat raw or undercooked eggs. Avoid consuming raw or unpasteurized milk or other dairy products. Produce should be thoroughly washed before consuming.
Shigella (over 30 types)	Person-to-person by fecal-oral route; fecal contamination of food and water. Most outbreaks result from food, especially salads, prepared and handled by workers using poor personal hygiene.	Disease referred to as "shigellosis" or bacillary dysentery. Diarrhea (watery or bloody), fever, abdominal cramps; 1–2 days from ingestion of bacteria and usually resolves in 5–7 days.	Hand washing is a very important step to prevent shigellosis. Always wash your hands with warm water and soap before handling food and after using the bathroom, changing diapers, or having contact with an infected person.

(continues)

TABLE 10-1 *(continued)*

BACTERIA	ASSOCIATED FOODS	SYMPTOMS AND POTENTIAL IMPACT	PREVENTION
Staphylococcus aureus	Commonly found on the skin and in the noses of up to 25% of healthy people and animals. Person-to-person through food from improper food handling. Multiply rapidly at room temperature to produce a toxin that causes illness. Contaminated milk and cheeses.	Severe nausea, abdominal cramps, vomiting, and diarrhea occur 30 minutes to 6 hours after eating; recovery from 1 to 3 days—longer if severe dehydration occurs.	Because the toxins produced by this bacterium are resistant to heat and cannot be destroyed by cooking, preventing the contamination of food before the toxin can be produced is important. Keep hot foods hot (over 140°F) and cold foods cold (40°F or under); wash your hands with warm water and soap and wash kitchen counters with hot water and soap before and after preparing food.
Vibrio vulnificus	Uncooked or raw seafood (fish or shellfish); oysters.	In healthy persons symptoms include diarrhea, stomach pain, and vomiting. May result in a blood infection and death for those with a weakened immune system particularly with underlying liver disease.	Do not eat raw oysters or other raw shellfish; cook shellfish (oysters, clams, mussels) thoroughly. Prevent cross-contamination by separating cooked seafood and other foods from raw seafood and its juices. Refrigerate cooked shellfish within 2 hours after cooking.

Source: United States Departments of Agriculture. Food Safety and Inspection Service. Foodborne Illness: What Consumers Need to Know. May 24, 2011. http://www.fsis.usda.gov

The spores are extremely heat resistant and must be boiled for 6 hours before they will be destroyed. Such a lengthy time will, of course, destroy the food they have infected. Home canned goods should be boiled for 10 minutes to ensure safety. **Botulism** is perhaps the rarest but most deadly of all food poisonings. Symptoms usually appear within 18–36 hours after eating and include double vision, speech difficulties, inability to swallow, and respiratory paralysis. The disease can be fatal in 5–10% of cases. Great care must be taken to prevent botulism when canning foods at home. The Centers for Disease Control and Prevention (CDC) reported that an average of 145 cases of botulism occur annually. If a can bulges, *Clostridium botulinum* may be present and can be fatal. A good rule of thumb is "If in doubt, throw it out" where children and animals cannot reach it.

 botulism
deadliest of food poisonings; caused by the bacteria *Clostridium botulinum*

Clostridium perfringens

Clostridium perfringens is often called the "cafeteria" or "buffet germ" because it tends to infect those who eat food that has been standing on buffets or steam tables for long periods. *C. perfringens* is found in soil dust, sewage, and the intestinal tracts of animals. It is a spore-forming pathogen that needs little oxygen. The bacteria are destroyed by cooking, but the spores can survive it.

Clostridium perfringens is transmitted by eating heavily contaminated food. Symptoms include nausea, diarrhea, and inflammation of the stomach and intestines. Symptoms may appear within 6–24 hours of ingestion and last approximately 24 hours. The CDC estimates that about 10,000 actual cases occur annually in the United States.

To best prevent it, hot foods should be kept at or above 140°F and cold foods below 40°F. Leftovers should be heated to 165°F before serving. Foods should be stored at temperatures of 40°F or lower. People with compromised immune systems should be very cautious concerning *C. perfringens*.

Cryptosporidium

Cryptosporidium is a parasite that causes cryptosporidiosis in the intestines of humans and animals. It can live outside of the body for long periods of time and is commonly found in infected stool of animals or humans. "Crypto" is commonly found in contaminated soil, food, and water, as well as in recreational water sources including swimming pools, lakes, rivers, and hot tubs.

The most common symptom of Crypto is watery diarrhea. Other symptoms include stomach cramps, fever, nausea, vomiting, and dehydration. Symptoms usually begin 2–10 days after becoming infected with the parasite and may last 1–2 weeks. Practicing good hygiene such as washing hands after going to the bathroom and handling raw meat can prevent infection. Contaminated water from wells, lakes, springs, and ponds should also be avoided.

Escherichia coli (E. coli 0157:H7)

Escherichia coli, commonly called *E. coli,* is a group of bacteria that can cause illness in humans. *E. coli* 0157:H7 is a highly infectious strain of this group. These bacteria can be found in the intestines of some mammals (including humans and animals used for food), in raw milk, and in water contaminated by animal or human feces.

Escherichia coli are transmitted to humans through contaminated water, unpasteurized milk or apple juice, raw or rare ground beef products, unwashed fruits or vegetables, and directly from person-to-person. Plant foods can be contaminated by fertilization with raw manure or irrigation with contaminated water. The CDC estimates 70,000 cases of infection with *E. coli* 0157:H7 occur in the United States every year.

Symptoms include severe abdominal cramps, diarrhea that may be watery or bloody, and nausea. Symptoms may occur within 3–8 days of ingestion with most people recovering within 10 days. Sometimes, however, *E. coli* 0157:H7 can cause hemorrhagic colitis (inflammation of the colon). This in turn can result in *hemolytic uremic syndrome* (HUS) in children, which can damage the kidneys.

Escherichia coli can be controlled by careful choice and cooking of foods. All meats and poultry should be cooked thoroughly. Ground beef, veal, and lamb should be cooked to 160°F and ground poultry to at least 165°F. Fruits and vegetables should be carefully washed, and unpasteurized milk and other dairy products and vegetable and fruit juices should be avoided. People with compromised immune systems should be especially vigilant.

Listeria monocytogenes

Listeria monocytogenes is a bacteria often found in human and animal intestines and in milk, leafy vegetables, and soil. It can grow in the refrigerator and can be transmitted to humans by unpasteurized dairy foods such as milk, soft cheeses, and ice creams and via raw leafy vegetables and processed meats.

Listeria monocytogenes can affect a person from 12 hours to 8 days after ingestion. Symptoms include fatigue, fever, chills, headache, backache, abdominal pain, and diarrhea. It can develop into more serious conditions and cause respiratory distress, spontaneous abortion, or meningitis.

To prevent infection by *Listeria monocytogenes,* meats and poultry should be thoroughly cooked and salad greens carefully washed. Attention must be paid to all dairy products—especially the unfamiliar from new sources—to be certain they have been pasteurized.

Salmonellosis

Salmonellosis (commonly called Salmonella) is an infection caused by the *Salmonella* bacteria. **Salmonella** can be found in raw eggs, poultry, and meat; unpasteurized milk and juice; cheese and seafood; and contaminated fruits and vegetables. It is transmitted by eating contaminated food or by contact with a carrier. Salmonellosis is characterized by headache, vomiting, diarrhea, abdominal cramps, and fever. Symptoms generally begin from 12–72 hours after eating. In severe cases, it can result in death. One species of *Salmonella* causes typhoid fever. Those who suffer the most severe cases are typically the very young, the elderly, and the weak or incapacitated.

 Salmonella
an infection caused by the *Salmonella* bacteria

Refrigeration (40°F or lower) inhibits the growth of these bacteria, but they can remain alive in the freezer and in dried foods. Heating foods to 145–165°F will render *Salmonella* bacteria, making it safe to ingest. To prevent contamination, thaw poultry and meats in the refrigerator or microwave and cook immediately. Avoid cross-contamination of raw and cooked foods by carefully cleaning utensils and counter surfaces that were in contact with raw food. Raw or undercooked eggs, or foods that contain them, should not be eaten. Even a taste of raw cookie dough or Caesar salad dressing made with raw egg yolk can cause contamination. People with compromised immune systems should be especially careful.

Shigella

Shigella bacteria are found in the intestinal tract and thus the feces of infected individuals. The disease they cause is called *shigellosis.* These bacteria are typically passed on by an infected food handler who did not practice proper hand washing after using the toilet. They are also found on plants that were fertilized with untreated animal feces or given contaminated water. According to The Association for Dressings and Sauces, research has found that commercially prepared mayonnaise is not the common culprit for foodborne illnesses in cold salads. *Shigella* are destroyed by heat, but infected cold foods such as tuna, chicken, or egg salads are common carriers and should be kept on ice when served.

Shigellosis can occur from 1 day to 1 week following infection. Symptoms include diarrhea (sometimes with blood and mucus), fever, chills, headache, nausea, and abdominal cramps and can lead to dehydration. Some people, however, experience no symptoms. Foods must be cooked to 145–165°F to make them safe for consumption.

Staphylococcus aureus

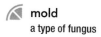
Staphylococcus (staph)
genus of bacteria causing food poisoning called "staph" or "staphylococcal poisoning"

Staphylococcus aureus bacteria are found on human skin, in infected cuts and pimples, and in noses and throats. Staphylococcal poisoning is commonly called **Staphylococcus (staph)**. These bacteria grow in meats; poultry; fish; egg dishes; salads such as potato, egg, macaroni, and tuna; and cream-filled pastries. This poisoning is transmitted by carriers and by eating foods that contain the toxin these bacteria create.

Symptoms, which include vomiting, diarrhea, and abdominal cramps, begin within 30 minutes to 6 hours after ingestion of the toxin and last from 24–72 hours. Staph is considered a mild illness.

The growth of these bacteria is inhibited if foods are kept at temperatures above 140°F or below 40°F. Their toxin can be destroyed by boiling the food for several hours or by heating it in a pressure cooker at 240°F for 30 minutes. Both of these methods would destroy both the appeal and nutrient content of the infected foods. It is more practical to safely discard foods suspected of being contaminated.

OTHER SUBSTANCES THAT CAUSE FOOD POISONING

mold
a type of fungus

Mold is a type of fungus. Its roots go down, into the food, and it grows a stalk upward on which spores form. The green "fuzzy" part that can be seen by the naked eye is where the spores are found. Some spores cause respiratory problems and allergic reactions for some people. For this reason, moldy food should never be smelled.

Some molds produce a dangerous mycotoxin called aflatoxin that can cause cancer. It can develop in spoiled peanuts and peanut butter, soybeans, grains, nuts, and spices. Symptoms of such an infection include abdominal pain, vomiting, and diarrhea, and may occur from 1 day to several months after ingestion. It can cause liver and skin damage and, ultimately, cancer.

The Food and Drug Administration observes the aflatoxin content of foods closely, and although this toxin cannot as yet be totally eradicated, foods containing more than a very minute amount of it cannot be sold by one state to another.

Neither cooking nor refrigeration destroys this toxin. Cheese may develop mold, and that part should be cut away to a depth of at least 1 inch. (Cheeses such as bleu or Roquefort that were intentionally ripened by harmless molds are safe to eat.) Fruits and vegetables showing signs of mold should not be purchased.

Trichinella spiralis is a parasitic worm that causes **trichinosis**. This disease is transmitted by eating inadequately cooked pork from pigs that are infected with the *T. spiralis* parasite. Symptoms include abdominal pain, vomiting, fever, chills, and muscle pain. Symptoms occur about 24 hours after ingesting infected pork. Cooking all pork to an internal temperature of at least 170°F kills the organism and prevents this disease. It can also be destroyed by freezing.

Dysentery is a disease caused by protozoa (tiny, one-celled animal). The protozoa are introduced to food by carriers or contaminated water. They cause severe diarrhea that can occur intermittently until the client is treated appropriately.

trichinosis
disease caused by the parasitic roundworm *Trichinella spiralis;* can be transmitted through undercooked pork

dysentery
disease caused by microorganism; characterized by diarrhea

PREVENTION OF FOODBORNE ILLNESSES

Strict federal, state, and local laws regulate the commercial production of food in the United States, and dairies, canneries, bakeries, and meatpacking plants are all subject to government inspection. Nevertheless, errors and accidents can and do occur, and illness can result. *Most foodborne illnesses occur because of the ignorance or carelessness of people who handle food.* People can introduce pathogens to food, prevent them from reaching it, or kill them with appropriate cooking temperatures.

Cleanliness is especially important in preventing foodborne illness. When kitchen equipment such as a cutting board, meat grinder, or countertop is used for preparing pathogen-infected foods and not cleaned properly afterward, noninfected food that is subsequently prepared with this equipment can become infected by the same pathogen(s). This is called cross-contamination. Dishes used to hold uncooked meat, poultry, fish, or eggs must always be washed before cooked foods are placed on them.

EXPLORING THE WEB

Choose one of the pathogens in the text that causes foodborne illness. Research this pathogen using the Web. What sources can you find on the pathogen? Create a fact sheet listing the signs and symptoms of the illness, the foods commonly infected with the pathogen, assessment of the client for the presence of the illness, and treatment. Also include tips on prevention of the illness.

In The Media

Eating Raw Cookie Dough

Anyone who has ever baked homemade cookies knows how tempting it can be to munch on the batter. A new study investigated the cause of a large outbreak of *E. coli* in 2009 and blamed raw chocolate chip cookie dough. The 2009 outbreak sickened at least 80 people across 30 states, 35 of whom had to be hospitalized. But what ingredient in the dough was to blame for the outbreak and how did it become contaminated? Investigations ruled out *Salmonella* from the eggs and other raw products, and found that the culprit in this case was likely not the eggs but flour. Flour does not undergo any specific processing to kill pathogens so it was the most likely suspect for contamination of the cookie dough. In the study, published in the *Journal of Clinical Infectious Diseases*, several people who were sickened bought the cookie dough with the sole intention of eating it raw and not baking. Studies conducted in 2008 found that 53% of college students admitted to eating unbaked cookie dough. The bottom line to consumers is to not eat raw cookie dough and to safely follow the four basic messages of food safety, which are clean, separate, cook, and chill.

(Source: Adapted from O'Connor, Anahad. Beware of Raw Cookie Dough. *The New York Times*. 2011. http://www.well.blogs.nytimes.com)

When food workers fail to wash their hands after blowing their noses or using the toilet, they can "share" their germs very easily. Mucus and feces are favorite breeding areas of pathogens.

Food workers who have even small cuts on their hands must wear gloves because a wound could carry a pathogen. Foods must be covered and stored properly to keep dust, insects, and animals from reaching and possibly contaminating them. Water from unknown sources should not be used for cooking because it, too, can carry pathogens.

Temperatures during preparation and storage of food must be carefully observed. When infected foods are undercooked, the pathogen is not destroyed and can be passed to consumers (Table 10-2). Foods allowed to stand at temperatures between 40°F and 140°F provide an ideal breeding place for pathogens (Figure 10-1).

Leftover food should always be refrigerated as soon as the meal is finished and covered when it is cold. It should not be allowed to cool to room

TABLE 10-2 Cooking Temperatures

PRODUCT	FAHRENHEIT
Eggs and Egg Dishes	
• Eggs	Cook until yolk and white are firm
• Egg dishes	160°
Fresh Beef, Veal, Lamb	
• Ground products like hamburger (prepared as patties, meatloaf, meatballs, etc.)	160°
• Roasts, steaks, and chops	
• Medium rare	145°
• Medium	160°
• Well done	170°
Fresh Pork	
• All cuts including ground product	145°
Poultry	
• Ground chicken, turkey	165°
• Whole chicken, turkey (well done)	180°
• Whole bird with stuffing (stuffing must reach 165°)	180°
• Poultry breasts, roasts	170°
• Thighs, wings	Cook until juices run clear
Ham	
• Fresh (raw)	160°
• Fully cooked, to reheat	140°

Source: U.S. Department of Agriculture, Food Safety and Inspection Service, Washington, DC. http://www.fsis.usda.gov.

temperature before it is refrigerated. Frozen food should be either cooked from the frozen state or thawed in the refrigerator. (When cooked from the frozen state, cooking time will generally increase by at least 50%.) Frozen food should not be thawed at room temperature. Food must always be protected from dust, insects, and animals.

Carriers are people (or animals) capable of transmitting infectious (disease-causing) organisms. Often the carrier suffers no effects from the organism and therefore is unaware of the danger she or he represents. Food

 carriers
those who are capable of transmitting an infectious organism

FIGURE 10-1 Temperatures of food for control of bacteria.

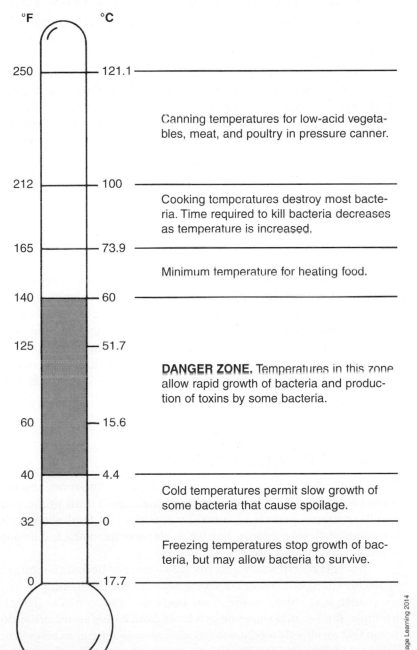

°F   °C

250 — 121.1

Canning temperatures for low-acid vegetables, meat, and poultry in pressure canner.

212 — 100

Cooking temperatures destroy most bacteria. Time required to kill bacteria decreases as temperature is increased.

165 — 73.9

Minimum temperature for heating food.

140 — 60

125 — 51.7

DANGER ZONE. Temperatures in this zone allow rapid growth of bacteria and production of toxins by some bacteria.

60 — 15.6

40 — 4.4

Cold temperatures permit slow growth of some bacteria that cause spoilage.

32 — 0

Freezing temperatures stop growth of bacteria, but may allow bacteria to survive.

0 — 17.7

© Cengage Learning 2014

EXPLORING THE WEB

Search the website of the Food Safety and Inspection Service of the U.S. Department of Agriculture (http://www.fsis.usda.gov). Look for information about eliminating pathogens and keeping food safe during preparation and storage. What helpful tips can you find? Create a fact sheet on maintaining the safety of food during preparation and storage in the home environment using the tips you find here.

> ### TABLE 10-3 Ways to Prevent Food Poisoning
>
> - Keep kitchen and equipment thoroughly clean.
> - Wash hands after blowing nose or using bathroom.
> - Wear gloves if cooking with a wounded hand
> - Cover and store foods to prevent microbes or animals from reaching it.
> - Cook foods to appropriate temperatures.
> - Limit standing time at temperatures between 40°F and 140°F.
> - Prevent known carriers from preparing foods.
> - Select only packages and jars that were sealed by the manufacturer.
> - Avoid bulging cans, foods that look or smell odd, and foods showing signs of mold.

insecticides
agents that destroy insects

allergy
sensitivity to specific substance(s)

hypersensitivity
abnormally strong sensitivity to certain substance(s)

allergens
substance causing allergy

urticaria
hives; common allergic reaction

dermatitis
inflammation of the skin

allergic reactions
adverse physical reactions to specific substances

workers should be tested regularly to confirm that they are not carriers of communicable diseases.

Selection of food should be made with great care. Packages and jars should be properly sealed. Cans should not bulge. Foods that look or smell at all unusual and foods showing signs of mold should be left in the store. Only pasteurized milk and dairy products should be used (Table 10-3).

MISCELLANEOUS FOOD POISONINGS

Occasionally, food poisoning is caused by ingesting certain plants or animals that contain poison. Examples are plants such as poisonous mushrooms, rhubarb leaves, and fish from polluted water.

Poisoning also can result from ingesting cleaning agents, **insecticides**, or excessive amounts of a drug. Children may swallow cleaning agents or medicines. The cook may mistakenly use a poison instead of a cooking ingredient. Sometimes insecticides cling to fresh fruits and vegetables. It is essential that all potential poisons be kept out of the reach of young children and kept separate from all food supplies. Fresh fruits and vegetables should be thoroughly washed before being eaten.

FOOD ALLERGIES

An **allergy** is an altered reaction of the tissues of some individuals to substances that, in similar amounts, are harmless to other people. The substances causing **hypersensitivity** are called **allergens**. Some common allergens are pollen, dust, animal dander (bits of dried skin), drugs, cosmetics, and certain foods. This discussion will be limited to allergic reactions to foods. A food allergy occurs when the immune system reacts to a food substance, usually a protein. When such a reaction occurs, antibodies form and cause allergic symptoms. An altered reaction to a specific food that does not involve the immune system is called (the specific food) *intolerance.* Approximately 6–8% of children and 3.7% of adults are known to have food allergies; many of these allergies began in the first year of life.

Types of Allergic Reactions

Sometimes allergic reactions are immediate, and sometimes several hours elapse before signs occur. Allergic individuals seem most prone to allergic reactions during periods of stress. Typical signs of food allergies include hay fever, **urticaria**, edema, headache, **dermatitis**, nausea, dizziness, and asthma (which causes breathing difficulties).

Allergic reactions are uncomfortable and can be detrimental to health. When breathing difficulties are severe, they are life-threatening.

Allergic reactions to the same food can differ in two individuals. For example, the fact that someone gets hives from eating strawberries does not mean that an allergic reaction to strawberries will appear as hives in another member of the same family. Allergic reactions can even differ from time to time with the same individual.

Treatment for Allergies

The simplest treatment for allergies is to remove the item that causes the allergic reaction. However, because of the variety of allergic reactions, finding the allergen can be difficult.

When food allergies are suspected, it is wise for the client to keep a food diary for several days and to record all food and drink ingested as well as allergic reactions and the time of their onset. Such records can help pinpoint specific allergens. Some common food allergens are listed in Table 10-4. It is common for other foods in the same class as the allergens to cause allergic reactions as well. Cooking sometimes alters the foods and can eliminate allergic reactions in some people.

Blood tests may be used to find the allergen or allergens. **Skin tests** are sometimes used to detect allergies. However, food allergies can be difficult to determine from skin tests.

After completion of the allergy testing, the client is usually placed on an **elimination diet**. For 1 or 2 weeks the client does not eat any of the tested compounds that gave a positive reaction. The client includes in the diet the foods that almost no one reacts to, such as rice, fresh meats and poultry, noncitrus fruits, and vegetables. Sometimes, these diets allow only a limited number of foods and can be nutritionally inadequate. If that is the case, vitamin and mineral supplements may be prescribed.

When relief is found from the allergic symptoms, the client is continued on the diet, and gradually other foods are added to the diet at a rate of only one every 4–7 days. Those foods most likely to produce allergic reactions are added last until an allergic reaction occurs. The allergy can then be pinpointed, and the offending foods eliminated from the diet. Knowing the cause of the allergy enables the client to lead a healthy, normal life, provided that eliminating these foods does not affect her or his nutrition.

If the elimination of the allergen results in a diet deficient in certain nutrients, suitable substitutes for those nutrients must be found. For example,

skin tests
allergy tests using potential allergens on scratches on the skin

elimination diet
limited diet in which only certain foods are allowed; intended to find the food allergen causing reaction

TABLE 10-4 Common Food Allergens

Milk
Wheat
Corn
Eggs
Citrus fruit
Strawberries
Tomatoes
Legumes
Tree nuts
Peanuts
Chocolate
Soybeans
Pork
Fish
Shellfish

© Cengage Learning 2014

SPOTLIGHT *on Life Cycle*

In 2011, The National Institute of Allergy and Infectious Disease published *Guidelines for the Diagnosis and Management of Food Allergy in the United States* for physicians and other health care professionals as well as clients, families, and caregivers. Families with children who have food allergies can access the guideline summary to learn more about how to manage the disorder and start conversations with their doctors about allergy care options for their children. The guidelines provide the following information:

- Definitions of food allergy and disorders associated with food allergy
- Descriptions of the development of food allergy and conditions associated with food allergy
- Recommendations on how to diagnose, manage life-threatening reactions and food-induced anaphylaxis, and other acute reactions

Definitions, common food allergens, how food allergies develop, and ways to manage food allergies after diagnosis are some of the numerous topics discussed within the guidelines. Being knowledgeable about allergies and the care for them will make discussions with a health professional more understandable and easier.

(Source: Adapted from National Institute of Allergy and Infectious Diseases, Department of Health and Human Services, National Institutes of Health. May 2011)

EXPLORING THE WEB

Go to the website for the International Food Information Council Foundation (http://www.ific.org). Search for information on allergic reactions and foods. What types of illnesses can be caused by food allergies? How are these allergies detected? Can you locate a recipe source online for individuals with food allergies?

desensitized
having gradually reduced the body's sensitivity (allergic reaction) to specific items

abstinence
avoidance

if a client is allergic to citrus fruits, other foods rich in vitamin C to which the client is not allergic must be found. If the allergy is to milk, soybean milk may be substituted.

The client must be taught the food sources of the nutrient or nutrients lacking so that other foods can be substituted that are nutritionally equal to those causing the allergy. It is essential that the client be taught to read the labels on commercially prepared foods and to check the ingredients of restaurant foods carefully. Baked products, mixes, meat loaf, or pancakes may contain egg, milk, or wheat that may be responsible for the allergic reaction.

Sometimes, however, the allergies require such a restriction of foods that the diet does become nutritionally inadequate. As in all cases of allergy, and particularly in such cases, it is hoped that the client can become **desensitized** to the allergens so that a nutritionally balanced diet can be restored. The client is desensitized by eating a minute amount of food allergen after a period of complete **abstinence** from it. The amount of the allergen is gradually increased until the client can tolerate it.

HEALTH AND NUTRITION CONSIDERATIONS

Some clients will need simple instructions from the health care professional about avoiding microbial contamination of food supplies at home. Many, if not most, should be warned not to thaw food at room temperature. Others should be reminded that leftover foods should *not* be cooled at room temperature before being refrigerated.

Clients with food allergies will require careful training to avoid their specific allergens. They must be taught to read food labels carefully and to ask for the ingredients of foods in restaurants and at friends' homes. Role-playing is an effective way to help such clients.

Supersize **USA**

Camden is eating lunch for the first time at school. He will be given a choice of white or chocolate milk, a "hot pack" containing chicken nuggets and tator tots, and a "cold pack" containing fruit and graham crackers. Camden chose to eat the chicken nuggets, two tator tots, a bite of fruit, one graham cracker, and chocolate milk. He is not a big eater, so he will be hungry when he gets home from school. Once home from school, he dives into potato chips and soda for a snack while watching television. He continues to snack for about an hour, consuming half a large bag of chips and two sodas. If his behavior continues over time, Camden will increase his risks of becoming obese.

One in three children is obese or overweight. To encourage healthy eating, Camden should have fresh fruits and vegetables available after school for a snack. Instead of watching television for an hour after school, increasing physical activity could reduce possible weight gain. Replace sugary drinks such as soda and fruit beverages with milk and 100% fruit juice. If calorie-dense foods are not purchased, a child will not have access to them. Therefore, it is important to offer nutrient-dense, healthy snacks such as string cheese, ½ a peanut butter sandwich, and yogurt for growing children.

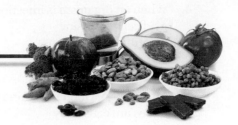

SUMMARY

Infection or poisoning traced to food is usually caused by human ignorance or carelessness. The serving of safe meals is essentially the responsibility of the cook. Food should not be prepared by anyone who has or carries a contagious disease. All fresh fruits and vegetables should be washed before being eaten. Meats, poultry, fish, eggs, and dairy products should be refrigerated. Pork should always be cooked to the well-done stage. Food should be covered to prevent contamination by dust, insects, or animals. Garbage should also be covered so that it does not attract insects. Hands that prepare foods should be clean and free of cuts or wounds. Kitchen equipment should be spotless. Finally, the food itself should be safe. People should avoid foods containing natural poisons.

Food allergies can cause many different and unpleasant symptoms. Elimination diets are used to determine their causes. Some of the most common food allergens have been found to be milk, chocolate, eggs, tomatoes, fish, citrus fruit, legumes, strawberries, and wheat.

DISCUSSION TOPICS

1. Name four types of foodborne illness. If any class member has suffered from one, ask the person to describe the symptoms.
2. How does food become contaminated?
3. Why should foods be refrigerated?
4. What are allergies? What can cause them?
5. What are some common allergic reactions to food? How can they be avoided?
6. Do people inherit allergies? Explain.
7. Of what use is a food diary in relation to allergies? What are elimination diets, and when are they used? What is the most difficult part of treating food allergies?
8. How can an allergic client be desensitized?
9. Is an elimination diet always nutritious? Explain.

10. Explain how eggs, wheat, or milk may be hidden in each of the following foods: mayonnaise, bread, rye crackers, potato salad, gravy, meat loaf, breaded veal cutlet, bologna, malted milk.

SUGGESTED ACTIVITIES

1. Ask a doctor or registered nurse to explain skin tests to the class. Discuss these tests after the lecture.
2. Ask someone with food allergies to speak to the class. Follow this talk with questions from the audience.
3. Visit a restaurant kitchen. Look for practices that may lead to potential food poisoning. Note the practices and uses of equipment designed to prevent food poisoning.
4. Ask the class if anyone has had a foodborne illness. What food caused the illness? What were the symptoms? How long were you sick?

REVIEW

Multiple choice. Select the *letter* that precedes the best answer.

1. A microorganism is
   a. a unit of measurement
   b. sometimes pathogenic
   c. a component of a microscope
   d. an individual human cell
2. Which of the following refrigeration temperatures inhibits the growth of *Salmonella*?
   a. 42°F
   b. 41°F
   c. 39°F
   d. 50°F
3. Someone who is capable of spreading an infectious organism but is not sick is called a
   a. food handler
   b. carrier
   c. transport
   d. fomite

4. When an organism is infectious, it is
   a. disease-causing
   b. prone to infections
   c. not contagious
   d. always fatal

5. Most cases of food poisoning in the United States are caused by
   a. careless processing in commercial factories
   b. lack of government inspection
   c. careless handling of food in the kitchen
   d. house pets

6. Food poisoning symptoms generally include
   a. joint pain
   b. constipation
   c. abdominal upset and headache
   d. swelling of the feet

7. Salmonella infections and staphylococcal poisoning are caused by
   a. a virus   c. protozoa
   b. bacteria   d. parasites

8. The deadliest of the bacterial food poisonings is
   a. staphylococcal poisoning
   b. salmonellosis
   c. botulism
   d. perfringens poisoning

9. The disease caused by a parasite sometimes found in pork is
   a. tularemia   c. avitaminosis
   b. dysentery   d. trichinosis

10. The disease caused by a protozoan and characterized by severe diarrhea is
    a. salmonellosis
    b. botulism
    c. dysentery
    d. infectious hepatitis

11. Foods may be contaminated by
    a. people
    b. overcooking them
    c. refrigeration
    d. all of the above

12. The temperatures in the danger zone that encourage bacterial growth are from
    a. 0–32°F
    b. 32–60°F
    c. 40–140°F
    d. 125–212°F

13. Leftover foods should be
    a. put in the refrigerator immediately after meals
    b. cooled to room temperature before refrigerating
    c. cooled in the refrigerator for at least an hour before freezing
    d. stored unwrapped in the refrigerator

14. Frozen foods should be
    a. thawed at room temperature
    b. refrozen if not used immediately after thawing
    c. thawed in the refrigerator
    d. any of the above

15. An adverse physical reaction to a food is called a food
    a. refusal
    b. allergy
    c. symptom
    d. allergen

16. Substances that cause altered physical reactions are called
    a. symptoms
    b. allergies
    c. allergens
    d. abstinence

17. One of the typical symptoms of food allergies is
    a. hives
    b. colitis
    c. dry mouth
    d. diarrhea

18. The simplest treatment for a food allergy is
    a. a skin test
    b. allergy shots
    c. elimination of the allergen
    d. the use of penicillin

19. In cases of food allergy, an elimination diet may be prescribed to
    a. desensitize the client
    b. avoid medication
    c. avoid surgery
    d. find the allergen

20. Some foods that frequently cause an allergic reaction are
    a. milk, eggs, and wheat
    b. lamb, rice, and sugar
    c. chocolate and strawberries
    d. rice and pears

Case In Point

ALAMEDA: LISTERIA INFECTION DURING PREGNANCY

Alameda is 8 months pregnant with her second child. She has been very busy trying to get ready for the new baby and balance life with a toddler. She has been very tired lately. In an effort to save money and free up a little extra time, she has not been cooking as she usually does. Alameda and her husband are Native Americans and she still loves to cook many of the same foods they ate growing up. While she knows her children will probably be influenced by many American customs and foods, she likes to keep the Native American culture and cuisine within their home. Recently, Alameda and her family have been eating quite a number of simple meals such as lunchmeat sandwiches, raw vegetables with ranch dressing, salads, and fresh fruit. Cutting down on food prep and cooking has given Alameda time for an extra nap here and there, too.

This morning Alameda awoke to flu-like symptoms. She aches all over her body and also has a stiff neck. Since she is currently 32 weeks pregnant she thought she should give her doctor a call. After examining Alameda, the doctor runs a blood test to confirm his suspicions. After the blood work is completed, the doctor tells Alameda she has Listeria. He tells Alameda that pregnant women are 20 times more susceptible to Listeria infections than the average population. He explains that raw meats such as lunchmeats, raw fruits and vegetables, and unpasteurized products often cause Listeria infections. He prescribes an antibiotic for Alameda and requests that she follow up with him again next week. He also instructs Alameda to make sure she heats any meats and vegetables she consumes thoroughly.

ASSESSMENT

1. What is Listeria?
2. What food sources may contain Listeria?
3. What are the symptoms of Listeria?
4. How can Listeria infection be prevented?

DIAGNOSIS

5. Write a nursing diagnosis for Alameda.

PLAN/GOAL

6. What should Alameda know about Listeria infections during pregnancy?
7. Are there any medications that are recommended for Listeria infection?

IMPLEMENTATION

8. Why is it important for Alameda to follow the recommended guidelines for preventing Listeria?

EVALUATION/OUTCOME CRITERIA

9. How will Alameda's doctor know she is following the recommended guidelines?

THINKING FURTHER

10. Aside from pregnant women, who may also be at increased risk for Listeria infections?

rate this **plate**

Alameda takes the doctor's advice and takes extra precaution when eating luncheon meats and fresh produce. Alameda's family recently hosted a baby shower for her, where a lunch buffet was prepared by friends and family. The buffet consisted of the following items.

Cold cut tray consisting of turkey, ham, roast beef, and cheeses (served over ice)

Relish tray with pickles, olives, and condiments

Baked cheesy potato salad

Green salad with egg and tomato

Macaroni salad

Pretzels and potato chips

Cold cheese ball with crackers

Previously baked crab dip

Vegetable tray

Fruit salad

Cupcakes and cookies

Make a plate that would be safe for Alameda to eat, telling why you chose what you did.

Case In Point

CARSON: DISCOVERING A SHELLFISH ALLERGY

Carson is a 9-year-old boy from Indiana. He is very excited about the long-awaited summer vacation his family has been planning. His family is headed to Bar Harbor, Maine, to relax and enjoy some deep-sea fishing. Carson has often been fishing with his grand-parents at their lake home, but he has never been deep-sea fishing. He is very excited and anxious to try his hand at helping to clean and cook his catch! Many of the local restaurants allow people to clean and cook their catch on site.

Carson and his Dad are very excited the time for their fishing trip is here. While at sea, Carson caught many fish and even caught a lobster, some clams, and a few oysters. Carson had never had seafood other than fish. Fresh seafood in Indiana is a little harder to come by. Carson really enjoyed trying the seafood he caught on the boat that day. He loved the lobster in butter sauce and of course the fried clams. The oysters weren't his favorite, but he liked getting to try them anyway. Later that evening they returned to the hotel. During the night, Carson awoke with severe stomach pains. He was nauseous and dizzy as well. He woke up his parents to inform them of his situation. When he began having difficulty breathing, his parents rushed him to the ER at the local hospital for assessment.

ASSESSMENT

1. What complaints did Carson have during the night?
2. What would you expect to be the problem?
3. Which foods are most likely the cause of the problem?

DIAGNOSIS

4. Carson's abdominal pain and nausea could have been caused by _____.
5. What information should be gathered during his initial assessment?

PLAN/GOAL

6. What is the immediate goal for Carson?
7. What is the long-range goal?

IMPLEMENTATION

8. In the ER, what should Carson and his parents discuss with the physicians?
9. Does it appear that Carson may have a food allergy?
10. Is the doctor able to verify that this is an allergy?
11. What is the most likely recommendation for Carson?
12. What should Carson be cautioned about in the future about dining out?

EVALUATION/OUTCOME CRITERIA

13. When the intervention is complete, how will Carson know it has been effective?

THINKING FURTHER

14. What information could be obtained on the Internet?

rate this **plate**

Carson was so excited about his catch of the day and wanted to try everything for dinner. Is this a good idea? Rate this plate.

- **2 oz. lobster in butter sauce**
- **3 oz. fried clams**
- **1 oz. oysters on the half shell**
- **1 small order of French fries**
- **1 small Caesar salad made with homemade dressing containing a raw egg**
- **12 oz. regular soda**

Since Carson had not tried shellfish before should he have been given so many different choices to taste? Would it have been better for Carson to have been served only one shellfish item and no raw eggs?

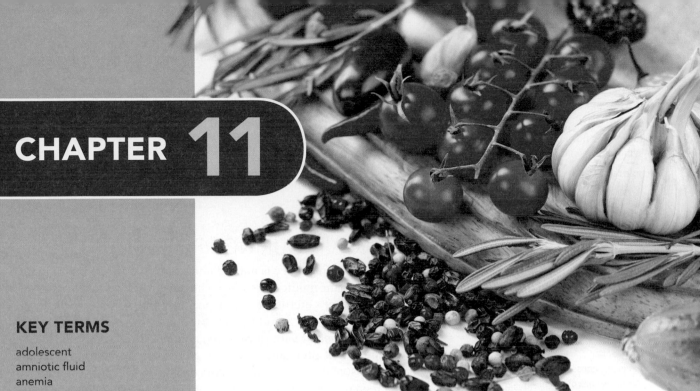

KEY TERMS

NUTRITION DURING PREGNANCY AND LACTATION

OBJECTIVES

After studying this chapter, you should be able to:

- Identify nutritional needs during pregnancy and lactation
- Describe nutritional needs of pregnant adolescents
- Modify the normal diet to meet the needs of pregnant and lactating women

Good nutrition during the 38–40 weeks of a normal pregnancy is essential for both mother and child. In addition to her normal nutritional requirements, the pregnant woman must provide nutrients and calories for the **fetus**, the **amniotic fluid**, the **placenta**, and the increased blood volume and breast, uterine, and fat tissue.

fetus
infant in utero

amniotic fluid
surrounds fetus in the uterus

placenta
organ in the uterus that links blood
supplies of mother and infant

retardation
delayed in mental development

trimester
3-month period; commonly used to
denote periods of pregnancy

adolescent
person between the ages of 13 and 20

Studies have shown a relationship between the mother's diet and the health of the baby at birth. It is also thought that the woman who consumed a nutritious diet before pregnancy is more apt to bear a healthy infant than one who did not. Malnutrition of the mother is believed to cause decreased growth and mental **retardation** in the fetus. Low-birth-weight infants (less than 5.5 pounds) have a higher mortality (death) rate than those of normal birth weight.

WEIGHT GAIN DURING PREGNANCY

Weight gain during pregnancy is natural and necessary for the infant to develop normally and the mother to retain her health. In addition to the developing infant, the mother's uterus, breasts, placenta, blood volume, body fluids, and fat must all increase to accommodate the infant's needs (Table 11-1).

The average weight gain during pregnancy is 25–35 pounds. During the first **trimester** of pregnancy, there is an average weight gain of only 2–4 pounds. Most of the weight gain occurs during the second and third trimesters of pregnancy, when it averages about 1 pound a week. This is because there is a substantial increase in maternal tissue during the second trimester, and the fetus grows a great deal during the third trimester.

Weight gain varies, of course. A pregnant **adolescent** who is still growing should gain more weight than a mature woman of the same size. Underweight women should gain 28–40 pounds. Women of average weight should avoid excessive weight gain and try to stay within the 25–35-pound average gain. If the woman is pregnant with twins, then the recommended weight gain is 35–45 pounds. Overweight women can afford to gain less than the average woman, but not less than 15 pounds.

No one should lose weight during pregnancy, because it could cause nutrient deficiencies for both mother and infant. On average, a pregnant adult requires no additional calories during the first trimester of pregnancy, 340 additional calories during the second trimester, and 450 additional calories for the third trimester.

In The Media

Shaping Food Habits

What if a mother could predispose her child to like green vegetables and nutrient-rich foods by what she ate during pregnancy? The concept known as *prenatal flavor learning* asserts that a child's food preferences could be developed from what the mother eats during pregnancy. Studies show that fetal taste buds mature in utero by 13–15 weeks, and flavors from foods can be transferred through the amniotic fluid to the fetus. Researchers say that prenatal flavor learning may have the potential to reduce the risks of diabetes and obesity.

(Source: Adapted from The Journal Gazette. Food habits begin in womb, researchers say. *Washington Post.* November 24, 2011.)

TABLE 11-1   **Components of Weight Gain during Pregnancy, with Approximate Amounts of Gain**

COMPONENT	AMOUNT OF GAIN
Fetus	7.5 pounds
Placenta	1 pound
Amniotic fluid	2 pounds
Uterus	2 pounds
Breasts	1–3 pounds
Blood volume	4 pounds
Maternal fat	4+ pounds

© Cengage Learning 2014

NUTRITIONAL NEEDS DURING PREPREGNANCY

Ideally when couples decide to have a child, they should make an appointment with their physician to discuss any health concerns or needed changes to the woman's diet. At that time, the physician needs to emphasize the importance of the woman taking a folic acid supplement at least 1 month prior to conception. During the 1990s, researchers established a correlation between taking folic acid before pregnancy and during the first trimester and having babies with brain and spinal cord defects. The results of this research led the U.S. government to require the addition of folic acid to grain products. The U.S. Public Health Service and the March of Dimes recommend that all women of child-bearing age take a multivitamin or 400 mcg of folic acid daily.

Lifestyle and habits also need to be taken into consideration before becoming pregnant. Certain medications, smoking, illegal drugs, and alcohol can all be detrimental to the embryo. Good nutrition is essential before becoming pregnant and during pregnancy.

EXPLORING THE WEB

Search the website of the American College of Obstetricians and Gynecologists (http://www.acog.org) for information regarding pregnancy and nutrition. What information can you find related to nutritional needs before, during, and after pregnancy? How does lactation affect caloric needs?

NUTRITIONAL NEEDS DURING PREGNANCY

Some specific nutrient requirements are increased dramatically during pregnancy, as can be seen in Table 11-2. These figures are recommended for the general U.S. population; the physician may suggest alternative figures based on the client's nutritional status, age, and activities.

The protein requirement is increased to 60 grams of protein per day during pregnancy. Proteins are essential for tissue building, and protein-rich foods are excellent sources of many other essential nutrients, especially iron, copper, zinc, and the B vitamins.

TABLE 11-2 RDA and AI for Pregnancy and Lactation

				FAT-SOLUBLE VITAMINS				WATER-SOLUBLE VITAMINS		
Age	Weight (kg) (lb)	Height (cm) (in)	Protein (gm/kg/day)	Vitamin A (µg RE)	Vitamin D (µg)	Vitamin E (mg α-TE)	Vitamin K (µg) (AI)	Vitamin C (mg)	Thiamine (mg)	Riboflavin (mg)
Pregnant			1.1	750; 700*	15	15	75; 90	80; 85	1.4	1.4
Lactating			1.3	1,200; 1,300*	15	19	75; 90	115; −120	1.4	1.6

WATER-SOLUBLE VITAMINS				MINERALS							
Niacin (mg)	Vitamin B₆ (mg)	Folate (µg)	Vitamin B₁₂ (µg)	Calcium (mg)	Phosphorus (mg) (AI)	Magnesium (mg)	Fluoride (mg) (AI)	Iron (mg)	Zinc (mg)	Iodine (µg)	Selenium (µg)
18	1.9	600	2.6	1,300; 1,000	1,250; 700	360; 310	3	27	12; 11	220	60
17	2.0	500	2.8	1,300; 1,000	1,250; 700	360; 310	3	10	13; 12	290	70

*First value is for females 14–18 years old; second value is for females 19 years old and above.

Reprinted with permission from the National Academies Press, Copyright © 2006, National Academy of Sciences. *Dietary Reference Intakes: The Essential Guide to Nutrient Requirements and the National Academies Press, Copyright © 2011, National Academy of Sciences. Dietary Reference Intakes Calcium and Vitamin D.*

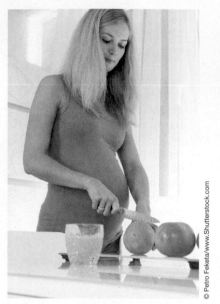

FIGURE 11-1 Healthy nutrition for a pregnant woman.

Current research indicates there is no need for increased vitamin A during pregnancy. Excess vitamin A (more than 3,000 RE) has been known to cause birth defects such as hydrocephaly (enlargement of the fluid-filled spaces of the brain), microcephaly (small head), mental retardation, ear and eye abnormalities, cleft lip and palate, and heart defects. The required amount of vitamin D is 5 mcg. The requirement for vitamin E is 15 mg α-TE. The amount of vitamin K required is given as AI of 75–90 mcg, depending upon age. See Chapter 7 for specifics about the need for fat-soluble vitamins.

The requirements for all the water-soluble vitamins are increased during pregnancy. Additional vitamin C is needed to develop collagen and to increase the absorption of iron. The B vitamins are needed in greater amounts because of their roles in metabolism and the development of red blood cells.

The requirements for the minerals calcium, iron, zinc, iodine, and selenium are all increased during pregnancy. Calcium is, of course, essential for the development of the infant's bones and teeth as well as for blood clotting and muscle action. If the mother is not consuming adequate calcium in her diet, the baby will get its calcium from her bones.

The need for iron increases because of the increased blood volume during pregnancy. In addition, the fetus increases its hemoglobin level to 20–22 grams per 100 ml of blood. This is nearly twice the normal human hemoglobin level of 13–14 mg per 100 ml of blood.

The infant's hemoglobin level is reduced to normal shortly after birth as the extra hemoglobin breaks down. The resulting iron is stored in the liver and is available when needed during the infant's first few months of life, when the diet is essentially breast milk or formula. Therefore, an iron supplement is commonly prescribed during pregnancy. However, if the pregnant woman's hemoglobin remains at an acceptable level without a supplement, the physician will not prescribe one.

FULFILLMENT OF NUTRITIONAL NEEDS DURING PREGNANCY

To meet the nutritional requirements of pregnancy, the woman should base her diet on MyPlate. Special care should be taken in the selection of food so that the necessary calories are provided by nutrient-dense foods (Figure 11-1).

Supersize **USA**

I was having dinner with a friend who was expecting a baby and when she picked up the menu she said, "I am eating for two now!" I looked at her and proceeded to tell her that she was misinformed. In the first trimester, a woman needs no additional calories. In the second and third trimesters, calorie needs increase only by about 300 calories per day. Three hundred calories is equal to ½ a chicken sandwich, or ¼ cup of dried fruit plus ¼ cup of nuts. You need extra nutrients though, which means you need to eat smarter while you are pregnant. Choosing healthy, nutrient-dense snacks over junk food or calorie-dense foods is a better alternative for the mother and growing baby. There are too many empty calories in soda and other junk food—80 oz of soda equals 1,000 calories. Increasing whole grains, fiber, fruits, vegetables, and milk intake will help provide the additional calories and nutrients needed throughout the pregnancy.

One of the best ways to consume extra calories during pregnancy is by drinking an additional two servings of milk each day. The extra milk will provide protein, calcium, phosphorus, thiamine, riboflavin, and niacin. If whole milk is used, it will also contribute saturated fat and cholesterol and provide 150 calories per 8 oz of milk. Fat-free milk contributes no fat and provides 90 calories per 8 oz serving and thus is the better choice.

To be sure that the vitamin requirements of pregnancy are met, **obstetricians**, nurse midwives, and physician's assistants (PAs) may prescribe a prenatal vitamin supplement in addition to an iron supplement. However, it is *not* advisable for the mother to take any unprescribed nutrient supplement, as an excess of vitamins or minerals can be toxic to mother and infant.

The unusual cravings for certain foods during pregnancy do no harm unless eating them interferes with the normal balanced diet or causes excessive weight gain.

obstetricians
doctors who care for mothers during pregnancy and delivery

CONCERNS DURING PREGNANCY
Nausea

Sometimes nausea (the feeling of a need to vomit) occurs during the first trimester of pregnancy. This type of nausea is commonly known as **morning sickness**, but it can occur at any time. It typically passes as the pregnancy proceeds to the second trimester. The following suggestions can help relieve morning sickness:

- Eat dry crackers or dry toast before rising.
- Eat small, frequent meals.
- Avoid foods with offensive odors.
- Avoid liquids at mealtime.

In rare cases, the nausea persists and becomes so severe that it is life threatening. This condition is called **hyperemesis gravidarum**. The mother may be hospitalized and given **parenteral nutrition**, meaning she is given nutrients via a vein (see Chapter 22 for further discussion). Such cases are difficult, and these clients need emotional support and optimism from their caregivers.

morning sickness
early morning nausea common to some pregnancies

hyperemesis gravidarum
nausea so severe as to be life threatening

parenteral nutrition
nutrition provided via a vein

Constipation

Constipation and hemorrhoids can be relieved by eating high-fiber foods, getting daily exercise, drinking at least eight glasses of liquid each day, and responding immediately to the urge to defecate.

Heartburn

Heartburn can result from relaxation of the cardiac sphincter and smooth muscles related to progesterone. Heartburn is a common complaint during pregnancy. As the fetus grows, it pushes on the mother's stomach, which may cause stomach acid to move into the lower esophagus and create a burning sensation there. Heartburn may be relieved by eating small, frequent meals; avoiding spicy or greasy foods; avoiding liquids with meals;

waiting at least an hour after eating before lying down; and waiting at least 2 hours before exercising.

Excessive Weight Gain

If weight gain becomes excessive, the pregnant woman should reevaluate her diet and eliminate foods (except for the extra pint of milk) that do not fit within MyPlate. Examples include candy, cookies, rich desserts, chips, salad dressings (other than fat free), and sweetened beverages. In addition, she might drink fat-free milk, if not doing so, which would reduce her calories but not her intake of proteins, vitamins, and minerals. Except in cases in which the woman cannot tolerate lactose (the sugar in milk), it is not advisable to substitute calcium pills for milk because the substitution reduces the protein, vitamin, and mineral content of the diet.

A bowl of clean, crisp, raw vegetables such as broccoli or cauliflower tips, carrots, celery, cucumber, zucchini sticks, or radishes dipped in a fat-free salad dressing or salsa can provide interesting snacks that are nutritious, filling, satisfying, and low in calories. Fruits and custards made with fat-free milk make nutritious, satisfying desserts that are not high in calories. Broiling, baking, or boiling foods instead of frying can further reduce the caloric intake.

Pregnancy-Induced Hypertension

pregnancy-induced hypertension (PIH)
typically occurs during late pregnancy; characterized by high blood pressure, albumin in the urine, and edema

proteinuria
protein in the urine

eclamptic stage
convulsive stage of toxemia

Pregnancy-induced hypertension (PIH) was formerly called *toxemia* or *preeclampsia*. It is a condition that sometimes occurs during the third trimester, and is characterized by high blood pressure, the presence of albumin in the urine (**proteinuria**), and edema. The edema causes a somewhat sudden increase in weight. If the condition persists and reaches the **eclamptic** (convulsive) **stage**, convulsions, coma, and death of mother and child may occur. The cause of this condition is not known, but it occurs more frequently in first-time pregnancies, in multifetal pregnancies, in those women with morbid obesity, and among pregnant women on inadequate diets, especially protein-deficient diets. Pregnant adolescents have a higher rate of PIH than do pregnant adults.

Pica

pica
abnormal craving for nonfood substance

Pica is the craving for nonfood substances such as starch, clay (soil), or ice. The reasons people get such a craving are not clear. Although both men and women are affected, pica is most common among pregnant women. Some believe it relieves nausea. Others think the practice is based on cultural heritage. The consumption of soil should be highly discouraged. Soil contains bacteria that would contaminate both mother and fetus. Ingesting soil can lead to an intestinal blockage, and substances in the soil would bind with minerals, preventing absorption by the body and thus leading to nutrient deficiencies. If any of the nonfood substances replaces nutrient-rich foods in the diet, this will result in multiple nutrient deficiencies. Eating laundry starch, in addition to a regular diet, will add unneeded calories and carbohydrates.

Anemia

Anemia is a condition caused by an insufficiency of red blood cells, hemoglobin, or blood volume. The patient suffering from it does not receive sufficient oxygen from the blood and consequently feels weak and tired, has a poor appetite, and appears pale. *Iron deficiency* is its most common form. During pregnancy, the increased volume of blood creates the need for additional iron. When this need is not met by the diet or by the iron stores in the mother's body, iron deficiency anemia develops. This may be treated with a daily iron supplement.

Folate deficiency can result in a form of megaloblastic anemia that can occur during pregnancy. It is characterized by too few red blood cells and by large immature red blood cells. The body's requirement for folic acid increases dramatically when new red blood cells are being formed. Consequently, the obstetrician might prescribe a folate supplement of 400–600 mcg a day during pregnancy.

 anemia
condition caused by insufficient number of red blood cells, hemoglobin, or blood volume

Alcohol, Caffeine, Drugs, and Tobacco

Alcohol consumption is associated with subnormal physical and mental development of the fetus. This is called **fetal alcohol syndrome (FAS)**. Many infants with FAS are premature and have a low birth weight. Physical characteristics may include a small head, short eye slits that make eyes appear to be set far apart, a flat midface, and a thin upper lip. There is usually a growth deficiency (height, weight), placing the child in the lowest tenth of age norms. There is also evidence of central nervous system dysfunction, including hyperactivity, seizures, attention deficits, and microcephaly (small head) (Figure 11-2). Another condition caused by ingesting alcohol while

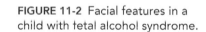 **fetal alcohol syndrome (FAS)**
subnormal physical and mental development caused by mother's excessive use of alcohol during pregnancy

FIGURE 11-2 Facial features in a child with fetal alcohol syndrome.

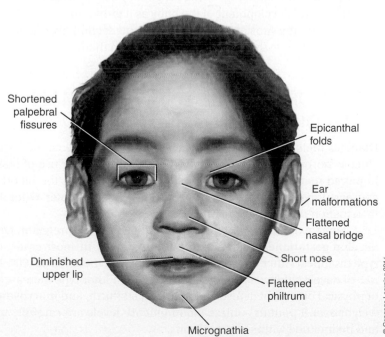

Shortened palpebral fissures

Epicanthal folds

Ear malformations

Flattened nasal bridge

Short nose

Diminished upper lip

Flattened philtrum

Micrognathia

© Cengage Learning 2014

pregnant is fetal alcohol effect (FAE). Children with FAE are born with less dramatic or no physical defects but with many of the behavioral and psychosocial problems associated with FAS. Those with FAE are not able to lead normal lives due to deficits in intelligence and behavioral and social abilities. When the mother drinks alcohol, it enters the fetal bloodstream in the same concentration as it does the mother's. Unfortunately, the fetus does not have the capacity to metabolize it as quickly as the mother, so it stays longer in the fetal blood than it does in the maternal blood. Abstinence is recommended.

Caffeine is known to cross the placenta, and it enters the fetal bloodstream. Birth defects in newborn rats whose mothers were fed very high doses of caffeine during pregnancy have been observed, but there are no data on humans showing that moderate amounts of caffeine are harmful. As a safety measure, however, it is suggested that pregnant women limit their caffeine intake to 2 cups of caffeine-containing beverages each day, or less than 300 mg/day.

Drugs vary in their effects, but self-prescribed drugs, including vitamins and mineral supplements and dangerous illegal drugs, can all damage the fetus. Drugs derived from vitamin A can cause **fetal malformations** and **spontaneous abortion**. Illegal drugs can cause the infant to be born addicted to whatever substance the mother used and, possibly, to be born with the human immunodeficiency virus (HIV). If a pregnant woman is known to be infected with HIV, her physician may prescribe AZT in an attempt to prevent the spread of the disease to the developing fetus.

Tobacco smoking by pregnant women has for some time been associated with babies of reduced birth weight. The more the mother smokes, the smaller her baby will be because smoking reduces the oxygen and nutrients carried by the blood. Other risks associated with smoking include sudden infant death syndrome (SIDS), fetal death, spontaneous abortion, and complications at birth. Smoking during pregnancy may also affect the intellectual and behavioral development of the baby as it grows up.

Because the substances discussed in this section may cause fetal problems, it is advisable that pregnant women avoid them.

DIET FOR THE PREGNANT WOMAN WITH DIABETES

Diabetes mellitus is a group of diseases in which one cannot use or store glucose normally because of inadequate production or use of insulin. This impaired metabolism causes glucose to accumulate in the blood, where it causes numerous problems if not controlled. (See Chapter 17 for additional information on diabetes mellitus.)

Some women have diabetes when they become pregnant. Others may develop **gestational diabetes** during pregnancy. In most cases, this latter type disappears after the infant is born; however, there is a 35–60% increased risk of developing type 2 diabetes later in life. Either type increases the risks of physical or mental defects in the infant, stillbirth, and **macrosomia** (birth weight over 9 pounds) unless blood glucose levels are carefully monitored and maintained within normal limits.

fetal malformations
physical abnormalities of the fetus

spontaneous abortion
occurring naturally; miscarriage

gestational diabetes
diabetes occurring during pregnancy; usually disappears after delivery of the infant

macrosomia
birth weight over 9 pounds

Every pregnant woman should be tested for diabetes between 24 and 28 weeks of gestation. Those found to have the disease must learn to monitor their diets to maintain normal blood glucose levels and to avoid both hypoglycemia and hyperglycemia.

In general, the nutrient requirements of the pregnant woman with diabetes are the same as for the normal pregnant woman. The diet should be planned with a registered dietitian or a certified diabetes educator because it will depend on the type of insulin and the time and number of injections. Patients with either gestational diabetes or preexisting diabetes who do not normally require insulin, may require insulin during their pregnancy to control blood glucose levels. A few of the oral hypoglycemic agents have also been approved for use during pregnancy. Between-meal feedings help maintain blood glucose at a steady level. Artificial sweeteners have been researched extensively and found to be safe for use during pregnancy.

Learning to eat healthy during pregnancy is important for any woman. Those with gestational diabetes not only need to learn the basics of healthy nutrition, but must also learn how to plan their meals throughout the day. It may mean that the carbohydrate sources they typically consume must be distributed into smaller, more frequent amounts over the course of the day. Three meals and two to three snacks is typically the best way for the carbohydrates to be planned. These meals and snacks may be consumed 2–3 hours apart throughout the day. The breakfast meal is typically the most carbohydrate restrictive. Early morning rises in hormone levels make controlling the morning blood sugars more difficult. It is recommended that no more than 45 grams of carbohydrate be consumed for breakfast and that simple carbohydrates, such as fruits or refined cereals, should be avoided until after lunch. It should be emphasized to these clients that healthy carbohydrates such as whole grains, fruits, and milk should not be eliminated. They are essential for fetal growth and brain formation. However, when reducing the amount of carbohydrates consumed during pregnancy, it is best to reduce the more highly processed and refined carbohydrates such as sweets and snack foods.

PREGNANCY DURING ADOLESCENCE

Teenage pregnancy is an increasing concern. The nutritional, physical, psychological, social, and economic demands on a pregnant adolescent are tremendous. With the birth of the infant, they increase. Young women who are themselves still in need of nurturing and financial support are suddenly responsible for a helpless newborn. If the mother does not have sufficient help, the total effect on her and the child can be devastating.

The young woman may need prenatal health care, infant care, and psychological, nutritional, and economic counseling, as well as help in locating appropriate housing. And at this time, the young woman's family may or may not be supportive.

At such a time, nutritional habits can seem to some as being of slight importance. They are, however, of primary importance. An adolescent's eating habits may not be adequate to fulfill the nutritional needs of her own growing body. When the nutritional burden of a developing fetus is added, both are put at risk. Adolescents are particularly vulnerable to pregnancy-induced

lactation
the period during which the mother is nursing the baby

lactation specialist
expert on breastfeeding

hypertension (PIH) and premature delivery. PIH can cause cardiovascular and kidney problems later. Premature delivery is a leading cause of death among newborns. Inadequate nutrition of the mother is related to both mental and physical birth defects.

These young women will need to know their own nutritional needs and the additional nutritional requirements of pregnancy (see Table 11-2). The government-funded Women, Infants, and Children (WIC) program can help with prenatal care, nutrition education, and adequate food for the best outcome possible. Pregnant teenagers will need much counseling and emotional support from caring, experienced people before nutritional improvements can be suggested.

LACTATION

A woman needs to decide whether to breastfeed before her infant is born. Almost all women can breastfeed; breast size is no barrier. **Lactation**, the production and secretion of breast milk for the purpose of nourishing an infant, is facilitated by an interplay of various hormones after delivery of the infant. Oxytocin and prolactin instigate the lactation process. Prolactin is responsible for milk production, and oxytocin is involved in milk ejection from the breast. The infant's sucking initiates the release of oxytocin, which causes the ejection of milk into the infant's mouth. This is called the let-down reflex. It is a supply-and-demand mechanism. The more an infant nurses, the more milk the mother produces.

It will take 2–3 weeks to fully establish a feeding routine; therefore, it is recommended that no supplemental feedings be given during this time. Human milk is formulated to meet the nutrient needs of infants for the first 6 months of life. Iron content in breast milk is very low, but it is very well absorbed; therefore, no iron supplement is needed for breast-fed babies.

Lactation Specialist

A **lactation specialist** is an expert on breastfeeding and helps new mothers who may be having problems such as the baby not latching on properly. This could cause the breast to become sore and could be discouraging to first-time mothers. Since the best first food for babies is breast milk, a lactation specialist can teach the proper techniques for successful breastfeeding.

Benefits of Breastfeeding

There are many positive reasons to breastfeed. The primary benefit of breast milk is nutritional. Breast milk contains just the right amount of lactose; water; essential fatty acids; and amino acids for brain development, growth, and digestion. No babies are allergic to their mother's milk, although they may have reactions to something their mother eats. Human milk contains at least 100 ingredients not found in formula.

Breast-fed babies have a lower incidence of ear infections, diarrhea, allergies, and hospital admissions. Breast-fed babies receive immunities from their mothers for the diseases that the mother has had or has been exposed to.

When a baby becomes ill, the bacteria causing the illness is transmitted to the mother while the baby is breastfeeding; the mother's immune system will start making antibodies for the baby.

Sucking at the breast promotes good jaw development because it is harder work to get milk out of a breast than a bottle, and the exercise strengthens the jaws and encourages the growth of straight, healthy teeth. Breastfeeding facilitates bonding between mother and child. The skin-to-skin contact helps a baby feel safe, secure, and loved. Many companies provide areas for mothers to pump breast milk while they are at work. Pediatricians encourage mothers of premature babies to hold their babies on their chests—skin to skin. This is called "kangaroo care," which has been shown to soothe and calm a baby and help maintain the baby's temperature. Fathers too can participate in kangaroo care by placing their infants against their bare chests.

Benefits for mother include help in losing the pounds gained during pregnancy and stimulating the uterus to contract to its original size. Resting is important for a new mother, and breastfeeding gives her that opportunity. Breastfeeding is economical, always the right temperature, and readily available—especially in the middle of the night.

There is no need to stop breastfeeding when returning to work; a breast pump can be used to express milk for feedings when the mother is not available. Breast milk will keep 8–10 hours at room temperature (66–72°F), 8 days in the refrigerator, 3–4 months in the refrigerator freezer, and 12 months in a deep freezer. Previously frozen milk must be used within 24 hours after defrosting in the refrigerator. Breast milk should not be heated in the microwave or directly on the stove. Those methods of heating breast milk will kill its immune-enhancing ability.

Calorie Requirements during Lactation

The mother's calorie requirement increases during lactation. The caloric requirement depends on the amount of milk produced. Approximately 85 calories are required to produce 100 ml (3.3 oz) of milk. During the first

SPOTLIGHT *on Life Cycle*

Being diagnosed with cancer during pregnancy can be a scary possibility. Although cancer during pregnancy is rare, occurring in approximately 1 out of every 1,000 pregnancies, some cancer treatments have been proven safe during pregnancy. Having a baby later in life can lead to a higher chance of cancer during pregnancy since age is the most significant risk factor for cancer development. If cancer is suspected during pregnancy, diagnostic tests such as x-rays may still be used, but with the woman using a lead shield to protect the abdomen from radiation. Because some treatments and tests may be harmful to the fetus, most doctors delay treatment until the second or third trimester when the baby is more developed. During this stage in the pregnancy, some types of chemotherapy may be given without harming the fetus. Some effects of chemotherapy during pregnancy include malnutrition, anemia, early labor, and low birth weight. Surgery to remove cancerous tissue is considered the safest cancer treatment option during pregnancy. If chemotherapy continues after the baby is born, doctors will advise women not to breastfeed as the treatment can be transferred to the infant through breast milk.

(Source: Adapted from American Society of Clinical Oncology. *Pregnancy and Cancer.* May 16, 2011. http://www.cancer.net)

6 months, average daily milk production is 750 ml (25 oz), and for this the mother requires approximately an extra 640 calories a day. During the second 6 months, when the baby begins to eat food in addition to breast milk, average daily milk production slows to 600 ml (20 oz), and the caloric requirement is reduced to approximately 510 extra calories a day.

The Institute of Medicine suggests an increase of 500 calories a day for the first 6 months of breastfeeding and 400 calories a day for 7–9 months. This is less than the actual need because it is assumed that some fat has been stored during pregnancy and can be used for milk production. The precise number of calories the mother needs depends on the size of the infant and its appetite and on the size and activities of the mother. Each ounce of human milk contains 20 calories.

If the mother's diet contains insufficient calories, the quantity of milk can be reduced, as seen in many Third World countries. Thus, lactation is not a good time to go on a strict weight loss diet. There will be some natural weight loss caused by the burning of the stored fat for milk production.

Nutrient Requirements during Lactation

In general, most nutrient requirements are increased during lactation. The amounts depend on the age of the mother (see Table 11-2). Protein is of particular importance because it is estimated that 10 grams of protein are secreted in the milk each day.

MyPlate will be helpful in meal planning for the lactating mother. She should be sure to include sufficient fruits and vegetables, especially those rich in vitamin C. Extra fat-free milk will provide many of the additional nutrients and calories required during lactation. Chips, sodas, candies, and desserts provide little more than calories. Vegetarians will need to be especially careful to be sure they have sufficient calories, iron, zinc, copper, protein, calcium, and vitamin D. A vitamin B_{12} supplement can be prescribed for them.

It is important that the nursing mother have sufficient fluids to replace those lost in the infant's milk. Water and real fruit juice are the best choices.

The mother should be made aware that she must reduce her caloric intake at the end of the nursing period to avoid adding unwanted weight.

Medicines, Caffeine, Alcohol, and Tobacco

Most chemicals enter the mother's milk, so it is essential that the mother check with her obstetrician before using any medicines or nutritional supplements. Caffeine can cause the infant to be irritable. Alcohol in excess, tobacco, and illegal drugs can be very harmful. Illegal drugs, such as marijuana or cocaine, and prescription medication, such as methadone and oxycodone, can cause the baby to be excessively drowsy and to feed poorly. Stimulant drugs can cause the baby to be irritable. The biggest concern is addiction of the mother and baby.

HEALTH AND NUTRITION CONSIDERATIONS

Good nutrition during pregnancy can make the difference between a healthy, productive life and one shattered by health and economic problems—for both mother and child.

Most pregnant women will want the best nutrition for themselves and their children. They also will be concerned about their weight during and after pregnancy. It is essential that they receive advice from a properly trained health care professional. Articles in newspapers and magazines or in pamphlets from health food stores may or may not be correct and should not be taken at face value unless approved by a professional in the dietetic field.

Nutrition is currently a popular topic, and people are inclined to believe what is printed. It can be difficult to persuade people that the information they read is incorrect. As always, the health care professional must use great patience in reeducating those clients who may require it.

The pregnant teenager can present the greatest challenge. Her needs are vast, but her experience, and thus her perspective, is limited. Teaching pregnant adolescents about good nutrition may be difficult but, if successful, can help not only that particular client but also her child and her friends.

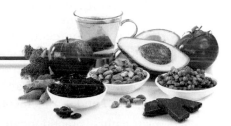

SUMMARY

A pregnant woman is most likely to remain healthy and bear a healthy infant if she follows a well-balanced diet. Research has shown that maternal nutrition can affect the subsequent mental and physical health of the child. Anemia and pregnancy-induced hypertension (PIH) are two conditions that can be caused by inadequate nutrition. Caloric and most nutrient requirements increase for pregnant women (especially adolescents) and women who are breastfeeding. The average weight gain during pregnancy is 25–35 pounds.

DISCUSSION TOPICS

1. Discuss the statement, "A pregnant woman must eat for two."

2. Why is it especially important for a pregnant woman to have a highly nutritious diet?

3. Discuss weight gain during pregnancy from the first month through the ninth. Why is an excessive weight gain during pregnancy undesirable? Is pregnancy a good time to lose weight? Explain.

4. Why are protein-rich foods important during pregnancy?

5. It is common for an iron supplement to be prescribed during pregnancy. Why? What may happen if the mother-to-be does not receive an adequate supply of iron? How might such a condition affect her baby? Discuss the advisability of the pregnant woman's taking a self-prescribed iron or vitamin supplement in addition to that prescribed by the obstetrician.

6. Discuss why the obstetrician regularly checks the pregnant woman's blood pressure, urine, and weight during pregnancy.

7. What is morning sickness, and how can it be helped? If any class member has been pregnant, ask her questions regarding morning sickness. Can this be a truly serious problem? Explain.

8. Why is it a good idea for a pregnant woman to include a citrus fruit or melon with every meal?

9. Why is the average weight gain 25–35 pounds during pregnancy when the infant weighs approximately 7–8 pounds?

10. Describe pica. Why is it undesirable?

11. Discuss the dangers to the fetus if the mother uses drugs.

12. How can the mother's diabetes affect the fetus?

SUGGESTED ACTIVITIES

1. Ask a dietitian to speak to the class on the importance of adequate nutrition before and during pregnancy. Ask the speaker questions regarding the effects of good and poor nutrition on the health of the mother, prenatal development, infant mortality, and the growth and development of the child. Ask the speaker's opinion regarding the use of alcohol, caffeine, and tobacco during pregnancy and during lactation.

2. Invite a nurse practitioner to speak to the class on the symptoms and dangers of PIH.

3. Invite a certified diabetes educator to speak to the class on the problems that can occur during the pregnancy of a diabetic mother.

4. Visit the International Breastfeeding Centre (http://www.nbci.com) and search for breast-feeding help videos to learn more about feeding techniques and benefits.

REVIEW

Multiple choice. Select the *letter* that precedes the best answer.

1. The infant developing in the mother's uterus is called the
   a. sperm
   b. fetus
   c. placenta
   d. ovary

2. A common form of anemia is caused by
   a. pica
   b. an excess of vitamin A
   c. a lack of iron
   d. a lack of B vitamins

3. High blood pressure, edema, and albumin in the urine are symptoms of
   a. calcium deficiency
   b. anemia
   c. not enough sodium
   d. pregnancy-induced hypertension

4. A common name given nausea in early pregnancy is
   a. morning sickness
   b. pica
   c. pregnancy-induced hypertension
   d. mortality

5. Folate and vitamin B_{12} requirements increase during pregnancy because of their roles in
   a. building strong bones and teeth
   b. fighting infections in the placenta
   c. building blood
   d. enzyme action

6. The additional daily energy requirement for the pregnant woman during the second trimester is
   a. 100 calories
   b. 340 calories
   c. 520 calories
   d. 1,000 calories

7. The additional calories required during pregnancy can be met by
   a. eating steak each day
   b. drinking a malted milk each day
   c. using an additional 2 servings of fat-free milk each day
   d. using an iron supplement

8. Craving nonfood substances during pregnancy is known as
   a. anemia
   b. megaloblastic anemia
   c. nausea
   d. pica

9. During pregnancy, the average weight gain is
   a. 15–24 pounds
   b. 25–35 pounds
   c. 11–24 kilograms
   d. 15–24 kilograms

10. Which of the following is *not* a known benefit of breastfeeding?
    a. lower incidence of allergies or infections in the baby
    b. strengthens the bonding between mother and child
    c. fathers can't participate
    d. helps mother to lose weight

11. Some appropriate substitutes for milk include
    a. orange juice and tomato juice
    b. cheese and yogurt
    c. breads and cereals
    d. vegetables and fruit juices

12. The DRI for additional calories for a nursing mother during the first 6 months is
    a. 100
    b. 300
    c. 500
    d. 1,000

13. The daily diet during pregnancy and lactation should
    a. be based on MyPlate
    b. include at least 2 quarts of milk
    c. be limited to 1,900 calories
    d. all of the above

14. Appropriate snacks for pregnant and lactating women include
    a. fruits and raw vegetables
    b. potato chips and pretzels
    c. sodas
    d. hard candies

15. The duration of a normal pregnancy is
    a. 34–36 weeks
    b. 36–38 weeks
    c. 38–40 weeks
    d. 40–42 weeks

16. The fluid surrounding the fetus in the uterus is the
    a. parenteral fluid
    b. intracellular fluid
    c. amniotic fluid
    d. synovial fluid

17. During pregnancy, parenteral nutrition may be necessary for clients
    a. with excessive weight gain
    b. suffering from hyperemesis gravidarum
    c. who cannot tolerate milk
    d. who do not eat meat

18. Heartburn may be prevented by
    a. eating small, frequent meals
    b. lying down immediately after eating
    c. taking an aspirin
    d. increasing fluids at meals

19. Pregnancy-induced hypertension
    a. is relieved with salty food
    b. may occur when diets contain insufficient protein
    c. tends to be a precursor of iron deficiency
    d. causes megaloblastic anemia

20. Gestational diabetes
    a. tends to cause low-birth-weight babies
    b. always develops into type 1 insulin-dependent diabetes mellitus
    c. usually disappears after the baby is born
    d. presents no danger to mother or child

21. Maternal malnutrition
    a. has little effect on the fetus
    b. may cause an increase in the fetal hemoglobin level
    c. often causes macrosomia
    d. can lead to developmental or mental retardation

22. The need for iron increases during pregnancy because
    a. it prevents maternal goiter
    b. it is essential to bone development
    c. it is necessary to fetal metabolism
    d. of the increased blood volume

23. Nutrient-dense foods provide substantial amounts of
    a. vitamins, minerals, and proteins
    b. calories per gram of food
    c. carbohydrates, fats, and water
    d. sodium, chloride, and water

24. Excessive vitamin A should be avoided during pregnancy because it may
    a. cause birth defects
    b. cause gestational diabetes
    c. contribute to gallstones in the fetus
    d. reduce the mother's appetite

Case In Point

JESSICA: TEENAGE PREGNANCY

Jessica always had a strong desire to fit in with her peers and often found herself doing things she didn't want to just to be accepted by her friends. Now that she is in high school it seems she is particularly concerned with fitting in. She is a good student with a 3.8 GPA, but her biggest concern is gaining approval from her friends. Since her freshman year, Jessica has been a cheerleader and on the dance team. She is now a junior, and has a boyfriend. She has been dating Ryan for most of her junior year. When Ryan asked her to prom, Jessica was very excited. She and Ryan attended prom and after-prom activities, then stayed over at another friend's house that night. Jessica felt she was in love with Ryan and was easily persuaded to do anything he requested to ensure he would not break up with her.

After her junior year, Jessica worked at a local coffee shop during the summer break. She often felt sick to her stomach when she arrived for her morning shift. She began noticing that many of the scents of the flavored coffees were making her feel nauseated. She was often invited to hang out with her friends after work, but rarely felt up for it. She often went home and slept. Finally, she confided in Ryan that she had missed two monthly periods and she was concerned she could be pregnant. He insisted she take a pregnancy test to confirm her suspicions. Jessica indeed was pregnant. She and Ryan were both scared and decided to confide in Jessica's mother. Jessica's mother made an appointment for Jessica to see a doctor.

The doctor confirmed Jessica's pregnancy. Jessica was given prenatal vitamins. She expressed to the doctor that she did not want to become fat during her pregnancy. The doctor discussed with her the importance of weight gain and the appropriate amount for her size. Jessica was afraid if she gained weight, Ryan would break up with her. Jessica's mother was very concerned for her daughter. She tried to talk to her about her nutrition and eating habits, but Jessica would not listen. She was eating like a bird and gaining no weight. At her next appointment, Jessica's doctor notes she has lost 2 pounds. After discussing this with Jessica and her mother, he decides she should see a dietitian to discuss appropriate foods for a healthy pregnancy. He also encourages Jessica to bring Ryan to the appointments so that he also understands what is happening to Jessica during the pregnancy.

ASSESSMENT

1. What objective data do you have about Jessica?
2. What caused Jessica to eat the way she did?
3. What was the cause of Jessica's noncompliance?
4. Which prenatal behaviors of Jessica were helpful? Which were not?

DIAGNOSIS

5. Complete the following diagnosis statement: Jessica's deficient knowledge about a healthy pregnancy and infant health is demonstrated by her lack of _____ .
6. Write a nursing diagnosis for Jessica that would be appropriate for her situation.

PLAN/GOAL

7. What is your plan for Jessica's health after the birth?

8. What is your goal for the baby's health related to reducing the risk of SIDS and delayed development?

IMPLEMENTATION

9. What topics does Jessica need to be taught about her baby's health and development? What does she need to know about apnea and SIDS? What does she need to learn about normal infant growth and development?
10. Who else needs to be present for the teaching?
11. As a teenage mother, Jessica needs what type of medical and nursing follow-up? Would home health care nursing visits help?
12. What is your primary concern for the baby?

EVALUATION/OUTCOME CRITERIA

13.   At the next visit, what criteria will the nurse practitioner be using to see if Jessica is eating healthy and caring for herself?

THINKING FURTHER

14.   What other issues make this situation more difficult for a teen mother to be successful?

15.   What other types of support may be helpful to a teenage mother?

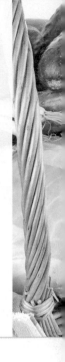

rate this **plate**

Jessica and Ryan meet with a registered dietitian to learn about adequate nutrition during pregnancy and proper weight gain to support a healthy baby. The dietitian emphasized the importance of eating a nutrient-rich diet containing good sources of protein and iron. Rate the meal that Jessica purchased for her lunch while working at the coffee shop.

1 medium raisin bagel

2 Tbsp low-fat cream cheese

½ cup mixed fruit

10 oz. regular coffee with cream and sugar

How many calories, grams of protein, and iron did Jessica consume in this meal? Is it enough for a pregnant teen? Why or why not?

Case In Point

AH MAR MO: MANAGING GESTATIONAL DIABETES

Ah Mar Mo is currently 28 weeks pregnant with her first child. She has migrated to the United States from Myanmar and is just beginning English language lessons. During her pregnancy she has been receiving prenatal care and a translator has attended her appointments with her. Ah Mar is 5 feet 3 inches tall. Her weight prior to pregnancy was 149 pounds. Her current weight is 174 pounds. Today at her appointment her doctor informed her that she has developed gestational diabetes. He tells her that her body is not processing the sugar in her foods well enough and he wants her to meet with a certified diabetes educator to discuss some of the changes she will need to make in her diet.

The educator explains to Ah Mar Mo what is happening in her body and discusses possible complications both she and the baby could develop. She shows her how to monitor her blood sugar and instructs Ah Mar Mo on the types of foods that will raise her blood sugar. Rice and noodles are staples in Ah Mar Mo's

meals and she rarely has a meal that does not contain one or the other. She also drinks large amounts of fruit juice with and between meals.

The educator discusses with Ah Mar Mo that she needs to have smaller, more frequent meals throughout the day and suggests three small meals and three snacks. She talks to Ah Mar Mo about replacing her consumption of juices with water and asks about her food preparation. Ah Mar Mo states that many of the foods she prepares are fried. Since the oils are very high in calories and eating fried foods could be contributing to her weight gain, they discuss alternative ways to prepare her foods. Ah Mar Mo also learns that she is eating much larger portions of rice and noodles than she should. The educator tells Ah Mar Mo that she was overweight prior to her pregnancy and is now at the high end of the weight gain recommendations for her prepregnancy weight. Ah Mar is not thrilled with changing her eating habits, but knows it is best for her and the baby.

ASSESSMENT

1. Why are elevated blood sugars during pregnancy a problem?
2. What are the consequences of high blood sugars during pregnancy on the baby?
3. What are the consequences of high blood sugars during pregnancy on mom?
4. All pregnant women should be screened for gestational diabetes at what point during their pregnancy?

DIAGNOSIS

5. Write a nursing diagnosis for Ah Mar Mo related to her gestational diabetes.
6. Write a nursing diagnosis for Ah Mar Mo related to her nutrition.

PLAN/GOAL

7. Ah Mar Mo needs to be educated regarding her gestational diabetes. What would be the two most important things to instruct Ah Mar Mo about?
8. How often may the nurse practitioner or educator need to see Ah Mar Mo?

IMPLEMENTATION

9. What steps might the dietitian take to ensure that Ah Mar Mo is following the guidelines she was instructed on?

EVALUATION/OUTCOME CRITERIA

10. How could the physician, nurse practitioner, and dietitian be assured their goals were met?

THINKING FURTHER

11. What are some of the considerations necessary when using a translator to speak to a client?

rate this **plate**

Rate the plate that Ah Mar has chosen for lunch.

⅔ cup rice

1 cup pork stirfry made of bok choy, snow peas, and broccoli

8 oz. mango juice

½ cup tapioca pudding with coconut

Can you determine if her carbohydrates are correct for her meal? Yes or no and why? What changes if any should be made to lower her caloric intake?

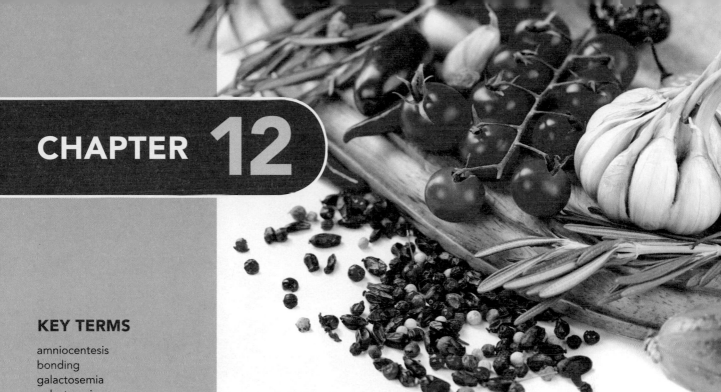

CHAPTER 12

NUTRITION DURING INFANCY

OBJECTIVES

After studying this chapter, you should be able to:

- State the effect inadequate nutrition has on an infant
- Discuss positive aspects of breastfeeding and bottle feeding
- Describe when and how foods are introduced into the baby's diet
- Describe inborn errors of metabolism and their dietary treatment

Food and its presentation are extremely important during the baby's first year. Physical and mental development are dependent on the food itself, and **psychosocial development** is affected by the time and manner in which the food is offered.

Infants react to their parents' emotions. If food is forced on a child, withheld until the child is uncomfortable, or if the food is presented in a tense manner the child reacts with tension and unhappiness. If the parent is relaxed, an infant's mealtime can be pleasurable for both parent and child (Figure 12-1).

FIGURE 12-1 Food is better accepted and digested in a happy and relaxed atmosphere.

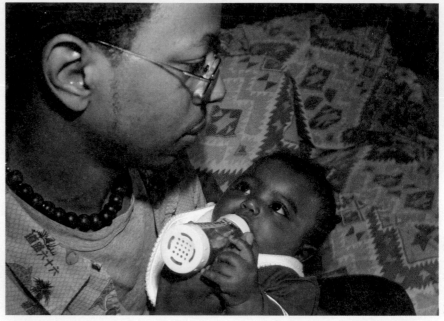

 psychosocial development
relating to both psychological and social development

 on demand
feeding infants as they desire

Although babies have been fed according to prescribed time schedules in the past, it is preferable to feed infants **on demand**. Feeding on demand prevents the frustrations that hunger can bring and helps the baby realize that his or her needs are being met. The newborn may require more frequent feedings, but normally the demand schedule averages approximately every 4 hours by the time the baby is 2 or 3 months old.

NUTRITIONAL REQUIREMENTS

The first year of life is a period of the most rapid growth in one's life. A baby doubles its birth weight by 6 months of age and triples it within the first year. This explains why the infant's energy, vitamin, mineral, and protein requirements are higher per unit of body weight than those of older children or adults. It is important to remember, however, that growth rates vary from child to child. Nutritional needs will depend largely on a child's growth rate.

During the first year, the normal child needs 98–108 calories per kilogram of body weight each day—approximately two to three times the adult requirement. Low-birth-weight infants and infants who have suffered from malnutrition or illness require more than the normal number of calories per kilogram of body weight. The nutritional status of infants is reflected by many of the same characteristics as those of adults (see Table 1-2).

The basis of the infant's diet is breast milk or formula. Either one is a highly nutritious, digestible food containing proteins, fats, carbohydrates, vitamins, minerals, and water.

It is recommended that infants up to 6 months of age have 2.2 grams of protein per kilogram of weight each day, and from 6–12 months, 1.6 grams of protein per kilogram of weight each day. This is satisfactorily supplied by human milk or by infant formulas (Figure 12-2).

Infants have more water per pound of body weight than adults. Thus, they usually need 1.5 ml of water per calorie. This is the same ratio of water to calories as is found in human milk and in most infant formulas. Babies receive enough water in both breast milk and formula; additional water is not needed. Essential vitamins and minerals can be supplied in breast milk, formula, and food. Except for vitamin D, breast milk provides all the nutrients an infant needs for the first 4–6 months of life. An infant is born with a 3–6-month supply of iron. When the infant reaches 6 months of age, the pediatrician usually starts the infant on iron-fortified cereal.

Human milk usually supplies the infant with sufficient vitamin C. Iron-fortified formula is available, and its use is recommended by the American Academy of Pediatricians if the baby is not being breastfed. The pediatrician can prescribe a vitamin D supplement for infants who are nursed and who are not exposed to sunlight on a regular basis. Newborns lack intestinal bacteria to synthesize vitamin K, so they are routinely given a vitamin K supplement shortly after birth. In addition, some pediatricians prescribe fluoride for breastfed babies or for formula-fed babies living in areas where the water, such as well water, contains little fluoride.

Care must be taken that infants do not receive excessive amounts of either vitamin A or D because both can be toxic in excessive amounts. Vitamin A can damage the liver and cause bone abnormalities, and vitamin D can damage the cardiovascular system and kidneys.

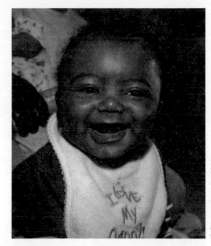

FIGURE 12-2 A happy, healthy, well-fed infant.

BREASTFEEDING

Although babies will thrive whether nursed or formula-fed, breastfeeding provides advantages that formulas cannot match. Breastfeeding is nature's way of providing a good diet for the baby. It is, in fact, used as the guide by which nutritional requirements of infants are measured (Figure 12-3).

Breast milk provides the infant with temporary **immunity** to many infectious diseases. It is economical, nutritionally perfect, and sanitary, and it saves time otherwise spent in shopping for or preparing formula. It is **sterile**, is easy to digest, and usually does not cause gastrointestinal disturbances or allergic reactions. Breastfed infants have fewer infections (especially ear infections) during the first few months of life than formula-fed babies; and because breast milk contains less protein and minerals than infant formula, it reduces the load on the infant's kidneys. Breastfeeding also promotes oral motor development in infants and decreases the infant's risk of obesity and diabetes.

Within the first several weeks of life the infant will nurse approximately every 2–4 hours. As the infant grows and develops, a stronger sucking ability will allow more milk to be extracted at each feeding, and the frequency of nursing sessions will decrease. It is recommended that an infant nurse at each breast for approximately 5–10 minutes each session. Growth spurts occur at about 10 days, 2 weeks, 6 weeks, and 3 months of age. During this time, the infant will nurse more frequently to increase the supply of nutrients needed to support growth.

One can be quite confident the infant is getting sufficient nutrients and calories from breastfeeding if (1) there are six or more wet diapers a day,

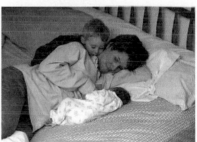

FIGURE 12-3 Breastfeeding offers many nutritional benefits to the newborn.

 immunity
ability to resist certain diseases

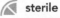 **sterile**
free of infectious organisms

bonding
emotional attachment

regurgitation
vomiting

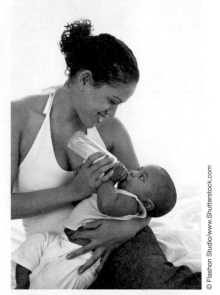

FIGURE 12-4 Feeding is a good time to provide the infant with love and attention.

FIGURE 12-5 To burp a baby, hold in one of the two positions shown and gently stroke the back.

(2) there is normal growth, (3) there are one or two mustard-colored bowel movements a day, and (4) the breast becomes less full during nursing.

From the mother's perspective at least, the **bonding** that occurs during breastfeeding is unmatched. In addition, breastfeeding helps the mother's uterus return to normal size after delivery, controls postpartum bleeding, and helps the mother more quickly return to her prepregnancy weight. Research has shown a correlation between breastfeeding and a decreased risk of breast cancer and osteoporosis in premenopausal women.

Breastfeeding had been on the decline for many years, but a growing number of mothers are now nursing their babies. If the mother works and cannot be available for every feeding, breast milk can be expressed earlier, refrigerated or frozen, and used at the appropriate time, or a bottle of formula can be substituted. Never warm the breast milk in a microwave because the antibodies will be destroyed.

BOTTLE FEEDING

Many parents will choose to bottle-feed their babies. Some women fear they will be unable to produce enough breast milk. Some lack emotional support from their families, and some simply find breastfeeding foreign to their culture. Others who are employed or involved in many activities outside the home find bottle feeding more convenient. Either way of feeding is acceptable provided the infant is given love and attention during the feeding.

The infant should be cuddled and held in a semi-upright position during the feeding (Figure 12-4). It appears that babies fed this way are less inclined to develop middle ear infections than those fed lying down. It is believed that the upright position prevents fluid from pooling at the back of the throat and entering tubes from the middle ear. During and after the feeding, the infant should be burped to release gas in the stomach, just as the breastfed infant should be burped (Figure 12-5). Burping helps prevent **regurgitation**.

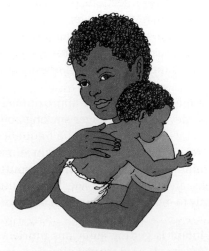
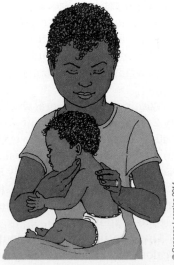

If the baby is to be bottle-fed, the pediatrician will provide information on commercial formulas and feeding instructions. Formulas are usually based on cow's milk because it is abundant and easily modified to resemble human milk. It must be modified because it has more protein and mineral salts and less milk sugar (lactose) than human milk. Formulas, such as soy formula, are developed so that they are similar to human milk in nutrient and caloric values.

When an infant is extremely sensitive or allergic to infant formulas, a synthetic formula may be given. Synthetic milk is commonly made from soybeans. Formulas with predigested proteins are used for infants unable to tolerate all other types of formulas.

Formulas can be purchased in ready-to-feed, concentrated, or powdered forms. Sterile or boiled tap water must be mixed with the concentrated and powdered forms. The most convenient type is also the most expensive.

If the type of formula purchased requires the addition of water, it is essential that the amount of water added be correctly measured. Too little water will create too heavy a protein and mineral load for the infant's kidneys. Too much water will dilute the nutrient and calorie value so that the infant will not thrive, and also it could lead to brain edema or seizures.

Infants under the age of 1 year should not be given regular cow's milk. Because its protein is more difficult and slower to digest than that of human milk, it can cause gastrointestinal blood loss. The kidneys are challenged by its high protein and mineral content, and dehydration and even damage to the central nervous system can result. In addition, the fat is less bioavailable, meaning it is not absorbed as efficiently as that in human milk.

Formula may be given cold, at room temperature, or warmed, but it should be given at the same temperature consistently. To warm the formula for feeding, place the bottle in a saucepan of warm water or a bottle warmer. The bottles should be shaken occasionally to warm the contents evenly. Warming the bottle in the microwave is not advisable because milk can heat unevenly and burn the infant's mouth. The temperature of the milk can be tested by shaking a few drops on one's wrist. The milk should feel lukewarm.

Infants should not be put to bed with a bottle. Saliva, which normally cleanses the teeth, diminishes as the infant falls asleep. The milk then bathes the upper front teeth, causing tooth decay. Also, the bottle can cause the upper jaw to protrude and the lower to recede. The result is known as the *baby bottle mouth* or *nursing bottle syndrome*. It is preferable to feed the infant the bedtime bottle, cleanse the teeth and gums with some water from another bottle or cup, and then put the infant to bed.

SUPPLEMENTARY FOODS

The age at which infants are introduced to solid and semisolid food has varied considerably over the years. At the beginning of the last century, doctors advocated that children be fed only breast milk during their first 12 months. By the 1950s, in response to parental demand, some pediatricians advised the introduction of solid food before the age of 1 year. Now, the general recommendation is that the infant's diet be limited to breast milk or formula until

SPOTLIGHT *on Life Cycle*

The Women, Infants, and Children (WIC) program is federally funded and provides nutritious foods, nutrition education, and referrals to health, and other social services to participants at no cost. Pregnant, postpartum, and breastfeeding women, infants, and children up to age 5 are eligible. Eligibility is based on income and nutritional risk including conditions such as anemia, underweight or overweight, history of pregnancy complications, poor pregnancy outcomes, or dietary risks. Different food packages are offered including infant cereal, iron-fortified adult cereal, vitamin C–rich fruit or vegetable juice, eggs, milk, cheese, peanut butter, dried and canned beans/peas, and canned fish. Vegetarian options are also available to accommodate the needs of the participants. Mothers can receive breastfeeding support and education as well as receive breast pumps to aide in the continuation of breastfeeding. Within the first 8 months of the year 2011, states have reported a monthly average of 9 million participants.

(Source: Adapted from Food and Nutrition Service, United States Department of Agriculture. WIC. *WIC fact sheet*. August 2011. Accessed February 15, 2012 from http://www.fns.usda.gov)

Supersize **USA**

We, the United States, have already supersized our population. One in three children is now considered overweight or obese. Educating parents about proper portion sizes for their child(ren) will be the first step in the fight against obesity. Overweight and obese parents may struggle with portion control when everything seems to have been supersized—plates, serving bowls, silverware, and glasses. Food comes in large packages, and chicken really is a *big* bird before processing. This big bird will yield boneless chicken breasts that will weigh 9–12 oz raw—a so-called single serving by those who are overeating and are no longer able to discern a normal serving of 3–4 oz. The easiest way to master portion sizes is to buy meat already prepared as such or ask the butcher to cut exactly what you need. Be sure and allow 1 oz for shrinkage from cooking. Also, get out the measuring cups and spoons—keep a set clean at all times just for measuring.

Here are some steps to prevent *supersizing children*:

- Breastfeed babies. Breastfeeding is the first step to preventing an overweight child.
- Select the right foods, and take the time to eat them. Kids fail to eat enough meats, fruits, and vegetables. Kids should have at least 15–20 minutes to eat.
- Set goals for activity—not only for kids, but for parents as well. Limit time for television, video games, and computers. The recommendation for exercise is 60 minutes per day.
- Work with other parents to remove junk food and soda from school vending machines.
- Do not reward children with food.

the age of 4–6 months and that breast milk or formula remain the major food source until the child is 1 year old. With the appropriate supplements of iron and vitamin D and possibly vitamin C and fluoride, breast milk or formula fulfills the nutritional requirements of most children until they reach the age of 6 months.

The introduction of solid foods before the age of 4–6 months is not recommended. The child's gastrointestinal tract and kidneys are not sufficiently developed to handle solid food before that age. Further, it is thought that the early introduction of solid foods may increase the likelihood of overfeeding and the development of food allergies, particularly in children whose parents suffer from allergies.

An infant's readiness for solid foods will be demonstrated by (1) the physical ability to pull food into the mouth rather than always pushing the tongue and food out of the mouth (extrusion reflex disappears by 4–6 months), (2) a willingness to participate in the process (Figure 12-6), (3) the ability to sit up with support, (4) having head and neck control, and (5) the need for additional nutrients. If the infant is drinking more than 32 oz of formula or nursing 8–10 times in 24 hours and is at least 4 months old, then solid food should be started.

Solid foods must be introduced gradually and individually. One food is introduced and then no other new food for 4 or 5 days. If there is no allergic reaction, another food can be introduced, a waiting period allowed, then another, and so on. The typical order of introduction begins with cereal, usually iron-fortified rice, then oat, wheat, and mixed cereals. Cooked and pureed vegetables follow, then cooked and pureed fruits, egg yolk, and, lastly, finely ground meats. A good rule of thumb for feeding during the first year of life is 2–4 tablespoons (1–2 oz) of each variety of food per meal. Between 6 and 12 months, toast, zwieback, teething biscuits, and Cheerios can be added in small amounts. Honey should never be given to an infant because it could be contaminated with *Clostridium botulinum* bacteria. When the infant learns to drink from a cup, juice can be introduced (Figure 12-7). Juice should never be given from a bottle because babies will fill up on it and not get enough calories from other sources. Pasteurized apple juice is usually given first. It is recommended that only 4 oz per day of 100% juice products be given because they are nutrient-dense.

Babies differ in the amount of food they eat from day to day. An infant will let you know when he or she is full in the following ways:

- Playing with the nipple on a bottle or a breast
- Looking around and no longer opening his or her mouth to solid food
- Falling asleep while eating
- Playing with food and not eating

Adults may try to overfeed infants when solid food is introduced. The guidelines in Table 12-1 may be helpful.

By the age of 1 year, most babies are eating foods from all of the MyPlate groups and may have almost any food that is easily chewed and digested. However, precautions must be taken to avoid offering foods on which the child can choke. Examples include hotdogs, nuts, whole peas, grapes, popcorn, small candies, and small pieces of tough meat or raw vegetables. Foods should be selected according to the advice of the health care provider or pediatrician. It is not necessary to use the commercially prepared "third" foods. Table foods generally can be used, though they may need to first be mashed or run through a blender.

MyPlate provides excellent help in determining the baby's menu. Its use will help supply the appropriate nutrients and develop good eating habits. It is particularly important at this time to avoid excess sugar and salt in the

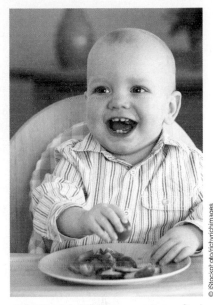

FIGURE 12-6 Infants sometimes find more pleasure in touching their food than tasting it.

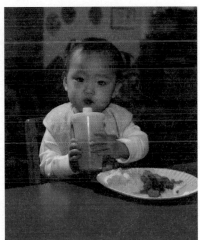

FIGURE 12-7 Juice should be served in a cup, not a bottle.

TABLE 12-1   Guidelines to Prevent Overfeeding of Infants

FEEDING	4–5 MONTHS	5–7 MONTHS
Early morning	Breast milk or 5–6 oz formula[*]	Breast milk or 5–6 oz formula[*]
Breakfast	Breast milk or 5–6 oz formula[*] 1–2 Tbsp infant cereal[†] (optional)	Breast milk or 5–6 oz formula[*] 3–4 Tbsp infant cereal[†]
Lunch	Breast milk or 5–6 oz formula[*]	Breast milk or 5–6 oz formula[*] 1–2 Tbsp vegetables
Late afternoon	Breast milk or 5–6 oz formula[*]	Breast milk or 5–6 oz formula[*]
Supper	Breast milk or 5–6 oz formula[*]	Breast milk or 5–6 oz formula[*] 3–4 Tbsp infant cereal[†] 1–2 Tbsp vegetables
Evening	Breast milk or 5–6 oz formula[*]	Breast milk or 5–6 oz formula[*] (optional)

Babies differ in the amounts of food they eat. Expect your baby's appetite to vary from day to day.

FEEDING	7–9 MONTHS	9–12 MONTHS
Breakfast	Breast milk or 6–8 oz formula[*] 4 Tbsp infant cereal[†] 2–3 Tbsp fruit	Breast milk or 6–8 oz formula[*] 4–6 Tbsp infant cereal[†] 2–3 Tbsp fruit
Lunch	Breast milk or 6–8 oz formula[*] 1–3 Tbsp meat or meat alternative 2–3 Tbsp vegetables 2–3 Tbsp fruit	Breast milk or 6–8 oz formula[*] 2–4 Tbsp infant cereal[†] 1–2 Tbsp meat or meat alternative 3–5 Tbsp vegetables 3–4 Tbsp fruit
Late afternoon	Breast milk or 6–8 oz formula[*]	Breast milk or 6–8 oz formula[*]
Supper	Breast milk or 6–8 oz formula[*] 4 Tbsp infant cereal[†] 2–3 Tbsp vegetables 2–3 Tbsp fruit	Breast milk or 6–8 oz formula[*] 2–3 Tbsp meat or meat alternative 3–5 Tbsp vegetables 2–3 Tbsp fruit
Evening	Breast milk or 6–8 oz formula[*] (optional)	Breast milk or 6–8 oz formula[*] (optional)

[*]If baby is not breastfed, iron-fortified, commercial infant formula is recommended for the first 9–12 months.
[†]Iron-fortified infant cereal is recommended for babies during the first 2 years.

infant's diet so that the child does not develop a taste for them and, consequently, overuse them throughout life.

weaning
training an infant to drink from the cup instead of the nipple

Weaning actually begins when the infant is first given food from a spoon (Figure 12-8). It progresses as the child shows an interest in and an ability to drink from a cup. The child will ultimately discard the bottle or refuse the breast. If the child shows great reluctance to discard the bottle or still seeks the breast, then parents should discuss this with their health care provider.

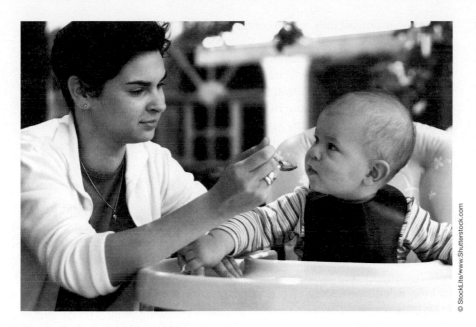

FIGURE 12-8 Solid foods are introduced at 4–6 months. Breast milk or formula continues to be the main source of calories at this age.

© StockLite/www.Shutterstock.com

In The Media

Taste Preference for Salt

A small new study suggests that taste preferences for high-sodium foods can be formed during infancy. Researchers found that 6-month-old babies are more likely to enjoy the taste for salt if they have been given starchy snack foods such as crackers and cereal. Infants that stayed on baby food in their first 6 months and were only given fruit in addition were likely to be indifferent to salt as they grew. Findings published in the *American Journal of Clinical Nutrition* suggest that delaying exposure to salt can create an adult population that is less fond of high-sodium foods. Reducing sodium intake can therefore decrease the chances of high blood pressure, heart disease, and stroke in the adult population.

(Source: Adapted from Gardner, Amanda. *Taste for Salt May Be Shaped During Infancy*. December 21, 2011. www.cnn.com)

SPECIAL CONSIDERATIONS FOR INFANTS WITH ALTERED NUTRITIONAL NEEDS
Premature Infants

An infant born before 37 weeks' gestation is considered to be premature. These babies have special needs. The sucking reflex is not developed until 34 weeks of gestation, and infants born earlier must be fed by total parenteral nutrition, tube feedings, or bolus feedings (Figure 12-9). The best food for a premature infant

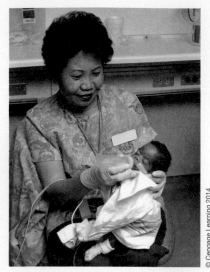

FIGURE 12-9 This premature infant receives a specially designed formula to meet his nutritional needs; note placement of nasogastric tube.

inborn errors of metabolism
congenital disabilities preventing normal metabolism

mutations
changes in the genes

EXPLORING THE WEB

Visit the cystic fibrosis website (http://www.cff.org). Search for information related to nutrition and the care of infants with cystic fibrosis. Are there any new therapies or research on the needs in this area? What should you tell new parents whose child is about to undergo newborn screening for cystic fibrosis?

is its mother's breast milk, which contains more protein, sodium, immunologic properties, and some other minerals than does the milk produced by mothers of full-term infants. Other concerns in preterm infants are low birth weight, underdeveloped lungs, immature GI tract, inadequate bone mineralization, and lack of fat reserves. Many specialized formulas are available for premature infants, but breast milk is best because its composition is made just for the baby, and it changes according to the baby's needs. Mothers of premature babies should be encouraged to pump their milk until the infant is able to nurse.

Cystic Fibrosis

Cystic fibrosis (CF) is an inherited disease that causes the body to produce abnormally thick, sticky secretions (mucus) within cells lining organs such as the lungs and pancreas. The thick mucus also obstructs the pancreas, preventing enzymes from reaching the intestines to help break down and digest food. Of those children with CF, 85% have exocrine pancreatic insufficiency (PI) and are at nutritional risk due to decreased production of digestive enzymes. Malabsorption of fat is also associated with CF; therefore, the recommendation is for 35–40% of total calorie intake to be fat. Digestive enzymes are taken in capsule form when food is eaten, and supplementation of fat-soluble vitamins should also be done at mealtime. There is also a water-miscible form of fat-soluble vitamins that can be administered if normal levels cannot be maintained with the use of only fat-soluble vitamins. It is not unusual for those having CF to be malnourished, even with supplementation, due to malabsorption of nutrients and increased needs. One possible solution would be nighttime tube feedings to supplement oral intake if adequate nutrition and weight cannot be maintained.

Failure to Thrive

Failure to thrive (FTT) can be determined by plotting the infant's growth on standardized growth charts (Figure 12-10); consideration must be made for genetic and ethnic variations. Weight for height is the first parameter affected when determining FTT. Later, height and head circumference are affected. Other signs might be slow development or lack of physical skills such as rolling over, sitting, standing, and walking. Mental and social skills will also be delayed. Babies grow the most in the first 6 months of life, and this is when their brain undergoes crucial development, which can affect the rest of their lives. Failure to thrive can have many causes, such as watered-down formula, congenital abnormalities, AIDS, lack of bonding, child abuse, or neglect.

SPECIAL CONSIDERATIONS FOR INFANTS WITH METABOLIC DISORDERS

Some infants are born with the inability to metabolize specific nutrients. These congenital disabilities are called **inborn errors of metabolism**. They are caused by **mutations** in the genes. There is great variation in the seriousness of the conditions caused by these defects. Some cause death at an early

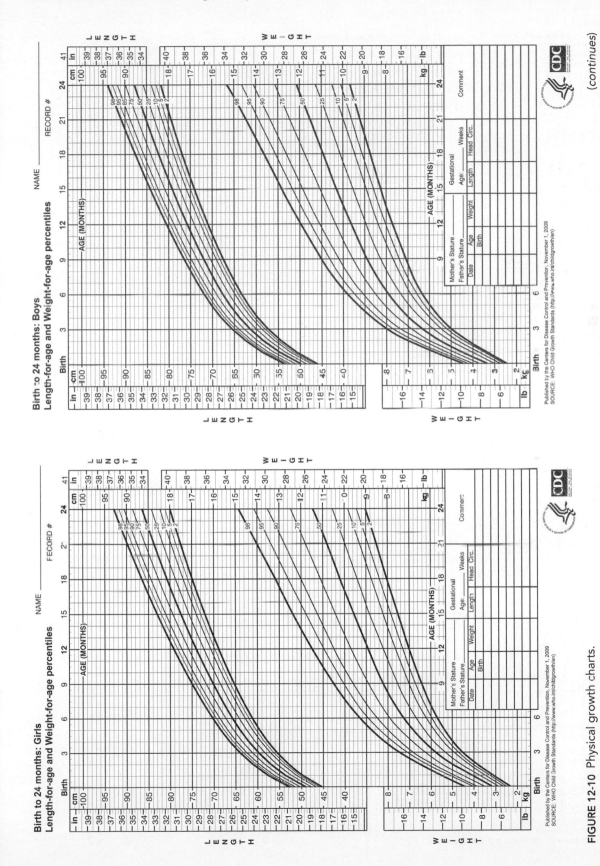

FIGURE 12-10 Physical growth charts.

Source: Centers for Disease Control and Prevention, National Center for Health Statistics in collaboration with the National Center for Chronic Disease Prevention and Health Promotion. 2000 CDC Growth Charts: United States. http://www.cdc.gov/growthcharts, updated November 1, 2009. Additional clinical growth charts with the 3rd and 97th percentiles can be found or the CDC website.)

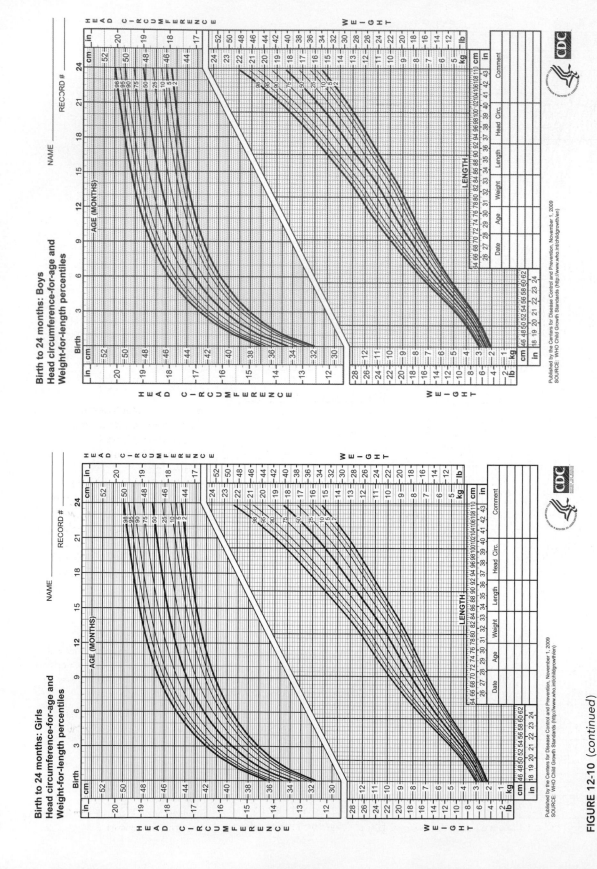

FIGURE 12-10 (continued)

Source: Centers for Disease Control and Prevention, National Center for Health Statistics in collaboration with the National Center for Chronic Disease Prevention and Health Promotion. 2000 CDC Growth Charts: United States. http://www.cdc.gov/growthcharts, updated November 1, 2009. Additional clinical growth charts with the 3rd and 97th percentiles can be found on the CDC website.)

age, and some can be minimized so that life can be supported by adjustments in the normal diet. Children born with these defects, however, face the common danger of damage to the central nervous system because of their abnormal body chemistry. This results in mental retardation and sometimes retarded growth. Early diagnosis of these inborn errors, combined with diet therapy, increases the chances of preventing retardation. Hospitals test newborns for some of these disorders as a matter of course. If there is a family history of a certain genetic disorder, genetic screening can be done. In addition, some of these abnormalities can be discovered by **amniocentesis**.

Galactosemia

Galactosemia is a condition that affects 1 in 30,000 live births, caused by the lack of the liver enzyme **transferase**. Transferase normally converts galactose to glucose. (Galactose is the simple sugar resulting from the digestion of lactose, the sugar found in milk; see Chapter 4). When an infant who lacks transferase ingests anything containing galactose, the amount of galactose in the blood becomes excessive. As a result of this toxic level, the newborn suffers diarrhea, vomiting, edema, and abnormal liver function. Cataracts may develop, **galactosuria** occurs, and mental retardation ensues.

Diet Therapy

Diet therapy for galactosemia is the exclusion of anything containing milk from any mammal. During infancy, the treatment is relatively simple because parents can feed the baby lactose-free, commercially prepared formula and can provide supplemental minerals and vitamins. As the child grows and moves on to adult foods, parents must be extremely careful to avoid any food, beverage, or medicine that contains lactose. Nutritional supplements of calcium, vitamin D, and riboflavin must be given so that the diet is nutritionally adequate. This restricted diet may be necessary throughout life, but some physicians allow a somewhat liberalized diet as the child reaches school age. This may mean only small amounts of baked or processed foods that contain small amounts of milk. Even this restricted diet must be accompanied by careful and regular monitoring for galactosuria.

Phenylketonuria

In **phenylketonuria (PKU)**, infants lack the liver enzyme **phenylalanine hydroxylase**, which is necessary for the metabolism of the amino acid **phenylalanine**. Infants seem to be normal at birth, but if the disease is not treated, most of them become hyperactive, suffer seizures between 6 and 18 months of age, and become mentally retarded. Public health law requires most hospitals today to screen newborns for phenylketonuria. PKU babies typically have light-colored skin and hair.

Diet Therapy

There is a special, nutritionally adequate, commercial infant formula available for PKU babies, called **Lofenalac**, with 95% of phenylalanine removed

 amniocentesis
a test to determine the status of the fetus in utero

 galactosemia
inherited error in metabolism that prevents normal metabolism of galactose

 transferase
liver enzyme that converts galactose to glucose

 galactosuria
galactose in the urine

EXPLORING THE WEB

Search the Galactosemia Information and Resources website (http://www.galactosemia.com) for content related to diet and control of the disorder galactosemia. How could you help parents of an infant with galactosemia begin to make the transition to solid foods for their baby? Create a list of safe foods that can be passed along to clients.

 phenylketonuria (PKU)
condition caused by an inborn error of metabolism in which the infant lacks an enzyme necessary to metabolize the amino acid phenylalanine

 phenylalanine hydroxylase
liver enzyme necessary to metabolize the amino acid phenylalanine

 phenylalanine
amino acid

 Lofenalac
commercial infant formula with 95% of phenylalanine removed

maple syrup urine disease (MSUD)
disease caused by an inborn error of metabolism in which the body cannot metabolize certain amino acids

leucine
an amino acid

isoleucine
an amino acid

valine
an amino acid

from its protein source. It provides just enough phenylalanine for basic needs, but no excess. The specific amount depends on the infant's size and growth rate. Regular blood tests determine the adequacy of the amounts. Diets are carefully monitored for calorie and nutrient content and are adjusted frequently as needs change. Except for fats and sugars, all foods contain some protein; and of that protein, some is phenylalanine, so diets for the growing child eating normal food must be carefully planned.

The two varieties of synthetic milk available for older children include *Phenyl-free* and *PKU-1, -2,* or *-3.* None of these contains any phenylalanine. They can be used as beverages or in puddings and baked products. Diets should be monitored throughout life to avoid mental retardation and to control hyperactivity and aggressive behavior (Table 12-2).

Maple Syrup Urine Disease

Maple syrup urine disease (MSUD) is a congenital defect resulting in the inability to metabolize three amino acids: **leucine**, **isoleucine**, and **valine**. It is named for the odor of the urine of these infants and affects 1 in 100,000–300,000 live births. When the infant ingests food protein, there are increased blood levels of these amino acids, causing ketosis. Hypoglycemia, apathy, and convulsions occur very early. Depending on the extent of the disease, if not treated promptly, the child can die from acidosis. Mild forms of the disease, if left untreated, will cause mental retardation and bouts of acidosis.

Diet Therapy

The diet must provide sufficient calories and nutrients but with extremely restricted amounts of leucine, isoleucine, and valine. A special formula and

---

TABLE 12-2   Acceptable and Unacceptable Foods for Those with PKU

FOODS ALLOWED FOR PEOPLE WITH PKU	FOODS NOT ALLOWED FOR PEOPLE WITH PKU
Special low-phenylalanine formulas	Meats
The following contain no phenylalanine:	Fish
• Fats	Poultry
• Sugars	Eggs
• Jellies	Milk
• Some candies	Cheese
The following contain some phenylalanine:	Nuts
• Fruits	Dried beans and peas
• Vegetables	Commercially prepared products made from regular flour
• Cereals	

low-protein foods are used. Diet therapy appears to be necessary throughout life.

HEALTH AND NUTRITION CONSIDERATIONS

Although the physical and mental development of infants depends on the nutrients and calories they receive, their psychosocial development depends on *how and when* these nutrients and calories are provided. Some new parents will have a solid knowledge of the nutrition information needed but lack a real understanding of the importance of how and when food should be presented to infants. They may hold the infant during feedings but focus instead on the television or newspaper.

Other parents may know instinctively how important cuddling and attention are to an infant, but they lack accurate knowledge of infant nutrition.

Parents from both groups are apt to have opinions that may or may not be correct. The health care professional will help these parents most by listening carefully to them. The parents are more inclined to listen to advice when a two-way discussion follows.

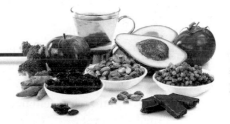

SUMMARY

It is particularly important that babies have adequate diets so that their physical and mental development are not impaired. Breastfeeding is nature's way of feeding an infant, although formula feeding is quite acceptable. Cow's milk is primarily used in formulas because it is most available and is easily modified to resemble human milk. The young child's diet is supplemented on the advice of the pediatrician. Added foods should be based on MyPlate.

Inborn errors of metabolism cause various problems, ranging from mental retardation to death, if not properly treated. In these conditions, diet therapy is the primary tool in maintaining the client's health.

Infants who are premature, have cystic fibrosis, or failure to thrive have special nutritional needs.

DISCUSSION TOPICS

1. Do any of the students know a woman who has breastfed her baby? If so, what were her reactions to the experience?

2. Why is breastfeeding not always possible?

3. Discuss the possible effects of regularly propping the baby's bottle instead of holding the baby during feeding.

4. Why is a rigid time schedule for feeding a baby not advisable? Explain why feeding infants on demand the first few months can lead to a regular feeding schedule.

5. How may weaning be accomplished?

6. What is meant by inborn errors of metabolism? What causes them? How might they affect infants?

7. Discuss PKU. Include its cause, symptoms, effects, and treatment.

8. Why should the mother give her baby special attention during feedings?

9. How is a bottle warmed? Is it always necessary to warm the bottle? Explain. Why is a microwave oven not recommended?

10. Why is it not advisable to give peanuts to an 8-month-old child?

SUGGESTED ACTIVITIES

1. Hold a panel discussion on the advantages and disadvantages of breastfeeding. Invite lactation specialists, doctors, and parents as panelists.
2. Observe a demonstration of the actual feeding and burping of a baby.
3. Visit a store that carries prepared infant formulas and compare their prices and nutritional values.
4. Invite a physician or nurse practitioner to give a talk on inborn errors of metabolism.

REVIEW

Multiple choice. Select the *letter* that precedes the best answer.

1. The most rapid growth in a child's life occurs during
   a. its first month
   b. the month following weaning
   c. the first 6 months
   d. its first year

2. The amount of protein needed by a child during its first year
   a. is greater during the first 6 months than during the second
   b. is greater during the second 6 months than during the first
   c. does not change over the course of the year
   d. increases on a weekly basis

3. After the initial supplement of vitamin K following birth, breast milk provides all the nutrients an infant needs during the first 4–6 months except for
   a. vitamin A
   b. vitamin B
   c. vitamin C
   d. vitamin D

4. The vitamin in question 3 might be provided
   a. by injection
   b. in diluted orange juice
   c. by regular walks in the sunshine
   d. in pasteurized apple juice

5. Breastfed babies are more resistant to infection than are bottle-fed babies because mother's milk provides
   a. sterile environment
   b. synthetic antibiotics
   c. leucine
   d. immunity

6. The development of emotional attachment to a child is called
   a. transferase
   b. bonding
   c. psychosocial development
   d. immunity

7. It is recommended that, at each feeding, a newborn nurse at each breast for approximately
   a. 3–5 minutes
   b. 5–10 minutes
   c. 10–15 minutes
   d. 20 minutes

8. It can be said that infant formulas
   a. are usually based on cow's milk
   b. have the same protein content as cow's milk
   c. contain fewer minerals than cow's milk
   d. contain no sugar

9. Infants with sensitivities to infant formulas may be given
   a. goat's milk
   b. synthetic milk, often made from soybeans
   c. formula with predigested carbohydrates
   d. any of the above

10. By the age of 6 months, a child
    a. may be introduced to a new formula
    b. is usually completely weaned
    c. is usually introduced to solid foods
    d. is no longer given milk

Case In Point

Bonita's youngest child Diego was born 4 weeks ago and was 7 pounds 14 ounces and 20 inches long at birth. Bonita was unable to take 6 weeks off work after Diego was born. Bonita is 34 years old. She and her husband are from Colombia and own a restaurant that serves authentic Columbian cuisine. Their head chef resigned shortly before Diego was born and Bonita was going to have to fill in as chef until a new one could be hired and trained. Diego was born during the height of the summer tourism season in their town and Bonita was desperately needed back at work. Bonita had hired the neighbor girl to care for Diego while she was working. The neighbor reported that Diego was often very cranky and would refuse his bottle. Bonita wasn't terribly concerned. Her first child had been very colicky so it wouldn't surprise her that Diego was as well. Finally, Bonita and her husband were able to find a new chef for the restaurant and Bonita was able to take some much needed time off. By now Diego was 4 months old. Bonita began realizing she never saw Diego smile like her other babies did. He also seemed unable to track objects such as toys when she would play with him. Bonita thought he seemed smaller than her other children at this age, but she wasn't sure how much smaller. At Diego's next well-baby check, his weight was 10 pounds 14 ounces and he only measured 21 inches long. The doctor explained to Bonita that Diego was not growing adequately and diagnosed him with failure to thrive (FTT).

ASSESSMENT

1. What data do you have about Bonita?
2. What data do you have about Diego?
3. What factors contributed to Diego's problem?
4. Using the growth charts in Figure 12-10, determine a baby's normal weight and height at 4 months. What should Diego weigh, and how long should he be?
5. What should Diego be doing developmentally at 4 months?
6. How severe is Diego's failure to thrive?

DIAGNOSIS

Complete the following nursing diagnoses:

7. Diego's failure to thrive is related to
   _____

8. Diego's imbalanced nutrition, less than body requirements, is secondary to
   _____

9. Bonita's ineffective feeding is a result of
   _____

PLAN/GOAL

10. What is your immediate goal for Diego?
11. What is your long-term goal for Diego?
12. What is your short-term goal for Bonita?
13. What is your long-term goal for Bonita?

IMPLEMENTATION

14. What changes need to occur for Diego to thrive?
15. What does the NP need to teach Bonita?
16. How else can the NP help Bonita?
17. Who else needs to be involved in Diego's care?

EVALUATION/OUTCOME CRITERIA

18. After the plan has been in place for 6 weeks, what changes should Bonita see in Diego?
19. What will the NP measure and observe in Diego and Bonita if the plan is successful?

THINKING FURTHER

20. Why is it important for infants to have a good start in life? Why is their nutrition so critical? What future complications can be avoided as a result?

rate this plate

Diego is now 6 months old and Bonita will have to experiment with different foods to get him back on track. He has only been getting formula, but now it's time to try solid foods. Rate this plate for lunch:

5 oz. infant formula

2 Tbsp infant rice cereal

2 Tbsp pureed green beans

1 Tbsp pureed applesauce

Are the servings correct for a 6-month-old infant? If not, what corrections should be made to this meal?

Case In Point

Ann is a new mom. Her son Caden was born 4 months ago. Up until this time, she has been exclusively breast-feeding him. She is reading about introducing solid foods into his diet. As she begins to feed Caden cereal, she notices that he spits each bite back out of his mouth. She is concerned that he does not like the cereal. She is afraid he is a picky eater and will not continue to gain weight if he doesn't like cereal. Her mother suggests she try the cereal in a bottle for him, but she remembers the pediatrician saying that is not how cereal should be introduced. Caden has a well-baby exam this week, so she decides to wait and see what the doctor has to say. During the visit, Ann expresses her concerns about Caden's refusal of cereal. She tells him that Caden seems to spit back every bite she feeds him with his tongue. The doctor tells Ann that when Caden pushes the cereal out of his mouth with his tongue it is not because he doesn't care for the food. This is a reflex infants have called the *extrusion reflex*. It gradually disappears between 4 and 6 months of age. He assures it is perfectly normal and even suggests she wait another month or two to try again. He graphs Caden's length of 25 inches, and weight of 15 pounds, on the age-appropriate chart. He reassures Ann that Caden is growing just fine. He suggests to Ann that she attend a class offered by the dietitians at a local hospital. The class is designed to educate new moms on how and when to introduce foods. Ann is very relieved that Caden is growing well. She makes plans to attend the next class offered by the dietitians.

ASSESSMENT

1. What are the benefits of breastfeeding?
2. Use Figure 12-10 to assess Caden's growth percentile for length and weight.
3. How many ounces of breast milk or formula would you expect a baby Caden's age to need? Use Table 12-1.
4. What would you expect Caden's calorie and protein needs to be at his age?

DIAGNOSIS

5. Write a nursing diagnosis for Caden.

PLAN/GOAL

6. What is the immediate goal for Caden?
7. What is your long-term goal for Caden?
8. What is your short-term goal for Ann?
9. What is your long-term goal for Ann?

IMPLEMENTATION

10. What does Ann need to learn from the dietitian's class?
11. Who else needs to be involved in Caden's care?

EVALUATION/OUTCOME CRITERIA

12. What might you expect of Caden by the time he is 1 year old?

THINKING FURTHER

13. The American Dietetic Association has a new webpage for children. Check out http://www.eatright.org/kids and see the information offered. How would a website like this be helpful for Ann as Caden grows?

rate this **plate**

Since Caden is not ready for solid foods, it would be recommended to wait and try again every week to see when his extrusion reflex disappears. At 10 months, Caden is now able to eat solid foods. Rate the meal that Bonita has prepared for his lunch.

- **6 oz. formula**
- **4 Tbsp infant cereal**
- **1 Tbsp baby chicken**
- **3 Tbsp pureed sweet potatoes**
- **4 Tbsp pureed pears**

Does this meal meet the recommendations? If not, what can be changed?

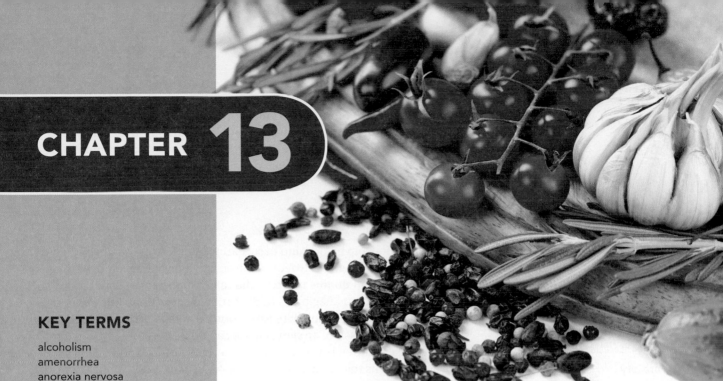

CHAPTER 13

KEY TERMS

alcoholism
amenorrhea
anorexia nervosa
anxiety
body mass index (BMI)
bulimia
cirrhosis
depression
fermentation
glycogen loading (carb-loading)
growth spurt
menses
neophobic
peers
self-esteem

NUTRITION FOR CHILDREN AND ADOLESCENTS

OBJECTIVES

After studying this chapter, you should be able to:

- Identify nutritional needs of children ages 1–12 and of adolescents
- State the effects of inadequate nutrition during the growing years
- Describe eating disorders that can occur during adolescence
- Explain the growing concern over obesity, pre-diabetes, and type 2 diabetes in youth
- Discuss nutrition basics for the athlete

Although specific nutritional requirements change as children grow, nutrition always affects physical, mental, and emotional growth and development. Studies indicate that the mental ability and size of an individual are directly influenced by nutrition during the early years. Children who have an inadequate supply of nutrients—especially of protein—and calories during their early years may be shorter and less intellectually able than children who receive an adequate diet. Parents and caregivers have the all-important task of producing the blueprint for healthy eating. When a good foundation is laid, children will maximize their learning and growth potential.

CHILDREN AGED 1–12

A child's relationship to food and basic eating habits develops in early childhood. The caregiver's goal is to feed children age-appropriate food that meets nutrition needs and do this in a way that allows adequate support and encouragement. Micromanaging a child's eating or providing little support or chaotic feeding methods can increase emotional and physical problems such as irritability, **depression**, **anxiety**, fatigue, and illness.

Because children learn partly by imitation, learning good eating habits is easier if parents role model those habits. Nutritious foods should be available at mealtime as well as snack time. Meals should include a wide variety of foods to ensure good nutrient intake. Families do best with structured meals and snacks, eaten at the kitchen table. When children are allowed constant food handouts and free rein of the kitchen, nutrition usually suffers and meal intake is suboptimal.

Eating together as a family should always be encouraged (Figure 13-1). Studies show that children who eat together with their family have healthier bodies, do better in school, have less risk-taking behaviors with drugs and alcohol, and have improved self-esteem. It is hard to dispute that it is one of the simplest and most effective ways for parents to be engaged in their children's lives.

Parents should be aware that it is not uncommon for children's appetites to vary. The rate of growth is not constant. As the child ages, the rate

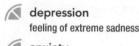

depression
feeling of extreme sadness

anxiety
apprehension

FIGURE 13-1 A family sitting down for a meal together.

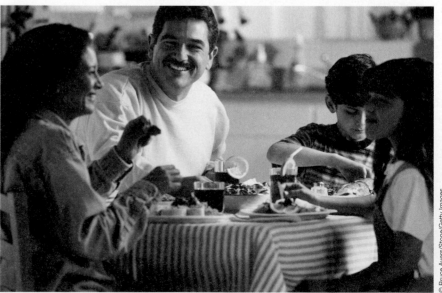

© Bruce Ayers/Stone/Getty Images

of growth actually slows. The approximate weight gain of a child during the second year of life is only 5 pounds. In addition, children's attention is increasingly focused on their environment rather than their stomachs. Consequently, their appetites and interest in food commonly decrease during the early years. Children between the ages of 1 and 3 undergo vast changes. Their legs grow longer, they develop muscles, they lose their baby shape, they begin to walk and talk, and they learn to feed and generally assert themselves (Figure 13-2). A 2-year-old child's statement "No!" is his or her way of saying "Let me decide!"

As children continue to grow and develop, they are anxious to show their growing independence. Parents should respect this need within safe and loving limits. Children's likes and dislikes may change. New foods should be introduced gradually, in small amounts, and made attractive to the eye. Parents need to understand very young children are generally **neophobic** and that it can easily take up to 10 times of exposure before a new food is eaten. Allowing a child to assist in purchasing and preparing a new food is often a good way of arousing interest in the food and a desire to eat it. Children should be offered nutrient-dense foods because the amount eaten often will be small. Fats should not be limited before the age of 2 years, but still avoid fat-laden meals and snacks. Whole milk is recommended until the age of 2 as extra fat is needed for brain development. Low-fat or fat-free milk should be served from age 2 and beyond. It is recommended that children not salt their food at the table or have foods prepared with a lot of salt. The same can be said for sugary foods or use of sugar at the table. Young children are especially sensitive to and reject hot (temperature) foods, but they will like crisp textures, mild flavors, and familiar foods. They may be wary of foods covered in sauce or gravy. Table 13-1 details serving sizes needed of the various food groups according to a child's age. Calorie needs will depend on rate of growth, activity level, body size, metabolism, and health.

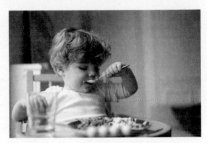

FIGURE 13-2 Children learn best by doing.

© PhotoAlto/ Sandro Di Carlo Darsa/ PhotoAlto Agency RF Collections/Getty Images

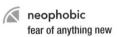 **neophobic**
fear of anything new

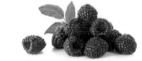

TABLE 13-1 Food Plan for Preschool and School-Age Children Based on MyPlate

FOOD GROUP	APPROXIMATE SERVING SIZES PER DAY			
	AGES 1–2	**AGES 3–4**	**AGES 5–6**	**AGES 7–12**
Milk	1½–2 cups	2½ cups	3 cups	3 cups
Protein	1–2 oz	3–4 oz	5 oz	5–6 oz
Vegetable	½–1 cup	1½ cups	2 cups	2–3 cups
Fruit	½–1 cup	1½ cups	1½ cups	1½–2 cups
Grains	1½–3 oz	4–5 oz	5 oz	5–7 oz

Oils and fats are not represented as one of the major food groups, but you need some for good health. Appropriate ranges are provided here. Plant-based fats are recommended as the major fat source.

Oils/Fat	3 tsp	4 tsp	4 tsp	5 tsp

Discretionary calorie allowance can range from 100–200 cal/day.

Source: Adapted from United States Departments of Agriculture. Daily Food Plans. 2011. http://www.choosemyplate.gov

Children can have food jags, such as eating only one or two foods, or rituals, such as not letting foods touch on the plate or using a different spoon for each food eaten. Choking is prevalent in young children. To prevent choking, do not give children under 4 years of age peanuts, grapes, hotdogs, raw carrots, hard candy, or thick peanut butter.

Often young children need a snack every 2–3 hours for continued energy. Children often prefer finger foods for snacks. Snacks should be nutrient-dense and as nutritious as food served at mealtime. Fruit, a fiber-rich unsweetened cereal, and low-fat cheese make good snacks. Mealtime should be pleasant, and food should not be forced on the child. *The parents' primary responsibility is to provide nutritious food in a pleasant setting, and the child's responsibility is to decide how much food to eat or whether to eat,* according to child expert Ellyn Satter (1995). When a child is hungry, he or she will eat. Forcing a child to eat can cause disordered eating and, ultimately, chronic overeating, **anorexia nervosa**, or **bulimia** (discussed later in this chapter).

 anorexia nervosa
psychologically induced lack of appetite

 bulimia
condition in which client alternately binges and purges

Calorie and Nutrient Needs

The *rate* of growth diminishes from the age of 1 until about 10 years; thus, the caloric requirement per pound of body weight also diminishes during this period. For example, at 6 months, a girl needs about 54 calories per pound of body weight, but by the age of 10, she will require only 35 calories per pound of body weight. See Table 13-2 for estimated calorie needs of young children.

Nutrient needs, however, do not diminish. From the age of 6 months to 10 years, nutrient needs actually *increase* because of the increase in body size. Therefore, it is especially important that young children are given nutritious foods *that they will eat.* The Dietary Reference Intake (DRI) tables show the amount of macronutrients (carbohydrates, protein, and fat) needed for children at different ages. The micronutrients (vitamins, minerals, and trace elements) are shown on the other DRI tables by life stage. Choose MyPlate (Figure 13-3) as a good foundation for developing meal plans that, with

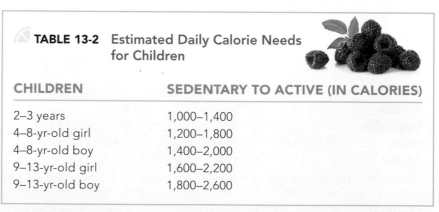

TABLE 13-2   Estimated Daily Calorie Needs for Children

CHILDREN	SEDENTARY TO ACTIVE (IN CALORIES)
2–3 years	1,000–1,400
4–8-yr-old girl	1,200–1,800
4–8-yr-old boy	1,400–2,000
9–13-yr-old girl	1,600–2,200
9–13-yr-old boy	1,800–2,600

Source: U.S. Department of Agriculture and U.S. Department of Health and Human Services. *Dietary Guidelines for Americans, 2010* (7th ed.). Washington, DC: U.S. Government Printing Office. December 2010. http://www.cnpp.usda.gov

adjustments, will suit all family members and allow consumers to view a customized daily food plan based on age, gender, size, and activity.

The new *Dietary Guidelines* published in 2010 address eating changes for individuals starting at age 2. Americans are encouraged to consume more of certain foods and nutrients such as fruits, vegetables, whole grains, fat-free and low-fat dairy products, and seafood. We are cautioned to consume fewer foods with sodium (salt), saturated fats, trans fats, cholesterol, added sugars, and refined grains.

High-nutrition vegetables include choices in the broccoli family, orange vegetables, and green leafy vegetables. High-nutrition fruits include citrus and berries. These have been coined the "powerhouse fruits and vegetables." Researchers believe that if Americans ate more of these nutrient-rich plant foods, a significant impact in public health would occur with disease prevention.

Children also need water and fiber in their diet. Generally fluid requirements are estimated at 1 ml of water for every calorie consumed: 1,200 calorie

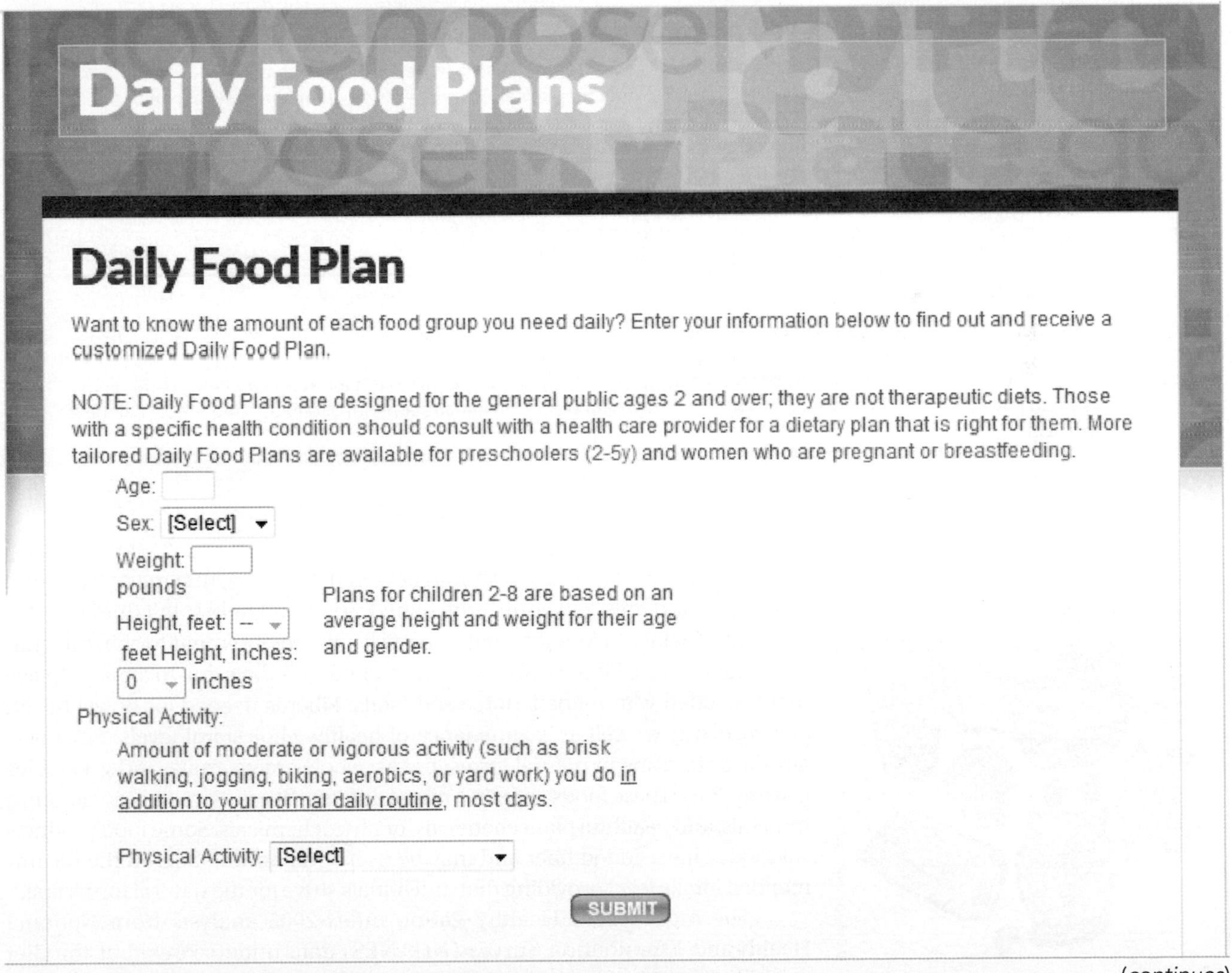

FIGURE 13-3 Use ChooseMyPlate to view a customized daily food plan.

(continues)

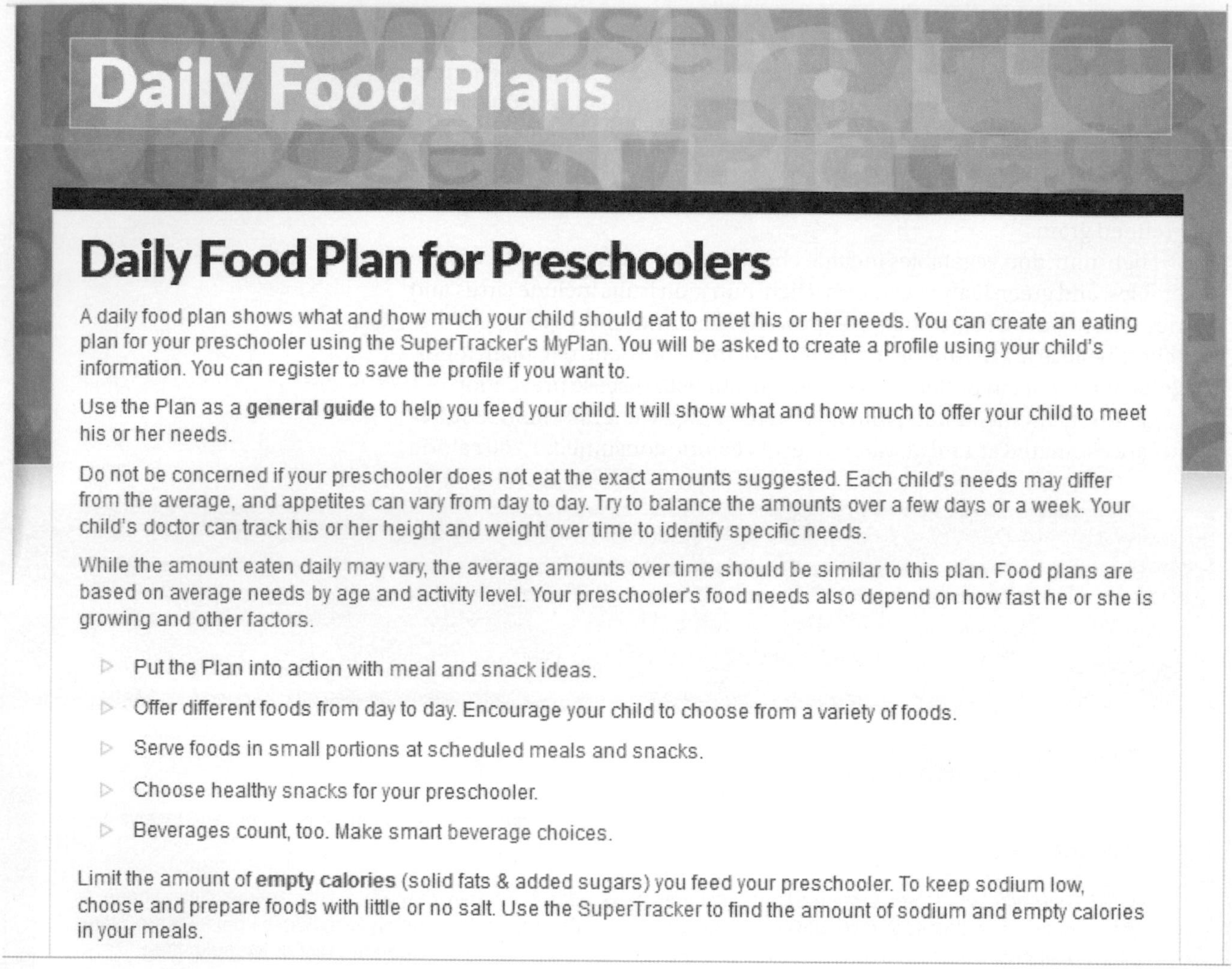

Daily Food Plans

Daily Food Plan for Preschoolers

A daily food plan shows what and how much your child should eat to meet his or her needs. You can create an eating plan for your preschooler using the SuperTracker's MyPlan. You will be asked to create a profile using your child's information. You can register to save the profile if you want to.

Use the Plan as a **general guide** to help you feed your child. It will show what and how much to offer your child to meet his or her needs.

Do not be concerned if your preschooler does not eat the exact amounts suggested. Each child's needs may differ from the average, and appetites can vary from day to day. Try to balance the amounts over a few days or a week. Your child's doctor can track his or her height and weight over time to identify specific needs.

While the amount eaten daily may vary, the average amounts over time should be similar to this plan. Food plans are based on average needs by age and activity level. Your preschooler's food needs also depend on how fast he or she is growing and other factors.

▷ Put the Plan into action with meal and snack ideas.

▷ Offer different foods from day to day. Encourage your child to choose from a variety of foods.

▷ Serve foods in small portions at scheduled meals and snacks.

▷ Choose healthy snacks for your preschooler.

▷ Beverages count, too. Make smart beverage choices.

Limit the amount of **empty calories** (solid fats & added sugars) you feed your preschooler. To keep sodium low, choose and prepare foods with little or no salt. Use the SuperTracker to find the amount of sodium and empty calories in your meals.

FIGURE 13-3 (*continued*)

U.S. Department of Agriculture. Daily Food Plans. 2012. http://www.choosemyplate.gov

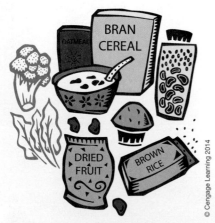

FIGURE 13-4 Foods rich in fiber.

© Cengage Learning 2014

intake = 1,200 ml or 5 cups. It should be noted, however, that many fruits and vegetables and milk will contribute to hydration and help fulfill fluid needs.

The Dietary Reference Intake charts list the requirement for fiber in children (Table 13-3). Fiber is often lacking in children's diets due to a marketplace that is flooded with refined, processed foods. Fiber is needed for bowel health and regularity as well as maintenance of healthy cholesterol levels. Fiber ideally needs to come in natural forms: beans, whole grains, fruits, and vegetables (Figure 13-4). These foods contain a mix of different fibers as well as key vitamins, minerals, and healthful plant chemicals, or phytochemicals. Some food products sold today have added fiber and may be useful in boosting fiber to the recommended intake level providing that individuals strive for the natural forms first.

The most recent Healthy Eating Index-2005 analysis from National Health and Examination Survey (NHANES) data underscores that the diet of children 2–17 years of age needs improvement. Data suggest that children's consumption falls short in whole fruit, whole grains, green and orange

TABLE 13-3	Fiber Needs for Children
AGE	**ADEQUATE INTAKE (AI) (IN GRAMS)**
1–3 yr	19
4–8 yr	25
9–13 yr male	31
14–18 yr male	38
9–13 yr female	26
14–18 yr female	26

Reprinted with permission from the National Academies Press, Copyright © 2006, National Academy of Sciences. *Dietary Reference Intakes: The Essential Guide to Nutrient Requirements.*

vegetables, and legumes. For children 2–5 years of age, only 22% are meeting government guidelines for vegetable consumption; 16% of children aged 6–11 meet requirements; and 11% of children aged 12–18 meet recommendations. One third of vegetable consumption was fried potatoes (French fries or potato chips) and a little more than one third of fruit consumption was juice.

As children get older, the following also occurs:

- Reduction in regular breakfast consumption
- Increase in foods prepared away from home
- Increase in snacking
- Increase in fried foods (especially French fries) and nutrient-poor food
- Increase in portion size
- Increase in sweetened beverages and sugar
- Decrease in dairy products

Poor diet patterns and imbalances can set children up for health issues such as obesity, cardiovascular disease, high blood pressure, and prediabetes. Positive nutrition education and practices therefore need to happen broadly—in primary care settings, schools, and homes across the nation and start at a young age.

As kids desire sweets and prefer these to nutrient-rich foods, sugar-laden dessert and snack foods should be given sparingly. Sweetened drinks and fruit juices should be limited. The gold standard is for health practitioners to suggest limiting juice to only 4–6 oz per day for children aged 1–6, and ensure that it is 100% juice. The appropriate range of juice for older children is 8–12 oz per day. Frequent exposure of teeth to sugary foods, especially sticky sweet foods, increases the likelihood of dental caries.

Assessing Growth

Pediatric growth charts from the Centers for Disease Control and Prevention (CDC) have been used by pediatricians, dietitians, nurses, and parents to track

In The Media

Kids Prefer Veggies With Cool Names

A new study by Cornell University shows that kids will eat more vegetables if they have "cool" names. Researchers tested 186 participants, offering these 4-year-olds "x-ray vision carrots" one day and plain old carrots on another. The kids ate twice as many "x-ray vision carrots." Other vegetables tested were "power peas" and "dinosaur broccoli trees."

(Source: Adapted from Eat Your Vegetables: Preschoolers Love Vegetables with Catchy Names Like "X-Ray Vision Carrots" and "Tomato Bursts." *ScienceDaily.* March 2, 2009. http://www.sciencedaily.com)

EXPLORING THE WEB

Visit the Centers for Disease Control and Prevention website (http://www.cdc.gov) to learn more about how to use growth charts. Search and use the BMI calculator to calculate your BMI and learn how it affects growth trends. What are some of the additional resources available at this site?

Supersize **USA**

Vending machines are everywhere! Have you visited your vending machine today? Hopefully you've pushed the button for a healthy choice. To prevent supersizing yourself, here is a list to help you when choosing a snack from a vending machine.

Healthy Choices	Poor Choices
Water	Breakfast pastries
Baked chips	Chips (nacho cheese)
Granola bars	Candy bars
Sunflower seeds	Cookies
Honey roasted nuts	Doughnuts
Pretzels	Sandwich crackers
Fig bars	Fruit pies
Skim milk	Whole milk
Reduced-fat popcorn	Snack cakes
Tea (unsweetened or diet)	Soda
Dried fruit	Sugary juice or punch

The poor choices contain too much sugar and saturated and trans fats. As a once-in-awhile treat they are alright, but not on a daily basis.

the growth of infants, children, and adolescents in the United States since 1977 (Figure 13-5). It is recommended that health care providers use the following:

- World Health Organization (WHO) growth standards to monitor growth for infants and children 0–2 years of age in the United States
- CDC growth charts for children 2 years of age and older in the United States

The growth charts for youth 2–20 years of age measure stature-for-age, weight-for-age, and body mass index-for-age and consist of a series of percentile curves that illustrate the distribution of these measurements in children. **Body mass index (BMI)** is a number calculated from a person's weight and height and is a fairly reliable indicator of body fatness for most people. A BMI calculator is available on the MyPlate website (http://www.choosemyplate.gov), under the SuperTracker tab.

Growth charts are not intended to be used as the only diagnostic instrument but can contribute to forming an overall clinical impression for the child being measured. Clinicians find it useful to track children's growth over time to see if growth is happening in a predictable way. Changes in the growth chart alert practitioners to delve further into current health practices that have been affecting growth.

body mass index (BMI)
a number calculated from a person's weight and height as a fairly reliable indicator of body fatness for most people

SPECIAL HEALTH CONCERNS DURING CHILDHOOD
Heart Health

Proper nutrition is vital to heart health. Recent studies have shown that children with one or both parents who have had heart disease before age 60 were

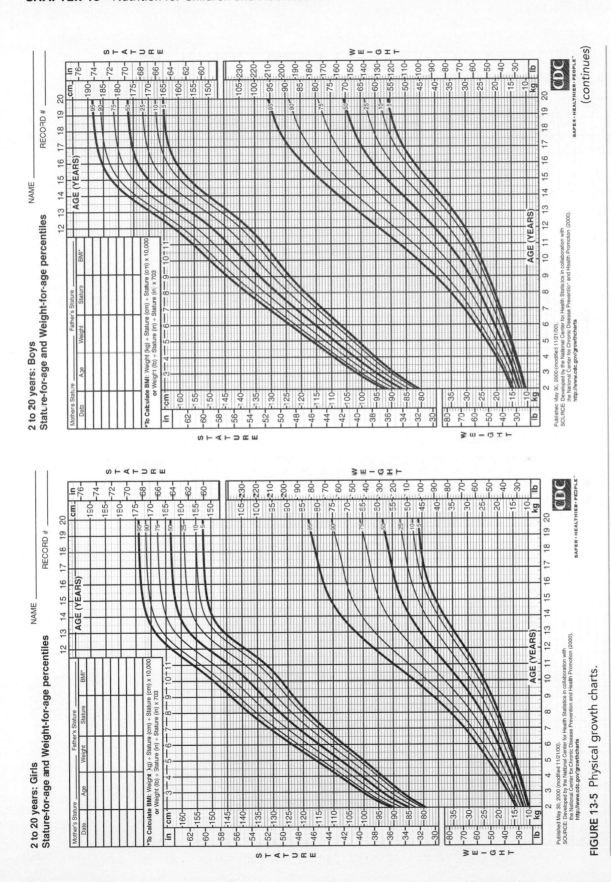

FIGURE 13-5 Physical growth charts.

Centers for Disease Control and Prevention, National Center for Health Statistics in collaboration with the National Center for Chronic Disease Prevention and Health Promotion. 2000 CDC Growth Charts: United States. http://www.cdc.gov/growthcharts, retrieved June 23, 2009. Additional clinical growth charts with the 3rd and 97th percentiles can be found on the CDC website.

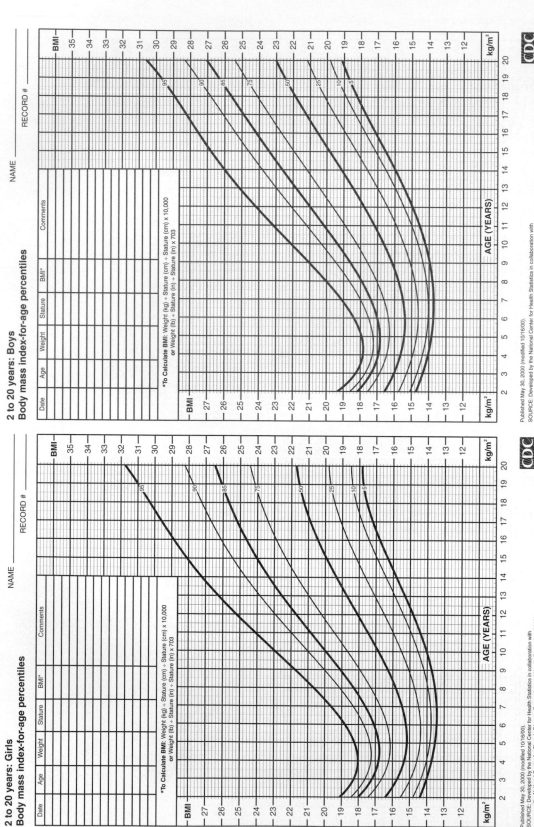

FIGURE 13-5 (continued)

Centers for Disease Control and Prevention, National Center for Health Statistics in collaboration with the National Center for Chronic Disease Prevention and Health Promotion. 2000 CDC Growth Charts: United States. http://www.cdc.gov/growthcharts, retrieved June 23, 2009. Additional clinical growth charts with the 3rd and 97th percentiles can be found on the CDC website.

more likely to have atherosclerosis themselves. Further, researchers know the risk of coronary artery disease increases progressively with age. Because it has been demonstrated that the atherosclerotic process can begin in youth, good nutrition, a physically active lifestyle, and absence of tobacco use are of utmost importance. These factors can contribute to lower risk prevalence and either delay or prevent the onset of cardiovascular disease.

Many health practitioners screen children at age 2 for high cholesterol. The National Cholesterol Education Program and American Academy of Pediatrics (AAP) has suggested that acceptable total cholesterol for youth should be less than 170 mg/dl (LDL less than 110 mg/dl).

Fat intake for children should follow the American Heart Recommendations: ages 1–3 should receive 30–40% of total daily calories from fat, and youth ages 4–18 should receive 25–35% of total calories from fat. If aiming for no more than 30% total calories from fat, an ideal fat distribution would be saturated at no more than 7%, polyunsaturated fat at no more than 8% and monounsaturated fat at 15% of total calories.

Bone Health

Optimizing bone health in youth results in stronger and denser bones in adulthood. Consumption of adequate calcium in the formative years is critical for the development of peak bone mass. Nutrient intake data, however, suggests that the majority of children and teens do not consume enough daily calcium and may have less than ideal bone health. In fact, bone fracture incidences have risen. According to *The Journal of the American Medical Association*, the incidences of bone fractures in U.S. youth were seen to be 32% higher in boys, and 56% higher in girls from the late 1960s through the 1990s.

Vitamin D is also a significant nutrient required for bone health. As described elsewhere in this text, many children and adolescents may be lacking this important nutrient. Other nutrients needed for bone strengthening are protein, phosphorus, magnesium, potassium, vitamin B_{12}, and zinc.

Genetics and physical activity also influence bone health. Regarding physical activity, lower levels of activity among our youth, especially weight-bearing types, have been linked to greater fracture risk. Overweight and obesity have also been linked to compromised bone health in children.

Anemia

Anemia (low hemoglobin or low hematocrit) is an indicator of iron deficiency. Iron deficiency, according to the WHO, is the most common nutritional disorder in the world. It is currently affecting millions of children in developing countries. Anemia is associated with developmental delays and behavior problems in children. The CDC reports that anemia occurs in 14% of U.S. toddlers (age 1–2 years). At this time of life, toddlers transition from their iron-rich infant foods to table food and cow's milk which contains less iron.

The incidence of anemia is slightly higher in low-income children and varies by racial and ethnic groups, with highest prevalence among African

American children. The AAP recommends screening for anemia between the ages of 9 and 12 months with additional screening between the ages of 1 and 5 years for clients at risk. Red meat, poultry and seafood, egg yolk, and iron-fortified breads and cereals can help meet iron needs. Vegetables and fruits such as spinach and other greens, peas, broccoli, dried beans, and dried fruit (raisins, dates, apricots) are iron rich as well. Vitamin C–containing foods eaten along with iron-rich foods enhance absorption of the iron.

Medicines that Increase or Decrease Appetite

Certain medications (psychostimulants) used to treat attention deficit and hyperactivity disorder (ADHD) in children cause marked decrease in appetite. According to the CDC, in the United States, 9.5% or 5.4 million children aged 4–17 have an ADHD diagnosis, as of 2007. In practice, parents of the medicated ADHD child often see a compromised appetite especially at the lunch meal, when the medicine is most active.

If a child's appetite decreases after taking ADHD medicine, it is recommended to give the dose after breakfast so that he or she will eat better in the morning. A parent may then want to serve a large dinner in the evening, when the drug is beginning to wear off. Often the bedtime snack needs to turn into the "third meal." Parents will need to keep plenty of healthy snacks on hand; a balanced diet with nutritious, higher-calorie foods and drinks will help to offset any weight loss from the ADHD medication.

Some health care providers may see changes in the growth of a child on some of these stimulants. If the child's poor appetite lasts for a long period, the health care provider may reduce the dose or stop the drug on weekends or summer breaks to allow appetite to return to normal. The provider may reevaluate the medication chosen.

On the other end of the spectrum, children and adolescents who take some of the newer generation of antipsychotic medications for mood stabilization and behavior issues have increased appetite. Users of those medicines risk rapid weight gain and metabolic changes that could lead to diabetes, hypertension, and other illnesses. Some children on those medicines were recorded to have an average weight gain of 1–1.5 pounds a week. Doctors believe, however, these drugs still have their place in behavioral health as they can spare children from psychological suffering. But practitioners are learning that they must be prescribed more cautiously and that the benefits must be weighed against the risks.

Food Allergies

Researchers are now estimating that as many as 8% of children under age 18 have allergies to at least one food. Preschoolers (age 3–5 years) have been shown to have the highest prevalence of allergies. Allergies to peanuts were the most commonly reported, affecting 2% of children. Milk and shellfish allergies ranked second and third. Tree nuts, egg, fish, strawberry, wheat, and soy rounded out the top nine food triggers. Some children with food allergies have mild cases and they outgrow them in time; however, researchers are discovering 40% of children experience severe reactions including wheezing and anaphylaxis. The Food Allergy Network (http://www.foodallergy .org) has useful information for families that are experiencing allergies. See Chapter 10 for further discussion on food allergies.

OBESITY AND RELATED HEALTH COMPLICATIONS

In America today, unprecedented numbers of our youth are being diagnosed with overweight and obesity. This is leading to a cascade of serious illnesses including pre-diabetes, diabetes, hypertension, and cardiovascular disease.

Obesity

Childhood overweight and obesity is a result of an imbalance between the energy taken in from food and beverages and the energy expended for normal growth and development, as well as physical activity. No single factor causes obesity, rather researchers believe it can stem from many factors including genetic, behavioral, and environmental issues. The CDC estimates that approximately 17% (or 12.5 million) of children and adolescents aged 2–19 years are obese. Since 1980, obesity prevalence among children and adolescents has almost tripled.

There are significant racial and ethnic disparities in obesity prevalence among U.S. children and adolescents. In 2007–2008, Hispanic boys and African American girls stand out as the groups experiencing higher rates of obesity. Further discussion on childhood obesity occurs in the weight management chapter (Chapter 16).

Pre-Diabetes

In 2005–2006, one in six U.S. adolescents had pre-diabetes. Among overweight youth, the prevalence was nearly one in three. Pre-diabetes means that your blood sugar level is higher than normal, but not increased enough to be classified as type 2 diabetes. Pre-diabetes is defined as a fasting blood sugar between 100 and 126 mg/dl. Another name associated with pre-diabetes is *metabolic syndrome* or *insulin resistance*. Besides the elevated blood sugar, other factors may sometimes be present: high waist circumference, increasing blood pressure, and impaired lipids such as high triglycerides and low HDL (high-density lipoprotein). In adults, researchers predict pre-diabetes may convert to type 2 diabetes within 10 years if interventions are not undertaken.

Exercise, diet, and weight changes are effective at turning around pre-diabetes. Specific to diet, research is beginning to show that fiber in addition to a high-phytochemical intake from plant foods helps improve pre-diabetes.

Acanthosis nigricans is a skin condition characterized by dark, thick, velvety skin in body folds and creases. Most practitioners see these skin changes around the neck during routine exams. This disorder is often associated with conditions that increase your insulin level, such as type 2 diabetes or being overweight. If your insulin level is too high, the extra insulin may trigger activity in your skin cells. This may cause the characteristic skin changes.

Diabetes

Type 2 diabetes in children and adolescents already appears to be a significant and growing problem among U.S. children and adolescents. Overall, diabetes is on the rise for all ages. In fact, the CDC states that one in three children born after the year 2000 will develop diabetes.

Children and adolescents diagnosed with type 2 diabetes are generally between 10 and 19 years old, obese, have a strong family history for type 2 diabetes, and have insulin resistance. Diabetes screening is recommended for all children and adolescents at high risk, even if they have no signs or symptoms of the condition.

Those affected with type 2 diabetes belong to all ethnic groups, but it is more commonly seen in non-white groups. CDC data indicates American Indian youths have the highest prevalence of type 2 diabetes. Diabetics are at higher risk of heart disease, kidney disease, and neuropathy, among others. Children with type 2 diabetes should see a certified diabetes educator to learn what to eat to control their diabetes. This specialist will also prescribe daily exercise and attention to fiber intake, both of which help control blood glucose.

Hypertension

High blood pressure in children may be the result of an underlying disease process or the early onset of hypertension. Hypertension among overweight or obese youth worsens with time if left untreated. Diagnosing hypertension in children is done using the National Heart Lung and Blood Institute's blood pressure tables for children and adolescents, which looks at age, gender, and height (http://www.nhlbi.nih.gov). Several blood pressure percentile readings over the 95th percentile suggest a diagnosis of hypertension. Regular aerobic activity, normalization of BMI, and watching sodium all improve blood pressure in youth.

Cardiovascular Disease

Children with the highest risks of developing cardiovascular disease are those who are sedentary and obese and may have diabetes or pre-diabetes. Youth that also have high blood pressure and high LDL cholesterol are at increased risk as well. Many children in late childhood or early adolescence already have fatty streaks in their coronary arteries. An overweight child who is sedentary, or one who consumes a diet high in saturated fat, should have routine cholesterol screenings throughout their youth.

A multipronged approach of sound health messaging will need to be communicated to youth. Parents hold the primary reigns for the change to begin. Health care providers, schools, daycare providers, government agencies though in tandem will also be required to change the culture, to turn the tide in obesity, pre-diabetes, and diabetes in our youth.

ADOLESCENTS

In general, a person between the ages of 13 and 20 is considered an adolescent. Adolescence is a period of rapid growth that causes major changes. It tends to begin between the ages of 10 and 13 in girls and between 13 and 16 in boys. The **growth spurt** may yield a height increase of 3 inches a year for girls and 4 inches a year for boys (Figure 13-6). Bones grow and gain density, muscle and fat tissue develop, and blood volume increases. Sexual maturity occurs: Boys' voices change, girls experience the onset of **menses**, and both may experience acne. Note that acne is not caused by eating specific foods but by having overactive sebaceous glands of the skin.

These changes are obvious and have a tremendous effect on an adolescent's psychosocial development. No two individuals will develop in the same way. One girl may become heavier than she might like, another may be thin, a boy may not develop the muscle or the height he desires, and some may develop serious complexion problems. Many teens will accept their changes, while others may need psychological counseling.

Food Habits

Adolescents, especially boys, typically have enormous appetites. When good eating habits have been established during childhood and there is nutritious food available, the teenager's food habits should present no serious problem.

Adolescents are imitators, like children, but instead of imitating adults, adolescents prefer to imitate their **peers** and do what is popular. Unfortunately, the foods that are popular often have low nutrient density such as potato chips, sodas, and candy. These foods provide mainly carbohydrates and fats and very little protein, vitamins, and minerals, except for salt, which is usually provided in excess. According to the Center for Science in the Public Interest, on average, teens get 13% of their calories from carbonated and noncarbonated soft drinks. It provides the average 12–19-year-old boy with about 15 tsp of refined sugars a day and the average girl with about 10 tsp a day—an amount that has public health officials concerned.

The concern of soda is not simply all the sugary calories, but for what soda pushes out of the diet. Youth used to consume twice as much milk as soft drinks. On average at present, boys and girls consume twice as much soda pop as milk (Figure 13-7).

Adolescents' eating habits can be seriously affected by busy schedules, part-time jobs, athletics, social activities, and the lack of an available adult to prepare nutritious food when they are hungry or have time to eat. When adolescents' food habits need improvement, it is wise for adults to tactfully inform them of nutritional needs and of the poor nutrition quality of their food choices. The adolescent has a natural desire for independence and may resent being told what to do.

Before attempting to change food habits, carefully check an adolescent's food choices for nutrient content. It is too easily assumed that because the adolescent chooses the food, the food is automatically a poor choice in regard to nutrient content. It might be a good choice. An adolescent who has a problem maintaining an appropriate weight may need some advice regarding diet.

 growth spurt
significant rapid gain in size near the onset of adolescence

 menses
another term for menstruation

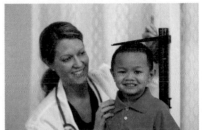

FIGURE 13-6 The doctor measures a child's height to record on the growth chart.

 peers
people who are approximately one's own age

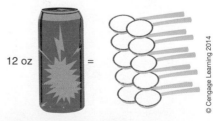

12 oz =

FIGURE 13-7 One 12 oz can of soda = 10 tsp of sugar.

EXPLORING THE WEB

Search the Web to learn about the Healthy, Hunger-Free Kids Act of 2010 and discuss the new rules that were passed for the National School Breakfast and Lunch program. Discuss why Congress did not pass all of the rulings and what the rationale was for amending the original proposal. Which celebrity chef was present when First Lady Michelle Obama made the announcement on January 25, 2012?

Calorie and Nutrient Needs

Because of adolescents' rapid growth, calorie requirements naturally increase. Boys' calorie requirements tend to be greater than girls' because boys are generally bigger, tend to be more physically active, and have more lean muscle mass than girls.

The requirement for energy-containing nutrients, vitamins, and minerals all dramatically increase more during adolescence than at any other time of life except pregnancy and lactation. The DRI table provides such changes by life stage. Because of menstruation, girls have a greater need for iron than boys. Calcium requirements are high to support peak bone mass. Optimizing calcium intake for bone health is particularly important during adolescence, as peak use of calcium for bone mineralization occurs on average at 12.5 years in girls and 14.0 years in boys. In a 3–4-year period in adolescence, 40% of total adult bone mass is accumulated. It has been understood that low calcium intake in adolescence is problematic in America. It has been reported that 85% of girls and 64% of boys age 12–19 years have too low of an intake. On average, boys only consume 2.4 servings of milk per day and girls only 1.7 servings of milk per day.

SPECIAL HEALTH CONCERNS DURING ADOLESCENCE

Adolescence is a stressful time for most young people. They are unexpectedly faced with numerous physical changes, an innate need for independence, increased work and extracurricular demands at school and jobs, and social and sexual pressures from their peers.

Anorexia Nervosa

While eating disorders may begin with an innocent attempt at dieting and losing weight, they are most often about much more than this. People with eating disorders often use food and the control of food in an attempt to compensate for difficult feelings and emotions that may seem overwhelming in their lives. Low self-esteem, troubled relationships, being teased about body issues, and stress are just some of the factors that play into the development of an eating disorder. Some may fear growing up. Many have overachieving personalities and are perfectionistic. Cultural factors also come into play as many want to resemble the slim fashion models exhibited in the media. As many as 10 million females and 1 million males are fighting a battle with an eating disorder. Some individuals switch from one eating disorder pattern to another, or have a mixture of disordered eating traits.

Anorexia nervosa is a serious, potentially life-threatening eating disorder characterized by self-starvation and excessive weight loss. Anorexia nervosa has four primary symptoms:

1. Failure to maintain body weight at or above a minimally normal weight for age and height; usually 85% of expected weight.
2. Intense fear of weight gain or being "fat," even though underweight.

3. Disturbance with body weight or shape.

4. Loss of menstrual periods in girls and women postpuberty.

Anorexia, a psychological disorder, is more common in women than men. It can begin as early as late childhood, but usually begins during the teen years or early 20s. The dramatic reduction in calories causes altered metabolism, hair loss, low blood pressure, weakness, **amenorrhea**, brain damage, and even death.

Individuals with anorexia usually set a maximum weight for themselves and become an expert at "counting calories" to attain their chosen weight. They also often exercise excessively to control or reduce their weight. Often once they achieve their weight goal, they are not satisfied and want to lose even more weight. If weight declines too far, organ failure will occur and the anorexic will ultimately die.

Treatment requires the following:

1. Development of a strong and trusting relationship between the client and the health care professionals involved in the case.

2. That the client learn and accept that weight gain and a change in body contours are normal during adolescence.

3. Nutritional therapy so the client will understand the need for both nutrients and calories and how best to obtain them.

4. Individual and family counseling by a licensed family therapist, ideally with a specialty in eating disorder counseling.

5. Medical monitoring by the health care professional.

6. Time and patience from all involved.

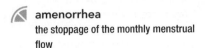

amenorrhea
the stoppage of the monthly menstrual flow

Bulimia

Bulimia is a syndrome in which an individual alternately binges on food then purges by inducing vomiting or using laxatives or diuretics, or overexercises, to compensate and "rid" oneself of ingested food. Bulimics are said to fear that they cannot stop eating. They tend to be high achievers who are perfectionistic, obsessive, and depressed. They generally lack a strong sense of self and have a need to seem special. They know their binge–purge syndrome is abnormal but also fear being overweight. This condition is more common among women than men and can begin any time from the late teens into the 30s.

A bulimic usually binges on high-calorie foods such as cookies, ice cream, pastries, and other "forbidden" foods. The binge can take only a few moments or can run several hours—until there is no space for more food. It occurs when the person is alone. Bulimia can follow a period of excessive dieting, and stress usually increases the frequency of binges. Bulimia is not usually life-threatening, but it can irritate the esophagus and cause electrolyte imbalances, malnutrition, dehydration, and dental caries.

Treatment involves helping the person learn how to live at peace with oneself and the food environment. Therapists, doctors, social workers, and dietitians are also involved with the treatments of this eating disorder. Returning to scheduled eating times, doing appetite awareness training and journaling, and developing alternate coping skills to destress are usual tactics that clients use to overcome bulimia.

Binge Eating Disorder

Another recognized eating disorder is binge eating, also known as compulsive overeating. This disorder manifests itself by periods of uncontrolled or impulsive eating beyond normal fullness. Individuals suffering from this do not purge; however, the binge may be precipitated by a fast or strict diet measure. Once a binge has occurred, feelings of guilt and shame usually occur. Individuals that compulsively overeat often struggle with anxiety, depression, and loneliness. While many binge eaters are obese, some may be only moderately overweight or even normal weight. Experts believe the binge eating disorder can easily start in the childhood or teen years.

Signs may include:

- A large amount of food missing from the refrigerator or pantry
- Visibly seeing a child eating a lot of food quickly
- A pattern of eating in response to emotional stress, such as family conflict, peer rejection, or poor academic performance
- A child feeling ashamed or disgusted by the amount eaten
- Finding food containers or wrappers hidden in a child's room
- An increasingly irregular eating pattern, such as skipping meals, eating lots of junk food, and eating at unusual times (such as late at night)

A parent must be coached on addressing this issue in a very gentle and loving way, so the child feels safe talking about the issue. Blaming, scolding, or punishing the child will only backfire. Mental health professionals can help address the underlying issues.

More and more health practitioners are seeing what is described as the female athletic triad. The symptoms of this are disordered eating, amenorrhea, and osteoporosis. Female athletes who exercise and train intensely have lower levels of estrogen. This combined with not eating enough calories (and commonly restricting fat) leads to menstrual irregularities or absence of menses, stress fractures, and early osteoporosis.

Eating disorder awareness and prevention is key. Parents of youth must model healthy body image and healthy self-esteem if their children are to develop these important attributes. It is clear that children are watching their parents at all times and observing the way they talk about themselves and their body. Respect and appreciation for what our bodies do for us must be part of the discussion we have with our youth. It's important we value ourselves based on character, talent, and accomplishments, rather than what we look like or what we weigh (Figure 13-8).

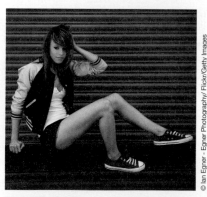

© Ian Egner - Egner Photography/ Flickr/Getty Images

FIGURE 13-8 The average model is 5'10" and weighs 110 pounds; however, an average 5'5" teen is 125–130 pounds.

Overweight and Obesity in Teens

Being overweight during adolescence is particularly unfortunate because it is apt to diminish an individual's **self-esteem** and, consequently, can exclude her or him from the normal social life of the teen years, further

self-esteem
feelings of self-worth

diminishing self-esteem. Also, it tends to make the individual prone to over-weight as an adult.

Genetics may play a role in overweight, but it's the environment that triggers overweight or obesity. Overfeeding during infancy and childhood can be a contributing factor. Once someone is overweight, isolative behavior may ensue. For example, if a teenager becomes the center of his classmates' jokes, he or she may prefer to spend time alone, perhaps watching television and finding comfort in food. This behavior adds more calories, reduces activity, and thus worsens the condition. Overweight or obese youth are at more risk for depression. In fact, obese children who were surveyed about their quality of life rated it as being as low as children receiving chemotherapy for cancer treatment. The problem of being overweight during adolescence is especially difficult to solve until the individual involved makes the independent decision to change lifestyle habits. After making such a decision, the teenager should see a physician to ensure proper health. The health care provider can play an important role by offering guidance on changing eating habits, increasing exercise, and adopting a healthier lifestyle. This issue is further addressed in the weight management chapter (Chapter 16).

Fast Foods

Many Americans have become extremely fond of fast foods. Data from the mid-1990s has shown that one third of young people eat fast food. Portion sizes offered by fast-food restaurants also grew during this time period, with individual items from two to five times larger than they were when originally introduced. More recent data from 2003–2004 indicate that fast food now contributes 16–17% of adolescents' total caloric intake, and each meal consumed in a fast-food or other restaurant increases adolescents' daily intake by 108 calories.

Teenager favorites include hamburgers, cheeseburgers, French fries, milkshakes, pizza, sodas, tacos, fried chicken, and onion rings. These and other choices in fast-food restaurants are high in fat, especially saturated fats, sodium, and sugar, and high in total calories. Generally speaking, many menu choices in a fast-food restaurant are nutrient poor and energy dense. Vitamin, mineral, and fiber content are usually sorely lacking in these high-calorie foods.

Many fast-food companies have the nutrient content of their products available to help the public make better choices. The Federal Drug Administration (FDA) is proposing that nutrition labeling be mandatory for all. Most restaurants do offer some healthful and lower calorie choices on their menus such as salads, grilled chicken, oatmeal, and fruit cups. Children can substitute apple or orange slices in place of French fries. These items are not big sellers, however, and unhealthy options are usually chosen.

The fast-food industry spends more than $4 billion a year on media advertising to promote its products. Fast food has increasingly become inexpensive with the introduction of "dollar menu choices." Therefore, for a relatively small amount of money, we can become quite full. Health can suffer over the long term, however, with frequent fast-food choices. Table 13-4 shows the nutrient content of a sample day of fast-food eating for a teenage girl compared with the nutrients her body needs.

TABLE 13-4 Calorie and Nutrient Content of a Fast-Food Day of Eating Compared with Requirements for a Teenage Girl

SAMPLE DAY OF EATING FOR TEENAGE GIRL	AMOUNT	CALORIES	PROTEIN (g)	FAT (g)	CALCIUM (mg)	IRON (mg)	SODIUM (mg)	VITAMIN A (re)	VITAMIN C (mg)	FIBER (g)
Sausage Muffin with Egg	1	450	20	28	300	3	930	115	1	2
Hot Chocolate	16 oz	100	0	0	0	0	85	0	0	0
Hamburger	1	292	15	11	84	3	555	3	0	2
French Fries, medium		389	5	21	16	2	235	0	3	4
Chocolate shake	10 oz	379	9	12	280	2	167	74	1	2
Pizza, pepperoni	¼ of 12"	500	22	20	282	4	1,144	127	0	3
Soda	16 oz	182	0	0	10	0	20	0	0	0
Daily Total		2,292	71	92	972	14	3,136	127	5	13
DRI/RDA for teenage girl		2,200	44	73	1,200	15	2,300	800	60	26

Alcohol

In a process called **fermentation**, sugars and starches can be changed to alcohol. Enzyme action causes this change. Alcohol is typically made from fruit, corn, rye, barley, rice, or potatoes. It provides 7 calories per gram but almost no nutrients.

Alcohol is a substance that can have serious side effects. Initially, it causes the drinker to feel "happy" because it lowers inhibitions. This feeling affects the drinker's judgment and can lead to accidents and crime. Ultimately, alcohol is a depressant; continued drinking leads to sleepiness, loss of consciousness, and, when too much is consumed in a short period, death.

Abuse (overuse) of alcohol is called **alcoholism**. Alcoholism can destroy the lives of families and devastate the drinker's nutritional status and thus health. It affects absorption and normal metabolism of glucose, fats, proteins, and vitamins. When thiamine and niacin cannot be absorbed, the cells cannot use glucose for energy. Blood cells, which depend on glucose for energy, are particularly affected. Over time, if alcohol abuse continues, fat will accumulate in the liver, leading to **cirrhosis**. Alcohol causes kidneys to excrete larger-than-normal amounts of water, resulting in an increased loss of minerals. In a poor nutritional state, the body is less able to fight off disease.

In addition, excessive, long-term drinking can cause high blood pressure and can damage the heart muscle. It is associated with cancer of the throat and the esophagus and can damage the reproductive system.

The risks to the drinker are obvious. When a pregnant or lactating woman drinks, however, she puts the fetus or the nursing infant at risk as well. Alcohol can lower birth weight and cause fetal alcohol syndrome or fetal alcohol effect, with related developmental disorders (see Chapter 11).

Unfortunately, many teenagers ignore the dangers of alcohol and use it in an effort to appear adult. The 2009 Youth Risk Behavior Survey from the CDC found that among high school students, during the past 30 days: 42% drank some amount of alcohol and 24% binge drank. In addition to the damage to their own health, potential accidents, and the random acts of violence caused by their drinking, teenagers' behavior sets a poor example for younger children who emulate them. The health professional is in a good position to spread the message that alcohol is a substance and can cause severe economic and family problems, as well as addiction, disease, and death.

Marijuana

Marijuana use among teens rose in 2011 for the fourth straight year. There had been a decline in use in the preceding decade. Daily marijuana use unfortunately is now at a 30-year peak among high school seniors. One marijuana cigarette is as harmful as four or five tobacco cigarettes, because the marijuana smoke is held in the lungs for a longer period of time. As a person smokes marijuana, the lungs absorb the fat-soluble active ingredient, delta-9-tetrahydrocannabinol (THC), and store it in the fat (Indiana Prevention Resource Center, 2003). Experts believe that the use of marijuana can lead to the use of other drugs such as cocaine. Some common names for marijuana are *pot, grass, herb, weed, Mary Jane, reefer, skunk, boom, gangster, kif, chronic,* and *ganja.*

fermentation
changing of sugars and starches to alcohol

alcoholism
chronic and excessive use of alcohol

cirrhosis
generic term for liver disease characterized by cell loss

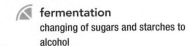

In The Media

Binge Drinking and Teens

One in four teens and young adults binge drinks. It is reported that 90% of the alcohol consumed by high school students is consumed in the course of binge drinking. MRI brain scans of teens who drank heavily showed damaged nerve tissues compared to nondrinking teens. Binge drinking is a huge public health problem among our youth that has largely gone unnoticed.

(Source: Adapted from Reinberg, Steven. 1 in 4 U.S. Teens and Young Adults Binge Drink. *USA Today.* October 8, 2010. http://www.usatoday.com)

Cocaine

Cocaine is highly addictive and extremely harmful. It causes restlessness, heightened self-confidence, euphoria, irritability, insomnia, depression, confusion, hallucinations, loss of appetite, and a tendency to withdraw from normal activities. Cocaine can cause cardiac irregularities, heart attacks, and cardiac arrests resulting in death. Weight loss is very common, mostly because it decreases appetite; addicts would give up food for the drug. The smokable form of cocaine is *crack*, which is more addictive than any other drug. It is estimated that half of all crimes against property committed in major cities are related to the use of crack cocaine and the addict's need for money to buy the drug.

Tobacco

Cigarette smoking is addictive. CDC data show that cigarette smoking by teenagers is prevalent, with 17.2% of high school students reporting that they are smokers. Further, 5.2% of middle schoolers report smoking. Teenagers smoke to "be cool," to look older, to lose weight, or to impress peers. Smoking can influence appetite, nutrition status, and weight. Smokers need the DRI for vitamin C plus 35 mg, because smoking alters their metabolism. Low intakes of vitamin C, vitamin A, beta-carotene, folate, and fiber are common in smokers. Smoking increases the risk of lung cancer and heart disease.

Other Addictive Drugs

Methamphetamine, also known as crystal meth, is the most potent form of amphetamines. Amphetamines cause heart, breathing, and blood pressure rates to increase. The mouth is usually dry, and swallowing is difficult. Urination is also difficult. Appetite is depressed. The users' pupils become dilated, and reflexes speed up. As the drug wears off, users experience feelings of fatigue or depression. Street names include *crank, speed, crystal, meth, zip*, and *ice*. Ecstasy, a slang term for MDMA, is known as the "club drug." This drug is found in capsule or tablet form.

Inhalants are chemicals whose fumes are inhaled into the body and produce mind-altering effects. Some inhalants are gasoline, lighter fluid, tool-cleaning solvents, model airplane glue, and permanent ink in felt-tip pens. Inhalants are both physically and psychologically addictive. Individuals who inhale may risk depression and apathy, nosebleeds, headaches, eye pain, chronic fatigue, heart failure, loss of muscle control, and death. Drugs can affect food intake, body weight, and taste preferences.

Energy Drinks

Energy drinks are sold legally and are advertised to boost energy. They contain stimulants, usually caffeine, as well as sugar. The AAP has stated that these energy drinks have no place in the diet of a child or adolescent; however, energy drinks are quite popular, especially in some athletic circles. The danger is that youth may view these as performance enhancers and consider them in the same category as fluid replacement drinks, which they are not. Further, energy drinks may interact with prescription medicines, especially ADHD medicine children or adolescents might be taking.

Many energy drinks contain about 80 mg of caffeine per 8 oz serving. Most energy drinks, however, are often packaged in 20–24 oz containers, which offers a dose of 200–240 mg of caffeine. Mix-your-own powders or concentrates are in the marketplace as well and in strengths researchers say range from 50–500 mg per serving.

The FDA limits the amount of caffeine a cola can have, but because energy drinks are marketed as a supplement, no such regulation on caffeine exists as yet. Energy drinks have been known to cause insomnia, nervousness, nausea, rapid heartbeat, and even more severe reactions such as seizures, cardiac irregularities, and cardiac arrest.

Caffeine, regardless of its form, is a central nervous system stimulant and causes a transient rise in blood pressure. From a nutrition standpoint, caffeine may cause the body to lose small amounts of calcium and magnesium.

Nutrition for the Athlete

Good nutrition during the period of life when one is involved in athletics can prevent unnecessary wear and tear on the body as well as maintain the athlete in top physical form (Figure 13-9). The specific nutritional needs of the athlete are not numerous, but they are important. The athlete needs additional water, calories, thiamine, riboflavin, niacin, sodium, potassium, iron, and protein.

The body uses water to rid itself of excess heat through perspiration. This lost water must be regularly replaced during the activity to prevent dehydration. Athletes should be well hydrated before exercise and drink enough fluid during and after exercise to balance fluid levels. While plain water is the beverage of choice for light to moderate exercise lasting under 1 hour, other nutrition is needed when engaging in endurance activities lasting longer than that. Sports beverages containing carbohydrates and electrolytes may be consumed before, during, and after exercise to help maintain blood glucose concentration, provide fuel for muscles, and decrease risk of dehydration and hyponatremia. Fruit, carbohydrate gels, and energy bars can help fuel these workouts. Interestingly, a recent study found that drinking 16 oz of fat-free chocolate milk with its mix of carbohydrates and protein (compared to mainstream sports drinks) led to greater concentration of glycogen in muscles at 30 and 60 minutes post exercise.

The increase in calories depends on the activity and the length of time it is performed. The requirement could be double the normal, up to 6,000 calories per day. Because carbohydrates, not protein, are used for energy, the normal diet proportions of 50–55% carbohydrate, 30% fat, and 10–15% protein are advised during moderate physical activity.

There is an increased need for B vitamins because they are necessary for energy metabolism. They are provided in the breads, cereals, fruits, and vegetables needed to bring the calorie count to the total required. Some extra

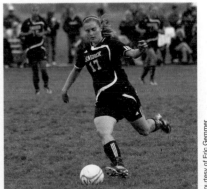

FIGURE 13-9 Participating in sports is great exercise for the mind and body.

Courtesy of Eric Gemmer

protein is used during training, when muscle mass and blood volume are increasing. Protein recommendations for endurance and strength-trained athletes range from 1.2–1.7 g/kg of body weight. These recommended protein intakes can generally be met through diet alone, without the use of protein or amino acid supplements. The minerals sodium and potassium are needed in larger amounts because of loss through perspiration. This amount of sodium can usually be replaced just by salting food to taste, and orange juice or bananas can provide the extra potassium. As stated, electrolyte replacement drinks may be needed for endurance activities lasting longer than 1 hour.

A sufficient supply of iron is important to the athlete, particularly to the female athlete. Iron-rich foods eaten with vitamin C–rich foods should provide sufficient iron. The onset of menstruation can be delayed by the heavy physical activity of the young female athlete, and amenorrhea may occur in those already menstruating.

When weight is a concern of the athlete, such as with wrestlers, care should be taken that the individual does not become dehydrated by refusing liquids in an effort to "make weight" for the class.

When weigh must be added, the athlete will need an additional 3,500 calories to develop 1 pound. The additional foods eaten to reach this amount of calories should contain the normal proportion of nutrients. A high-fat diet should be avoided because it increases the potential for heart disease. Athletes should reduce calories when training ends.

In general, the athlete should select foods using MyPlate. The pregame meal should be eaten 3 hours before the event and should consist primarily of carbohydrates and small amounts of protein and fat. Concentrated sugar foods are not advisable because they may cause extra water to collect in the intestines, creating gas and possibly diarrhea.

glycogen-loading (carb-loading) is sometimes used for endurance activities. To increase muscle stores of glycogen, the athlete begins 6 days before the events. For 3 days, the athlete eats a diet consisting of only 10% carbohydrate and mostly protein and fat as she or he performs heavy exercise. This depletes the current store of glycogen. The next 3 days, the diet is 70% carbohydrate, and the exercise is very light so that the muscles become loaded with glycogen. Carbohydrate loading isn't right for every endurance athlete and may not be as effective in women as it is in men. A carbohydrate-loading diet can cause some discomfort or side effects, such as:

1. *Weight gain.* Much of this gain is extra water, but if it hampers performance, it's recommended to skip the extra carbohydrates.

2. *Digestive discomfort.* It may be important to avoid or limit some high-fiber foods (e.g., beans, bran, broccoli) for 1–2 days before the event, as these can cause gassy cramps, bloating, and loose stools.

3. *Blood sugar changes.* Carbohydrate loading can affect your blood sugar levels. Some athletes monitor their blood sugar during training or practices.

A qualified sports dietitian or U.S. board certified specialist in sports dietetics can provide individualized nutrition direction as needed.

glycogen-loading (carb-loading)
process in which the muscle store of glycogen is maximized; also called carb-loading

Creatine is currently the most widely used ergogenic aid among athletes wanting to build muscle and enhance recovery. Creatine has been shown to be effective in repeated short bursts of high-intensity activity in sports such as sprinting and weightlifting but not for endurance sports such as distance running. Ergogenic aids that are dangerous, banned, or illegal are anabolic or androgenic steroids, ephedra, and human growth hormone, among others. Steroid drugs can affect the fat content of the blood, damage the liver, change the reproductive system, and even alter facial appearance. Good diet, good health habits and practice, combined with innate talent remain the essentials for athletic success.

HEALTH AND NUTRITION CONSIDERATIONS

The health care professional who works with young children may encounter poor appetites and eating habits in clients. Compounding this problem will be the anxiety of the clients' parents. They will understandably be concerned about their children's appetites and physical conditions. The health care professional can be most helpful to all concerned by exhibiting patience and understanding and by listening to parents and the client.

Adolescence is a rapid time of change. Sound nutrition is needed to optimize growth and health during these years, which may be tumultuous. As some teens are experiencing issues with overweight and obesity, a supportive health practitioner can serve as a gateway for positive nutrition and exercise messages. As many teens try to diet, some will be at risk for disordered eating. Screening tools will be valuable assets to determine if an eating disorder is developing or has developed. A team of professionals will need to be called upon to provide the best medical care.

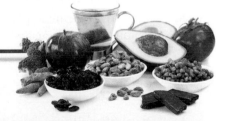

SUMMARY

Children's nutritional needs vary as they grow and develop. The rate of growth slows between the ages of 1 and 10, and the child's calorie requirement per pound of body weight slows accordingly. However, nutrient needs gradually increase during these years. During adolescence, growth is rapid, and nutritional and calorie requirements increase substantially. A positive feeding environment with sound, reliable nutrition will set the stage for optimum learning, growth, and development.

Unfortunately, health issues surface during childhood and adolescence. Many of our youth fall short with their nutrition quality. Anemia is a disorder seen in children worldwide. Overweight and obesity are on the rise. More of our youth experience pre-diabetes and type 2 diabetes, which was once considered adult-onset. Eating disorders experienced by youth are complex and underdiagnosed. Alcohol can be a serious problem for adolescents, and it is essential that they understand its potential dangers. The nutrition needs of athletes need to be carefully planned for maximum performance.

DISCUSSION TOPICS

1. Discuss how parents' anxieties about children's food habits may affect those habits.

2. In what ways does being overweight affect an adolescent's self-esteem?

3. Why can it be especially difficult for a parent to influence her or his adolescent's attitudes about food?

4. Discuss the nutrient content and food value of average fast-food choices. Discuss healthier options available and go online to find a fast-food restaurant's nutrition facts.

5. What could result if a 30-year-old lawyer continued to eat as he did as a 17-year-old football player?

6. Describe anorexia nervosa. Ask if anyone in the class knows of someone who has suffered from it. Ask that individual for descriptions of the person's attitude, physical condition, possible causes, and today's condition.

7. Discuss the use of growth charts in the primary care physician setting. What deviations in the growth chart of a child would raise cause for concern?

8. Why is it important to spot pre-diabetes in youth? What screening methods are used?

9. When do significant deposits in bone mass occur in youth? Discuss why this is especially critical and name the key nutrients involved.

SUGGESTED ACTIVITIES

1. List your favorite snack foods. List nutritious snack foods. Check the calorie values of these foods and compare lists for nutrition and taste. Discuss possible improvements in your list of favorite snacks.

2. Plan a talk for fourth-grade students on the importance of good food habits. Research major nutrients, calories, fiber, and food needs to meet requirements of a 9-year-old boy and girl. Begin with an outline and develop it into a

narrative that 9-year-old children will understand. If possible, ask permission of a fourth-grade teacher to deliver this talk to the class.

3. Role-play a situation in which your younger sister, who is somewhat overweight, has just asked you to help her get in shape. Ask her what food and lifestyle habits she believes have led to her feeling less healthy. Brainstorm three simple changes with her regarding food and exercise habits. Be positive and nonjudgmental and let her voice her realistic changes she wants to make both short and long term.

4. Invite a registered dietitian to speak to the class on sports nutrition. Seek out a dietitian that has this as a special interest or practice and ideally one that is a certified sports nutrition professional. Often large universities or fitness centers know of these individuals. The Academy of Nutrition and Dietetics (http://www.eatright.org) may be able to get you in touch with a local dietetic association.

5. Invite a counselor who specializes in adolescent eating disorders to speak to the class.

6. Hold a panel discussion on alcohol and drugs. Assign the following topics to individual class members. They should prepare themselves by doing outside research before the panel discussion.
   What is alcohol?
   What are some commonly abused drugs?
   Why do people use alcohol or drugs?
   How do alcohol and drugs affect the human body?
   How can alcohol and drug abuse affect one's nutritional status?
   What are the dangers of drinking or using drugs during pregnancy?

REVIEW

Multiple choice. Select the *letter* that precedes the best answer.

1. Anorexia nervosa
   a. is characterized by binges and purges
   b. causes severe acne
   c. is a psychological disorder
   d. typically causes overweight

2. A child's eating habits
   a. can reflect his or her desire to assert self
   b. seldom change after the child reaches the age of 1 year
   c. usually improve when parents force the child to try new foods
   d. have no relation to the child's growth rate

3. Children's appetites
   a. vary
   b. are static
   c. are irrelevant to their nutritional status
   d. are entirely dependent on the size of the child

4. The Healthy Eating Index from NHANES data indicates that
   a. generally children are meeting nutrition needs, except for protein
   b. generally children are meeting nutrition needs, except for eating too many fried foods
   c. consumption of fruit, whole grains, green and orange vegetables, and legumes is lacking
   d. consumption of adequate fiber is the only nutrient lacking

5. At what age should children be screened for high cholesterol, especially if there is a family history of heart disease?
   a. 5 years
   b. 12 years
   c. 2 years
   d. 16 years

6. Children's iron requirement is high because iron is needed for
   a. healthy bones and teeth
   b. fighting infections
   c. prevention of night blindness
   d. carrying oxygen

7. As a child grows, his or her calorie requirement per pound of body weight
   a. remains unchanged
   b. increases
   c. becomes less
   d. doubles each year

8. What age group has the highest prevalence of food allergies?
   a. toddlers
   b. preteens
   c. preschoolers
   d. midteens

9. A teenager who consumes frequent fast food
   a. is at risk for becoming overweight
   b. likely has a diet high in salt and fat, which could contribute to disease later in life
   c. is influenced to some degree by fast-food marketers when making food choices
   d. experiences all of the above

10. Although adolescent boys usually need more calories than adolescent girls, the girls usually need more
    a. protein
    b. vitamin C
    c. iron
    d. vitamin D

Case In Point

ELIZABETH: IDENTIFYING ANOREXIA NERVOSA

Elizabeth loves hanging out with her friends. She also loves to read. In addition to books, she loves to read magazines. She loves to look at the latest fashion trends in hair, makeup, and clothing. She would like to be a fashion designer when she is older. She is currently 5 feet 2 inches tall and weighs 80 pounds. She has gotten taller over the past year, but her waist and hip measurements have changed only slightly.

Elizabeth and her family rarely have a night where they are all home together for supper. Elizabeth's Dad works second shift and is always gone in the evenings. Now that Elizabeth is 14 years old, her mother decided to pick up a second job as a waitress a few nights a week to help make ends meet. Elizabeth is in charge of her younger sister on the evenings when her parents are both gone. Elizabeth's mom would typically have something easy for the girls to fix for supper while she was working. Elizabeth's sister, Hannah, is 12 years old.

She started noticing that Elizabeth is no longer eating supper with her. At first, she thought Elizabeth was taking food to her room because she just wanted to be alone. But now, she is realizing that Elizabeth isn't eating much, if at all. Lately, Elizabeth has complained about being tired and told Hannah to eat supper without her. She often naps on the weekend and after school instead of playing with her friends. Her after-school snacks have gone from choices such as cheese and crackers or granola bars, to no more than a small piece of fruit.

One night Hannah confronted Elizabeth and asked why she wasn't eating. Elizabeth admitted to Hannah that she was hungry, but wasn't going to eat because she did not want to gain weight. Her sister immediately informed her parents of this and her parents are now watching her eating habits and behaviors more closely.

ASSESSMENT

1. What objective information do you have about Elizabeth?
2. What subjective information do you have about Elizabeth?
3. Which psychological issues are having an effect on Elizabeth's understanding of proper nutrition?
4. What are the psychological needs of preteens?
5. What would lead you to believe Elizabeth may be having appearance issues?

DIAGNOSIS

6. Complete the following statement: Elizabeth's imbalanced nutrition is secondary to _____.
7. What signs of anorexia nervosa does Elizabeth exhibit?

PLAN/GOAL

8. What is the major nutritional goal for Elizabeth?
9. What is the priority for Elizabeth's physical development?

IMPLEMENTATION

10. What should Elizabeth and her mother be taught about good nutrition?
11. What needs to be taught about anorexia nervosa? Who else needs this information?

rate this **plate**

Elizabeth may be feeling pressured by the media she reads in her magazines to look a certain way and be a particular weight. As she continues to grow throughout her teen years, her calorie and nutrient needs will increase. Elizabeth needs nutrient-dense foods. Rate the plate she ate for dinner:

2 chicken nuggets

¼ cup instant mashed potatoes

½ cup diced pineapple

8 oz. fruit punch drink

Are any of these foods nutrient dense? Are any of these foods calorie dense? If so, which one(s)? How could this meal be improved to provide Elizabeth with adequate calories and nutrients to support growth throughout her teenage years?

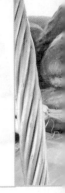

12. Would a counselor be of assistance to Elizabeth and her mother?
13. What can be done to prevent anorexia nervosa in her sister? Does anorexia nervosa have an age limit?

EVALUATION/OUTCOME CRITERIA

14. What criteria could be used to demonstrate that her anorexia nervosa was under control?
15. Can anorexia nervosa be cured?

THINKING FURTHER

16. How can parents, teachers, and coaches help pre-teens who have eating disorders?
17. Will Elizabeth's younger sister be at risk for anorexia nervosa?

Case In Point

JORDAN: CHILDHOOD OBESITY

Jordan's parents divorced 2 years ago when she was 4 years old. She spends the majority of her time at her mother's house. Her father sees her every other weekend and on Wednesday nights for supper. Her mother used to stay home with her, but was forced to go back to work full time after the divorce. Jordan is often shuffled between different babysitters when her parents are working. Her parents are so busy that many of the meals they provide for Jordan have become fast foods and convenience foods. Every Wednesday night Jordan and her Dad go to a fast food resturant for supper. Jordan loves that she gets a new toy each week!

Jordan used to take dance lessons and play soccer, but she has had to give both activities up because her parents simply can't afford them since the divorce. Jordan started kindergarten this fall and her mother is hoping that will fill the void of friendship she lost since discontinuing her activities. Jordan is a very smart girl, but she tells her mom she hates school. She cries each morning when she gets up and complains that she does not want to go. Finally she reveals to her mother that the other kids are making fun of her. She says that they tell her she is fat. Jordan's mom is heartbroken. She knows Jordan has gained a lot of weight, but she had no idea it was affecting her at school. Jordan's mom makes an appointment for Jordan with her pediatrician. She asks Jordan's dad to attend the appointment as well. At the doctor's office, Jordan measures 45 inches tall and weighs 61 pounds. The doctor informs her parents that he is concerned about her weight and would like them to meet with a registered dietitian to discuss a plan for Jordan and to set some goals for her weight. Despite their differences, Jordan's parents are both concerned about Jordan's weight. Both Jordan's parents have struggled with their weight through the years and have made numerous attempts to lose weight. They are concerned that Jordan is headed down the same path. They both agree to meet with the dietitian and work on this together for Jordan. They have also discussed ways to encourage Jordan to increase her activity and decrease the amount of less nutritious foods and snacks she consumes.

ASSESSMENT

1. What objective data do you have about Jordan?
2. Using Figure 13-5, what percentile weight and height is Jordan in for a 6-year-old girl?
3. How do diet, activity, heredity, and family lifestyle impact her current weight?
4. How significant is this problem?

DIAGNOSIS

Complete the following diagnostic statements:

5. Imbalanced nutrition; more than body requirements related to _____.
6. Deficient knowledge related to _____.

PLAN/GOAL

7. State two reasonable and measurable goals for Jordan.
8. At Jordan's checkup, the doctor agreed with her mom and referred them to a dietitian. As a dietitian, what personal goals are appropriate for Jordan and her parents, including their activities and foods?

IMPLEMENTATION

9. What information does the dietitian need to know to help Jordan?
10. Who needs to be involved in the plan for it to be successful?
11. What are the two big changes that need to occur to help Jordan stop gaining weight?
12. What strategies could you suggest so Jordan would be successful but have fun in the process?
13. How can playing outdoors with friends be helpful?
14. How can her family help?

EVALUATION/OUTCOME CRITERIA

15. How often should Jordan be weighed?
16. What outcome is reasonable in 3 months? In 6 months?

THINKING FURTHER

17. Why is it important to intervene with Jordan's weight now? What are the future consequences of a lifetime of being overweight? Why is this a community health issue in America now?
18. What would the Internet be able to provide?
19. In March 2012, the National Nutrition Standards for school lunches were revised. You can read the current guidelines by visiting http://www.fns.usda.gov/cnd/governance/regulations.htm.

rate this plate

Jordan still enjoys the occasional treats from a fast-food restaurant when she visits her father on Wednesday nights. Rate the meal that her father ordered for her.

1 kids-size cheeseburger

1 small order French fries

4 oz. vanilla yogurt

½ cup apple slices

12 oz. orange juice drink

Check a fast food menu online to determine total calories. Is this too much food? If so, where can calories be decreased in this meal?

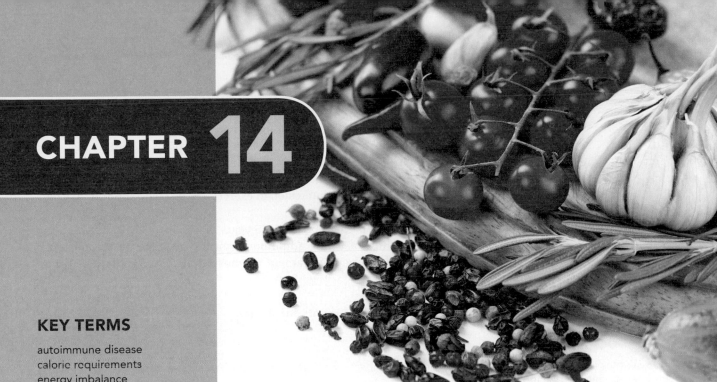

CHAPTER 14

KEY TERMS

autoimmune disease
caloric requirements
energy imbalance
menopause
nutrient requirements

NUTRITION DURING YOUNG AND MIDDLE ADULTHOOD

OBJECTIVES

After studying this chapter, you should be able to:

- Identify the nutritional needs of young and middle-age adults
- Explain sensible, long-range weight control for this age group
- Discuss the importance of exercise in weight control
- Discuss diet-related diseases that can be prevented by good nutrition at this age: osteoporosis, heart disease, diabetes

Adulthood can be broadly divided into three periods: young, middle, and late adulthood. The first two periods will be discussed in this chapter. Late adulthood is discussed in Chapter 15.

YOUNG AND MIDDLE ADULTS

Young adulthood is a time of excitement and self-exploration. The age range spans 18–40 years of age. Individuals are alive with plans, desires, and energy as they begin searching for and finding their place in the mainstream of adult life. They appear to have boundless energy for both social and professional activities. They are often interested in exercise for its own sake and may participate in athletic events as well.

The middle period spans 40–65 years of age. This is a time when the physical activities of young adulthood typically begin to decrease, resulting in lowered caloric requirement for most individuals. Table 14-1 shows

---

 TABLE 14-1　Equations to Estimate Energy Requirements for Adults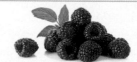

IRETON-JONES

For resting energy expenditure (REE) or resting metabolic rate (RMR), where weight (W) in kilograms (kg), height (H) in centimeters, and age (A) in years.

- Spontaneously breathing: $629–11(A)+25(W)–609(O)$
- Ventilator-dependent (original, 1992): $1925–10(A)+5(W)+281(S)+292(T)+851(B)$
- Ventilator-dependent (revised, 2002): $1784–11(A)+5(W)+244(S)+239(T)+804(B)$
- B = Diagnosis of burn (present = 1, absent = 0)
- O = Obesity, body mass index (BMI) > 27 kg/m² (present = 1, absent = 0)
- S = Sex (male = 1, female = 0)
- T = Diagnosis of trauma (present = 1, absent = 0)

MIFFLIN–ST JEOR

According to the American Academy of Nutrition and Dietetics, if it is not possible to measure RMR, then the Mifflin–St Jeor equation using actual weight is the most accurate for estimating RMR for overweight and obese individuals.

- Men: $(9.99 \times W)+(6.25 \times H)–(4.92 \times A)+5$
- Women: $(9.99 \times W)+(6.25 \times H)–(4.92 \times A)–161$

HARRIS–BENEDICT EQUATION

- Men: RMR = $66.47+(13.75 \times W)+(5 \times H)–(6.75 \times A)$
- Women: RMR = $655.09+(9.56 \times W)+(1.84 \times H)–(4.67 \times A)$

Total energy requirements (TEE) = REE × (activity factor) × (injury factor) ± 500 calories (for desired weight loss or weight gain, if applicable) + fever factor

ACTIVITY FACTORS	INJURY FACTORS
• Comatose: 1.1	• Surgery
• Confined to bed: 1.2	◦ Minor: 1.0–1.2
• Confined to chair: 1.25	◦ Major: 1.1–1.3
• Out of bed: 1.3	• Skeletal trauma: 1.1–1.6
• Normal activities of daily living (ADLs): 1.5	• Head trauma: 1.6–1.8

FEVER FACTOR	INJURY FACTORS		
Fahrenheit scale: add 7% of REE for every 1° over normal	• Pressure ulcers	• Infection	• Burns (% body surface area)
Centigrade scale: add 13% of REE for every 1° over normal	◦ Stage I: 1.0–1.1	◦ Mild: 1.0–1.2	◦ <20% BSA: 1.2–1.5
	◦ Stage II: 1.2	◦ Moderate: 1.2–1.4	◦ 20%–40% BSA: 1.5–1.8
	◦ Stage III: 1.3–1.4	◦ Severe: 1.4–1.8	◦ >40% BSA: 1.8–2.0
	◦ Stage IV: 1.5–1.6		

Source: Adapted from *Estimating Energy Requirements for an Obese Patient Professional Refresher*. Accessed May 9, 2012 from http://www.rd411.com.

equations Registered Dietitians use in assessing energy (calorie) requirements. For a person who simply wants an estimate of one's calorie intake, he or she can assess information from www.choosemyplate.gov. During these years, people seldom have young children to supervise, and the strenuous physical labor of some occupations may be delegated to younger people. Middle-agers may tire more easily than they did when they were younger. Therefore, they may not get as much exercise as they did in earlier years. Because appetite and food intake may not decrease, there is a common tendency toward weight gain during this period.

During young to middle adulthood, the beginnings of osteoporosis may also be evident. A diet rich in calcium, vitamin D, magnesium, and fluoride is thought to help prevent osteoporosis.

The onset of rheumatoid arthritis (RA), an **autoimmune disease**, usually occurs between the ages of 30 and 50 and will affect approximately 1.3 million Americans of which about 70% are women. RA affects the wrists, joints of the fingers other than those closest to the fingernail, hips, knees, ankles, elbows, shoulders, feet, and necks. Although researchers have determined that diet changes have no effect on rheumatoid arthritis, it is still important to maintain a healthy diet that includes adequate calcium and protein. A multiple vitamin containing vitamin D and a calcium supplement should be taken daily. Many studies suggest that a diet high in fruits, vegetables, and vitamin C may be linked to a lower risk of RA. Rheumatoid arthritis is less severe in some Mediterranean countries such as Greece and Italy, as the main diet consists of large amounts of fruits, vegetables, olive oil, and fatty fish high in omega-3s. More recent findings show that the higher intake of omega-3 fatty acids with the Mediterranean diet may be linked to the improvement in RA symptoms.

NUTRITIONAL REQUIREMENTS

Growth is usually complete by age 25 years. Consequently, except during pregnancy and lactation, the essential nutrients are needed only to maintain and repair body tissue and to produce energy. During these years, the **nutrient requirements** of healthy adults change very little.

The iron requirement for women throughout the child-bearing years remains higher than that for men. Extra iron is needed to replace blood loss during menstruation and to help build both the infant's and the mother's extra maternal blood needed during pregnancy. After menopause, this requirement for women matches that of men.

Protein needs for healthy adults are thought to be 0.8 gram per kilogram of body weight. To determine the specific amount, one must divide the weight in pounds by 2.2 to obtain the weight in kilograms and then multiply the weight in kilograms by 0.8.

The current requirement for calcium for adults age 19–50 is 1,000 mg, and for vitamin D, 15 µg per day (or 600 IUs). Both calcium and vitamin D are essential for strong bones, and both are found in milk. Bone loss begins slowly, at about age 35–40, and can later lead to osteoporosis. Therefore, it is wise for young people, especially women, to consume foods that provide more than the requirements for these two nutrients. Three glasses of milk a day nearly fulfill the requirement for calcium, however the level of vitamin D in three glasses of milk still falls short of the newer recommended allowance.

autoimmune disease
an illness that occurs when the body tissues are attacked by its own immune system

nutrient requirements
amounts of specific nutrient needed by the body

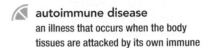
SPOTLIGHT *on Life Cycle*

Individuals aged 50 and older may find it difficult to meet their nutritional needs through food alone. As a person ages, multiple medications can be prescribed that may interact with nutrient absorption and appetite. The market currently offers numerous multivitamin/ mineral supplements that are aimed toward meeting the nutritional needs of the aging population. Most multivitamin supplements include higher levels of vitamin C, folic acid, vitamin D, vitamin E, vitamins B_1, B_2, B_6, and B_{12}. Elderly clients should be referred to their physician for advice before starting a multivitamin supplement. Pharmacists can also assess the client's need and refer clients to a registered dietitian if possible food and drug interactions are present.

(Source: Adapted from Terrie, Y.C. Multivitamins for the Senior Population. *Pharmacy Times.* January 1, 2009. http:// www.pharmacytimes.com)

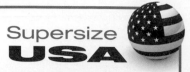

Supersize USA

Pizza is probably the food most consumed by young and middle-age adults. Especially popular is the buffet—all the salad and pizza, pasta, cinnamon sugar pizza strips, and dessert pizza you can eat. Wow, what a feast! Let's see how much can be eaten in one sitting—the way most people approach a buffet. This is how we as Americans have supersized ourselves. How should a buffet be handled?

Tune in on hunger upon arrival—how hungry are you? Head for the salad bar first, and choose vegetables, ignoring the cheese, eggs, pasta, bacon bits, seeds, and regular dressing. Enjoy a vegetable salad or drink a glass of water or milk before the meal, to help fill you almost up. At this point, tune in to "full." Are you full yet? If not, then the pizza buffet awaits. Choose one slice of a pizza topped with vegetables (mushrooms, peppers) over a pizza topped with sausage or pepperoni. Walk back to your seat. Eat slowly and enjoy. Ask yourself again, are you still hungry? If you're comfortable, then it's time to stop eating. The pizza will be there the next time you want it. Some adults can eat two to three times their caloric needs in one sweep of the pizza buffet, so instead of piling on the food at the first pass and feeling compelled to clear your plate, choose smaller portions and walk back up to the buffet if you are still hungry. Again, how do *you* handle pizza buffets?

Most people will need to include other vitamin D sources, or more likely add a supplement of vitamin D. Increasing this amount could prevent osteoporosis. Fat-free milk or foods made from fat-free milk should be consumed to limit the amount of fat in the diet.

CALORIE REQUIREMENTS

Calorie requirements begin to diminish after age 25, as basal metabolism rates decrease. After age 25, a person will gain weight if the total calories are not reduced according to actual need, which will be determined by activity, BMI (REE), and amount of lean body mass. Those who are more active will require more calories than those who are less active.

SPECIAL CONSIDERATIONS RELATED TO NUTRITION CONCERNS

It is especially important to maintain good eating habits during young and middle adulthood. Those who may be concerned about weight, cost of food, or time can easily develop nutrient deficiencies. For example, a woman who settles for a piece of pie at lunchtime while her husband eats a hamburger and salad is not obtaining adequate nutrients. If she continues to eat like this, she will jeopardize her health.

A hamburger can have 250–400 calories. The salad will contain less than 50 calories without dressing, and the dressing could be limited to 1 Tbsp, or approximately 100 calories, for a total intake of 400–550 calories. Pies average 100 calories per 1-inch slice. Most slices are about 3.5 inches. A scoop of ice cream on the pie would bring the total to at least another 100 calories.

Although the calorie intakes of the husband and wife would be comparable, the nutrient intakes would differ. The wife's would be inadequate. If the woman is of child-bearing age and plans to have children, she or her children could suffer from such habits. It would have been better to have ordered a grilled chicken sandwich instead of a hamburger along with a side salad. Replacing the hamburger and pie choices with healthier, more nutrient-dense items such as mixed fruit or a side salad with assorted vegetables will result in lower calorie intake and higher nutrient intake.

In general, people today are concerned about nutrition and want to limit fats, cholesterol, sugar, salt, and calories and increase fiber. Many know the sources of these items; others do not. Unfortunately, both groups tend to select their food because of convenience and flavor rather than nutritional content. It is easier to drive through a fast-food restaurant or heat a prepared frozen dinner than it is to shop for individual food items, cook them, and clean up after the meal. Consequently, many people ingest more fats, sugar, salt, and high-calorie foods and less fiber and other nutrients than they should.

Many physical changes also take place during middle adulthood. For women, **menopause** is a time where it is important to incorporate healthy lifestyle choices such as reducing calories and increasing physical activity to make the transition into middle adulthood easier. On average, women meet menopause at age 51. As a woman ages, the two main hormones essential in reproduction, called estrogen and progesterone, begin to decrease. As hormone levels decrease, menstrual periods become shorter and eventually cease. Due to the lessening of hormone levels, weight maintenance during the 40s and 50s may be a challenge. Research shows that to maintain weight in the mid to late 40s, women need about 200 fewer calories per day. Eating smaller meals throughout the day along with participating in physical activity will maintain metabolism and prevent significant weight gain. For the adult male, a diet that supports reducing the risk for heart disease is especially important because males develop heart disease at a younger age than women. Both regular exercise and weight-bearing exercise are important to promote bone health.

Adults will not outgrow their need for essential vitamins and minerals as they age. Although calcium is necessary for growing bones, it's also needed to help keep bones strong throughout adulthood. Three servings of dairy foods per day provide adequate calcium for adults. Fiber is also an essential nutrient for overall health. Fiber is known best for maintaining bowel regularity and preventing intestinal conditions such as diverticular disease, but research has also proven that fiber can lower risks of heart disease, high blood pressure, cancer, and type 2 diabetes. Fiber can also help lower cholesterol levels by absorbing fat and cholesterol from the blood. Fiber is also relatively low in calories and increases satiety, therefore controlling weight. Whole-grain products as well as beans, fruits, and vegetables are rich sources of fiber. Women of childbearing age need adequate intake of folic acid and iron in order to prevent birth defects and iron-deficiency anemia during pregnancy. Food sources of folate include lentils, spinach, broccoli, and other leafy green vegetables. Other vitamins and minerals of concern during adulthood include magnesium, potassium, and vitamins E, A, and C. Magnesium contributes to bone strength, immunity, and numerous body functions. Potassium plays a critical role in muscle contractions, nerve impulses, and maintaining fluid balance in the body. Eating a variety of green vegetables, beans, and dairy products will provide potassium. Vitamins A, E, and C contain powerful antioxidant properties that offer a variety of health benefits including maintaining eye health and vision, combating free radicals, and repelling germs to achieve a healthy immune system. Consuming a diet balanced with fruits, vegetables, whole grains, lean protein, and dairy will provide essential nutrients needed through young and middle adulthood.

WEIGHT CONTROL

Weight control is one of the top concerns of U.S. adults. Whether for reasons of vanity, health, or both, most people are interested in controlling their weight. It is advisable because overweight can introduce health problems. Cases of diabetes mellitus, metabolic syndrome, and hypertension are more numerous among the overweight than among those of normal weight. Overweight individuals are poor risks for surgery, and their lives are generally shorter than others who are not overweight. They are prone to social and emotional problems because overweight and obesity can reduce self-esteem.

The causes of overweight are not always known, but the most common cause appears to be **energy imbalance**. In other words, if one is overweight, chances are that more calories have been taken in than were needed for energy.

An intake of 3,500 calories more than the body needs for maintenance and activities will result in a weight gain of 1 pound. An individual who overeats by only 200 calories a day can gain 20 pounds in 1 year. Obviously,

 calorie requirements
number of calories required daily to meet energy needs

 menopause
the end of menstruation

EXPLORING THE WEB

Search the Web for information related to diet and disease or disorders. What conditions are directly affected by diet? Can these conditions be prevented by changing one's nutritional status? How can this be done? What resources are available for individuals experiencing a nutrition-related disorder?

Supersize USA

My husband and I went out for dinner and he ordered a 10 oz. ribeye steak, a loaded baked potato (butter, sour cream, cheese, and bacon), a small loaf of crusty bread and butter, a salad with eggs, cheese, and bacon bits along with a heaping side of honey mustard dressing, and two 16 oz. sodas. Eating this tasty meal equals about 2,200 calories and 98 grams of fat. Way too much for one meal! The grams of fat are over 3 days' worth and the calories are above his average daily need for an adult man.

 energy imbalance
eating either too much or too little for the amount of energy expended

when nutrient requirements remain static but calorie requirements decrease, people must select their foods carefully to fulfill their nutrient requirements (Table 14-2). Genetics and a hypothyroid condition, although rare, can also contribute to overweight.

Individuals who are overweight simply because of energy imbalance can solve the problem by eating less and increasing physical exercise. Exercise will increase the number of calories burned. However, unless the exercise is sufficient to burn more calories than the ingested food contains, exercise alone will not solve the problem. By far the most effective method of weight loss is increased exercise combined with reduced calories. This will help tone the muscles as excess fat is lost. Exercise may also increase lean body mass in such a way that weight loss will not be necessarily significant; in this case, a decrease in clothing size may be a better indicator of fat loss.

When weight reduction is necessary, clients should confirm with their physician that they are in good health. Then, with the help of a registered dietitian, they can develop a healthy eating plan to fit their lifestyle. A healthy eating plan is easiest to follow when it is based on MyPlate. This plan will aid dieters in obtaining needed nutrients, will help change previously unsatisfactory eating habits, and will allow them to adapt and thus enjoy meals anywhere—at home, parties, or in restaurants. For additional information about weight loss diets, see Chapter 16.

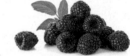

TABLE 14-2   2,000-Calorie Daily Menu

BREAKFAST	LUNCH
Cold cereal	**Tuna salad sandwich**
• 1 cup ready-to-eat oat cereal	• 2 slices rye bread
• 1 medium banana	• 2 oz tuna
• ½ cup fat-free milk	• 1 tbsp mayonnaise
• 1 slice whole-wheat toast	• 1 tbsp chopped celery
• 1 tsp tub margarine	• ½ cup shredded lettuce
Beverage: 1 cup prune juice	• 1 medium peach
	Beverage: 1 cup fat-free milk
DINNER	**SNACKS**
Roasted chicken	• ¼ cup dried apricots
• 3 oz cooked chicken breast	• 1 cup flavored yogurt (chocolate)
• 1 large sweet potato, roasted	
• ½ cup succotash (limas and corn)	
• 1 tsp tub margarine	
• 1 oz whole-wheat roll	
• 1 tsp tub margarine	
Beverage: 1 cup water, coffee, or tea	

Source: U.S. Department of Agriculture. *Sample Menus for a 2000 Calorie Food Pattern.* Retrieved November 2011 from http://www.choosemyplate.gov

HEALTH AND NUTRITION CONSIDERATIONS

The young and middle years of life are busy. Most people feel they have too many things to do and too little time to accomplish them. Most have families, jobs, and social obligations and, thus, more responsibilities. In their fast paced world drive-thru meals become common place. This can lead to obesity not only in young and middle aged adults but in their children as well.

SUMMARY

Although calorie requirements diminish after the age of 25, most nutrient requirements do not. Consequently, food must be selected with increasing care as one ages to ensure that nutrient requirements are met without exceeding the calorie requirement.

Overweight can cause health problems. If it is caused by energy imbalance, a program of weight loss, which includes exercise, should be undertaken. The diet should be based on MyPlate, and eating habits should be taught so that the lost weight will not be regained later.

DISCUSSION TOPICS

1. Why do calorie requirements tend to diminish after the age of 25? Why do nutrient requirements not diminish at the same time?

2. How can an extra 200 calories a day result in overweight?

3. Why does a 40-year-old road constructor require more calories than a 40-year-old administrative assistant?

4. Why are middle-age adults more inclined to be overweight than young adults?

5. Why is 35-year-old Vera putting on weight even though she doesn't eat any more than she did as a 17-year-old cheerleader?

6. What are the health and psychological consequences of being overweight?

SUGGESTED ACTIVITIES

1. Keep a food diary for a day and check off each food under MyPlate headings, as shown in the form provided.

	Fat/ Sweet	Dairy	Meats	Veg.	Fruit	Bread/ Grain
Recommended servings/day	Use sparingly	2–3	2–3	3–5	2–4	6–8
Breakfast						
Lunch						
Dinner						
Total						

© Cengage Learning 2014

a. Total the entries in the vertical columns. Which columns have the highest totals?
b. Discuss the shortages or excesses and the possible dangers of each.
c. Discuss realistic ways of improving your diet.
d. Repeat this exercise in a week. Evaluate for improvements.

2. Interview a person with RA and discover how she or he performs activities of daily living. Does the person use adaptive equipment?

3. Interview a relative or neighbor with osteoporosis. What is this person doing to prevent future pain and degeneration associated with the disease?

4. Research various autoimmune diseases. Is there any nutrition component that may help in these conditions?

REVIEW

Multiple choice. Select the *letter* that precedes the best answer.

1. The number of calories one needs each day is called the
   a. nutrient requirement
   b. calorie intake
   c. calorie requirement
   d. nutritional requirement

2. Overweight during middle age is often due to
   a. obesity
   b. hypertension
   c. adipose tissue
   d. energy imbalance

3. The measure of energy in foods eaten is one's
   a. calorie requirement
   b. calorie intake
   c. nutrient requirement
   d. energy imbalance

4. Because of menstruation and pregnancy during the young and middle years, women have a greater need than men for
   a. proteins
   b. B vitamins
   c. iodine
   d. iron

5. Calorie requirements
   a. increase with age
   b. decrease with age
   c. remain unchanged throughout adult life
   d. none of the above

6. To lose 1 pound of weight, one must reduce calorie intake by
   a. 1,000 calories
   b. 800 calories
   c. 3,500 calories
   d. none of the above

7. Daily protein needs of adults are thought to be
   a. 0.5 gram per kilogram of body weight
   b. 0.8 gram per kilogram of body weight
   c. 10 grams per kilogram of body weight
   d. 8 mg per day regardless of body weight

8. Exercise
   a. is more important to men than to women
   b. has no effect on muscles after the age of 40
   c. eliminates the need for postmenopausal women to drink milk
   d. helps to burn calories as it tones the muscles

9. Nutrient requirements during adult life generally
   a. increase with age
   b. decrease with age
   c. change very little
   d. none of the above

10. Women's calorie requirements as compared with men's are generally
   a. lower
   b. higher
   c. the same
   d. none of the above

11. The protein needs for a 35-year-old male weighing 192 pounds is
   a. 60.2 grams
   b. 72.4 grams
   c. 69.8 grams
   d. 87.3 grams

Case In Point

NIKOLAI: CHANGING BEHAVIORS TO ACHIEVE WEIGHT LOSS

Nikolai has been very active working in a bakery for the past 4 years while completing his college degree. He is studying business and will graduate next spring. He is a 36-year-old married man with one daughter, and his parents are immigrants to the United States from Romania. His mother is a wonderful cook. His dream is to open his own bakery and restaurant that will serve many of the same recipes his mother made for his family when he was growing up. His wife and daughter are both very excited about his upcoming graduation. They know that Nikolai has been trying to balance work and school for a very long time. They are happy that he will have more free time to spend with them in the near future. Over the past 4 years, however, Nikolai has developed some bad habits. Due to his long hours and rushing between work and classes, he will often eat only food from the bakery. It has become common for his lunch to be a large cinnamon roll and his supper to be a handful of cookies. He has rarely had time to exercise and even when he does have time, he is too exhausted. Nikolai has gained 25 pounds over the past 4 years. He is now 235 pounds and 6 feet 1 inch tall. He is not happy with his current body weight. He would like to improve his eating habits and resume an exercise program before he graduates.

ASSESSMENT

1. What do you know about Nikolai?
2. What value has he acted on for several years?
3. What values does he want to act on in the future?
4. What do you suspect Nikolai had been eating?

DIAGNOSIS

5. What are possible causes of Nikolai's weight problem?
6. What education is needed to help Nikolai lose weight?

PLAN/GOAL

7. What is a reasonable goal for weight loss for Nikolai once he graduates? Assume a loss of 1–2 pounds per week.

IMPLEMENTATION

8. What are the two most important changes that Nikolai needs to make to lose weight?
9. How could a 24-hour food diary help?
10. What does he need to do about exercise?
11. How can his family help?
12. How can strategies like packing his lunch help?
13. Would he be more successful losing weight alone or in a group?

EVALUATION/OUTCOME CRITERIA

14. One month after starting the new plan, what changes will be in place?

15. If the plan is successful, what changes will Nikolai report in 3 months?

THINKING FURTHER

16. Even though Nikolai's short-term goal is to lose weight, how could he maintain his new habits so he won't regain the weight?
17. Why is it important to control excess weight in middle age?

rate this **plate**

Nikolai has begun making healthy decisions in an effort to lose weight. He knows that eating baked goods for his meals is not the best choice. Nikolai decides to pack a lunch that he can eat between school and work. Rate the plate that he prepared:

6 inch Italian sub sandwich on white bread including:

2 oz. salami, 2 oz. ham, 2 oz. pepperoni, 1 oz. cheddar cheese, red onion, tomatoes, lettuce, black olives, and mayonnaise sauce

1 medium apple

1 cup raw baby carrots

1 chocolate chip cookie

32 oz. regular soda

What ingredients need to be changed? Is white bread his best choice for good nutrition? What would be a better option instead of a soft drink? Could he really eat just one chocolate chip cookie? Is this a good choice for dessert?

Case In Point

ALAINA: PREPARING FOR HER BIG DAY

Alaina is so excited! Her boyfriend Eric just proposed to her! She has been dating Eric for the past 2 years. Now that they are both 24 years old and college graduates, Alaina can hardly wait to become Eric's wife.

During high school, Alaina was an active member of the gymnastics team and cheerleader squad, and served on the yearbook committee. During her college days she worked out at least 3 days a week and ate healthier than most college students. She even managed to avoid gaining "the freshman 15."

A few months before the wedding, Alaina decides she needs to go on a strict diet. She is worried that the holiday celebrations she attended caused her to gain weight. She is afraid her wedding dress won't fit when she goes to pick it up. She doesn't want to "look fat" for her wedding photos so she is determined to lose some weight. Several weeks later, Alaina's longtime friend, Lillie, notices that Alaina doesn't have her typical "glow" about her. Alaina is of Asian descent and has always had beautiful, glowing skin, but now she appears pale and sickly, tired, irritable, and quite thin. Lillie noticed during a recent luncheon that Alaina ate only a few bites of food. Lillie questioned Alaina about the changes, and Alaina admitted she hadn't been eating. She agreed to Lillie's suggestion to make an appointment with her doctor.

ASSESSMENT

1. Identify changes in Alaina that suggest she was getting into trouble.
2. What information would be important to share with the physician?
3. In which category of nutritional assessment would you list Lillie's observations?
4. Which observation would you consider significant to cause concern?
5. Is there any other information that would be helpful in identifying Alaina's condition?

DIAGNOSIS

6. Write a nursing diagnosis that most likely applies to Alaina's problem.
7. What contributed to the development of the problems?

PLAN/GOAL

8. Who can help with the plan?
9. What two changes are most significant for Alaina?

IMPLEMENTATION

10. Name three methods that could be used to improve Alaina's nutrition.
11. How could friends and family help?
12. How could a food diary help?

EVALUATION/OUTCOME CRITERIA

13. What can the doctor assess at the next appointment to see if the plan is working?
14. What observations could Alaina's friend Lillie offer about the success of the plan?
15. What information from Alaina would benefit the success of the plan?

THINKING FURTHER

16. Who else could be at risk for a similar problem?
17. How could information from the Internet be useful?

rate this **plate**

Like all brides, Alaina would like to look her best on her wedding day. Rate this plate. For lunch Alaina has fixed herself:

1 small side salad with tomatoes, cucumbers, broccoli, and carrots

2 Tbsp Italian dressing

1 cup tomato soup

1 cup tea with 1 tsp of sugar

What macronutrients are lacking in this meal? Was the amount of dressing on her salad sufficient? Are there any foods that you would like to add to this meal? What would they be, and why?

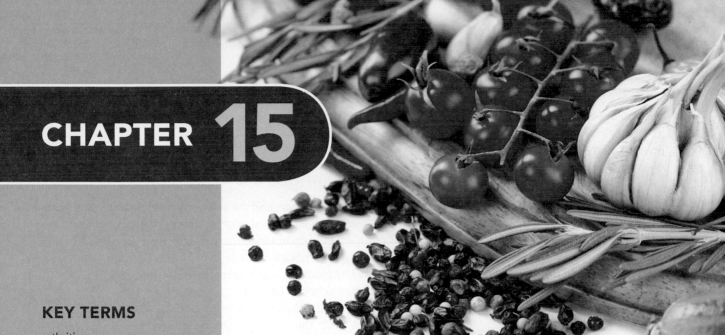

CHAPTER 15

KEY TERMS

arthritis
dentition
estrogen
food faddists
geriatrics
gerontology
occlusions
periodontal disease
physiological
skeletal system

NUTRITION DURING LATE ADULTHOOD

OBJECTIVES

After studying this chapter, you should be able to:

- Explain the nutritional and calorie needs of people 65 and over
- Explain the development of given chronic diseases
- Identify physiological, economic, and psychosocial problems that can affect an older adult's nutrition

Currently, the fastest-growing age group in the United States is that of people age 85 and older. The average life expectancy in this country is now 80 years for women and 75 years for men (National Center for Health Statistics, 2010). In the year 2000, people 65 and older represented 12.4% of the population. This percentage is expected to grow to 19% of the population by the year 2030. Consequently, **gerontology**, the study of aging, is of increasing importance.

The rate of aging varies. Each person is affected by heredity, emotional and physical stress, and nutrition. Research continues to reveal more about the causes of aging and the role of nutrition in the aging process.

THE EFFECTS OF AGING

gerontology
the study of aging

physiological
relating to bodily functions

dentition
arrangement, type, and number of teeth

As people age, **physiological**, psychosocial, and economic changes occur that affect nutrition.

Physiological Changes

The body's functions slow with age, and the ability of the body to replace worn cells is reduced. The metabolic rate slows; bones become less dense; lean muscle mass is reduced; eyes do not focus on nearby objects as they once did, and some grow cloudy from cataracts; poor **dentition** is common; the heart and kidneys become less efficient; and hearing, taste, and smell are less acute. If poor nutrition has been chronic, the immune system may be compromised.

Osteoarthritis and its debilitating effects are of great concern to the elderly. Arthritis can limit the ability to perform activities of daily living (ADLs). The role that diet plays in arthritis has been of increasing interest to researchers. Excessive weight, certain vitamin deficiencies, and the type of diet being followed may influence some types of arthritis. Eating a healthy, well-balanced diet that includes the "5 a day" fruits and vegetables, along with grain products, and sugar and salt in moderation, may be beneficial for arthritis sufferers. Your physician or dietitian may also recommend taking a multiple vitamin daily.

There appears to be no direct connection between a specific kind of food and a specific symptom of arthritis. Neither is there a special diet that is consistently beneficial for arthritis sufferers; however, the best advice is to eat a healthy diet that includes a variety of foods and to exercise.

Digestion is affected because the secretion of hydrochloric acid and enzymes is diminished. This in turn decreases the intrinsic factor synthesis, which leads to a deficiency of vitamin B_{12}. The tone of the intestines is reduced, and the result may be constipation or, in some cases, diarrhea.

Psychosocial Changes

Feelings do not decrease with age. In fact, psychosocial problems can increase as one grows older. Age does not diminish the desire to feel useful, appreciated, and loved by family and friends. Retirement years may not be "golden" if one suffers a loss of self-esteem from feelings of uselessness. Grief over the loss of a spouse or close friend, combined with the resulting loneliness, can be devastating. Physical disabilities that develop in the senior years and prevent one from going out independently can destroy a social life. Becoming a fifth wheel in a grown child's home or a resident of a nursing home can lead to severe depression. Problems such as these can diminish a person's appetite and ability to shop and cook.

Economic Changes

Retirement typically results in decreased income. Unless one has carefully prepared for it, this can affect one's quality of life by reducing social activities, adding worry about meeting bills, and causing one to select a less than healthy diet by choosing foods on the basis of cost rather than nutrient content.

Sidestepping Potential Problems

Healthy eating habits throughout life, an exercise program suited to one's age, and enjoyable social activities can prevent or delay physical deterioration and psychological depression during the senior years. The benefits can be said to be circular. The first two contribute largely to one's physical condition, and social activities can prevent or diminish depression. Healthy eating habits and a suited exercise program give purpose to the day, happiness to life, and zest to the appetite. Whenever an elderly person is depressed, his or her nutrition and lifestyle should be carefully reviewed.

Food–drug interactions must be monitored closely in the elderly. Frequently, specific foods will prevent, decrease, or enhance the absorption of a particular drug. Dairy products should not be consumed within 2 hours of taking the antibiotic tetracycline, or it will not be absorbed. A person taking a blood clot–reducing drug such as coumadin or warfarin (often called a blood thinner) needs to consume vitamin K–rich food in moderation as it counteracts blood thinners. Even vitamin supplements can cause interactions. The antioxidant vitamins are not to be taken with blood clot–reducing medications because they also have a tendency to thin the blood.

Drug–drug interactions as well as food–drug interactions can contribute to decreased nutritional status. These interactions could affect appetite as well as absorption of nutrients from the food eaten. Careful monitoring is recommended. (See Appendix E.)

NUTRITIONAL REQUIREMENTS

Although the nutritional needs of growth disappear with age, the normal nutritional needs for maintaining a constant state of good health remain throughout life. Good nutrition can speed recovery from illness, surgery, or broken bones and generally can improve the spirits and quality, and even the length, of life.

Despite the physical changes the body undergoes beyond age 50, only a few of the DRIs and AIs in this age category are less than those for younger people.

The protein requirement remains at the average 50 grams per day for women and 63 grams for men. This is based on the estimated need of 0.8 gram per kilogram of body weight. After age 65, it may be advisable to increase one's daily protein intake to 1.0 gram per kilogram of body weight. In general, vitamin requirements do not change after the age of 51, except for a slight decrease in the DRIs for thiamine, riboflavin, and niacin. The need for these three vitamins depends largely on the calorie intake, and calorie requirement is reduced after the age of 51. The need for iron is decreased after age 51 in women because of menopause.

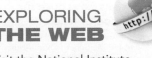

EXPLORING THE WEB

Visit the National Institute on Aging (http://www.nia .nih.gov) for guidelines on good nutrition throughout life. What are some of the challenges and concerns facing older adults in relation to healthy eating?

Supersize USA

Are you aware that 70% of adults over age 60 are overweight or obese? Research has shown that an extra 10–15 pounds is beneficial in case of illness or surgery but, in order to prevent diabetes and other weight-related diseases, it is best to maintain a near normal, healthy weight. Type 2 diabetes has doubled in the United States in the past 15 years and is highest among adults over age 65, according to the Centers for Disease Control and Prevention. Consequences of diabetes include blindness, heart disease, kidney disease, stroke, and other serious medical conditions. Besides eating well, even light physical activity can significantly contribute to a healthier life for many elderly adults. The National Institute on Aging recommends four types of exercises that Americans should include in their workout: endurance activities, such as walking, biking, or swimming; strength training, such as light weightlifting, to reduce age-related muscle loss; stretching, to maintain flexibility; and balance exercises, to reduce the likelihood of falls.

(Source: Adapted from Salahi, Laura. Staying Fit: Majority of Older Adults Struggle with Weight. *ABC News*. June 23, 2010.)

The calorie requirement decreases approximately 2% per decade after age 20, because metabolism slows and activity is reduced. If the calorie intake is not reduced, weight will increase. This additional weight would increase the work of the heart and put increased stress on the **skeletal system**. It is important that the calorie requirement not be exceeded and just as important that the nutrient requirements be fulfilled to maintain good nutritional status. An exercise plan appropriate for one's age and health can be helpful in burning excess calories and toning and strengthening the muscles.

FOOD HABITS

A lifetime of poor food habits are more likely to continue as one ages. These habits will not be easy to change. Poor food habits that begin during old age can also present problems. Decreased income during retirement, lack of transportation, physical disability, and inadequate cooking facilities may cause difficulties in food selection and preparation. Anorexia caused by grief, loneliness, boredom, depression, or difficulty in chewing can decrease food consumption. Dementia and Alzheimer's may cause the elderly to think they have eaten when in fact they have not.

Studies indicate that many senior citizens consume diets deficient in protein; vitamins C, D, B_6, B_{12}, and folate; and the minerals calcium, zinc, iron, and sometimes calories.

An elderly client's diet plan should be based on MyPlate and the nutrients should be checked against the DRIs and AIs. Older persons' needs can vary considerably, depending on their conditions, so each person should be examined by a physician to determine specific requirements. If the client consumes less than 1,500 calories a day, a multivitamin-mineral supplement is recommended.

Variety and nutrient-dense foods should be encouraged, as should water. Water is important to help prevent constipation, to maintain urinary volume, to prevent dehydration, and to prevent urinary tract infections (UTIs). When there is serious protein energy malnutrition (PEM), the reason may be economic or psychosocial. Elderly people who have long hospital stays can develop PEM in the hospital. They may dislike the food, drugs may dull the appetite, and they may be lonely and depressed. Sometimes poor or missing teeth can make eating protein foods difficult. In such cases, protein-rich supplements can be used.

If overweight is a problem, it may be caused by overeating, lack of exercise, drugs, or alcohol.

Any adjustment in food habits will require thorough explanation, and plans for changes must be based on the individual's total situation.

FOOD FADS

Some older people are consciously or unconsciously searching for eternal life, if not youth. Consequently, they are frequently susceptible to the claims of **food faddists** who seek to profit from their ignorance. Senior citizens spend money on unnecessary vitamins, minerals, and special honey, molasses, bread, milk, and other foods that may be guaranteed by the salesperson to prevent or cure various diseases. This money could be much more effectively

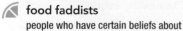

skeletal system
body's bone structure

food faddists
people who have certain beliefs about particular foods or diets

used on ordinary foods from MyPlate that would cost considerably less. It would be better to spend money on foods that represent MyPlate than on food supplements.

APPROPRIATE DIETS

The diets of older adults should be planned around MyPlate (Table 15-1). When special health problems exist, the normal diet should be adapted to meet individual needs (see Section 3, Medical Nutrition Therapy).

The federal government provides the states with funds to serve hot meals at noon in senior centers across the country. These senior centers become social clubs and are immensely beneficial to the elderly. They

EXPLORING THE WEB

Search the Web for information on food fads. What makes the elderly vulnerable to food fads? Are these types of diets and fads geared toward the elderly population? Why? What advice would you provide to an elderly client inquiring about one of these fads?

TABLE 15-1 1,500-Calorie Daily Menu

BREAKFAST	CALORIES
½ cup oatmeal	145
1 Tbsp brown sugar	45
1 orange	60
1 cup 1%-milk	100
Total Calories	350

LUNCH	
4 ounces roast beef	300
4 ounce baked potato	80
½ cup cooked carrots	25
1 slice of apple pie (1/8 of 8-inch pie)	130
1 cup coffee	
1 cup water	
Total Calories	535

DINNER	
½ cup chicken salad	208
1 cup vegetable soup	145
6 crackers	80
17 grapes	60
1 cup unsweetened iced tea	0
Total Calories	493

SNACKS	
½ cup custard	116
Total Calories	116
TOTAL CALORIES	**1,494**

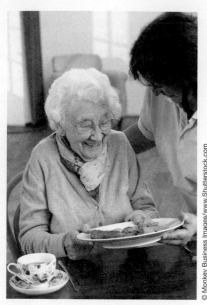

FIGURE 15-1 A volunteer delivers a warm meal to a homebound elderly woman.

 geriatrics
the branch of medicine involved with diseases of the elderly

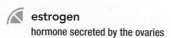 **estrogen**
hormone secreted by the ovaries

provide companionship in addition to nutritious food. Frequently the noon meal at "the center" becomes the focal point of an older person's day (Figure 15-1).

The federal government also provides transportation for those who are otherwise unable to reach the senior center for the meal. When individuals are completely homebound, arrangements can be made for the meals to be delivered to their homes. Some communities have Meals-on-Wheels projects. Participating people pay according to ability. In addition, food stamps are available and can sometimes be used for the Meals-on-Wheels programs.

SPECIAL CONSIDERATIONS FOR THE CHRONICALLY ILL OLDER ADULT

The CDC reports approximately 80% of older adults have one chronic condition and 50% have at least two. Examples include osteoporosis, arthritis, cataracts, cancer, diabetes mellitus, hypertension, heart disease, and periodontal disease. The branch of medicine that is involved with diseases of older adults is called **geriatrics**.

Osteoporosis

Osteoporosis is a condition in which the amount of calcium in bones is reduced, making them porous. The International Osteoporosis Foundation estimates that osteoporosis and low bone mass are currently a major public health threat for almost 44 million U.S. women and men aged 50 and older. Those at higher risk for osteoporosis are small-boned women, Caucasian, smokers, those who drink more than moderately, and those who do little or no exercise. Men are also at risk due to the same factors as women. A bone density scan (DEXA scan) can be done with a special X-ray to diagnose osteoporosis. It is typically unnoticed at its onset, which occurs at approximately age 45, and it may not be noticed at all until a fracture occurs. One of its symptoms is a gradual reduction in height.

Doctors are not certain of its cause. It is thought that years of a sedentary life coupled with a diet deficient in calcium, vitamin D, and fluoride contribute to it, as does **estrogen** loss, which occurs after menopause. Physicians are recommending estrogen replacement therapy (ERT) to help prevent osteoporosis. Some doctors are also advising clients to consume 1,500 mg of calcium, which would require the daily consumption of over 1 quart of milk or its equivalent. Calcium tablets, preferably calcium carbonate, could be used instead, but the client would also require supplementary vitamin D if sunshine was unavailable year-round or if the client was homebound. A diet with sufficient calcium and vitamin D plus an appropriate exercise program begun early in the adult years is thought to help prevent this disease.

Another possible cause of osteoporosis may be a diet containing excessive amounts of phosphorus, which can speed bone loss. It is known that Americans are ingesting increasing amounts of phosphorus. Sodas and processed foods contain phosphorus, and their consumption is increasing as milk consumption is decreasing in the United States. Soda intake is linked to osteoporosis in so far as it is replacing milk consumption. Some believe that **periodontal disease** may be linked to osteoporosis. Periodontal disease is characterized by bone loss in the jaw, which can lead to loosened teeth and infection in the gums.

Arthritis

Arthritis is a disease that causes the joints to become painful and stiff. It results in structural changes in the cartilage of the joints. A client with arthritis should be especially careful to avoid overweight because the extra weight adds stress to joints that are already painful. If the client is overweight, a weight reduction program should be instituted.

The regular use of aspirin by these clients may cause slight bleeding in the stomach lining and subsequent anemia, so their diets may require additional iron. Arthritis can greatly complicate one's life because it may partially or completely immobilize one so much that shopping, moving around, and cooking become difficult.

Aspirin and other anti-inflammatory drugs do help relieve the pain of arthritis, but there is as yet no cure. Clients should be well informed of this to prevent them from wasting their money on so-called miracle cures recommended by health food faddists or quacks.

Cancer

Research about the role of nutrition in cancer development continues. The American Cancer Society has indicated that diets consistently high in fat or low in fiber and vitamin A may contribute to cancer (see Chapter 21).

Diabetes Mellitus

Diabetes mellitus is a chronic disease. It develops when the body does not produce sufficient amounts of insulin or does not use it effectively for normal carbohydrate metabolism. Diet is very important in the treatment of diabetes. Chapter 17 discusses this treatment in detail.

Hypertension

Hypertension, or high blood pressure, can lead to strokes. It is associated with diets high in salt or possibly low in calcium. Most Americans ingest from two to six times the amount of salt needed each day. It is thought that the earlier a person reduces salt intake, the better that person's chances of avoiding hypertension, particularly if there is a family history of it. Hypertension is discussed in detail in Chapter 18.

Heart Disease

Heart attack and stroke are the major causes of death in the United States. They occur when arteries become blocked (occluded), preventing the normal passage of blood. These **occlusions** (blockages) are caused by blood clots that

SPOTLIGHT on Life Cycle

The "silent disease" known as osteoporosis is most common in postmenopausal women; however, in the past few years, osteoporosis has been recognized as a public health issue in a number of men over the age of 70. In men, bone loss starts later in life and progresses slowly compared to women who begin to experience bone loss after the hormonal changes associated with menopause. By age 65–70, however, both men and women begin losing bone mass at similar rates and the absorption of calcium decreases. Men are also more likely to die from hip fracture complications compared to women. Another population at risk for osteoporosis is women of Hispanic descent. An estimated 10% of Hispanic women aged 50 and older have osteoporosis, and 49% are estimated to have low bone mass. Decreased calcium intake within this culture and age group could be a contributor to the diagnosis of osteoporosis. Prevention of osteoporosis begins in childhood with eating a well-balanced diet rich in calcium and vitamin D, exercising regularly, not smoking, and drinking alcohol in moderation.

(Sources: Adapted from NIH Osteoporosis and Related Bone Diseases National Resource Center. National Institute of Arthritis and Musculoskeletal and Skin Diseases. *Osteoporosis and Hispanic Women.* June 2012; Osteoporosis and Men. January 2011. http://www.niams.nih.gov)

 periodontal disease
disease of the mouth and gums

 arthritis
chronic disease involving the joints

 occlusions
blockages

form and are unable to pass through an unnaturally narrowed artery. Arteries are narrowed by plaque, a fatty substance containing cholesterol that accumulates in the walls of the artery. This condition is called atherosclerosis. It is believed that excessive cholesterol and saturated fats in the diet over many years contribute to this condition. The therapeutic diet appropriate for atherosclerosis is discussed in Chapter 18.

Effects of Nutrition

Current research about the role of nutrition in preventing or relieving these chronic diseases continues. The effects of nutrition are cumulative over many years. The effects of a lifetime of poor eating habits cannot be cured overnight. When diets have been poor for a long time, prevention of these chronic diseases may not be possible. It may be possible, however, to use nutrition to help stabilize the condition of such a client. The prevention of many of the diseases of the elderly should begin in one's youth (Figure 15-2).

HEALTH AND NUTRITION CONSIDERATIONS

It is essential that the health care professional remember that each client is an individual with unique needs. It is easy for someone working exclusively with geriatric clients to group them together, but doing so diminishes the quality of the care they receive and adds to their unhappiness. The 80-year-old client is just as pleased to see a smile on the face of a nurse as is an 18-year-old client. The 70-year-old overweight arthritic client deserves as much help with a weight loss program as the 45-year-old client. The 85-year-old client suffering from senility still enjoys a bright hello and a gentle pat on the back. People's feelings must never be forgotten. The incapacitation that can accompany old age is a terrible indignity, and these clients deserve special care.

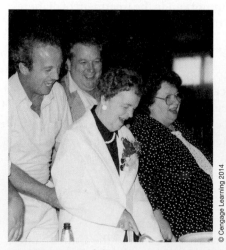
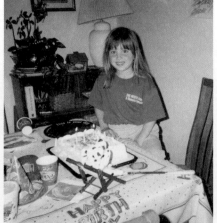

FIGURE 15-2 Celebrating an 80th birthday is as much fun as turning 8—when health is good, of course.

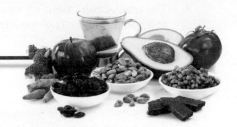

SUMMARY

The elderly are becoming an increasingly large segment of the U.S. population, and their nutritional needs are of growing concern. It is becoming apparent that many of the chronic diseases of the elderly could be delayed or avoided by maintaining good nutrition throughout life. Most nutrient requirements do not decrease with age, but calorie requirements do. When food habits of senior citizens must be changed, adjustments require great tact and patience on the part of the dietitian. Older people are easily attracted to food fads that promise good health and prolonged life.

DISCUSSION TOPICS

1. Why does the iron requirement usually diminish for women after the age of 50?
2. Why might elderly people suffer from anorexia?
3. How might arthritis affect one's eating habits?
4. In what ways can emotional stress affect eating habits? What kinds of emotional **stress** do the elderly sometimes suffer?
5. Why are older people inclined to believe food faddists' stories?
6. What is osteoporosis? Name the risk factors involved. Which risk factors do you or a close relative have for osteoporosis?
7. Why do calorie requirements diminish as people age?

SUGGESTED ACTIVITIES

1. Arrange a talk on nutrition for senior citizens at a congregate meal site.
2. If possible, visit a nursing home at mealtime. Write your evaluation of the food and a description of resident's reactions to it and to you, the visitor.
3. Describe an appropriate response to your 65-year-old aunt, who has just become captivated by a salesperson in a local health food store and has announced that she is buying a 6-month supply of vinegar-honey tablets that are guaranteed to cure arthritis.
4. Research current food fads and pick one to discuss with the class, stating whether this product would help or hinder nutritional health.

REVIEW

Multiple choice. Select the *letter* that precedes the best answer.

1. Gerontology is of increasing interest because it is
   a. the branch of medicine involved with diseases of older people
   b. the study of nutrition
   c. hoped that experimentation in this field will explain the causes of aging
   d. the study of heart disease
2. Nutrient requirements for the elderly generally
   a. increase
   b. decrease
   c. remain unchanged
   d. none of the above
3. Calorie requirements for the elderly generally
   a. increase
   b. decrease
   c. remain unchanged
   d. none of the above

4. The iron requirement for women after the age of approximately 51 generally
   a. increases
   b. decreases
   c. remains unchanged
   d. none of the above

5. As the metabolic rate slows with age,
   a. the calorie requirement is increased
   b. the calorie requirement is decreased
   c. there is a decreased need for vitamins A, D, and K
   d. cataracts can develop

6. Osteoporosis is a disease that causes
   a. poor appetite
   b. a reduction in the number of red blood cells
   c. joints to become painful and stiff
   d. bones to become porous

7. Arthritis is a disease that causes
   a. poor appetite
   b. a reduction in the number of red blood cells
   c. joints to become painful and stiff
   d. bones to become porous

8. Hypertension is related to diets high in
   a. cholesterol
   b. vitamin D
   c. calcium
   d. salt

9. Diets high in cholesterol content are thought to contribute to
   a. diabetes mellitus
   b. hypertension
   c. heart disease
   d. cataracts

10. Which of the following may cause depression in the elderly?
    a. loss of a family member
    b. lack of social ability
    c. physical disability
    d. all of the above

Case In Point

MARY: DISCOVERING OSTEOPOROSIS

Fred and Mary have been married for 52 years. Throughout the years they have been a very active and healthy couple. They have always tried to eat healthy, exercise, and see their doctor routinely. After Fred retired, he and Mary began playing tennis with a group at their local country club. They particularly enjoyed the doubles tennis and even participated in some senior tournaments. In one particularly exciting match, Mary fell and injured her wrist. She wasn't in too much pain at the time, but by the next morning her wrist was swollen, bruised, and painful to move. She decided see a doctor to have it x-rayed. The x-ray revealed that her wrist had a small fracture. The doctor also noted that her bones didn't look quite as dense as they should on the x-ray film. The doctor explained to Mary that it is possible she had developed osteoporosis. Mary never liked to take pills and so she did not take an estrogen replacement therapy after menopause. In addition, she was now 2 inches shorter than she was in her younger days. Her doctor informed her that these were both risk factors for developing osteoporosis. The doctor asked Mary to have a bone density scan done as well. The doctor wanted further assessment of Mary's situation in hopes to prevent future fractures.

ASSESSMENT

1. What do you know about Mary's health?
2. What did the doctor suspect about Mary?
3. How significant is this problem?
4. How common is this problem in the elderly?

DIAGNOSIS

5. Write a diagnosis for Mary's alteration in health maintenance and its cause.
6. Write a diagnosis for Mary's deficient knowledge and the type of education she needs.

PLAN/GOAL

7. What must change in Mary's diet?

IMPLEMENTATION

8. What additions or alterations in Mary's diet would prevent further osteoporosis? What are the best sources of calcium?
9. What information does Mary need to make this change?
10. Who can help her learn?
11. How can regular exercise help?
12. How could information from the National Osteoporosis Foundation (http://www.nof .org) help Mary?

EVALUATION/OUTCOME CRITERIA

13. At her next office visit with the doctor what will Mary report?

14. How long will it take before the doctor can measure an improvement in a DEXA scan?

THINKING FURTHER

15. From your review of the National Osteoporosis Foundation website (http://www.nof.org), what kind of information is available there?
16. Aside from calcium, how could other medications for osteoporosis help?
17. Why is it important to intervene with a person at any age who suffers from osteoporosis?
18. How can you use this lesson in other situations?

rate this **plate**

Mary's problem was first noticed when she injured her wrist on the tennis court. She will need further testing to properly diagnose osteoporosis. Even though Mary has tried to eat healthy and live an active life, adequate calcium and vitamin D may not have been eaten to develop dense bones. Rate this plate on calcium content:

1 cup clam chowder

6 whole-wheat crackers

1 medium peach

½ cup tapioca pudding

Water with lemon

Will this meal give Mary a serving of calcium? How many milligrams of calcium is considered a serving? List foods that are good sources of calcium.

Case In Point

MAX: DECREASING APPETITE

Max is a 95-year-old man. His wife of 64 years, Sophia, suffered a stroke 12 years ago and died. Max misses Sophia dearly, but tries to remain active and busy to keep his mind off of the sadness that he now has in his life. Max had been a salesman for many years and had a love for people and a gift for conversation. After Sophia's death, he decided to volunteer at the local hospital. For several years he helped transport clients at discharge, offer books and magazines to clients, and deliver flowers and mail. About a year ago, the volunteer work began to be too much for him physically, so he decided to stop.

Max's daughter, Avery, and her children live nearby. Avery would often stop to visit with her dad in the evenings, and cook meals and bring food to him on a regular basis. Max wasn't much of a cook. After Sophia died, he depended on Avery or restaurants for any hot meals. Recently, Avery noticed that her Dad was eating less of the food she put in his refrigerator. Max stated he didn't have much of an appetite. Avery also noticed her father's hygiene practices were in decline, as he was not the neatly dressed, clean-shaven man she knew, but was bearded and usually dressed in pajamas. Avery was concerned because her father looked very pale and thin. Max also reported feeling weak and dizzy. Avery decided it was time to take her father to the doctor.

ASSESSMENT

1. What do you know about Max and his health?
2. What do you know is a barrier in Max's life to maintaining health?
3. What nutrients are missing from Max's diet, and why?
4. How significant is the problem? What are the long-term consequences of the problem?

DIAGNOSIS

5. Complete the following statement: Imbalanced nutrition; less than body requirements related to _____.
6. What nutrition education does Avery need, to help Max?

PLAN/GOAL

7. What are your goals for Max's diet?

IMPLEMENTATION

8. Identify how each of the following resources can help Max solve this problem and prevent further problems.

EVALUATION/OUTCOME CRITERIA

9. At Max's next NP appointment, what changes would the NP expect to note? What would the NP expect Avery to report?

THINKING FURTHER

10. Why it is so important in older persons to ensure there is a balance between nutrition, medication, and chronic illness?
11. What would be the benefits of an assisted living setting for Max?
12. How can you use this lesson in other situations?

rate this plate

Max's lack of energy and weakness could be directly related to his poor appetite. Avery brought Max a warm meal to encourage her father to eat. This is the plate she brought for Max:

4 oz. meatloaf

1 small baked potato with butter and sour cream

½ cup of green beans and corn

1 dinner roll

½ cup custard

Coffee

Are these choices good or does any food need to be changed or added? Will this meal provide enough calories and nutrients for Max?

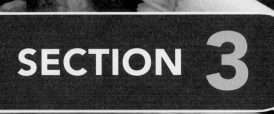

SECTION 3

MEDICAL NUTRITION THERAPY

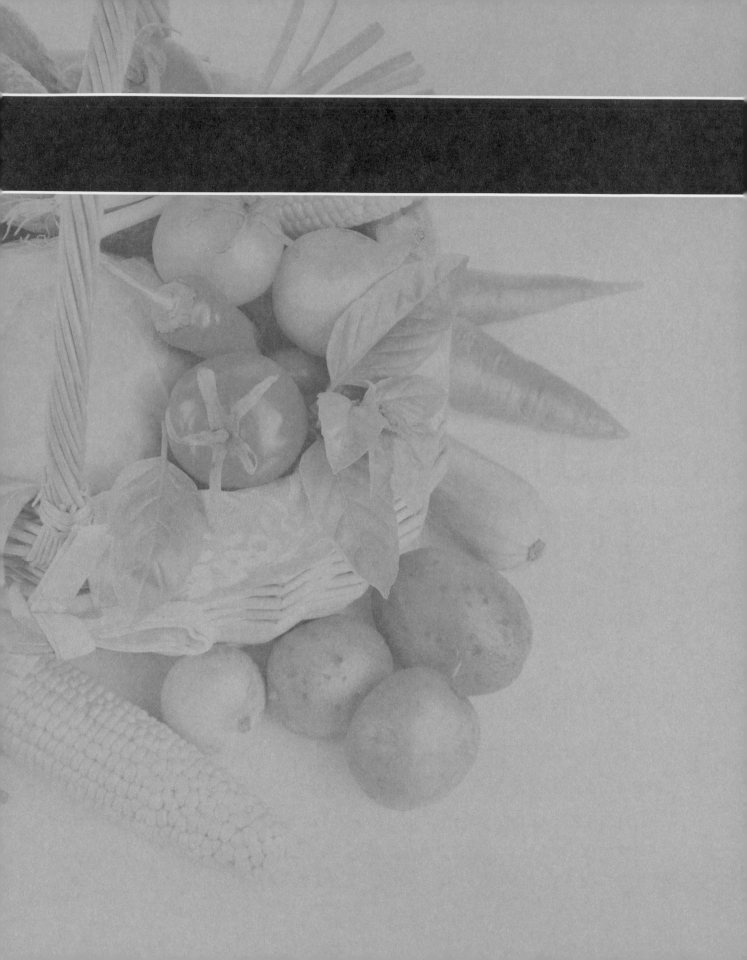

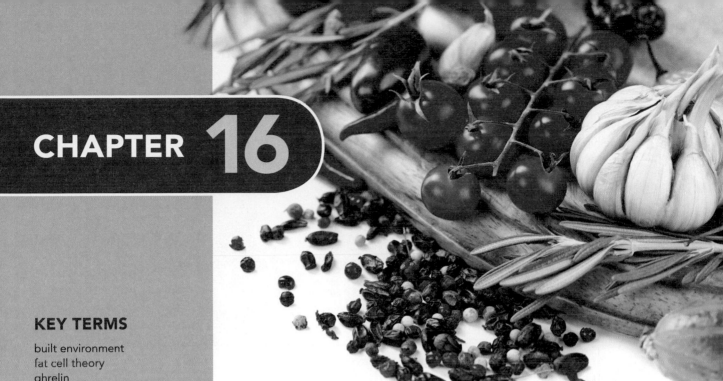

CHAPTER 16

WEIGHT MANAGEMENT ACROSS THE LIFE CYCLE

OBJECTIVES

After studying this chapter, you should be able to:

- Describe factors that contribute to energy balance and weight
- Describe changes in environment that have influenced obesity rates
- Understand medical complications of obesity for children and adults
- Explain treatment methods for overweight and obesity for children and adults and where to find resources
- Discuss prevention strategies and national efforts to reign in the obesity epidemic

FIGURE 16-1 The places where you store your body fat affect your health. "Pear" shapes tend to store fat in the hips and buttocks. "Apple" shapes store fat around the waist, which may be associated with more health issues.

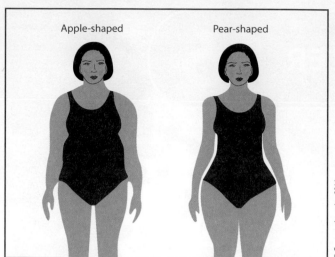

© Cengage Learning 2014

We are all born with the innate ability to regulate our eating so that we grow and develop properly and meet our energy needs over the life cycle. Our body's appetite regulation system is designed to guide us on the proper amount of food to consume, which in turn regulates our weight. But weight regulation is complex and influenced by many factors. Our genetics and physiology play key roles in how our body turns out—its shape, size, and weight distribution as well as susceptibility to disease (Figure 16-1). Our environment and lifestyle choices also exert considerable influence on our weight and health as well.

The very young are excellent food regulators; however, research shows that children can, starting at about age 5, respond more to external influences and learn to bypass internal fullness cues.

TRIGGERS FOR OVEREATING

If more food is set before us, overconsumption happens. If we smell or see appetizing food, we may eat it whether we were hungry or not. Boredom or stress are other external factors that can trigger eating. For many of us, we are not conscious of these effects. These habits can become ingrained and continue habitually throughout life. Pair these factors with a world of rich, plentiful, and highly marketed food, then sprinkle in liberal amounts of media time and low physical activity and here lies the recipe for emerging obesity.

Parents can disrupt the natural flow of feeding by putting pressure on children to either eat more or eat less at meals, therefore pulling them away from natural feeding cues. Underweight children who are coerced to eat tend to back away from food. Children who are restricted in their diets, to lose weight, are prone to overeat in the absence of hunger. Some end up managing their eating well; others become distressed eaters, which then can follow into adulthood.

Many individuals struggle with balancing their weight in a healthy fashion. Obesity is commonplace in today's society. Some feel obesity is a result of the "thrifty" gene. The genes that helped our ancestors survive occasional shortages of food may now be working against us in a supply that is abundantly plentiful year round. Some researchers believe that genes may have a role in those who suffer from poor appetite regulation and those who have an easily stimulated capacity to store body fat. Likely, it is not one gene that predisposes a person to obesity, but a cluster of genes; and many researchers today believe obesity has strong ties to insulin resistance.

While genetics predisposes a person to obesity, it's really the environment and lifestyle factors that tip the scale in its favor. Our modern world has efficiently engineered the art of movement out of the culture: sedentary desk jobs, remote controls, elevators, cars, escalators, and more. Time- and energy-saving gadgets abound. Food is available 24 hours a day, around every corner, at every venue imaginable. The shifts are dramatic; higher fast-food and soft drink consumption, reduced frequency of family meals, and increased portion sizes. Children and adults gravitate to television, video games, computers, and smart phones and, consequently, engage in little physical activity.

EATING REGULATION AND ENERGY BALANCE

Regulation of eating occurs primarily in the brain. In the hypothalamus, hunger and satiety chemicals work to regulate eating. The hormone **leptin** receives signals from fat and the intestine to make you feel full so eating will stop. The hormone **ghrelin** is released from the stomach and signals the hypothalamus that it's time to eat. Other key hormones and neurotransmitters are involved as well in food regulation.

Theories about weight gain have surfaced for decades, among them the **fat cell theory** and the **set point theory**. According to the fat cell theory, obesity is related to having too many fat cells and enlarged fat cells. Fat cells increase in number during youth, when growth occurs but then taper off in young adulthood. The premise of the set point theory is that we are programmed to carry a certain amount of weight. This complex weight regulation mechanism is governed by the hypothalamus. If you lose weight, your body tries to get back to its set point. Physical activity is the primary way to lower your set point if it's done at least 3–5 times per week.

The body needs a certain amount of energy (calories) from food to sustain basic life functions and, in children, growth. Body weight is maintained when calories eaten equal the number of calories the body expends,

 leptin
an appetite-suppressing hormone involved in maintenance of body composition

 ghrelin
a hormone from the stomach that signals the brain it's time to eat

 fat cell theory
a belief that fat cells have a natural drive to regain any weight lost

 set point theory
a belief that individuals have a natural weight (set point) at which the body is most comfortable

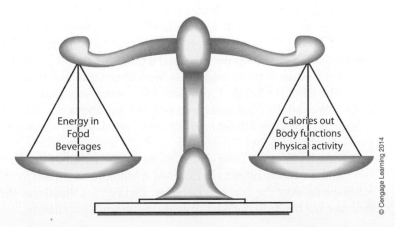

FIGURE 16-2 Balancing "energy in" and "energy out" will maintain weight.

© Cengage Learning 2014

FIGURE 16-3 Components of basal metabolic rate.

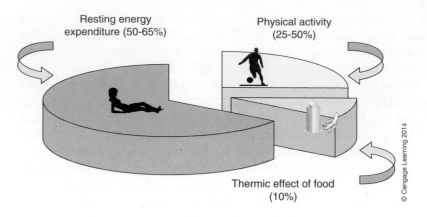

Resting energy expenditure (50-65%)

Physical activity (25-50%)

Thermic effect of food (10%)

© Cengage Learning 2014

or "burns" (Figure 16-2). When more calories are consumed than burned, energy balance is tipped toward weight gain, overweight, and obesity.

As referenced in Chapter 3, the components of our energy "out" are basal metabolic rate (BMR), physical activity, and the thermic effect of food. Figure 16-3 breaks down these components into percentages. Activity level and basal metabolic rate can vary greatly. Factors that affect BMR include age, height, growth cycle, and body composition. Other factors that affect BMR are temperature (body temperature as well as climate temperature) and fasting, or undereating. If an individual is underproducing thyroid hormone, BMR can decrease. This condition is called **hypothyroidism**.

Regarding physical activity, only 31% of U.S. adults report that they engage in regular leisure-time physical activity (150 minutes per week of light to moderate physical activity or 60 minutes of vigorous activity per week). About 40% of adults report no leisure-time physical activity. Interestingly when physical activity is measured by a device that detects movement, only about 3–5% of adults obtain 30 minutes of moderate or greater intensity physical activity on at least 5 days per week.

Without a doubt, many Americans are having a hard time balancing the "energy in" part of the equation. It appears that there has been a steady increase in calorie intake over the last few decades. Adults on average are consuming approximately 300 more calories a day as of 2008, than they did in 1985.

It has also been documented that Americans have a greater consumption of low-nutrition, energy-dense foods. Cost seems to be a factor in driving that change. Adjusted for inflation, prices for low-nutrient, energy-dense foods and beverages, such as soda and fast food, have declined sharply, which makes them appealing for consumers with smaller food budgets. Unfortunately on the flipside, research has documented a dramatic rise in price of more nutritious foods, such as fruits, vegetables, lean meats, and low-fat dairy products.

The CDC verifies that Americans are eating less fruits and vegetables. Only 32% of adults consumed fruit two or more times per day and only 26% consumed vegetables three or more times per day—far short of goals set for public health.

Obesity has risen to be one of the most serious public health concerns of our nation. Obesity rates have doubled in adults and tripled in children and adolescents over the last two decades. Figure 16-4 illustrates the dramatic increase in obesity in the past 20 years in the adult population.

⬦ **hypothyroidism**
a condition in which the thyroid gland secretes too little thyroxine and T3 resulting in a lower basal metabolic rate

---

In The Media

Too Fat to Fight?

The Pentagon has issued a statement saying there may be a shortage of qualified troops due to the mounting number of obese and unfit Americans wanting to qualify for military service. The Pentagon's director states "the major component of this is obesity and poor physical condition." There is a possibility that obese soldiers may not lose excess weight during basic training, even if they complete the program. National security may be at risk according to the "Mission: Readiness" group.

(Source: Adapted from McMichael, William. Most U.S. Youths Unfit to Serve, Data Show. *Army Times.* November 3, 2009. www.armytimes.com)

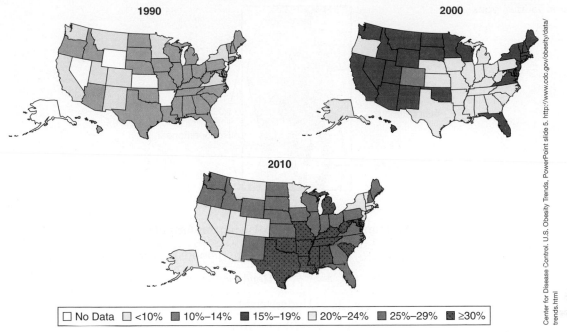

FIGURE 16-4 Obesity trends among U.S. adults over a 20-year period.

According to recent data from the CDC, about one third of U.S. adults (33.8%) are obese. Approximately 17% (or 12.5 million) of children and adolescents aged 2–19 years are obese. In 2010, no state had a prevalence of obesity less than 20%. Thirty-six states had a prevalence of 25% or more with 12 of these states having a prevalence of 30% or more. The obesity epidemic continues to be most dramatic in the South, which includes 9 of the 10 states with the highest adult obesity rates.

The obesity epidemic continues to overtake our country, especially among children, minorities, and the poor. Even though, on average, adult occurrences of obesity are no longer skyrocketing, men, teenage boys, and black and Mexican American women are gaining weight faster than ever before.

DEFINING OBESITY

On a basic level, obesity can be defined as excess fat accumulation under the skin and around the organs in the body. Fat accumulated in the lower body (the pear shape) is **subcutaneous fat** (Figure 16-5). Fat in the abdominal area (the apple shape) is mostly **visceral fat**. Abdominal fat correlates more with health risks such as cardiovascular disease and type 2 diabetes. In women, it also correlates with breast cancer risk and gallbladder disease. Where we deposit fat is influenced by hormones and heredity.

Body mass index (BMI) is a number calculated from a person's weight and height that provides a reliable indicator of body fatness for most people. It is used to screen for weight categories that may lead to health problems.

 subcutaneous fat
fat stored directly under the skin

 visceral fat
fat stored within the abdominal cavity

FIGURE 16-5 View of various types of fat tissue.

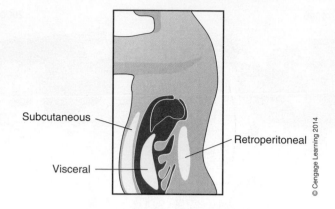

Subcutaneous

Retroperitoneal

Visceral

© Cengage Learning 2014

You can calculate your BMI using this formula:

$$BMI = \frac{weight\ (pounds) \times 703}{Height\ squared\ (inches^2)}$$

- Below 18.5 = Underweight
- 18.5–24.9 = Healthy weight
- 25.0–29.9 = Overweight
- 30.0 or higher = Obese

A BMI table is a useful tool to approximate BMI (Table 16-1). To use, follow height column vertically on left side until height is found. Trace column horizontally to the right until you find your client's closest weight. Once weight has been pinpointed, trace column upward in a straight line to find out the approximate BMI and classification of BMI.

You may also use a BMI calculator online such as the one provided on the National Institutes of Health website (http://www.nhlbisupport.com/bmi/) (Figure 16-6). Using this calculator, enter weight and height using standard or metric measures. Select "Compute BMI" and your BMI will appear there. Smart phone apps are also available for calculating BMIs.

Although BMI can be used for most men and women, it does have some limits:

- It may overestimate body fat in athletes and others who have a muscular build.
- It may underestimate body fat in older persons and others who have lost muscle.

Health Consequences of Obesity

Research has shown that as weight increases to reach the levels referred to as "overweight" and "obesity," the risks for the following conditions also increase:

- Coronary heart disease
- Insulin resistance and type 2 diabetes

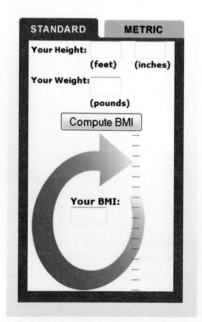

The National Heart Lung and Blood Institute, National Institutes of Health. www.nhlbisupport.com/bmi/

FIGURE 16-6 Body mass index calculator.

TABLE 16-1 BMI Table

BMI category																								
	NORMAL						OVERWEIGHT					OBESE										EXTREME OBESITY		
BMI	19	20	21	22	23	24	25	26	27	28	29	30	31	32	33	34	35	36	37	38	39	40	41	42
Height (Feet-Inches)	**Weight (Pounds)**																							
4' 10"	91	96	100	105	110	115	119	124	129	134	138	143	148	153	158	162	167	172	177	181	186	191	196	201
4' 11"	94	99	104	109	114	119	124	128	133	138	143	148	153	158	163	168	173	178	183	188	193	198	203	208
5' 00"	97	102	107	112	118	123	128	133	138	143	148	153	158	163	168	174	179	184	189	194	199	204	209	215
5' 01"	100	106	111	116	122	127	132	137	143	148	153	158	164	169	174	180	185	190	195	201	206	211	217	222
5' 02"	104	109	115	120	126	131	136	142	147	153	158	164	169	175	180	186	191	196	202	207	213	218	224	229
5' 03"	107	113	118	124	130	135	141	146	152	158	163	169	175	180	186	191	197	203	208	214	220	225	231	237
5' 04"	110	116	122	128	134	140	145	151	157	163	169	175	180	186	191	197	204	209	215	221	227	232	238	244
5' 05"	114	120	125	132	138	144	150	156	162	168	174	180	186	192	198	204	210	216	222	228	234	240	246	252
5' 06"	118	124	130	136	142	148	155	161	167	173	179	186	192	198	204	210	216	223	229	235	241	247	253	260
5' 07"	121	127	134	140	146	153	159	166	172	178	185	191	198	204	211	217	223	230	236	242	249	255	261	268
5' 08"	125	131	138	144	151	158	164	171	177	184	190	197	203	210	216	223	230	236	243	249	256	262	269	276
5' 09"	128	135	142	149	155	162	169	176	182	189	196	203	209	216	223	230	236	243	250	257	263	270	277	284
5' 10"	132	139	146	153	160	167	174	181	188	195	202	209	216	222	229	236	243	250	257	264	271	278	285	292
5' 11"	136	143	150	157	165	172	179	186	193	200	208	215	222	229	236	243	250	257	265	272	279	286	293	301
6' 00"	140	147	154	162	169	177	184	191	199	206	213	221	228	235	242	250	258	265	272	279	287	294	302	309
6' 01"	144	151	159	166	174	182	189	197	204	212	219	227	235	242	250	257	265	272	280	288	295	302	310	318
6' 02"	148	155	163	171	179	186	194	202	210	218	225	233	241	249	256	264	272	280	287	295	303	311	319	326
6' 03"	152	160	168	176	184	192	200	208	216	224	232	240	248	256	264	272	279	287	295	303	311	319	327	335
6' 04"	156	164	172	180	189	197	205	213	221	230	238	246	254	263	271	279	287	295	304	312	320	328	336	344

ADAPTED FROM: GEORGE BRAY, PENNINGTON BIOMEDICAL RESEARCH CENTER, CLINICAL GUIDELINES ON THE IDENTIFICATION, EVALUATION, AND TREATMENT OF OVERWEIGHT AND OBESITY IN ADULTS: THE EVIDENCE REPORT, NATIONAL INSTITUTES OF HEALTH, NATIONAL HEART, LUNG, AND BLOOD INSTITUTE, SEPTEMBER 1998.

Source: National Institute of Diabetes and Digestive and Kidney Diseases. Weight Control Information Network. (November 2008). *Understanding Adult Obesity.* Retrieved in January 2011 from http://win.niddk.nih.gov

- Cancers (endometrial, breast, and colon)
- Hypertension (high blood pressure)
- Dyslipidemia (e.g., high total cholesterol or high levels of triglycerides)
- Stroke
- Liver and gallbladder disease
- Sleep apnea and respiratory problems
- Osteoarthritis (a degeneration of cartilage and its underlying bone within a joint)
- Gynecological problems (abnormal menses, infertility)

Besides the physical consequences of obesity and overweight, emotional and social health is affected. Some overweight or obese individuals suffer from low self-esteem and negative body image. Often those who suffer from weight issues can be depressed and feel that they are the object of discrimination.

Financial issues are a concern as well. On average, people who are considered obese pay 42% more in health care costs than normal-weight individuals. Our nation as a whole is seeing the staggering economic effect. The cost of overweight and obesity in the United States is estimated at $270 billion per year. This cost is related to the increased need for medical care and the loss of productivity from disability and death.

Waist Circumference

Because of the science behind the health risk of visceral fat, it is useful to measure waist circumference, along with BMI, and correlate this to disease risk. Note that in Table 16-2, you can see the disease risk increase as waist circumference and BMI increase.

In The Media

Sitting is Hazardous to your Health

The medical community has recently been reporting that those who sit for prolonged periods have a higher risk of disease. Scientists at the Pennington Biomedical Research Center in Louisiana have discovered that people who sit for most of the day are 54% more likely to die of heart attacks. In addition, researchers at the American Cancer Society found that even if you exercise nearly every day, those health benefits can be undone if you spend the rest of your time sitting. Employers have a stake in keeping their employees healthy and productive. Some companies are retrofitting conference room and office areas with standing desks and treadmill desks. An elliptical machine office desk is now on the market.
(Source: Adapted from Cardoni, Salvatore. *Conference Room Cardio: Firm Stands Behind Walking Meetings.* December 6, 2011.)

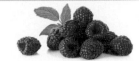

TABLE 16-2 Classification of Overweight and Obesity by BMI, Waist Circumference, and Associated Disease Risks

| | BMI (KG/M²) | OBESITY CLASS | DISEASE RISK* RELATIVE TO NORMAL WEIGHT AND WAIST CIRCUMFERENCE | |
			MEN (40 IN) OR LESS WOMEN (35 IN) OR LESS	MEN >40 IN WOMEN >35 IN
Underweight	< 18.5		—	—
Normal	18.5–24.9		—	—
Overweight	25.0–29.9		Increased	High
Obesity	30.0–34.9	I	High	Very high
	35.0–39.9	II	Very high	Very high
Extreme Obesity	40.0⁺	III	Extremely high	Extremely high

* Disease risk for type 2 diabetes, hypertension, and CVD. ⁺ Increased waist circumference also can be a marker for increased risk, even in persons of normal weight.

Source: The National Heart Lung and Blood Institute, National Institutes of Health. *Obesity and Physical Activity Information. Classification of Overweight and Obesity by BMI, Waist Circumference, and Associated Disease Risks.* Retrieved January 2012 from www.nhlbi.nih.gov

One important note is that BMI does not show the difference between fat and muscle. It does not always accurately predict when weight could lead to health problems. For example, when someone with a lot of muscle (such as a body builder or football player) has a higher BMI, they may still be healthy and have little risk of developing secondary complications from overweight or obesity. Studies do show it's the level of fitness that correlates to long-term survival better than one's level of obesity. Simply put, research tends to show overweight people who are fit have a lower risk of death than normal-weight individuals who are sedentary.

Body fat assessment is much more specific to your actual fat content and thus provides a more accurate picture. The two most common methods used are skinfold measurement and bioelectrical impedance analysis (BIA) machines or scales. In skinfold measurement, a trained specialist uses calipers to measure specific spots on the body. These measurements are compared to a chart that estimates fat percentage. However, the accuracy of this method varies greatly based on the user's abilities.

Bioelectrical impedance analysis is the technology behind the many fat percentage machines in use at fitness centers and in scales sold for home use. However, the error rates for these can be as high as 8%. Body fat measures that are more accurate are x-ray analysis (DEXA scan) and water displacement methods, which are largely used in research institutions.

According to the American Council on Exercise, acceptable body fat percentages for women are between 25% and 31%, and for men between 18% and 24%. To be considered in the "fitness" body fat percentage range, women should be between 21% and 24%, and men between 14% and 17%. Despite the multiple factors that influence weight, altered food intake and decreased physical activity play into the equation in a significant way.

EXPLORING THE WEB

How have portion sizes changed in restaurants over the past 20 years? Research what the calorie content was of a fast-food meal back in the 1970s. Compare that with a fast-food meal of today. The term "portion distortion" describes the phenomenon that is happening. Check out the National Heart Lung and Blood Institute's slide set on portion distortion by going to http://www.nhlbi.nih.gov and typing "Obesity Education Initiative (OEI) Slide Sets" into the search bar.

STRATEGIES FOR WEIGHT LOSS

When an individual begins the journey of weight loss, the road can begin to look very bumpy. There are numerous diet and self-help books available to the public. In fact, according to data from 2010, the diet industry overall is nearly a $61 billion industry.

Among America's 75 million dieters, 80% are trying to do it on their own. But the big question remains: What works and is it safe? Safe weight loss has been described in the medical literature for decades at 1–2 pounds per week, in order to preserve lean body mass. That equates to roughly decreasing your intake between 500 and 1,000 calories a day. For very obese individuals, some references state that they can safely lose 1% of their body weight per week (325-pound man = 3.25 pounds/week acceptable weight loss). Research has documented many benefits for persons losing as moderately as 5–10% of their body weight.

There are many eating styles that are healthy and safe and will yield weight loss. The Therapeutic Lifestyle Change (TLC) diet from the National Institute of Health is an all-around healthy plan aimed at improving heart health and lowering cholesterol. The same can be said of the Ornish diet and the Mediterranean diet. The DASH diet (Dietary Approaches to Stop Hypertension), also from the National Institutes of Health, works to improve hypertension and heart health. Common threads in these eating plans are consuming highly nutritious fruits, vegetables, high-fiber grains, heart-healthy protein foods such as seafood, beans, very lean poultry, low-fat dairy, nuts, seeds, and small amounts of oil (Figure 16-7).

A way to assemble your plate that naturally trims calories would be to estimate portions using hand size:

- Cup your hands—very lean protein would fit in one palm; a higher fiber grain or healthy starchy vegetable/starchy bean dish would fit in the other palm.

- Fill in the rest of your plate with non-starchy vegetables in the form of salads, soups, and steamed or lightly sautéed vegetables. Besides high nutrient value, they will add fullness and bulk to your eating and help keep your calories in check for weight loss. Examples of non-starchy vegetables include broccoli, spinach, tomatoes, green beans, cucumbers, mushrooms, carrots, cabbage, peppers, summer squash such as zucchini, lettuce, and onion.

FIGURE 16-7 Healthy eating for weight management.

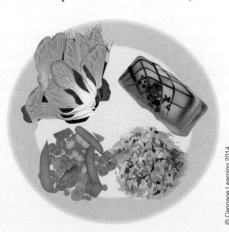

© Cengage Learning 2014

- Provide yourself a serving of fruit, skim milk, and a small allowance of healthy fat for optimal intake.

As discussed elsewhere in this text, Choose MyPlate (http://www .choosemyplate.gov) offers mainstream advice to the public about healthy eating plans. The website includes information for "dieters" and offers ways to track food intake using the SuperTracker. Other popular plans with focused weight loss goals include the Mayo Clinic Diet, the Volumetric Diet, Weight Watchers, and the Biggest Loser Diet. Some individuals desiring weight loss swear by simply counting calories or fat grams. Others learn to weigh and measure their food and follow an exchange-type meal plan. Table 16-3 shows "less conventional" approaches to weight loss and their advantages and disadvantages.

TABLE 16-3 **Less Conventional Approaches to Weight Loss**

DIET METHOD	PRO	CON
Low carbohydrate (<100 g/day) (Atkins, South Beach, Protein Power)	Rapid initial weight loss; low circulating glucose; may see drop in lipids	Much of initial weight loss is water; could cause poor stamina and ketosis; Atkins high in unhealthy fat; high protein taxes kidney; no higher weight loss shown with this eating vs. low-fat eating after 1 yr; artificial sweetener use touted; hard to follow long term
Extremely low fat (<20% calories from fat) (T-Factor, Pritikin)	Wide variety of wholesome foods allowed at normal portions; reduces risk of heart disease and cancer	Little satiety and palatability; decreased absorption of fat-soluble vitamins and minerals
Novel diets promoting certain nutrients, foods, or combinations	May promote rapid weight loss	Nutritionally inadequate; doesn't promote permanent change in food habits or body weight
Suzanne Sommer's Get Skinny	Reducing sweets and high-calorie starches may foster better glucose control in diabetics	Book teaches food combining which is not based on solid science; carbohydrate content of meals vary widely; glycemic index use eliminates some healthful food
Fit for Life	Encourages vegetables	Teaches food combining and diet is low in calcium, zinc, iron, and vitamins B_{12} and D
Enter the Zone	Six small eating sessions offer steady supply of energy	Low in fiber and marginal in some nutrients; portrays some high-glycemic foods as dangerous, even though they may have merit nutritionally
Very low calorie (<800 cal/day) or formula (Optifast, Medifast, Cambridge)	Quick weight loss Eliminates behavior cues and food decisions	Low-calorie diets can be dangerous if not monitored by a doctor; does not foster long-term behavior change
Premeasured (Jenny Craig, Nutrisystem)	Generally safe and effective Eliminates decision making from eating	Expensive, clients may have trouble transitioning to their own home-cooked meals

(Sources: Adapted from Zonya Health International. *Zonya's Diet Comparison Chart.* 2003, 2006. www.zonya.com; Bastin, Sandra. *Fad Diets.* UK Cooperative Extension Service. www.ca.uky.edu)

plateau period
period in which there is no change in weight

yo-yo effect
when a dieter's weight goes up and down over short periods due to swings in eating (from strict dieting to overconsumption)

Going on a rigid diet low in calories may result in an initial rapid weight loss. However, a higher portion of the weight loss may be lean body mass versus body fat. Sudden weight loss of this type lowers metabolic rate. Often individuals reach a **plateau period** as well in which weight does not decrease further. Due to the depriving nature of strict dieting, individuals are at risk for binge eating. Some may categorize food into "good" and "bad" categorizes and if something forbidden is eaten, they feel guilty. Swings in eating then can lead to weight gain, until another diet method is tried. This can have a **yo-yo effect** on weight and impact health.

Behavior Change Methods

Regardless of which type of eating pattern is chosen for weight loss, true behavior change is a must. It's interesting to note that although many people receive frequent information on healthy lifestyle and eating behavior, few (30%) reflect on what the information can mean for them and whether there are reasons to change their own behavior.

There are a multitude of behavior patterns that influence energy balance and contribute to obesity. Skipping breakfast, eating in front of the television, late-night snacking, lack of adequate sleep, being too rushed to exercise, or eating to help manage stress or difficult emotions are just some of the patterns we engage in. What drives our behavior patterns, however, are often not evident but need to be brought to the surface before permanent change can be made. Clients need to evaluate their habits around food and exercise and find the source of the obstacle. We must trace and address underlying issues. Behavior change requires coming to a stage of readiness and being open to readily accept it.

Here are behavioral strategies for weight loss clients:

- Set specific, realistic goals to address changes in eating and exercise and begin to establish new routines.

- Keep a record of food intake and amount of physical activity. Sometimes clients will have startling self-discovery and eat differently once they know they will be recording it. Individuals may think they exercise more than they really do, but their log may tell them a different story. Reflecting on a personal log can inspire clients as they learn new habits. Wellness habits increase over the long term as clients develop higher self-esteem and better health.

- On their food record, clients may want to include emotions surrounding their eating patterns, assessing their level of hunger and satiety when finished eating. Sometimes eating happens in the absence of hunger (external drivers), and clients may eat until the stuffed or too full stage. Sensing normal hunger and fullness cues is important, as are triggers for eating.

- Encourage clients to change their surroundings to avoid overeating. For example, they can avoid eating in front of the television. Instruct to keep a pantry full of healthy food, not tempting snack foods and sweets, and to take balanced portions of food to work for lunch and snacks.

- Clients should reward their success in a non-food way. Once they've met a goal, treating oneself to a movie, music CD, an afternoon off from work, a massage, or personal time is gratifying.

- Clients need support from a health care provider, friend, or spouse. A call, email, or even a text can boost support. Perhaps they should join a local support group for accountability.

- Instruct clients to weigh in only once a week for self-monitoring. Clients who are fearful of the scale may only want to measure themselves with a tape measure.

Physical Activity

Staying physically active to build and preserve muscle, in tandem with a healthier diet, are the ingredients for weight loss and healthy weight maintenance. The research on physical activity is compelling. Exercise provides these benefits:

- Lowers the risk of chronic disease (e.g., heart disease, diabetes, cancers) and can help improve blood pressure

- Strengthens lungs and helps them to work more efficiently

- Builds and strengthens muscles and keeps joints in good condition

- May slow bone loss

- Increases energy levels and builds self-confidence

- Helps in relaxation and coping skills by reducing stress and possibly lessening depression

- Helps provide solid sleep habits

- Boosts immunity

How much activity is needed?

- For good health and to reduce risk of disease, aim for at least 30 minutes of moderate physical activity most days of the week.

- To help manage body weight and prevent gradual weight gain, aim for 60 minutes of moderate-to-vigorous physical activity most days of the week.

- To maintain weight loss, aim for at least 60–90 minutes of daily moderate physical activity.

Breaking up exercise into 15-minute increments is useful for some people. If clients have been inactive for some time, they should start slowly and gradually increase their activity. For example, start walking for 10–15 minutes three times a week, then gradually build up to the recommended amount with brisk walking.

Some overweight individuals do not have success "going it alone" and may require formal instruction from a registered dietitian. A dietitian can meet with clients one-on-one for weight management counseling, or in a group setting. Group classes can offer participants moral support, enhanced learning, and significant accountability. Behavior therapy expertise as well

EXPLORING THE WEB

Go to the Mayo Clinic website (http://www.mayoclinic.com) for a critique of popular over-the-counter weight loss pills. Review the different products and consider their claims, effectiveness, and safety.

as instruction from an exercise scientist forms the basis for comprehensive programming for weight management. Oversight and medical monitoring from a physician is also an important variable.

With new health care reform, the primary care physician's office is now referred to as the "medical home." Primary care doctors are the gatekeepers and serve to organize overall care. Many overweight and obese individuals do receive initial coaching on health habits to help lower their weight in this setting. Since late 2011, individuals on Medicare with a BMI of 30 or more can receive weekly in-person weight management counseling visits for 1 month, followed by visits every 2 weeks for an additional 5 months. These are fully paid by Medicare with no co-pay.

Weight Loss Drugs

Some clients ask their physicians about prescription weight loss drugs. Often, doctors strongly encourage clients to use more natural methods first. Doctors understand that every medicine has inherent risks and should only consider the drugs in patients who are at increased medical risk, not simply because they want to lose weight for cosmetic reasons.

Prescription weight loss drugs are approved only for those clients with a BMI above 30, or a BMI of 27 and above with associated diseases such as hypertension, type 2 diabetes, or dyslipidemia. Appetite suppressants, approved by the FDA, are meant only to be used short term. They include phentermine, phendimetrazine, and diethylpropion. Amphetamines that suppress appetite are not recommended for use in the treatment of obesity as there is a strong potential for abuse and dependence.

In the late 1990s, the FDA approved the drug orlistat (Xenical). This drug reduces the body's ability to absorb fat from food by 33%. It can be viewed as a fat blocker, as it inhibits lipase. In 2007, orlistat was approved for over-the-counter use in adults age 18 and over. The dose then changed and it became known as "Alli." This drug is meant to be used in tandem with a reduced-calorie, low-fat diet, along with exercise and a daily multivitamin. Orlistat may cause intestinal discomfort, diarrhea, and leakage of oily stools (especially if a higher-fat food item is eaten); however, these reactions are usually mild and temporary.

In 1997, fenfluramine and dexfenfluramine were withdrawn from the market as they were linked to heart valve problems and primary pulmonary hypertension. In 2010, Abbott labs removed sibutramine (Meridia) as clinical trials showed an increased risk of heart attack and stroke in clients using this drug.

There are numerous over-the-counter weight loss pills and supplements promoting "fat burning." Most products have not been proven effective and some may be dangerous. Supplements and weight loss aids are not subject to the same rigid standards as prescription drugs, although the FDA does monitor their safety and can recall or ban a product if deemed necessary. Even of late, a new unconventional weight loss product is on the market, called Sensa. Sprinkling food with this **tastant** enhances the sense of smell and taste, and tells the brain when the stomach is full and satisfied.

tastant
a chemical that stimulates the sensory cells in the taste bud

Weight Loss Surgery

When sustainable weight loss efforts have failed, some obese individuals opt to have bariatric surgery. The four types of operations common in the United States are as follows (Figure 16-8):

- *Adjustable gastric band (AGB).* A small bracelet-like band is placed around the top of the stomach to restrict the size of the opening from the throat to the stomach, thereby reducing food intake. The size of the opening can be controlled via a balloon inside the band.

- *Roux-en-Y gastric bypass (RYGB).* Food intake is limited as surgeons create a small pouch for the stomach. This pouch is then connected to a different part of the intestine (bypassing the stomach and duodenum), thereby changing the way food is absorbed. The pouch is only about the size of a walnut.

- *Vertical sleeve gastrectomy (VSG).* This newer procedure involves removing much of the stomach in a vertical fashion, allowing only a tubular sleeve-shaped stomach which empties into the duodenum. Because so much stomach is removed, there is less ghrelin which reduces hunger more than banded gastroplasty.

- *Biliopancreatic diversion with duodenal switch (BPD-DS).* Sometimes this surgery is done 6–18 months after a sleeve surgery, as a "staged approach" to weight loss surgery. It involves rerouting the sleeve from much of the small intestine and diverting bile and gastric juices to change digestion and absorption.

Bariatric surgery may be an option for adults with a BMI ≥40, or a BMI ≥35 with a serious health problem linked to obesity (e.g., type 2 diabetes, heart disease, or severe sleep apnea). The FDA recently approved the use of the adjustable gastric band for patients with BMI ≥30 who also have at least one condition linked to obesity such as heart disease or diabetes.

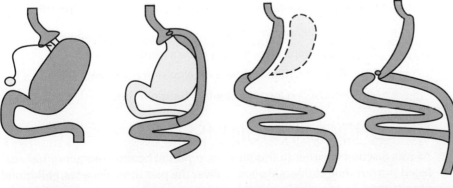

FIGURE 16-8 Four types of bariatric surgery.

Adjustable Gastric Band (AGB)

Roux-en-Y Gastric Bypass (RYGB)

Vertical Sleeve Gastrectomy (VSG)

Biliopancreatic Diversion with a Duodenal Switch (BPD-DS)

Before surgery is approved, clients must show proof they have tried traditional methods of weight loss and not found success. Often a psychological evaluation is done to determine if the client is a proper candidate and can respond well to the weight loss and change in body image. Surgeons require clients to demonstrate their full understanding of the undertaking and their motivation to follow extensive food, exercise, and medical guidance the rest of their lives. A surgeon, primary care doctor, psychologist, and dietitian are key people on the treatment team.

Side effects may include bleeding, infection, leaks from the site where the intestines are sewn together, diarrhea, and blood clots in the legs that can move to the lungs and heart. Side effects that may occur later include some nutrient deficiencies especially in clients who do not take their prescribed vitamins and minerals. Dumping syndrome may occur, in which clients may experience cramping, and weight gain over the long term. Complication rates among clients initially hospitalized for bariatric surgery is now 15%, which is lower than previous estimates. Many surgeries are now done laparoscopically.

Weight loss surgery is considered successful when 50% of excess weight is lost and the loss is sustained up to 5 years. Bariatric surgeries may cost $20,000–$25,000 and insurance coverage varies by state and insurance plan.

Many individuals struggle with being successful at weight loss. Some attempt weight loss multiple times. There is a lot of talk that 95% of diets fail, yet if individuals are ready to change their thinking, habits, and environment, a healthy weight can be within their grasp. Research has shown that approximately 20% of overweight individuals are successful at long-term weight loss when defined as losing at least 10% of initial body weight and maintaining the loss for at least 1 year. Newer research has shown 29.7% of obese individuals being successful at 1-year weight loss maintenance.

The National Weight Control Registry, established in 1994, serves as the largest prospective investigation of long-term successful weight loss maintainers. This registry, from Brown University School of Medicine, tracks over 10,000 people who have lost significant amounts of weight and kept it off for long periods of time.

Solid habits reported common among the participants include maintaining a low-calorie, low-fat diet and doing high levels of activity.

- 78% eat breakfast every day.
- 75% weigh themselves at least once a week.
- 62% watch less than 10 hours of television per week.
- 90% exercise, on average, about 1 hour per day.

CHILDHOOD WEIGHT ISSUES

As was discussed earlier in this chapter, a public health emergency has surfaced surrounding childhood obesity. Over the past three decades, childhood obesity rates in America have tripled. Today, nearly one in three children in America are overweight or obese. Unfortunately, childhood weight issues follow into adulthood—overweight adolescents have a 70% chance of becoming overweight or obese adults. This increases to 80% if at least one parent is overweight or obese.

In African American and Hispanic communities, nearly 40% of the children are overweight or obese. Nine of the 10 states with the highest rates of obese children are in the South, which also correlates to poverty rates.

Because of the rising obesity rates, researchers speculate this may be the first generation of children who live shorter lives than their parents. Current research has found that obesity, glucose intolerance, and elevated blood pressure during childhood and adolescence are associated with increased rates of early death.

Risk factors for heart disease, such as high cholesterol and high blood pressure, occur with increased frequency in overweight children and adolescents compared to children with a healthy weight. Also, type 2 diabetes, previously considered an adult disease, has increased dramatically in children and adolescents. As discussed in Chapter 13, overweight and obesity are closely linked to type 2 diabetes and its precursor, insulin resistance. Asthma, hepatic steatosis (fatty liver), and sleep apnea are other disorders sometimes associated with overweight youth. Polycystic ovarian syndrome (PCOS), a hormonal imbalance that may be associated with insulin resistance, is sometimes seen in overweight teen girls.

The most immediate consequence of overweight as perceived by the children themselves is social discrimination. Overweight children may feel they are viewed as lazy or lacking discipline. Many overweight children are teased or bullied, which is associated with poor self-esteem and depression. Low self-esteem, in turn, can hinder academic and social functioning, and persist into adulthood.

Children today lead different lives from their parents and grandparents, who as children played outdoors most of the time. Now neighborhoods may be less safe and outside play is limited. The walks to school have been replaced by car or bus rides. Gym class and after-school sports activities have been subject to program cuts. Researchers know that only 42% of children aged 6–11 obtain the recommended 60 minutes per day of physical activity and only 8% of adolescents achieve this goal.

Afternoons and evenings are filled with "screen" time—television, video games, online computing, and texting. The average media time per U.S. child is 7.5 hours/day. Today's families share fewer home-cooked meals. Snacking between meals is rampant as pantries are "fair game," so children can obtain out-of-control portion sizes any time of the day. It's no wonder researchers have used the term "toxic" to describe the food environment in America. Table 16-4 outlines key behaviors that contribute to childhood overweight and obesity.

The CDC and the American Academy of Pediatrics (AAP) recommend the use of BMI to screen for overweight and obesity in children beginning at age 2 years. BMI can be calculated for children and teens and the resulting number plotted on the CDC's "BMI-for-age" growth charts. These percentiles help practitioners assess growth relative to the averages set for children of the same sex and age. A BMI between the 85th and 95th percentile is considered overweight; one that falls above the 95th percentile is considered obese (Figure 16-9).

An important perspective for overweight and obese children and teens is to consider lifestyle changes that slow the rate of weight gain while allowing

TABLE 16-4 Contributors to Overweight and Obesity

- Skipping breakfast
- Low fruit and vegetable intake
- Sweetened beverage intake
- Excessive media time (especially TV in bedroom)
- Low physical activity level (sedentary behavior)
- Not eating meals together as a family
- Parental restriction of palatable foods

Source: Intermountain Health Care. *Primary Care Guide to Weight Management in Children and Adolescents.* 2007 (updated 2010). www.intermountainhealthcare.org.

FIGURE 16-9 CDC's growth chart shows different BMIs and their weight status in a sample of 10-year-old males.

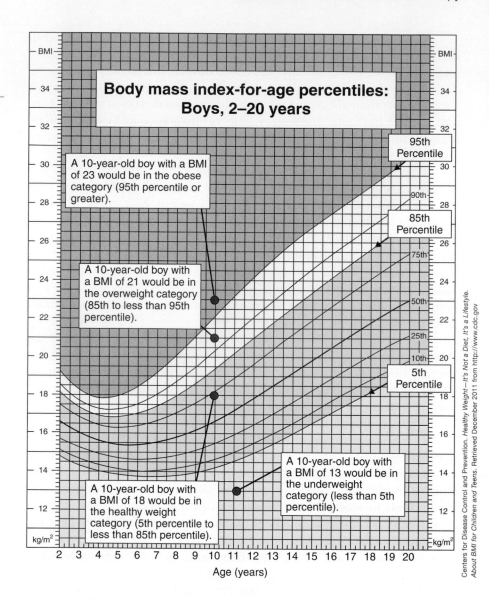

Centers for Disease Control and Prevention. *Healthy Weight—It's Not a Diet, It's a Lifestyle. About BMI for Children and Teens.* Retrieved December 2011 from http://www.cdc.gov

normal growth and development. If a child can simply slow or halt weight gain during the active growth years and allow their "height" to catch up, BMI can lower and normalize. However, if a child is experiencing other health complications such as high cholesterol, high blood pressure, high blood sugar, and is also overweight or obese, some weight loss is indicated. Table 16-5 shows weight management or loss guidelines for kids.

Strategies for Childhood Weight Loss

Treatment of the overweight or obese child or teen can happen with success. Parents can improve the food environment and keep their kids physically fit, especially if they serve as the role model. Measures are successful when surrounded with positive support and consistency. Important tactics would be to provide reliable meals and snacks at the table, with limits on food handouts at

TABLE 16-5 Weight Guidelines for Overweight or Obese Children

AGE RANGE	HEALTH	OVERWEIGHT (85TH–95TH PERCENTILE)	OBESE (>95TH PERCENTILE)
Age 2–7	Otherwise healthy	Maintenance	Maintenance
	Secondary complication*	Maintenance	Very slow weight loss (no more than 1 lb/mo)
Ages 7 and above	Otherwise healthy	Maintenance	Weight loss (2–4 lb/mo)
	Secondary complication*	Weight loss (2–4 lb/mo)	Weight loss (1–2 lb/week)

*Secondary complication could include high cholesterol, high blood pressure, insulin resistance, sleep apnea, fatty liver, joint problems, PCOS, or depression/anxiety.

Source: Intermountain Health Care. *Primary Care Guide to Weight Management in Children and Adolescents.* 2007 (updated 2010). www.intermountainhealthcare.org.

other times. Meals should be freshly prepared and balanced. Fiber and nutrient density are especially important for kids experiencing insulin resistance. Fun, home-based activity options need to be provided to children as well as encouragement of sporting activities. Parental limits on media time will naturally facilitate more activity as well.

When families of overweight children need additional support, the answer may lie within family-based treatment programs in a hospital, clinic, recreation center, or school. Those that are most successful are behavioral-based healthy eating and exercise programs. Popular programs that can improve fitness and health while halting weight gain or promoting weight loss, among others, are the CATCH program (Child and Adolescent Trial for Cardiovascular Health), LEAP (Lifestyle Education for Activity Program), Project Spark (Sports, Play and Active Recreation for Kids) and Shapedown, a treatment program from the University of California.

Bariatric surgery is sometimes used to treat very obese youth. Teens can lose weight after bariatric surgery; however, many questions exist about the long-term effects on their developing bodies and minds. Doctors suggest that, as with adults, families consider surgery for their teens only after they have tried for 6 months to lose weight and were unsuccessful. Candidates must meet three criteria: have extreme obesity with a BMI >40; have reached their adult height (age 13 or older for girls and age 15 or older for boys); and have serious health problems linked to weight (type 2 diabetes or sleep apnea, for example). Doctors also need to assess the candidate's emotional stability and his or her willingness to follow through with lifestyle changes. Gastric bypass surgery is the main operation used. Adjusted gastric banding has not been approved in those under age 18 in the United States.

To reverse nationwide obesity will require a long-term effort where many entities work together for the greater good. Individuals, families, communities, schools, businesses, government, and other groups will be needed to turn the tide. How we handle this health crisis will be this generation's defining moment. The stakes are high, as this epidemic will affect the health of generations to come. Policy change is needed to strengthen the ability to make healthy decisions and remove obstacles for change, especially for those whose options have been limited.

The Let's Move Initiative spearheaded by First Lady Michelle Obama, has put the childhood obesity issue on the forefront. This initiative is bringing together public officials, the food industry, advocacy groups, and others to join forces to save our youth (Figure 16-10).

On the Let's Move website (http://www.letsmove.gov), families can access information on how to eat healthy and get active. There is information for health professionals, elected officials, schools, chefs, children, parents, and community leaders to change the culture of health in our nation. Citizens are encouraged to sign the pledge for a healthier country and take part in the Let's Move movement across the United States.

The private sector, as well, is adding momentum to the fight against child obesity. The "LiVe" campaign, for example, is a public health media promotion developed by Intermountain Healthcare in Salt Lake City, Utah. The campaign promotes eight key health habits as its cornerstone (Figure 16-11). The eight habits have been thoroughly researched and provide remedy to the corresponding eight main contributors to childhood overweight (as discussed in Table 16-5). Three habits are about food, two are about activity, and three are about positive family support, which is highly critical in the overweight population.

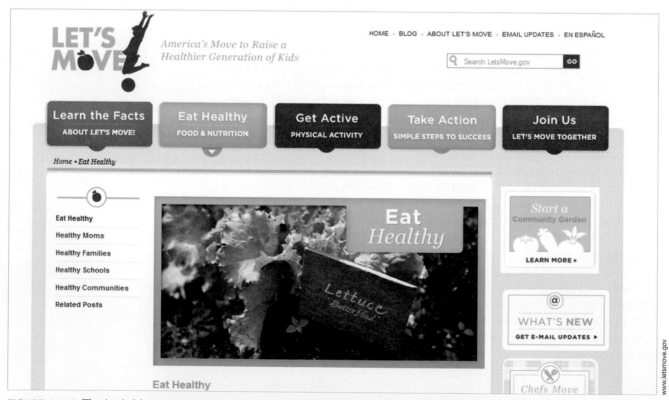

FIGURE 16-10 The Let's Move campaign strives to promote a healthier generation of children.

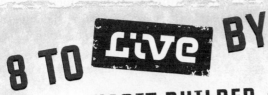

HABIT BUILDER for Kids, Teens, and Families

To reach and keep a healthy weight, build better habits together. The 8 habits prescribed below are the best place to start. Scientific studies show that these have the biggest impact on your weight, your health, and your outlook.

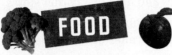

1 Always eat breakfast—and make it healthy

- Eating a healthy breakfast can improve your memory, boost your creativity, raise your test scores—and help you reach and keep a healthy weight.

- Aim for breakfasts that **include 3 of the 5 main food groups**. Try combos such as: (cereal + milk + juice) or (eggs + toast + milk) or (fruit + yogurt + bagel).

2 Eat more fruits and vegetables

- Fruits and vegetables are full of nutrients that help you learn and grow, prevent disease, and keep up your energy and mood. Studies show that they're important for a healthy body weight, too.

- Every day, aim to get **1 to 2 cups of fruit**, and **1½ to 3 cups of vegetables**.

3 Limit—or eliminate—sweetened drinks

- Studies suggest that America's weight problem is linked to America's "drinking problem"—that is, to our increasing intake of sweetened drinks like sodas and sports drinks. Sweetened drinks are also linked to weak bones and tooth decay.

- Aim for **less than 12 ounces per week** of soda, sports drinks, lemonade, and other sweetened drinks. Limit juice to less than 6 ounces per day. Drink water instead, and aim for 3 glasses of milk each day.

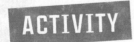

4 Limit screen time (TV, video games, Internet)

- Research links TV to a wide range of negative health effects in children and teens—including obesity.

- Make a rule of **no more than 1 to 2 hours a day** in front of a TV or computer screen. (Children age 2 and under shouldn't be watching at all.)

5 Increase your physical activity

- Everyone needs regular physical activity—regardless of their shape, size, health, or age. Physical activity gives you better energy, stronger muscles, less stress, and easier weight management.

- Aim for **at least 60 minutes of physical activity** every day. You can get most of this from daily playtime, walking or biking to school, or family activities. The rest can come from sports or other exercise.

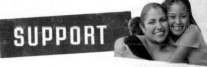

6 Eat meals together as a family—sitting down

- Many studies have shown that children and teens who eat regular meals with their parents are more likely to eat in a balanced way, do well in school, and maintain a healthy weight.

- Aim to **eat dinner together** most nights of the week. Sit down at the table, turn the TV off, and enjoy!

7 Be positive about food

- Experts agree that how you think and talk about food and bodies can have a big impact on your health now—and in the future.

- Forget "forbidden foods"—all foods can fit in a balanced diet. Don't give food as a reward or withhold it as a punishment. **Be food-friendly**, not food-phobic.

8 Don't criticize about weight

- If you, your friends, or your family obsess about food or weight, you're more likely to have unhealthy behaviors—and an unhealthy body weight.

- Watch what you say. **Don't criticize** your own body—even as a joke. **Don't compare** your own weight, size, or shape to anyone else's. Being healthy means being positive.

FIGURE 16-11 Eight key healthy habits from the LiVe campaign.

(Source: Intermountain Health Care. *Primary Care Guide to Weight Management in Children and Adolescents.* 2007 [updated 2010]. www.intermountainhealthcare.org)

The momentum is spreading to prevent and reduce obesity for the sake of America's health. Carrying this forward will be the challenge, as it will require increased and sustained efforts nationwide. The Robert Wood Johnson Foundation has the challenging but admirable goal of reversing childhood obesity by 2015. Through their vision and influence on both private and public sectors, they are leading efforts to:

- Ensure that all food and beverages served in school meet or exceed the 2010 Dietary Guidelines for Americans
- Increase access to high-quality and affordable food through new or improved grocery stores and healthier corner stores
- Increase the time, intensity, and duration of physical activity during the school day and in after-school programs
- Increase physical activity by improving the **built environment** in communities
- Using pricing strategies (incentives and disincentives) to promote the purchase of healthier food
- Reduce youth's exposure to the marketing of unhealthy foods through regulation policy and effective industry self-regulation

built environment
man-made resources and infrastructure designed to support health and activity (e.g., parks, walking and bike paths, access to healthy foods)

There are a multitude of health resources for clients who want to journey toward health and a better weight. Government websites such as the Weight Information Network, the CDC, and Let's Move are just a few of the many scientifically sound Web-based resources. Healthy eating tips and recipes and physical fitness information abound in our culture via TV shows and media, magazines, books, the Internet, medical literature, among others. There are online calorie and exercise calculators and counters, smart phone apps, and computerized fitness gear that can assist anyone's health pursuits. Check out the Alliance for a Healthier Generation (http://www.healthiergeneration.org) and the Action for Healthy Kids (http://www.actionforhealthykids.org) if you want to become involved.

UNDERWEIGHT

Although staying lean may be advantageous, being truly underweight could have its risks as well. Underweight status may be the result of a medical condition and/or compromised nutrition intake. Underweight is seen in anorexia, depression, and in those with cancer and a variety of other conditions. It can be the result of tissue wasting, poor absorption of nutrients, infection, excessive activity, or **hyperthyroidism**. Those who are underweight may have weaker immune systems. They may have lower muscle mass, compromised bone status, and substandard nutrition stores.

hyperthyroidism
condition in which the thyroid gland secretes too much thyroxine and T3 resulting in an unusually high metabolism

Adults with a BMI of ≤18.5 are considered underweight. Children who are at or below the 5th percentile on the BMI chart are considered underweight. In children, the inability to gain weight may be a condition called failure to thrive, which is referenced in chapter 12. This may be caused by an illness, or issues related to swallowing and digestion, lack of feeding support, or an imbalanced diet. Genetics can play a factor in underweight, but so can the environment.

Underweight is treated by a high-calorie diet. If the goal is to gain 1 pound per week, then 500 extra calories a day must be eaten. Often those who need to gain weight must begin slowly, and eat a bit more with every meal and snack. Some clients need an extra vitamin or mineral supplement if they are not absorbing their food well, or if they have food intolerances.

The foods not recommended on a high-calorie diet would be ones that add too much bulk, fiber, or water content to the diet, thereby filling up the individual without providing a high amount of energy. Items to limit when desiring a high-calorie diet would be salads, broth-based soups, raw vegetables, ultra-high-fiber cereals, and light or diet products made with artificial sweeteners. A high consumption of water would also be filling, especially just prior to a meal.

Tips that help with underweight include:

- Eat frequently (five or six small meals per day) to avoid feeling full.
- Eat foods that are dense in nutrients and calories (e.g., nuts, seeds, dried fruit, egg, avocado, yogurt). Limit heavy amounts of sugar or unhealthy fats.
- Add healthy fat to food in cooking such as olive or canola oil or mayonnaise. Butter, whole milk, and cheese have higher amounts of saturated fats and may need to be used with a little more discretion in those with cholesterol concerns.
- Pack foods to eat when away from home so there are no gaps in eating if a restaurant is not convenient.
- Check out high-calorie snack recipes to make at home such as milk shakes and puddings and dense foods such as a homemade peanut butter granola bar.
- Consider supplement drinks to boost calories as needed.
- Encourage parents of underweight children to provide support, but not threaten, bribe, or force-feed their child, as their child will engage in the opposite behavior and back away from the food.
- Fully investigate the root cause of the underweight status.
- Consult a doctor or dietitian for a full evaluation and treatment plan.

HEALTH AND NUTRITION CONSIDERATIONS

Weight regulation is complex and governed by many factors. Often multiple attempts at weight loss occur before success happens. What works for one individual may not work for another. A permanent lifestyle change is required whereby clients change their mindset about healthy eating and movement throughout their environment. If a lapse occurs, individuals need to learn how to spot it and set in motion new behaviors to get back on track. A state of readiness needs to be present for clients to begin to change. Positive weight management resources, based on current science and "best practices," need to be available to clients. The health care provider can support clients to help them voice realistic changes, to attain better health and weight. As a health care provider, support and encouragement can help pave the way for change.

SUMMARY

Genetics, the environment, and lifestyle factors all affect weight. We are all engineered to be good food regulators, but some respond more to external influences and begin to overeat. Nationally, we have an obesity crisis on our hands and it is causing serious health consequences. Children who are overweight tend to become overweight adults. Altered food intake and decreased physical activity are to blame. Americans go on and off various diets at an alarming rate to reduce, when a long-term view of health is what contributes to a normal weight. Realistic and dedicated changes in eating and exercise can be the winning ticket with weight control. Our nation is pulling together to start policy change that will affect adults and children in a positive way. Community groups, health care providers, schools, among others are forming the web of change to get adults and children in our nation healthy again. Health care providers play key roles in helping individuals of every shape and size to lead healthier lives.

DISCUSSION TOPICS

1. Discuss ways to determine body mass index. Note BMI ranges for underweight, overweight, and obesity, including the stages of obesity, in adults. How would you assess BMI in children and determine if they are underweight, overweight, or obese?

2. What is the value in knowing waist circumference and how is it related to disease risk? Discuss the health consequences of obesity.

3. Discuss criteria used for assessing whether children need weight maintenance or weight loss.

4. How might an overweight athlete be in better shape and healthier than a sedentary person at normal weight?

5. Describe a balanced eating approach for weight loss and compare this to a fad diet. Which is sustainable? What might be the consequences of a fad diet?

6. Name three food changes and three behavior changes an individual could make to help begin weight loss. Why is it important to have a long-term view of healthful weight maintenance?

7. Describe at least three positive benefits of physical activity. Why is it important to record exercise in a log? What might be some types of exercise suited for persons with mobility problems? Who would they go to for guidance and advice?

8. Why might individuals be underweight? Name ways they could change their diet to gain weight.

SUGGESTED ACTIVITIES

1. Do a 3-day food record on yourself, making sure one of the day's intake is on a weekend. Use the SuperTracker (http://www .choosemyplate.gov) to analyze your intake. Critique your eating based on MyPlate. If you needed to trim your eating for weight loss, what would you change?

2. The doctor you work for wants you to suggest to a client a weight management class taught by the office dietitian. Role-play this discussion with a fellow student. Begin with an assessment of the client's feelings, such as "How do you feel about your health and weight?" Be positive and supportive as you describe the weight management class and the referral. What happens if you hear resistance?

REVIEW

1. The complication rates for bariatric surgery
   a. have gone down from 40% to 30%
   b. are unchanged
   c. are less than 3%
   d. have gone down to 15%

2. If one or both parents are overweight or obese, an overweight child has a _____ chance that this will follow him or her into adulthood.
   a. 50%
   b. 25%
   c. 80%
   d. 70%

   C

3. In studies, contributors to overweight and obesity in children include
   a. eating an evening snack
   b. not making the sports team at school
   c. skipping breakfast, drinking pop, and overdoing media time
   d. underperforming in school

   C

4. A 13-year-old obese child with high blood pressure should
   a. maintain current weight and not gain any more
   b. lose 1–2 pounds per week
   c. lose 2–4 pounds per month
   d. engage in very slow weight loss of 1 pound per month

   B

5. If a man has a waist circumference of 42 inches and he has stage II obesity, what is he at increased risk of having, and what is his risk level?
   a. high level of risk for diabetes only
   b. increased risk for cardiovascular disease, hypertension, and/or diabetes
   c. high level of risk for reflux
   d. very high risk for cardiovascular disease, hypertension, and/or diabetes

   D

6. Approved weight loss drugs that are sometimes used short term when obese clients are at increased medical risk are
   a. phentermine and diethylproprion
   b. fenfluramine and dexfenfluramine
   c. sibutramine (Meridia)
   d. none of the above, as all amphetamines are good to use

   A

7. Policy changes than can reduce obesity would be
   a. scheduling an exercise session with a fitness trainer
   b. calculating the calories daily from the foods eaten
   c. requiring local governments to plan neighborhoods with walking and bike paths and easy accessibility to healthy grocery stores and farmers markets
   d. shopping the perimeter of the grocery store

   C

8. If an underweight child's goal is to gain 1.5 pounds per week, how many extra calories would he need to consume daily?
   a. 500
   b. 750
   c. 250
   d. 1,000

   B

9. What is an external factor that can trigger eating?
   a. packing lunch for work every day
   b. walking by the donut shop and you see and smell the aroma of donuts
   c. feeling weak and light-headed when your stomach is growling
   d. consuming caffeine

   B

10. According to 2010 data, obesity continues to climb
    a. only in those who live in the South
    b. in teen boys and Hispanic women
    c. in the entire United States
    d. in children, minorities, and the poor

    D

11. Factors that could affect BMR include
    a. quantity of vitamin C containing foods eaten daily
    b. your age, size, and body composition
    c. whether there is a diagnosis of hypertension
    d. distance to the nearest gym

    B

12. When an individual wants to find reliable resources to help with weight loss, she should
    a. talk to a local health food store representative
    b. talk to a health care provider and check out literature from the Weight Control Information Network and Choose MyPlate
    c. talk to a friend who lost 100 pounds on a liquid diet
    d. decrease her calories to no more than 1,000 per day

    B

Case In Point

RIDA: GAINING WEIGHT IN RETIREMENT

Rida had been a fifth-grade teacher for 38 years and just retired this past school year. She and her husband have two daughters who are grown and married, so it is just the two of them at home. Rida had always packed her lunch through the years when she was working. She usually spent many of her evenings grading papers and preparing lesson plans. She and her husband would usually eat a light supper in the evening so she wouldn't have to spend a lot of time cooking. Now at age 63, Rida is enjoying her new lifestyle and less-stressful routine. She finally has time for some hobbies and crafts. She has always loved to cook and bake, but never had quite enough time to enjoy that, either.

Since her retirement, Rida has been trying many new recipes. She enjoys cooking "fancier" meals for her husband now, including rich desserts.

In addition, Rida has been catching up with old friends. Many of the teachers she worked with through the years are also retired. Twice a week they meet for lunch to catch up and enjoy each other's company. Although she's enjoying her retirement, Rida gained 7 pounds almost immediately but she felt the weight gain was worth it and was no cause for worry. But after 4 months, Rida's weight was up 16 pounds. Then she decided it was time to make some changes.

ASSESSMENT

1. What information do you have about Rida's activity and eating habits before her retirement?
2. How did Rida's habits change after she retired?
3. How has the change affected her?
4. How long should Rida expect to take to lose the 16 pounds she gained?

DIAGNOSIS

5. Write a diagnosis for Rida's alteration in nutrition.
6. Write a diagnosis for Rida's activity level change.

PLAN/GOAL

7. What is a reasonable, measurable goal for Rida's weight loss?

IMPLEMENTATION

8. List some strategies that match Rida's new priorities.
9. What can her husband and friends do to help her lose weight?
10. How can she enjoy her new routine without gaining weight?

EVALUATION/OUTCOME CRITERIA

11. What criteria would Rida use to determine the success of the plan?

THINKING FURTHER

12. How can she maintain weight control for the rest of her life?
13. How can websites such as SparkPeople.com be helpful to Rida?

rate this **plate**

Rida has been enjoying retirement by visiting with friends over lunch a few times a week. Since her recent weight gain, Rida has decided to pay closer attention to the meals she orders while out with her friends. Rate this plate:

2 cups orange chicken stir-fry with broccoli, snow peas, and carrots

1 cup steamed white rice

1 garlic breadstick

12 oz. sweet iced tea

What questions could Rida ask the server before ordering the meal? What decisions could Rida make to improve the nutritional quality of her meal? What suggestions would you give Rida when choosing to eat out with friends?

Case In Point

BELLA: STAYING HEALTHY FOLLOWING GASTRIC BYPASS SURGERY

Bella has been overweight most of her life. She never thought much about it because her parents were both overweight as well. She is currently 5 feet 3 inches tall, 287 pounds, and 58 years old. Most of her life her weight has fluctuated between 200 and 220 pounds, but began gaining more weight after menopause. Bella's family immigrated from Italy, and she has always maintained a taste for the authentic Italian foods she grew up eating. She remembers her mother saying on more than one occasion, "When there is a problem, a great Italian meal is the answer!" Bella's diet has always included many varieties of pasta. Her favorite recipes are prepared with creamy alfredo or wine and butter sauce. She loved the richness of her mother's soups when she prepared them with cream as well. Bella enjoys vegetables, but prefers them in a cheese sauce. To truly complete an Italian meal, says her mother, you always need a good decadent dessert. Ice cream and sorbets have been Bella's favorites since childhood. Bella has tried different diets through the years in an attempt to lose weight, but unsuccessfully. She seems to regain the weight she lost and a little extra as soon as she stops dieting.

Bella has noticed recently some swelling in her legs. She also seems to be having headaches on a regular basis. Her physician requests she have some blood work completed before seeing him. At her appointment, her doctor informs her that her blood pressure is 212/102. Her total cholesterol is 347 with an LDL of 200 and HDL of 26. Her fasting glucose level is 114 mg/dl as well. Her doctor is very concerned. He prescribes both blood pressure and cholesterol reduction medications. In addition, he informs her that her blood sugar level is considered to be in the range of pre-diabetes. He states that she must lose weight to improve all of her conditions. Bella asks her doctor about gastric bypass surgery. He emphasizes the changes she would need to make to even be a candidate for the surgery.

Bella underwent gastric bypass surgery 6 months later. Bella has been under the supervision of her physician, surgeon, and dietitian during this time. Only after Bella met the presurgical requirements and was deemed safe for the surgery, could it be performed. Bella's daughter was her health coach postoperatively. She assisted Bella throughout the presurgical time as well. Bella and her daughter attended classes on eating healthy, weight loss, exercise, and behavior modification. Bella felt confident her surgery would improve her health and the quality of her life.

ASSESSMENT

1. What do you know about Bella?
2. What was her new priority?
3. What is her ideal weight?
4. How many pounds does she need to lose to be at the high end of her ideal body weight?
5. How long should it take to be done safely without the assistance of gastric bypass?
6. What is her current BMI and what are her risks for health problems on the basis of her BMI?
7. What are her known health problems?
8. At what weight will her health risk be reasonable?
9. How long will it take to reach that reasonable health-risk weight?

DIAGNOSIS

10. Write a complete nursing diagnostic statement for Bella's nutrition problem.
11. Write a diagnosis for her activity intolerance.

PLAN/GOAL

12. Write at least three goals for Bella that are reasonable and measurable.

IMPLEMENTATION

13. What class of obesity was Bella in when she weighed 287 pounds?
14. How much weight would Bella need to lose to move from category III obesity to the overweight category?
15. What topics are essential in Bella's nutrition classes?
16. Use the food items Bella liked to eat and list low-calorie, low-fat alternatives.
17. What are some behavior modification hints or tips related to where and when she eats that would help her?
18. Bella was instructed to turn in her home scale to the doctor's office and to see him every Friday

morning to weigh in and have her blood pressure checked. What is the rationale for these directions?

19. How would the obesity information on the National Heart Lung and Blood Institute's website (http://www.nhlbi.nih.gov) be helpful to Bella?

EVALUATION/OUTCOME CRITERIA

20. What changes should the doctor see, hear, and be able to measure that are indicative of success?

THINKING FURTHER

21. Why is it important for Bella to persevere at weight reduction?

22. What are some of the serious potential complications of this surgery?

rate this plate

After surgery, Bella allowed her stomach to start to heal by only consuming liquids and semisolid foods. She transitioned from semisolids to soft solid foods after a few weeks and by 8 weeks was ready to try solid foods. Four months after gastric bypass surgery, Bella returns to a normal, healthy diet following the advice of her health care team. She continues to meet with a registered dietitian to assist in planning her meals. Rate this plate:

2 oz. pork tenderloin

¼ cup sweet potatoes

¼ cup pears

¼ cup cottage cheese

6 oz. water

Does this meal meet the recommendations for diet after gastric bypass surgery? If not, what can be improved?

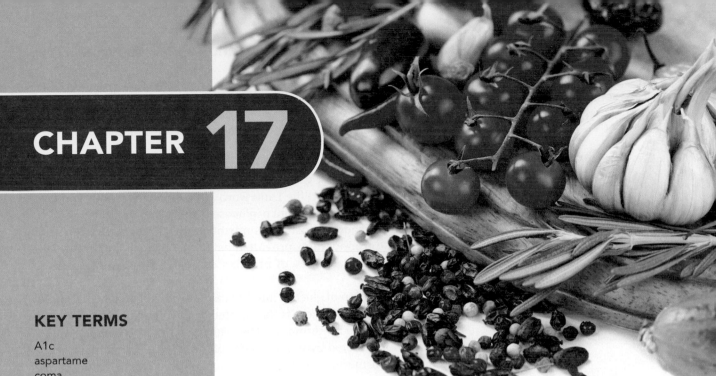

CHAPTER 17

KEY TERMS

A1c
aspartame
coma
diabetes mellitus
dyslipidemia
endogenous insulin
exchange lists
exogenous insulin
glycosuria
insulin reaction
ketoacidosis
ketonemia
ketonuria
nephropathy
neuropathy
oral diabetes medication
polydipsia
polyphagia
polyuria
renal threshold
retinopathy
sucralose
type 1 diabetes
type 2 diabetes
vascular system

DIET AND DIABETES MELLITUS

OBJECTIVES

After studying this chapter, you should be able to:

- Describe diabetes mellitus and identify the types
- Describe the symptoms of diabetes mellitus
- Explain the relationship of insulin to diabetes mellitus
- Discuss appropriate nutritional management of diabetes mellitus

Diabetes mellitus is the name for a group of serious and chronic (long-standing) disorders affecting the metabolism of carbohydrates. These disorders are characterized by hyperglycemia (abnormally large amounts of glucose in the blood). Diabetes insipidus is a different disorder. It also generates large amounts of urine, but it is "insipid," not sweet. This is a rare condition, caused by a damaged pituitary gland. It is not discussed in this chapter.

According to the American Diabetes Association (ADA), 25.8 million people in the United States have diabetes. An estimated 18.8 million people have been diagnosed with the disease, with 7 million more going undiagnosed.

diabetes mellitus
chronic disease in which the body lacks
the normal ability to metabolize glucose

There are approximately 79 million people with pre-diabetes, and 1.9 million new cases of diabetes in people aged 20 years and older diagnosed in 2010. It is a major cause of blindness; heart and kidney disease; amputations of toes, feet, and legs; infections; and death.

Hundreds of years ago, a Greek physician named the condition *diabetes*, which means "to flow through," because of the large amounts of urine generated by clients. Later, the Latin word *mellitus*, which means "honey," was added because of the amount of glucose in the urine.

The body needs a constant supply of energy, and glucose is its primary source. Carbohydrates provide most of the glucose, but about 10% of fats and up to nearly 60% of proteins can be converted to glucose if necessary.

The distribution of glucose must be carefully managed for the maintenance of good health. Glucose is transported by the blood, and its entry into the cells is controlled by hormones. The primary hormone is insulin.

Insulin is secreted by the beta cells of the islets of Langerhans in the pancreas. When there is inadequate production of insulin or the body is unable to use the insulin it produces, glucose cannot enter the cells and it accumulates in the blood, creating hyperglycemia. This condition can cause serious complications.

Another hormone, glucagon, which is secreted by the alpha cells of the islets of Langerhans, helps release energy when needed by converting glycogen to glucose. Somatostatin is a hormone produced by the delta cells of the islets of Langerhans and the hypothalamus. All actions of this hormone are inhibitory. It inhibits the release of insulin and glucagons.

The amount of glucose in the blood normally rises after a meal. The pancreas reacts by providing insulin. As the insulin circulates in the blood, it binds to special insulin receptors on cell surfaces. This binding causes the cells to accept the glucose. The resulting reduced amount of glucose in the blood in turn signals the pancreas to stop sending insulin.

ETIOLOGY

The etiology (cause) of diabetes is not confirmed. Although it appears that diabetes may be genetic, environmental factors also may contribute to its occurrence. For example, viruses or obesity may precipitate the disease in people who have a genetic predisposition.

The World Health Organization indicates that the prevalence of the disease is increasing worldwide, especially in areas showing improvement in living standards.

renal threshold
kidneys' capacity

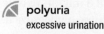

glycosuria
excess sugar in the urine

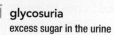

polyuria
excessive urination

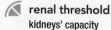

polydipsia
abnormal thirst

SYMPTOMS

The abnormal concentration of glucose in the blood of clients with diabetes draws water from the cells to the blood. When hyperglycemia exceeds the **renal threshold**, the glucose is excreted in the urine, a process known as **glycosuria**. With the loss of the cellular fluid, the client experiences **polyuria** (excessive urination), and **polydipsia** (excessive thirst) typically results.

The inability to metabolize glucose causes the body to break down its own tissue for protein and fat. This response causes **polyphagia** (excessive appetite), but at the same time a loss of weight, weakness, and fatigue occur. The body's use of protein from its own tissue causes it to excrete nitrogen.

The untreated client with diabetes cannot use carbohydrates for energy so, therefore, excessive amounts of fats are broken down, and consequently the liver produces ketones from the fatty acids. In healthy people, ketones are subsequently broken down to carbon dioxide and water, yielding energy. In clients with diabetes, fats break down faster than the body can handle. Ketone collection in the blood is known as **ketonemia**. Excretion of ketones in the urine, a necessary process, is known as **ketonuria**. Ketones are acids that lower blood pH, causing acidosis. Acidosis, caused by ketones, is known as **ketoacidosis**. Ketoacidosis can lead to loss of consciousness, which can result in death if the client is not treated quickly with fluids and insulin.

In addition to the symptoms previously mentioned, clients with diabetes are more likely to suffer from diseases of the **vascular system** such as hypertension and atherosclerosis. Atherosclerosis is a condition in which there is a buildup of fatty substances inside artery walls. This can reduce blood flow and is a major cause of death among clients with diabetes. **Neuropathy**, damage to the nervous system, occurs in 60–70% of clients with diabetes. Damage to the small blood vessels in the eye is known as **retinopathy**. Retinopathy is the leading cause of blindness in the United States. **Nephropathy**, damage to the kidneys, is also a complication of diabetes. Nephropathy is the number one cause of the need for kidney dialysis. It is also common for clients with diabetes to suffer from frequent infections such as urinary tract infections.

 polyphagia
excess hunger

ketonemia
ketones collected in the blood

ketonuria
ketone bodies in the urine

ketoacidosis
unconsciousness caused by a state of acidosis due to too much sugar or too little insulin

vascular system
circulatory system

neuropathy
nerve damage

retinopathy
damage to small blood vessels in the eyes

nephropathy
damage to the kidneys

DIABETES CLASSIFICATION

The types of diabetes are pre-diabetes, type 1, type 2, and gestational. Pre-diabetes, or impaired glucose tolerance, means that the cells in the body are not using insulin properly. The diagnosis is made by a fasting blood glucose, which is more than 100 mg/dl but less than 126 mg/dl. One's lifestyle will determine if pre-diabetes will advance to type 1.

Type 1 Diabetes

Type 1 diabetes, also known as juvenile diabetes, develops when the body's immune system destroys the pancreatic beta cells. These are the only cells in the body that make the hormone insulin that regulates blood glucose. Type 1 diabetes is usually diagnosed in children and young adults. It accounts for 5–10% of all cases of newly diagnosed diabetes. Some risk factors include genetics, autoimmune status, and environmental factors. Clients with type 1 diabetes must use exogenous insulin to survive. There are a variety of insulins that can be used to maintain control of blood sugars. Insulins vary in their actions. They differ in onset, peak, and duration of their effectiveness. Table 17-1 identifies the different insulins and their actions.

type 1 diabetes
diabetes occurring suddenly between the ages of 1 and 40; clients secrete little, if any, insulin and require insulin injections and a carefully controlled diet

TABLE 17-1 Insulin Actions

RAPID-ACTING	ONSET	PEAK	DURATION
Lispro (Humalog)	10–15 minutes	30–90 minutes	2–4 hours
Aspart (Novolog)	10–15 minutes	30–90 minutes	2–4 hours
Glulisine (Apidra)	10–15 minutes	30–90 minutes	3–5 hours
Short Acting			
Regular	30 minutes	2–4 hours	6–8 hours
Intermediate Acting			
NPH	1–2 hours	6–12 hours	16–24 hours
Long Acting			
Detemir (Levemir)	1–2 hours	Minimal	24 hours
Glargine (Lantus)	1–2 hours	Minimal	24 hours
Premixed			

Humulin or Novolin 70/30: follows the actions of both regular and NPH insulins
Novolog 70/30: follows the actions of both Novolog and NPH
Humalog 75/25: follows the actions of both Humalog and NPH
Humulin 50/50: follows the actions of both regular and NPH

© Cengage Learning 2014

Type 2 Diabetes

type 2 diabetes
diabetes occurring usually after age 40; onset is gradual and production of insulin gradually diminishes; can usually be controlled by diet and exercise

Type 2 diabetes was previously called adult-onset diabetes because it usually occurred in adults over the age of 40. Type 2 is associated with obesity, and obesity has become an epidemic, which has drastically increased the incidence of type 2 diabetes among adolescents and young adults. A family history of diabetes, prior history of gestational diabetes, impaired glucose tolerance, older age, physical inactivity, and race and ethnicity can predispose one to type 2 diabetes. African Americans, Hispanic and Latino Americans, Native Americans, some Asian Americans, and Native Hawaiians and other Pacific Islanders are at particularly high risk for type 2 diabetes. It is not uncommon for the client to have no symptoms of diabetes and to be totally ignorant of his or her condition until it is discovered accidentally during a routine urine or blood test or after a complication is discovered. In type 2 diabetes, hypertension may be present as part of the metabolic syndrome (i.e., obesity, hyperglycemia, and **dyslipidemia**) that is accompanied by high rates of cardiovascular disease. The American Diabetes Association recommends that blood pressure be controlled at <130/80 mm Hg for diabetics.

dyslipidemia
increased lipid in the blood

oral diabetes medication
oral hypoglycemic agent; medication that may be given to type 2 diabetes to lower blood glucose

Type 2 diabetes can usually be controlled by diet and exercise, or by diet, exercise, and an **oral diabetes medication**. Table 17-2 shows types of oral glucose-lowering medications. The goals of medical nutrition therapy for clients with type 2 diabetes include maintaining healthy glucose, blood pressure, and lipid levels. Also, because approximately 80% of type 2 clients are overweight, these clients may be placed on weight reduction diets to help achieve blood glucose levels that are within acceptable range. Thus, monitoring their weight loss also becomes part of their therapy.

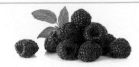

TABLE 17-2	Types of Oral Diabetes (Glucose-Lowering) Medications
Meglitinide	• Repaglinide (Prandin)
D-Phenylalanines	• Nateglinide (Starlix)
Thiazolidinedione	• Pioglitazone (Actos)
	• Rosiglitazone (Avandia)
Combination drugs	• Glyburide and metformin (Glucovance)
	• Glipizide and metformin (Metaglip)
	• Glyburide and metformin (Avandamet)
	• Pioglitazone and metformin (ACTOplus Met)
	• Rosiglitazon and glimiperide (Avandaryl)
	• Pioglitazone and glimiperide (Duetact)
	• Sitagliptin and metformin (Janumet)
	• Rapaglinide and metformin (PrandiMet)
	• Linigliptin and metformin (Jentadueto)
Nonsulfonylurea	• Metformin (Glucophage)
	• Melformin and a time-released controlling polymer (Glucophage XR)
Alpha-glucosidase inhibitor	• Acarbose (Precose)
	• Miglitol (Glycet)
Second-generation sulfonylureas	• Glyburide (DiaBeta, Micronase, Glynase Prestabs)
	• Glipizide (Glucotrol, Glucotrol XL)
	• Glimepride (Amaryl)
Class-bile acid sequestrants (primarily used to decrease cholesterol but also improves blood sugar control)	• Colesevelam (Welchol)
DPP-4 Inhibitors	• Sitagliptin (Januvia)
	• Saxagliptin (Onglyza)
	• Linagliptin (Tradjenta)

© Cengage Learning 2014

Noninsulin Injectable Medications

There is a new class of injectable medications used to improve blood sugar control, called incretin mimetics. The two incretin mimetics on the market are exenatide (Byetta) and liraglutide (Victoza). Incretin mimetics are injected the same as insulin, but they are not insulins. Another noninsulin injectable antihyperglycemic medication is pramlintide (Symlin). It is used in clients with type 1 diabetes. It works to lower blood sugars by assisting insulin injected at meals to lower postmeal blood sugar levels. It also suppresses postmeal glucagon release, slows gastric emptying, and decreases appetite.

When food is eaten, incretin hormones are released from cells located in the small intestine. In the pancreas, incretins will act on the beta cells to increase glucose-dependent insulin secretions to ensure an appropriate insulin response after a meal. This medication can be used in conjunction

In The Media

Paula Deen

Recently Food Network star Paula Deen announced that she had been diagnosed with type 2 diabetes. Paula is famous for her homestyle and southern cooking. She has been criticized by some, stating that her high-fat, high-carbohydrate, and high-calorie foods led her to develop her diabetes. Paula was quick to remind people that they are ultimately responsible for what they eat and that more than diet determines whether or not a person will develop diabetes. After being diagnosed, Paula wanted to develop a webpage that would assist clients with diabetes. She wanted to include educational information and suggestions on ways to make modifications to her recipes that would decrease the number of calories, refined and processed sugars, salt, and fat content. Paula's informational webpage is titled "Diabetes in a New Light" (http://www.diabetesinanewlight.com).

(Source: Adapted from *Paula Deen Announces She Has Type 2 Diabetes, Cooking Not to Blame.* ICTMN Staff. Indian Country: Today Media Network. January 17, 2012.)

SPOTLIGHT *on Life Cycle*

Years ago doctors were telling people with type 1 diabetes they couldn't compete in sporting events, but today there are many resources that make exercising with type 1 possible. Team Type 1 is a group of young cyclists that travel around the world racing in competitions, bringing hope and inspiration to those with diabetes. The team was cofounded in 2005 by two competitive bike racers that shared more than just cycling in common—they both had type 1 diabetes. In 2006, the team rode the 3,000-mile Race Across America, winning the eight-person division. Team Type 1 has expanded over the years to include Team Type 2, an eight-man team of type 2 athletes. Today, cyclists and athletes can manage their glucose levels by using small insulin pumps.

(Source: Adapted from Curry, Andrew. Team Type 1: Serious Competition. *Diabetes Forecast Magazine.* September 2009. www.forecast.diabetes.org)

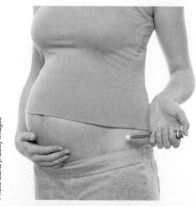

FIGURE 17-1 A pregnant woman can develop diabetes during her pregnancy that may need to be managed by insulin injections.

 A1c
a blood test to determine how well blood glucose has been controlled for the last 3 months

with oral medications to help clients lower their A1c to less than 7%. **A1c** is a blood test to determine how well blood glucose has been controlled for the last 3 months. The American Diabetes Association prefers the outcome to be less than 7% for a client with diabetes. The American College of Endocrinology has a target of less than 6.5% for clients with diabetes.

Gestational Diabetes

Gestational diabetes can occur in pregnancy between weeks 16 and 28. If it is not responsive to diet and exercise, insulin injection therapy will be used (Figure 17-1). It is recommended that a dietitian or a diabetic educator be consulted to plan an adequate diet that will control blood sugar for mother and baby.

Concentrated sugars should be avoided. Weight gain should continue, but not in excessive amounts. Usually, gestational diabetes disappears after the infant is born. Women who have gestational diabetes have a 35–60% chance of developing type 2 diabetes in the next 10–20 years.

Secondary diabetes occurs infrequently and is caused by certain drugs or by a disease of the pancreas. For example, steroid medications can increase blood sugars and a client can develop steroid-induced diabetes.

TREATMENT

The treatment of diabetes is intended to do the following:

1. Control blood glucose levels
2. Provide optimal nourishment for the client
3. Prevent symptoms and thus delay the complications of the disease

Treatment is typically begun when blood tests indicate hyperglycemia, impaired glucose tolerance, or when other previously discussed symptoms occur. Normal blood glucose levels (called fasting blood sugar, or FBS) range from 70–100 mg/dl.

Treatment can be by diet alone or by a diet combined with insulin or an oral glucose-lowering medication plus regulated exercise and the regular monitoring of the client's blood glucose levels.

The physician and dietitian can provide essential information and counseling and can help the client prevent complications. The ultimate responsibility, however, rests with the client. When a person with diabetes uses nicotine, eats carelessly, forgets insulin, ignores symptoms, and neglects appropriate blood tests, he or she increases the risk of developing permanent complications.

NUTRITIONAL MANAGEMENT

The dietitian will need to know the client's diet history, food likes and dislikes, and lifestyle at the onset. The client's calorie needs will depend on age, activities, lean muscle mass, size, and resting energy expenditure.

It is recommended that carbohydrates provide 50–60% of the calories. Approximately 40–50% should be from complex carbohydrates (starches). The remaining 10–20% of carbohydrates could be from simple sugars.

Research provides no evidence that carbohydrates from simple sugars are digested and absorbed more rapidly than are complex carbohydrates, and they do not appear to affect blood sugar control. It is the *total amount of carbohydrates eaten* that affects blood sugar levels rather than the type. Being able to substitute foods containing sucrose for other carbohydrates increases flexibility in meal planning for the person with diabetes.

Fats should be limited to 30% or less of total calories, and proteins should provide from 15–20% of total calories. Lean proteins are advisable because they contain limited amounts of fats.

EXPLORING THE WEB

Search the Web for additional information on gestational diabetes. What are the presenting signs and symptoms of gestational diabetes? What are the dangers of gestational diabetes to the mother and to the fetus if left untreated? Are there factors that put certain women at a higher risk for developing gestational diabetes? If yes, what are these risks?

Supersize **USA**

To prevent supersizing yourself and your meal and increasing your blood sugar, try the following tips when eating out:

- Ask, ask, ask. Ask your waitress the serving size of the entrée and how it is prepared. Special requests and substitutions to the menu can be made.
- Try to eat the same portion size you would at home. If portions are large, ask for a take-home container to save part of the meal for later.
- Eat slowly and pay attention to what you are eating and savor the flavor.
- Ask for sauces, gravies, and dressings on the side.
- Avoid any breaded and/or deep fried food.
- Ask for fresh fruit instead of chocolate cake for dessert.
- Limit alcohol consumption since it provides no nutrients, only additional calories.

Regardless of the percentages of energy nutrients prescribed, the foods ultimately eaten should provide sufficient vitamins and minerals as well as energy nutrients.

The client with type 1 diabetes needs a nutritional plan that balances calories and nutrient needs with insulin therapy and exercise. It is important that meals and snacks be composed of similar nutrients and calories and eaten at regular times each day. Small meals plus two or three snacks may be more helpful in maintaining steady blood glucose levels for these clients than three large meals each day. Medications and insulin dosing can help determine the number and timing of meals.

The client with type 1 diabetes should anticipate the possibility of missing meals occasionally and carry a few crackers and some cheese or peanut butter to prevent hypoglycemia, which can occur in such a circumstance.

The client with type 2 diabetes may be overweight. The nutritional goal for this client is not only to keep blood glucose levels in the normal range but also to lose weight. Exercise can help attain both goals.

Carbohydrate Counting

Carbohydrate counting is the newest method for teaching a client with diabetes how to control blood sugar with food. The starch and bread category, milk, and fruits have all been put under the heading "carbohydrates." This means that these three food groups can be interchanged within one meal. One would still have the same number of servings of carbohydrates, but it would not be the typical number of starches or fruits and milk that one usually eats. For example, a person is to have four carbohydrates for breakfast (2 breads, 1 fruit, and 1 milk). If there is no milk available, a bread or fruit must be eaten in place of the milk. The exchange lists are utilized in carbohydrate counting as well as in traditional meal planning. Protein, approximately 3–4 oz, is eaten for lunch and dinner. No more than 1 or 2 fat exchanges are recommended

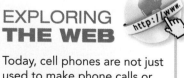

EXPLORING THE WEB

Today, cell phones are not just used to make phone calls or send messages. Smart phones are becoming more popular and there are numerous applications at our fingertips. Search the Web for nutrition, weight management, and meal tracker applications. What applications are available to assist clients with diabetes? How can these applications assist in diabetes management?

for each meal. Two carbohydrates and 1 oz of protein should be eaten for an evening snack. These are only beginning guidelines. A dietitian or diabetic educator can help tailor this to the individual client.

Diets Based on Exchange Lists

The method of diet therapy most commonly used for diabetic clients is based on **exchange lists**. These lists were developed by the American Diabetes Association in conjunction with the American Dietetic Association and are summarized in Table 17-3 and included completely in Appendix G.

exchange lists
lists of foods with interchangeable nutrient and calorie contents; used in specific forms of diet therapy

 TABLE 17-3 Summary of Exchange Lists

THE FOOD LISTS

The following chart shows the amount of nutrients in 1 serving from each list.

FOOD LIST	CARBOHYDRATE (GRAMS)	PROTEIN (GRAMS)	FAT (GRAMS)	CALORIES
Carbohydrates				
Starch: breads, cereals and grains, starchy and lentils vegetables, crackers, snacks, and beans, peas	15	0–3	0–1	80
Fruits	15	—	—	60
Milk				
Fat-free, low-fat, 1%	12	8	0–3	100
Reduced-fat, 2%	12	8	5	120
Whole	12	8	8	160
Sweets, desserts, and other carbohydrates	15	varies	varies	varies
Nonstarchy vegetables	5	2	—	25
Meat and Meat Substitutes				
Lean	—	7	0–3	45
Medium-fat	—	7	4–7	75
High-fat	—	7	8+	100
Plant-based proteins	varies	7	varies	varies
Fats	—	—	5	45
Alcohol	varies	—	—	100

Source: Reproduction of the Exchange Lists in whole or part, without permission of the American Dietetic Association or the American Diabetes Association, Inc., is a violation of federal law. This material has been modified from *Choose Your Foods: Exchange Lists for Diabetes,* which is the basis of a meal planning system designed by a committee of the American Diabetes Association and the American Dietetic Association. While designed primarily for people with diabetes and others who must follow special diets, the Exchange Lists are based on principles of good nutrition that apply to everyone. Copyright © 2008 by the American Diabetes Association and the American Dietetic Association. Academy of Nutrition and Dietetics (formerly the American Dietetic Association). Reproduced with permission.

Under this plan foods are categorized by type. The foods within each list contain approximately equal amounts of calories, carbohydrates, protein, and fats. This means that any one food on a particular list can be substituted for any other food on that *particular list* and still provide the client with the prescribed types and amounts of nutrients and calories.

The amounts of nutrients and calories on one list are not the same as those on any other list. Each list includes serving size by volume or weight and the calorie value of each food item, in addition to the grams of carbohydrates, and, when appropriate, proteins and fats. The number of calories a person needs will determine the number of items prescribed from any particular list. These lists also can be used to control calorie content of diets and are thus appropriate for low-calorie diets.

The total energy requirements for adult diabetic clients who are not overweight will be the same as for nondiabetic individuals. When clients are overweight, a reduction in calories will be built into the diet plans, typically allowing for a weight loss of 1 pound a week.

The diet is given in terms of exchanges rather than as particular foods. For example, the menu pattern for breakfast may include 1 fruit exchange, 1 meat exchange, 2 bread exchanges, and 2 fat exchanges. The client may choose the desired foods from the exchange lists for each meal but must adhere to the specific exchange lists named and the specific number of exchanges on each list. Vegetables (nonstarchy) are relatively free and can be eaten in amounts up to 1½ cups cooked or 3 cups raw. If more than this amount is eaten at one meal, count the additional amount as one more carbohydrate. Snacks are built into the plan. In this way, the client has variety in a simple yet controlled way.

When there are changes in one's physical condition, such as pregnancy or lactation, or in one's lifestyle, the diet will need to be modified. A change in job or in working hours can affect nutrient and calorie requirements. When such changes occur, the client should be advised to consult a physician or dietitian so that calorie and insulin needs can be promptly adjusted.

SPECIAL CONSIDERATIONS FOR THE CLIENT WITH DIABETES
Fiber

The therapeutic value of fiber in the diabetic diet has become increasingly evident. High-fiber intake appears to reduce the amount of insulin needed because it lowers blood glucose. It also appears to lower the blood cholesterol and triglyceride levels. "High fiber" may mean 25–35 grams of dietary fiber a day. Such high amounts can be difficult to include. High-fiber foods should be increased very gradually, as an abrupt increase can create intestinal gas and discomfort. When increasing fiber in the diet, one must also increase water intake. An increased fiber intake can affect mineral absorption. For clients dosing insulin based on the grams of carbohydrate they are consuming, a portion of fiber may be subtracted. When reading food labels, if the fiber content is greater than 5 grams, half the grams of fiber may be subtracted from the total carbohydrates for which the client is dosing.

Alternative Sweeteners

Sucralose is the newest sweetener to gain approval by the FDA. Sucralose is made from a sugar molecule that has been altered in such a way that the body will not absorb it. **Aspartame** is the generic name for a sweetener composed of two amino acids: phenylalanine and aspartic acid. The FDA removed the sweetener saccharine from its list of products that could cause cancer. Research indicates that all these sweeteners are safe. All have been approved by the FDA, and their use has been endorsed by the American Diabetes Association. Novel sweeteners, such as stevia (Truvia), are combination sweeteners. Truvia is a name brand product that contains highly refined stevia. The FDA does not approve whole-leaf stevia or crude stevia. However, the FDA does approve highly refined stevia preparations.

 sucralose
a sweetener made from a molecule of sugar

aspartame
artificial sweetener made from amino acids; does not require insulin for metabolism

Dietetic Foods

The use of diabetic or dietetic foods is generally a waste of money and can be misleading to the client. Often the containers of foods will contain the same ingredients as containers of foods prepared for the general public, but the cost is typically higher for the dietetic foods. There is potential danger for diabetic clients who use these foods if they do not read the labels on the food containers and assume that because they are labeled "dietetic," they can be used in larger quantities. In reality, their use should be in specified amounts only, as these foods will contain carbohydrates, fats, and proteins that must be calculated in the total day's diet.

It is advisable for the client with diabetes to use foods prepared for the general public but to avoid those packed in syrup or oil. The important thing is for the diabetic client to *read the label* on all food containers purchased.

Alcohol

Although alcohol is not recommended for diabetic clients, its limited use is sometimes allowed if approved by the physician. However, some clients with diabetes who use hypoglycemic agents cannot tolerate alcohol. Clients must be very careful to only consume alcohol while eating. If alcohol is consumed on an empty stomach the person may experience hypoglycemia. When used, alcohol must be included in the diet plan to account for the calories consumed.

Exercise

Exercise helps the body use glucose by increasing insulin receptor sites and stimulating the creation of glucagon. It lowers cholesterol and blood pressure and reduces stress and body fat as it tones the muscles. For clients with type 2 diabetes, exercise helps improve weight control, glucose levels, and the cardiovascular system.

However, for clients with type 1 diabetes, exercise can complicate glucose control. As it lowers glucose levels, hypoglycemia can develop. Exercise must be carefully discussed with a physician. If done, it should be on a regular

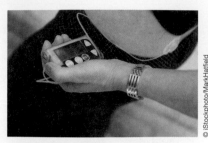

FIGURE 17-2 Insulin pump therapy may be used for better glucose control in clients with type 1 diabetes.

 exogenous insulin
insulin produced outside the body

endogenous insulin
insulin produced within the body

basis, and it must be considered carefully as the meal plans are developed so that sufficient calories and insulin are prescribed.

Insulin Therapy

Clients with type 1 diabetes must have injections of insulin every day to control their blood glucose levels (Figure 17-2). This insulin is called **exogenous insulin** because it is produced outside the body. **Endogenous insulin** is produced by the body.

Exogenous insulin is a protein. It must be injected because, if swallowed, it would be digested and would not reach the bloodstream as a complete hormone. After insulin treatment is begun, it is usually necessary for the client to continue it throughout life.

Human insulin is the most common insulin given to clients. This insulin does not come from humans but is made synthetically by a chemical process in a laboratory. Human insulin is preferred because it is very similar to insulin made by the pancreas. Animal insulin comes from cows or pigs and is called beef or pork insulin. These insulins are rarely used because they contain antibodies that make them less pure than human insulin.

Various types of insulin are available. They differ in the time it takes for them to peak (if at all) and in the duration they continue to act. This latter category is called insulin action. Consequently, they are classified as very rapid, rapid, intermediate, and long acting. Those most commonly used are the very rapid acting, dosed just before meals, and the long acting, which provide the background insulin (i.e., the amount needed regardless of meals). For type 1 diabetes, insulin is often given in two or more injections daily and may contain more than one type of insulin. Injections are given at prescribed times.

More clients with insulin-dependent diabetes are using insulin-pump therapy for better blood glucose control. Pumps deliver insulin in two ways: the basal rate and a pre-meal bolus. The basal rate is a small amount of very-rapid-acting insulin delivered continuously throughout the day. This insulin keeps blood glucose in check between meals and during the night. Pre-meal boluses of very-rapid-acting insulin are designed to cover the food eaten during a meal. This allows more flexibility as to when meals are eaten. Insulin pumps are not for everyone. An endocrinologist and diabetes educator can determine the best candidates for pump therapy.

Insulin Reactions

 insulin reaction
hypoglycemia leading to insulin coma caused by too much insulin or too little food

coma
state of unconsciousness

When clients do not eat the prescribed diet but continue to take the prescribed insulin, hypoglycemia can result. This is called an **insulin reaction**, or *hypo-glycemic episode,* and may lead to **coma** and death. Symptoms include sweating, shaking, light-headedness, headache, blurred vision, confusion, poor coordination, and eventual unconsciousness. Insulin reaction is dangerous because if frequent or prolonged, brain damage can occur. (The brain must have sufficient amounts of glucose in order to function.) The physician should be consulted if an insulin reaction occurs or seems imminent.

Conscious clients may be treated by giving them glucose tablets, a sugar cube, or a beverage containing sugar. This should be followed by a complex carbohydrate. If the client is unconscious, glucagon can be injected or an intravenous treatment of dextrose and water is given. It is advisable for the clients with diabetes to carry identification explaining the condition so that people do not think they are drunk when, in reality, they are experiencing an insulin reaction.

HEALTH AND NUTRITION CONSIDERATIONS

EXPLORING THE WEB

Search the Web for additional information on insulin therapies. What different types of therapies exist? Are there any experimental therapies currently being used and researched? What are some of the trial findings for these therapies?

It is important to point out to clients with diabetes that they can live a near-normal life by following their meal plan, taking medication as prescribed, and allowing time for sufficient exercise and rest. The dietitian must also stress the importance of eating all of the prescribed food, eating food at regular times to maintain the insulin–glucose balance, and carefully reading all labels on commercially prepared foods.

Adjustments must be made in shopping, cooking, and eating habits in order to follow the meal plan. Family meals can be simply adapted for the diabetic meal plan. The client with diabetes soon learns which exchange lists are to be included at each meal and at snack times and the foods within each exchange list. It is also important for the person's family to understand that the meal plan for diabetes is a very healthy way of eating. All members of the family could benefit from the portion control, lower fat content, and the awareness of everything being consumed.

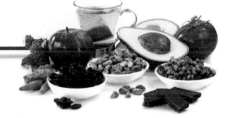

SUMMARY

The meal plan for diabetes is a key component in treating diabetes. Diabetes is a metabolic disease caused by the improper functioning of the pancreas that results in inadequate production or utilization of insulin. If the condition is left untreated, the body cannot use glucose properly, and then serious complications, even death, can occur. Treatment includes nutrition, medication, and exercise. Meal plans for diabetes are prescribed by the physician or dietitian in consultation with the client.

DISCUSSION TOPICS

1. Discuss the onset of type 1 and type 2 diabetes and list the symptoms.

2. Explain the difference between type 1 and type 2 diabetes.

3. Name the risk factors for developing type 1 and type 2 diabetes.

4. Discuss the treatment options for type 1 and type 2 diabetes.

5. Why would it be important for a client with diabetes to be educated about nutrition?

6. What are some of the complications that can occur if type 1 or type 2 diabetes is not well controlled or well managed?

7. True or False: It is necessary for clients with diabetes to purchase sugar-free and diabetic foods.

8. Discuss what the term "exchange" means in the meal plan for a client with diabetes.

9. Which of the following foods contain one carbohydrate exchange? More than one answer

may be correct. (See Appendix G for more information)

a. 1 slice of bread
b. ½ cup corn
c. ½ cup black beans
d. 1 Tbsp butter
e. 4 oz orange juice
f. 8 oz milk
g. 3 oz chicken
h. 1 tsp olive oil

10. How is gestational diabetes different from type 1 or type 2 diabetes?

11. Name the four major complications that can occur long term in clients with diabetes.

a. _____
b. _____
c. _____
d. _____

12. Name two tips that can be done to help reduce calories while eating out.

13. What percentage of the meal plan for someone with diabetes should come from carbohydrate sources? What portion could come from simple sugars?

SUGGESTED ACTIVITIES

1. Attend a local diabetes support group and listen to some of the topics the clients discuss. What are some of their difficulties, and how are they handling them?

2. Keep a food log for 1 week. Track in your log the time, the food, and the portion size of everything you eat. Use the respective food label to track calories, total carbohydrate, total fat, and protein consumed. If you don't have a food label, use the exchange list in Appendix G to estimate for those items consumed. At the week's end, answer these questions: How did you feel about writing down everything you ate? What difficulties did you encounter? Are there areas of your diet that could be modified to improve your health?

3. Visit a local grocery store. Find five foods that also offer a sugar-free option. Discuss the differences in the calories, carbohydrates, fats, and proteins in the regular verses the sugar-free version. What was the price difference between the two items? Did you find some foods where the sugar-free version would be better for a client with diabetes? Did you find some foods where it made little difference at all?

4. Identify someone you know who has diabetes. Ask to interview them. What are some of their challenges and frustrations in living with diabetes? What complications, if any, do they have? How often are they seeing their physician? Do they follow a meal plan? Have they ever had diabetes education or met with a registered dietitian or certified diabetes educator?

5. Investigate some of the resources available to clients with diabetes. Remember, we want clients to use credible and validated sources to obtain information about their health and caring for their diabetes. Make a list of some of the credible current resources. Can you find five books, five websites, five magazines/journals, and five smart phone applications that would be accurate, reliable, and helpful resources for clients with diabetes?

REVIEW

Multiple choice. Select the *letter* that precedes the best answer.

1. Which of the following statements is correct for type 1 diabetes?
   a. Most clients with diabetes (90–95%) have type 1.
   b. The pancreas continues to produce insulin; the body simply has difficulty using it.
   c. Clients with type 1 diabetes are often obese.
   d. Diabetes is caused by an autoimmune reaction.

2. Which of the following statements is correct for type 2 diabetes?
   a. Clients are usually diagnosed at a young age.
   b. Clients may not have obvious symptoms of type 2 diabetes.
   c. Insulin must be used to control blood sugars.
   d. The pancreas no longer produces any insulin.

3. Damage to the kidneys as a complication of diabetes is known as
    a. glycosuria
    b. polyuria
    c. nephropathy
    d. renal threshold

4. Insulin may be administered via which of the following routes?
    a. insulin pens
    b. insulin pumps
    c. insulin syringes
    d. by mouth
    e. Only a, b, and c
    f. All

5. Oral medications for diabetes help improve blood sugars in all of the following ways except
    a. stimulating the pancreas to make more insulin
    b. helping the body use insulin more efficiently
    c. increasing appetite
    d. preventing the liver from releasing stored glucose

6. The American Diabetes Association recommends the A1c level for clients with diabetes to be below
    a. 7%
    b. 9%
    c. 3%
    d. 5%

7. Which of the following is NOT true of gestational diabetes?
    a. Foods high in concentrated sugars should be avoided.
    b. It is a risk factor for developing type 2 diabetes.
    c. Weight gain during the pregnancy should stop.
    d. Insulin injections may be used to control blood sugar.

Case In Point

SIMONE: TYPE 2 DIABETES AND HEART HEALTH

Simone was diagnosed with type 2 diabetes 10 years ago. At the time of her diagnosis her doctor had her attend classes to learn about monitoring her blood sugars and eating healthy. She went to the classes, but really didn't believe she had diabetes. She felt fine and she didn't have any family history of diabetes. In fact, her parents immigrated to the United States from France. The French have a very low incidence of diabetes. Surely her doctor had made a mistake. So, for the most part, Simone ate what she wanted and she never worried about testing her blood sugars. She didn't have insurance to cover the cost of the test strips and they were just too expensive to purchase out of pocket. In addition, she decided not to go back to the doctor. She felt fine and he didn't know what he was talking about anyway.

Now that she is 50 years old, Simone has managed to all but forget about the diabetes. She is 5 feet and 5 inches tall and weighs 134 pounds. She is in her ideal body weight range and, up to this point, has no symptoms of diabetes. Then, while preparing breakfast one morning for her family, Simone experiences a sudden, sharp pain down her left arm and unbearable pressure on her chest. She falls to the floor and, in a state of panic, her husband calls 911.

Following emergent cardiac bypass surgery, Simone and her husband hear from the surgeon that she is lucky to be alive because the diabetes has greatly damaged her heart. The surgeon told Simone her A1c was 12.3%, and that if she didn't begin caring for her diabetes, she would certainly develop other complications in the near future.

ASSESSMENT

1. Why didn't Simone think she had diabetes?
2. Simone is 5 feet 5 inches and 134 pounds. Is she within her ideal body weight range?
3. Simone's A1c is 12.3%. What is the normal range and the recommendation for someone with diabetes?
4. Why does the doctor think the diabetes has caused damage to Simone's heart.

DIAGNOSIS

5. Write a nursing diagnosis for Simone.

PLAN/GOAL

6. What resources do you think Simone's doctor should refer her to?
7. Simone's family needs to understand the severity of the situation and be supportive of her efforts. What could they do to support her efforts in gaining control of her diabetes and her health?
8. What is a primary goal in Simone's care?

IMPLEMENTATION

9. What could Simone begin doing to show she is beginning to accept her diagnosis and move toward a healthier lifestyle?

EVALUATION/OUTCOME CRITERIA

10. How would you determine the effectiveness of the plan and the goals.

THINKING FURTHER

11. Go to the website for the American Diabetes Association (http://www.diabetes.org) and look particularly at the food and fitness tab. What are some of the recommendations and resources they have available to clients? What information did you find useful?

rate this **plate**

Simone has met with a diabetes educator to learn about the importance of monitoring her blood sugar levels and eating healthy. Simone decides that carbohydrate counting would be the easiest way to plan her meals. The diabetes educator recommends a 1,500–1,600 calorie meal plan, which allows 2–3 carbohydrate choices per meal. Rate the plate that Simone plans for her breakfast:

1 toasted whole-grain English muffin

1 tsp margarine

1 tsp grape jelly

1 egg cooked over-easy

1 medium banana

8 oz. low-fat milk

Does Simone have the correct number of carbohydrates for this meal? What should be added or subtracted from this plate?

Case In Point

MICHAEL: MANAGING NEW-ONSET TYPE 1 DIABETES

Michael, age 15, is a freshman in high school, where he is very involved in athletics. During the basketball season, he develops an insatiable appetite. His mother is amazed at how much he can eat. At first, she assumes the overeating is due to a growth spurt and the increased activity level at daily basketball practice and games. At his last doctor's appointment, Michael measured 5 feet 10 inches and weighed 166 pounds. Lately, however, his mother notices that Michael looks too thin, despite his increased food intake.

Michael has also been getting up frequently during the night to use the bathroom. When his mother questions him about this, Michael reports having a strong urge to go, but then can only void a small amount when in the bathroom. Michael is frustrated because the "false" urges are interrupting his sleep and, as a result, making him extremely tired throughout the school day. He states that he has been taking a water bottle to school daily and refilling it multiple times. He just thought he was dehydrated from basketball practice and his body just needed more water. He also assumed this was why he needed to get up in the night and go to the bathroom.

Michael and his mother are African American and have a strong family history of type 2 diabetes. His mother begins to piece together some of his symptoms and decides he needs to see his doctor. At the doctor's office, Michael's mother becomes very concerned. Michael only weighs 147 pounds! After completing blood and urine tests, the doctor diagnoses Michael with type 1 diabetes and admits him to the hospital where insulin will be initiated to bring his blood sugar down. He and his mother will then be educated on nutrition, insulin, and blood sugar monitoring.

ASSESSMENT

1. List all the subjective information you have about Michael related to diabetes.
2. What objective data do you have about Michael?
3. What tests are necessary to confirm the diagnosis of diabetes?

DIAGNOSIS

4. What education will be needed for Michael's diagnosis?
5. What nursing diagnoses apply to Michael?

PLAN/GOAL

Complete the following goal statements:

6. Michael will verbalize and demonstrate his self-care measures related to ____
   _____.
7. Michael will verbalize and demonstrate survival skills for persons with diabetes and information by _____
   _____.

IMPLEMENTATION

The doctor has prescribed a long-acting insulin injection for Michael at bedtime and a dose of rapid-acting insulin at meals based on the amount of carbohydrate Michael will consume and his current pre-meal blood sugar level.

8. What topics are essential for Michael to learn?
9. What skills does he need to master before he goes home?
10. Who else needs to be in class with Michael?
11. What information does Michael's mother need to know about emergency situations?
12. What does Michael need to know about exercise?

EVALUATION/OUTCOME CRITERIA

13. What should Michael's fasting blood sugar be at his 2-week follow-up appointment?
14. What should he be able to verbalize and demonstrate?
15. What should happen to his weight?

THINKING FURTHER

16. Why is it essential for Michael to manage his diabetes?
17. What challenges does Michael face in balancing between being a carefree teenager and managing a serious chronic disease?
18. What information will need to be provided to Michael's school, including his teachers and his coach?

rate this **plate**

During his stay at the hospital, Michael receives a visit by a registered dietitian. The dietitian provides education on carbohydrate counting and how carbohydrates will affect his blood sugar levels. She also explains to Michael that exercise will have an effect on his blood sugar levels and that it is important to check his blood sugar regularly when engaging in basketball practice and games. Since Michael is an active, growing teenager, the dietitian recommends a 2,800 calorie diabetic meal plan. This meal plan allows for 5–6 carbohydrate choices per meal and 2–3 carbohydrates choices for snacks between meals. Rate the snack that Michael plans to eat before basketball practice.

2 mozzarella string cheese sticks

1 medium apple

1 oz. cookie snack pack

8 oz. low-fat milk

Will this snack provide him with enough carbohydrate servings to maintain his blood sugar levels through basketball practice? Does the mozzarella cheese contain carbohydrates? Why is it recommended to consume a protein source with a carbohydrate choice as a snack for the diabetic meal plan?

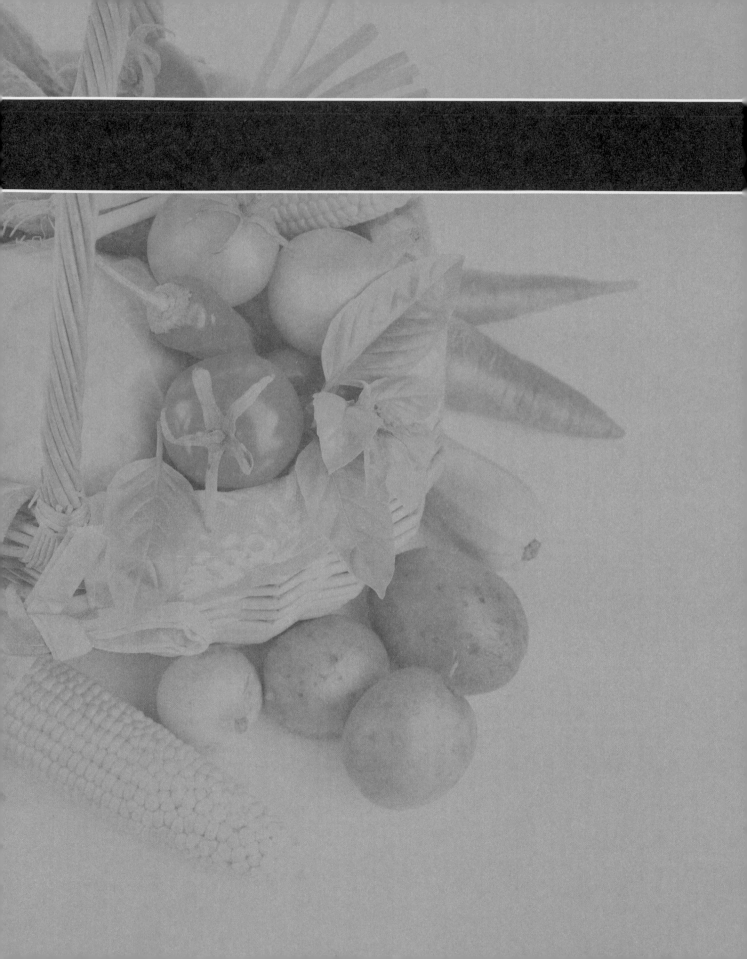

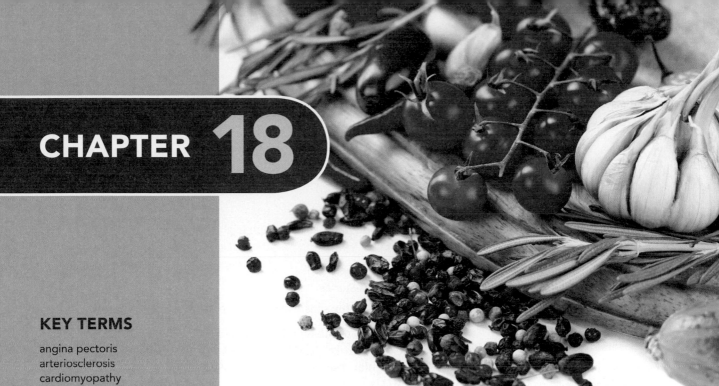

CHAPTER 18

DIET AND CARDIOVASCULAR DISEASE

KEY TERMS

angina pectoris
arteriosclerosis
cardiomyopathy
cardiovascular disease (CVD)
cerebrovascular accident (CVA)
compensated heart disease
congestive heart failure (CHF)
coronary artery disease (CAD)
decompensated heart disease
endocardium
essential hypertension
hyperlipidemia
infarct
ischemia
lumen
monosodium glutamate (MSG)
myocardial infarction (MI)
myocardium
pericardium
peripheral vascular disease (PVD)
primary hypertension
secondary hypertension
serum cholesterol
thrombus
vascular disease

OBJECTIVES

After studying this chapter, you should be able to:

- ◇ Identify factors that contribute to heart disease
- ◇ Explain why cholesterol and saturated fats are limited in some cardiovascular conditions
- ◇ Identify foods to avoid or limit in a cholesterol-controlled diet
- ◇ Explain why sodium is limited in some cardiovascular conditions
- ◇ Identify foods that are limited or prohibited in sodium-controlled diets

Cardiovascular disease (CVD) affects the heart and blood vessels. It is the leading cause of death and permanent disability in the United States today.

cardiovascular disease (CVD)
disease affecting heart and blood vessels

myocardial infarction (MI)
heart attack; caused by the blockage of an artery leading to the heart

compensated heart disease
heart disease in which the heart is able to maintain circulation to all body parts

decompensated heart disease
heart disease in which the heart cannot maintain circulation to all body parts

myocardium
heart muscle

endocardium
lining of the heart

pericardium
outer covering of the heart

arteriosclerosis
hardening of the arteries

vascular disease
disease of the blood vessels

lumen
the hollow area in a tube

ischemia
reduced blood flow causing an inadequate supply of nutrients and oxygen to, and wastes from, tissues

angina pectoris
pain in the heart muscle due to inadequate blood supply

thrombus
blood clot

infarct
dead tissue resulting from blocked artery

The grief and economic distress it causes are staggering. Organizations, especially the American Heart Association, are promoting programs designed to alert people to the risk factors for CVD and thereby reduce its frequency. A group of risk factors have been identified and are known as the metabolic syndrome, previously known as syndrome X. These risk factors apply to children as well as adults.

- Abdominal obesity
- High blood lipids such as high triglycerides, low HDL, and high LDL
- High blood pressure
- Insulin resistance
- Elevated highly sensitive C-reactive protein in the blood

Those diagnosed with metabolic syndrome are at increased risk of coronary heart disease, stroke, peripheral vascular disease, and type 2 diabetes.

Cardiovascular disease can be acute (sudden) or chronic. **Myocardial infarction (MI)** is an example of the acute form. Chronic heart disease develops over time and causes the loss of heart function. If the heart can maintain blood circulation, the disease is classified as **compensated heart disease**. Compensation usually requires that the heart beat unusually fast. Consequently, the heart enlarges. If the heart cannot maintain circulation, the condition is classified as **decompensated heart disease**, and congestive heart failure (CHF) occurs. The heart muscle (**myocardium**), the valves, the lining (**endocardium**), the outer covering (**pericardium**), or the blood vessels may be affected by heart disease.

ATHEROSCLEROSIS

Arteriosclerosis is the general term for **vascular disease** in which arteries harden (become thickened), making the passage of blood difficult and sometimes impossible. Atherosclerosis is the form of arteriosclerosis that most frequently occurs in developed countries. It is believed to begin in childhood and is considered one of the major causes of heart attack.

Atherosclerosis affects the inner lining of arteries (the intima), where deposits of cholesterol, fats, and other substances accumulate over time, thickening and weakening artery walls. These deposits are called plaque (Figure 18-1). Plaque deposits gradually reduce the size of the **lumen** of the artery and, consequently, the amount of blood flow. The reduced blood flow causes an inadequate supply of nutrients and oxygen delivery to and waste removal from the tissues. This condition is called **ischemia**.

The reduced oxygen supply causes pain. When the pain occurs in the chest and radiates down the left arm, it is called **angina pectoris** and should be considered a warning. When the lumen narrows so that a blood clot (**thrombus**) occurs in a coronary artery and blood flow is cut off, a heart attack occurs. The dead tissue that results is called an **infarct**. The heart muscle that should have received the blood is the myocardium. Thus, such an attack is commonly called an acute myocardial infarction (MI). Some clients who experience an MI will require surgery to bypass the clogged artery.

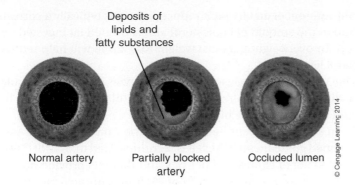

Deposits of
lipids and
fatty substances

Normal artery   Partially blocked   Occluded lumen
                          artery

© Cengage Learning 2014

FIGURE 18-1 Progression of atherosclerosis.

The procedure is a coronary artery bypass graft (CABG), which is commonly referred to as bypass surgery.

When blood flow to the brain is blocked in this way or blood vessels burst and blood flows into the brain, a stroke, or **cerebrovascular accident (CVA)**, results. When it occurs in tissue some distance from the heart, it is called **peripheral vascular disease (PVD)**.

Risk Factors

Hyperlipidemia, hypertension (high blood pressure), and smoking are major risk factors for the development of atherosclerosis. Other contributory factors are believed to include obesity, diabetes mellitus, male sex, heredity, personality type (ability to handle stress), age (risk increases with years), and sedentary lifestyle. Although some of these factors are beyond one's control, some factors are not.

It is known that dietary cholesterol and triglycerides (fats in foods and in adipose tissue) contribute to hyperlipidemia. Foods containing saturated fats and trans fats increase **serum cholesterol**, whereas unsaturated fats tend to reduce it.

Lipoproteins carry cholesterol and fats in the blood to body tissues. Low-density lipoprotein (LDL) carries most of the cholesterol to the cells, and elevated blood levels of LDL are believed to contribute to atherosclerosis. High-density lipoprotein (HDL) carries cholesterol from the tissues to the liver for eventual excretion. It is believed that low serum levels of HDL can contribute to atherosclerosis.

Diet can alleviate hypertension (discussed later in this chapter), reduce obesity, and help control diabetes mellitus. A sedentary lifestyle can be changed. Exercise can help the client lose weight, lower blood pressure, and increase the HDL ("good") cholesterol level. Exercise must be done in consultation with the physician and be increased gradually. Also, one can stop smoking. In sum, a person can considerably reduce the risk of atherosclerosis and thus an MI, CVA, and PVD.

MEDICAL NUTRITION THERAPY FOR HYPERLIPIDEMIA

Medical nutrition therapy is the primary treatment for hyperlipidemia. It involves reducing the quantity and types of fats and often calories in the diet.

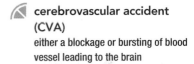

cerebrovascular accident (CVA)
either a blockage or bursting of blood vessel leading to the brain

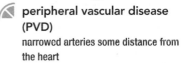

peripheral vascular disease (PVD)
narrowed arteries some distance from the heart

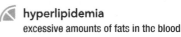

hyperlipidemia
excessive amounts of fats in the blood

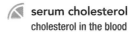

serum cholesterol
cholesterol in the blood

When the amount of dietary fat is reduced, there is typically a corresponding reduction in the amount of cholesterol and saturated fat ingested and a loss of weight. In overweight persons, weight loss alone will help reduce serum cholesterol levels.

The American Heart Association categorizes blood cholesterol levels of 200 mg/dl or less to be desirable, 200–239 mg/dl to be borderline high, and 240 mg/dl and greater to be high.

In an effort to prevent heart disease, the American Heart Association has developed guidelines in which it is recommended that adult diets contain less than 200 mg of cholesterol per day and that fats provide no more than 20–35% of calories, with a maximum of 7% from saturated fats and trans fat, a maximum of 8% from polyunsaturated fats, and a maximum of 15–20% of monounsaturated fats. Carbohydrates should make up 50–55% of the calories and proteins from 12–20% of them. Currently, it is believed that nearly 40% of the calories in the average U.S. diet come from fats.

One may find a fat-restricted diet to be difficult to accept. A diet very low in fat will seem unusual and highly unpalatable (unpleasant tasting). It takes approximately 2 or 3 months to adjust to a low-fat diet. If the physician will allow it, the change in the nutrient makeup of the diet should be made gradually (Table 18-1).

Information about the fat content of foods and methods of preparation that minimize the amount of fat in the diet are essential to the client. The client must be taught to select whole, fresh foods and to prepare them without the addition of any fat. Only lean meat should be selected, and all visible fat must be removed. Fat-free milk and fat-free milk cheeses should be used instead of whole milk and natural cheeses. Desserts containing whole milk, eggs, and cream are to be avoided.

In a fat-controlled diet, one must be particularly careful when using animal foods. Cholesterol is found only in animal tissue. Organ meats, egg yolks, and some shellfish are especially rich in cholesterol and should be used in limited quantities, if at all. Saturated fats are found in all animal foods and in coconut, chocolate, and palm oil. They tend to be solid at room temperature. Polyunsaturated fats are derived from plants and some fish and are usually soft or liquid at room temperature. Soft margarine containing mostly liquid vegetable oil is substituted for butter, and liquid vegetable oils are used in cooking.

Studies indicate that water-soluble fiber, such as that found in oat bran, legumes, and fruits, bind with cholesterol-containing substances and prevent their reabsorption by the blood. The recommendation for total fiber per day is 38 grams for men and 25 grams for women. Research published by the National Institute of Health shows that people who increased their soluble fiber intake by 5–10 grams each day had about a 5% drop in their LDL ("bad") cholesterol. This is a large amount of fiber and must be introduced gradually to the diet along with increased fluids, or flatulence may result. Table 18-2 lists foods to limit on a low-cholesterol diet.

Some clients will find the diabetic exchange lists useful for controlling the fat content of their diets. When fat-controlled diets are severely restricted, limiting calorie intake to 1,200, they may be deficient in fat-soluble vitamins. Consequently, a vitamin supplement may be needed.

EXPLORING THE WEB

Search the Web for additional information on cholesterol-lowering drugs. Create a table of these drugs and list the side effects of each drug, including any foods or medications that the drug reacts with and any contraindications for use of the drug.

TABLE 18-1   Foods to Include and Foods to Avoid on Fat-Restricted Diets

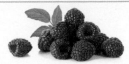

FOODS TO INCLUDE	FOODS TO AVOID
Breads and Cereals	
• Whole-grain breads and rolls	• Breads made with egg or cheese, croissants
• Plain buns, bagels, pita bread	• Bakery products
• Cereals without coconut	• Butter crackers
• Saltines, matzos, rusks	
• Rice, pasta	
Vegetables and Fruits	
Any fresh fruit or vegetable, except coconut	Coconut oil, palm oil
Meats, Poultry, and Fish	
After trimming fat and removing skin before eating:	Fatty or prime-grade meats, pastrami, spareribs, sausage, bacon, lunch meats, domestic ducks and geese, organ meats
• Fish, but limited shrimp or lobster	
• Lean beef, pork, lamb, veal	
• Egg whites, yolks (2–3 per week)	
Dairy	
• Fat-free milk or low-fat milk	• Milk with more than 1% fat, cream, nondairy creamers
• Dry curd or low-fat cottage cheese	• Most cheese, especially processed or blue
• Buttermilk	
• Puddings made with fat-free milk	
• Low-fat cheese	
Other Foods	
• Oils (canola, olive, peanut)	• Butter
• Syrup	• Lard
• Gelatin	• Bakery desserts
• Jelly	• Ice creams
• Honey	• Fried foods
• Fat-free broths	• Commercially prepared meals; salad dressings
• Margarine made from liquid corn, sesame, olive, or sunflower oil (in limited amounts)	• Cream soups
• Limited nuts (walnuts, almonds)	• Cream sauces; gravies
• Limited homemade salad dressings	
• Sherbet	
• Hard candy	

If appropriate blood lipid levels cannot be attained within 3–6 months by the use of a fat-restricted diet alone (see Table 18-3 for menus), the physician can prescribe a cholesterol-lowering drug such as atorvastatin (Lipitor) or simvastatin (Zocor). Food and/or drug interactions can occur with cholesterol-lowering drugs, as well as with other cardiac drugs. For example, Zocor and Lipitor interact with grapefruit and its juice; therefore, total avoidance is necessary.

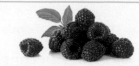

TABLE 18-2   Foods to Limit on a Low-Cholesterol Diet

Fats on meats and fish	Natural cheeses
Lard	Commercially fried foods
Organ meats	Commercially prepared baked goods
Bacon	
Lunch meats	Commercially prepared meatloaf
Prime-grade meats marbled with fat	Commercially prepared mayonnaise
	Quiche Lorraine
Duck	Chicken à la king
Skin-on chicken and turkey	Cheeseburgers
Crab meat	Chicken livers
Shrimp	Custard
Lobster	Soufflé
Egg yolks	Lemon meringue pie
Butter	Cheesecake
Cream	Ice cream
Whole milk	Eggnog

© Cengage Learning 2014

TABLE 18-3   Sample Menus for a Fat-Controlled Diet

BREAKFAST	LUNCH	DINNER
Orange	Tomato juice	3 oz salmon
Oatmeal	Uncreamed cottage cheese on fruit salad	Baked sweet potato
1 Tbsp sugar and		Baked acorn squash with 1 Tbsp honey
1 cup fat-free milk	2 slices wheat toast with	
1 slice whole-wheat toast	2 Tbsp honey	Lettuce salad
1 Tbsp jelly	Angel food cake	1 slice whole-wheat bread
Coffee	1 cup fat-free milk	1 Tbsp jelly
	Tea	Canned peaches
		1 cup fat-free milk
		Tea

© Cengage Learning 2014

MYOCARDIAL INFARCTION

Myocardial infarction is caused by the blockage of a coronary artery supplying blood to the heart. The heart tissue is denied blood because of this blockage and dies (see Figure 18-2). Atherosclerosis is a primary cause, but hypertension, abnormal blood clotting, and infection such as that caused by rheumatic fever (which damages heart valves) are also contributory factors.

© Cengage Learning 2014

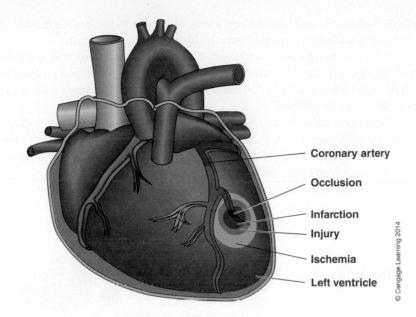

FIGURE 18-2 When a coronary artery is occluded, the heart muscle dies.

Coronary artery

Occlusion

Infarction

Injury

Ischemia

Left ventricle

After the attack, the client is in shock. This causes a fluid shift, and the client may feel thirsty. The client should be given nothing by mouth (NPO), however, until the physician evaluates the condition. If nausea remains after the period of shock, IV infusions are given to prevent dehydration.

After several hours, the client may begin to eat. A liquid diet may be recommended for the first 24 hours. Following that, a low-cholesterol–low-sodium diet is usually given, with the client regulating the amount eaten.

Foods should not be extremely hot or extremely cold. They should be easy to chew and digest and contain little roughage so that the work of the heart will be minimal. Both chewing and the increased activity of the gastrointestinal tract that follow ingestion of high-fiber foods cause extra work for the heart. The percentage of energy nutrients will be based on the particular needs of the client, but, in most cases, the types and amounts of fats will be limited. Sodium is usually limited to prevent fluid accumulation. Some physicians will order a restriction on the amount of caffeine for the first few days after an MI. The dual goal is to allow the heart to rest and its tissue to heal.

CONGESTIVE HEART FAILURE

Congestive heart failure (CHF) is an example of decompensation, or severe heart disease. Heart failure is caused by conditions that damage the heart muscle, including **coronary artery disease (CAD)**, heart attack, **cardiomyopathy**, valve disease, heart defects present at birth, diabetes mellitus, and chronic renal disease. Heart failure can also occur if several diseases or conditions are present. In this situation, when damage is extreme and the heart cannot provide adequate circulation, the amount of oxygen taken in is insufficient for body needs. Shortness of breath is common, and chest pain can occur on exertion.

Because of the reduced circulation, tissues retain fluid that would normally be carried off by the blood. Sodium builds up, and more fluid is retained, resulting in edema. In an attempt to compensate for this pumping

 congestive heart failure (CHF)
a form of decompensated heart disease

 coronary artery disease (CAD)
severe narrowing of the arteries that supply blood to the heart

 cardiomyopathy
damage to the heart muscle caused by infection, alcohol, or drug abuse

deficit, the heart beats faster and enlarges. This adds to the heart's burden. In advanced cases when edema affects the lungs, death can occur.

With the inadequate circulation, body tissues do not receive sufficient amounts of nutrients. This insufficiency can cause malnutrition and underweight, although the edema can mask these problems. In some cases, a fluid restriction may be ordered.

Diuretics to aid in the excretion of water and sodium and a sodium-restricted diet are typically prescribed. Because diuretics can cause an excessive loss of potassium, the client's blood potassium should be carefully monitored to prevent hypokalemia, which can upset the heartbeat. Fruits, especially oranges, bananas, and prunes, can be useful in such a situation because they are excellent sources of potassium and contain only negligible amounts of sodium (Table 18-4). When necessary, the physician will prescribe supplementary potassium.

TABLE 18-4   Potassium-Rich Foods

FRUITS

Apricots	Dates	Kiwifruit
Oranges	Figs	Peaches
Bananas	Raisins	Pineapple
Avocados	Honeydew melon	Prunes
Cantaloupe	Grapefruit	Strawberries

VEGETABLES

Asparagus	Squash
Broccoli	Tomatoes
Cabbage	Spinach
Green beans	Potatoes, sweet potatoes, yams
Pumpkin	

© Cengage Learning 2014

In The Media

Can Regular Teeth Cleaning Benefit your Heart?

Findings presented at the American Heart Association meeting in 2011 suggested that people who visit the dentist regularly may have a lower risk for heart attacks and strokes. Researchers from Taiwan followed 100,000 people for 7 years and found that those who had their teeth scraped and cleaned by a dentist at least twice a year had a 24% lower risk for a heart attack. Experts and numerous studies have shown the association between inflammation and heart disease. A separate study conducted in Sweden discovered how different types of gum disease may predict the risks of heart attacks, strokes, and even heart failure. Health care specialists continue to recommend good dental hygiene for all clients.

(Source: Adapted from Dallas, Mary Elizabeth. *Regular Teeth Cleanings Could Cut Heart Attack Risk: Study.* November 13, 2011. www.Health.com)

HYPERTENSION

When blood pressure is chronically high, the condition is called hypertension (HTN). In 90% of hypertension cases, the cause is unknown, and the condition is called **essential** or **primary hypertension**. The other 10% of the cases are called **secondary hypertension** because the condition is caused by another problem. Some causes of secondary hypertension include kidney disease, problems of the adrenal glands, and use of oral contraceptives.

The blood pressure commonly measured is that of the artery in the upper arm. This measurement is made with an instrument called the sphygmomanometer. The top number is the systolic pressure, taken as the heart contracts. The lower number is the diastolic pressure, taken when the heart is resting. The pressure is measured in millimeters of mercury (mm Hg). Hypertension can be diagnosed when, on several occasions, the systolic pressure is 140 mm Hg or more and the diastolic pressure is 90 mm Hg or more. The blood pressure categories are the following:

- Normal: less than 120/less than 80 mm Hg
- Prehypertension: 120–139/80–88 mm Hg
- Stage 1 hypertension: 140–159/90–99 mm Hg
- Stage 2 hypertension: 160/100 mm Hg

Hypertension contributes to heart attack, stroke, heart failure, and kidney failure. It is sometimes called the *silent disease* because sufferers can be asymptomatic (without symptoms). Its frequency increases with age, and it is more prevalent among African Americans than others.

Heredity and obesity are predisposing factors in hypertension. Smoking and stress also contribute to hypertension. Weight loss usually lowers the blood pressure and, consequently, clients are often placed on weight reduction diets.

Excessive use of ordinary table salt also is considered a contributory factor in hypertension. Table salt consists of over 40% sodium plus chloride. Both are essential in maintaining fluid balance and thus blood pressure. When consumed in normal quantities by healthy people, they are beneficial.

When the fluid balance is upset and sodium and fluid collect in body tissue, causing edema, extra pressure is placed on the blood vessels. A sodium-restricted diet, often accompanied by diuretics, can be prescribed to alleviate this condition. When the sodium content in the diet is reduced, the water and salts in the tissues flow back into the blood to be excreted by the kidneys. In this way, the edema is relieved. The amount of sodium restricted is determined by the physician on the basis of the client's condition.

Previous research focused primarily on sodium as a primary factor in the development of hypertension, but as research continues, the effects of chloride also are receiving increasing scrutiny. In addition, the particular roles of calcium and magnesium in relation to hypertension are being studied. Knowing that sodium raises blood pressure and that potassium lowers blood pressure, the NIH (National Institutes of Health)

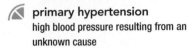

essential hypertension
high blood pressure with unknown cause; also called primary hypertension

primary hypertension
high blood pressure resulting from an unknown cause

secondary hypertension
high blood pressure caused by another condition such as kidney disease

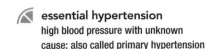

EXPLORING THE WEB

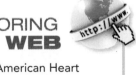

Visit the American Heart Association's website (http://www.americanheart.org). Look for information on hypertension. Create a list of factors that may predispose people to hypertension. List ways to alleviate these risks and prevent hypertension and other serious heart conditions. How can diet play a role in alleviating some of these risk factors?

monosodium glutamate (MSG)
flavor enhancer containing large
amounts of sodium

Supersize USA

"Love, love, love Chinese buffets! Lunch is eaten out since I am on the road as a sales representative. I have discovered that Chinese buffets are a good place to eat because I can get a lot of food and even desserts. I usually eat at the buffets at least three times a week. During my yearly checkup, my doctor told me that my blood pressure was really high. She also commented on the weight that I had gained. What could be causing my blood pressure to be high? What can I do to lower my blood pressure? Is there anything in the Chinese food that could raise my blood pressure and cause me to gain weight?"

Sodium intake and increased weight could be causing high blood pressure. To lower it, lose weight, exercise, and do not salt your food at the table. Chinese food may contain **monosodium glutamate (MSG)**. If you desire Chinese food, ask that the food be prepared with no MSG and order food in a clear sauce; brown sauces have soy sauce in them, which is high in sodium. Also check for a stir-fry grill where you can choose your own ingredients such as vegetables and meat. Try to go light on the sauce. Limit your visit to the buffet to one time per week.

created the DASH (Dietary Approaches to Stop Hypertension) eating plan. The DASH plan has been clinically shown to reduce high blood pressure while increasing the serving of fruits and vegetables to 8–12 servings per day, depending upon calorie intake (see Appendix C-1). Many fruits and vegetables are high in potassium levels, which will lower blood pressure. The newest guideline for potassium intake is 4.7 grams, or 4,700 mg, per day to lower blood pressure. It is recommended that a physician be consulted if the DASH eating plan is undertaken and one is already on blood pressure–lowering medication.

DIETARY TREATMENT FOR HYPERTENSION

As indicated, weight loss for the obese client with hypertension usually lowers blood pressure, and thus a calorie-restricted diet might be prescribed. A sodium-restricted diet frequently is prescribed for clients with hypertension. Certain ethnic groups, such as African Americans with new onset of HTN and those already diagnosed with HTN, should limit sodium intake to 1,500 mg/day. A discussion of this diet follows. When diuretics are prescribed together with a sodium-restricted diet, potassium may be lost via the urine and, thus, clients may be advised to increase the amount of potassium-rich foods in the diet (see Table 18-4). It is estimated that the average daily sodium intake for Americans is 3,400 mg.

Sodium-Restricted Diets

A sodium-restricted diet is a regular diet in which the amount of sodium is limited. Such a diet is used to alleviate edema and hypertension. Most people obtain far too much sodium from their diets. A committee of the

Food and Nutrition Board recommends that the daily intake of sodium be limited to no more than 2,300 mg (2.3 grams), and the board itself set a safe minimum at 500 mg/day for adults (see Table 8-6). Sodium is found in food, water, and medicine.

It is impossible to have a diet totally free of sodium. Meats, fish, poultry, dairy products, and eggs all contain substantial amounts of sodium naturally. Cereals, vegetables, fruits, and fats contain small amounts of sodium naturally. Water contains varying amounts of sodium. However, sodium often is added to foods during processing and cooking and at the table. The food label should indicate the addition of sodium to commercial food products. In some of these foods, the addition of sodium is obvious because one can taste it, as in prepared dinners, potato chips, and canned soups. In others, it is not. The following are examples of sodium-containing products frequently added to foods that the consumer may not notice:

- Salt (sodium chloride)—used in cooking or at the table and in canning and processing.
- Monosodium glutamate (MSG), sold under several brand names—a flavor enhancer used in home, restaurant, and hotel cooking and in many packaged, canned, and frozen foods.
- Baking powder—used to leaven quick breads and cakes.
- Baking soda (sodium bicarbonate)—used to leaven breads and cakes; sometimes added to vegetables in cooking or used as an "alkalizer" for indigestion.
- Brine (table salt and water)—used in processing foods to inhibit growth of bacteria; in cleaning or blanching vegetables and fruits; in freezing and canning certain foods; and for flavor, as in corned beef, pickles, and sauerkraut.
- Disodium phosphate—present in some quick-cooking cereals and processed cheeses.
- Sodium alginate—used in many chocolate milks and ice creams for smooth texture.
- Sodium benzoate—used as a preservative in many condiments such as relishes, sauces, and salad dressings.
- Sodium hydroxide—used in food processing to soften and loosen skins of ripe olives, hominy, and certain fruits and vegetables.
- Sodium propionate—used in pasteurized cheeses and in some breads and cakes to inhibit growth of mold.
- Sodium sulfite—used to bleach certain fruits in which an artificial color is desired, such as maraschino cherries and glazed or crystallized fruit; also used as a preservative in some dried fruit, such as dried plums.

Because the amount of sodium in tap water varies from one area to another, the local department of health or the American Heart Association affiliate should be consulted if this information is needed. Softened water always has additional sodium. If the sodium content of the water is high, the client may have to use bottled water.

Sodium restrictions are a popular lifestyle prescription to help prevent hypertension and heart disease. While there has been debate over different levels of sodium intake and the effect on developing heart conditions, numerous medical studies support that mild sodium restriction can lower blood pressure. The guidelines established by the 2010 Dietary Guidelines for Americans and supported by the American Heart Association recommend no more than 1,500 mg of sodium per day for most middle-aged and older Americans. The 2010 Dietary Guidelines for Americans list 2,300 mg as the upper limit for healthy individuals. While the recommendation for 1,500 mg seems unrealistic for many Americans, it is still something to strive toward. Limiting the amount of processed foods and eliminating the salt shaker from the dinner table will assist in achieving the recommendation.

In The Media

Is Salt in Your Diet a Problem?

Reducing your sodium intake can help prevent disease such as high blood pressure and stroke. Others ways to decrease sodium in your diet would be to cook with natural herbs and spices instead of table salt. Check food labels for sodium content and choose products that state "reduced sodium." Processed foods and snacks consistently have high sodium content. Fresh or frozen fruits and vegetables are the better choices when choosing a healthy snack. It will take approximately 3 months for your taste buds to get used to no or reduced salt.

(Source: Adapted from The National Heart Lung and Blood Institute, National Institutes of Health. *Tips for Reducing Sodium in Your Diet*. www.nhlbi.nih.gov)

Some over-the-counter medicines contain sodium. Anyone on a sodium-restricted diet should obtain the physician's permission before using any medication or salt substitute. Many salt substitutes contain potassium, which can affect the heartbeat.

The amount of sodium allowed depends on the client's condition and is prescribed by the physician. A very low restriction limits sodium to 2 grams a day. A moderate restriction limits sodium to 3–4 grams a day.

Adjustment to Sodium Restriction

Sodium-restricted diets range from "different" to "tasteless" because most people are accustomed to salt in their food. It can be difficult for one to understand the necessity for following such a diet, particularly if it must be followed for the remainder of his or her life. If the physician allows, it will help the client adjust if the sodium content of the diet can be reduced gradually.

A reminder of the numerous herbs, spices, and flavorings to be used in place of sodium will be beneficial (Table 18-5). It would also be useful to practice ordering from a menu so as to learn to choose those foods lowest in sodium content.

HEALTH AND NUTRITION CONSIDERATIONS

When one is given a new eating plan, it may take a long time for full compliance to be demonstrated. Asking one to make multiple changes at one time may result in poor compliance. Each task should be focused on separately, beginning with the most detrimental problem to you. The cardiac dietitian can help facilitate these changes and provide support along the way.

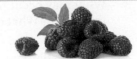

TABLE 18-5 Foods to Allow and Foods to Avoid on Sodium-Restricted Diets of 1–2 Grams

FOODS PERMITTED ON MOST SODIUM-RESTRICTED DIETS	FOODS TO LIMIT OR AVOID
Fruit juices without additives	Tomato juice and vegetable cocktail
Fresh fruits	Canned vegetables, if not salt-free
Fresh vegetables (except for those on the "Avoid" list)	Sauerkraut
Dried peas or beans	Frozen vegetables if prepared with salt
Fat-free milk	Dried, breaded, smoked, or canned fish or meats
Puffed-type cereals	Cheeses; salted butter or margarine
Regular, cooked cereals without added salt, sugar, or flavorings	Salt-topped crackers or breads
Plain pasta	Salty foods such as potato chips, salted nuts, peanut butter, pretzels
Rice	Canned fish, meats, or soups
Unsalted, uncoated popcorn	Ham, salt pork, corned beef, lunch meats, smoked or canned fish
Fresh fish	Prepared relishes, salad dressings, catsup, soy sauce
Fresh unsalted meats	Bouillon, baking soda, baking powder, MSG
Unsalted margarine	Commercially prepared meals
Oil	Fast foods
Vinegar	
Spices containing no salt, herbs, lemon juice	
Unsalted nuts	
Hard candy	
Jams, jellies, honey	
Coffee, tea	

© Cengage Learning 2014

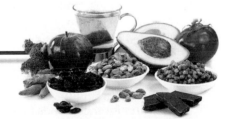

SUMMARY

Cardiovascular disease represents the leading cause of death in the United States. It may be acute, as in myocardial infarction, or chronic, as in hypertension and atherosclerosis. Hypertension may be a symptom of other disease. Weight loss, if the client is overweight, and a salt-restricted diet are typically prescribed.

Atherosclerosis is a vascular disease in which the arteries are narrowed by fatty deposits, reducing blood flow. Angina pectoris, myocardial infarction, or stroke can result. Because cholesterol is associated with atherosclerosis, a low-cholesterol diet or a fat-restricted diet might be prescribed.

By maintaining one's weight and activities at a healthy level, limiting salt and fat intake, and avoiding smoking, one reduces the risks of heart disease.

DISCUSSION TOPICS

1. Why are sodium-restricted diets prescribed for clients with hypertension or heart failure?

2. What precautions might one take to prevent hypertension? To prevent atherosclerosis? Explain your answers.

3. What may occur in severe myocardial infarction? What causes myocardial infarction?

4. What are diuretics? How could they be harmful? How could this danger be avoided?

5. What is edema? How is it related to cardiovascular disease?

6. Why is it impossible to prepare a diet absolutely free of salt?

7. Why might a sodium-restricted diet be unpleasant for a client?

8. Name four snack items that would not be allowed on sodium-restricted diets.

9. For what heart condition might a fat-controlled diet be ordered?

10. What is cholesterol? How is it associated with atherosclerosis?

11. What is hyperlipidemia? How is it related to atherosclerosis?

12. Discuss known risk factors for the development of atherosclerosis. Which could be avoided? Explain.

SUGGESTED ACTIVITIES

1. Make a list of the foods eaten yesterday. Circle those foods that would not be allowed on a low-cholesterol diet and suggest satisfactory substitutions. Underline those not allowed on moderate sodium-restricted diets. Are any both circled and underlined?

2. Visit a local supermarket and, only checking foods along the outside walls, list the foods containing sodium compounds. Suggest substitutes for these foods for clients on sodium-restricted diets.

3. Marita Jiminez was placed on a fat-restricted diet containing no more than 70 grams of fat. She wants to order the following breakfast:
   - Sliced avocado
   - Poached egg with ham in cheese sauce on English muffin
   - Coffee with cream

   Would this be acceptable? Explain your answer and, if necessary, suggest alternative foods that would be acceptable.

4. Justin Chen has been told that he has atherosclerosis and must follow a low-cholesterol diet. He is visiting his aunt who is serving the following meal:
   - Cream of broccoli soup
   - Roast chicken
   - Mashed potatoes with gravy
   - Lima beans with butter
   - Green salad with vinegar and oil dressing
   - Rolls and butter
   - Milk
   - Angel food cake with whipped cream and strawberries

   Which of the foods can Justin eat, and which must he avoid? Why? Can he eat certain parts of any of the foods? If so, which ones, and why?

5. Susan Smith has developed hypertension and has been placed on a mild sodium-restricted diet. She has planned the following dinner for her daughter's graduation party.
   - Fresh fruit cup
   - Baked ham
   - Potato chips
   - Fresh frozen broccoli chunks baked in canned cream of chicken soup
   - Homemade coleslaw
   - Rolls and butter
   - Dill pickles and olives
   - Chocolate cake with peppermint ice cream

   Which of the foods can she eat, and which must she avoid? Explain.

REVIEW

Multiple choice. Select the *letter* that precedes the best answer.

1. Metabolic syndrome has the following risk factors except
   a. abdominal obesity
   b. high blood pressure
   c. anemia
   d. insulin resistance

2. Sodium is commonly found in
   a. sugar
   b. fresh fruits
   c. baking soda and baking powder
   d. coffee and tea

3. A client with angina pectoris might be advised to follow a diet
   a. that contains limited sodium
   b. in which the calories are increased
   c. containing minimum amounts of proteins
   d. in which saturated fats are limited

4. Herbs, spices, and flavorings may
   a. be used in sodium-restricted diets
   b. never be used in sodium-restricted diets
   c. increase sodium in the diet
   d. be used only in the mild sodium-restricted diet

5. A sodium-restricted diet may be ordered for clients with
   a. mitral valve prolapse
   b. lipidemia
   c. congestive heart failure
   d. atherosclerosis

6. When water accumulates in body tissues
   a. the condition is called edema
   b. a fat-restricted diet may be prescribed
   c. it is a definite symptom of myocardial infarction
   d. salt is completely eliminated from the diet

7. It is thought that excessive fats in the blood over time contribute to
   a. congestive heart failure
   b. hypokalemia
   c. plaque
   d. edema

8. Table salt
   a. is 60% sodium
   b. is over 40% sodium
   c. contains only negligible amounts of sodium
   d. must be restricted in fat-restricted diets

9. In a low-cholesterol diet
   a. eggs are used freely
   b. vegetable oils are not permitted
   c. organ meats are permitted
   d. fat-free milk is used instead of whole milk

10. Cholesterol
    a. is found in food and in body tissue
    b. has no connection to lipoproteins
    c. is the primary cause of congestive heart failure
    d. is commonly found in fruits and vegetables

11. Foods allowed in a low-fat diet include
    a. cheese
    b. cooked vegetables
    c. sausage
    d. all soups

12. When preparing foods for the low-fat diet,
    a. small amounts of fat can be added
    b. visible fats must be removed from meats
    c. fat-free milk is never used
    d. butter is substituted for vegetable oil

13. On the low-cholesterol diet, saturated fats are
    a. reduced
    b. eliminated
    c. increased
    d. unchanged from the amount in the regular diet

14. Saturated fats are usually
    a. solid at room temperature
    b. liquid at room temperature
    c. found in fruits
    d. derived from plants

15. Polyunsaturated fats are usually
    a. solid at room temperature
    b. found in animal foods
    c. liquid at room temperature
    d. derived from dairy products

16. When the heart muscle reacts with pain because of inadequate blood supply after activity, the condition is called
    a. cerebral accident
    b. edema
    c. hypertension
    d. angina pectoris

17. Some examples of blood lipids are
    a. triglycerides
    b. polyunsaturated fats
    c. sterols
    d. plaques

18. Examples of foods particularly rich in potassium are
    a. milk and ice cream
    b. beef and lamb
    c. whole-grain breads and cereals
    d. bananas and oranges

Case In Point

AYVION: CONGESTIVE HEART FAILURE

Ayvion is a manager for a large electronics distributor. He has been working long hours in preparation for the holiday season. For the past few days, he has noticed some tightening in his chest. Thinking it was indigestion, Ayvion started an over-the-counter antacid. The antacid has not provided him with much relief and today the pain seems to be radiating down his left arm. He also seems to be having difficulty catching his breath and is extremely tired. When he gets home from work, Ayvion is having so much trouble breathing, he asks his wife to take him to the emergency room.

When he arrives at the hospital, the doctor orders nasal oxygen and a series of blood tests for Ayvion, and admits him to the telemetry unit for further monitoring and assessment. The admitting nurse learns from Ayvion that his father suffered his first heart attack at age 36. Ayvion is currently 47 years old, 5 feet 10 inches tall, and weighs 215 pounds. His current blood pressure is 208/98. The nurse knows that Ayvion's family history, age, weight, and African

American ethnicity put him at risk for heart disease. Ayvion's blood work reveals an elevated cholesterol and LDL. It also shows that Ayvion has indeed suffered a minor heart attack. The doctor tells Ayvion he has some damage to his heart that would indicate he has had a previous heart attack that went undetected. The doctor tells Ayvion he is going to survive, but he needs to make some changes. His current problems coupled by his previous heart attack have caused him to develop a condition known as congestive heart failure. He tells Ayvion that his heart is weakened by the damage and cannot pump as strongly as it used to. As a result, Ayvion has fluid in his lungs causing the shortness of breath and the fatigue. The doctor orders medications to lower both his blood pressure and cholesterol. He orders diuretics to help control the fluid overload. He also refers Ayvion to a cardiac rehabilitation program in order to learn how to eat properly and exercise safely. Ayvion knows he needs to follow the doctor's recommendations. However, he is worried that his time away from work will cost him his job.

ASSESSMENT

1. What subjective data do you have about Ayvion and his health?
2. What objective data do you have?
3. How significant is his problem?
4. What are the potential consequences if Ayvion ignores his doctor's advice?

DIAGNOSIS

5. Write a diagnostic statement about Ayvion's lack of knowledge regarding his cardiac condition and his new diet.
6. What education is needed to help achieve improvement in his health?

PLAN/GOAL

7. What are several reasonable goals for Ayvion?

IMPLEMENTATION

8. What issues must Ayvion begin to comply with regarding his new diet?

9. What cardiac topics does Ayvion need to learn to understand his new diet?
10. What two food categories can Ayvion use that have almost no restriction in his new diet?
11. What other problems may Ayvion be at risk for?
12. How could the information at the American Heart Association website (http://www.americanheart.org) be helpful to Ayvion?

EVALUATION/OUTCOME CRITERIA

13. If diet and exercise are successful, what changes will be measurable in 3–6 months?
14. What will the dietitian be able to assess in an interview with Ayvion?

FURTHER THINKING

15. What are the possible consequences of noncompliance for Ayvion?

rate this **plate**

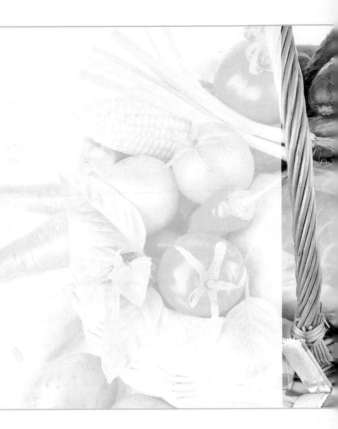

Ayvion attended the cardiac rehabilitation program with support from his wife, to learn about the importance of regular exercise, maintaining a healthy weight, and consuming meals that are low in cholesterol and sodium. Ayvion has decided to plan his meals on a weekly basis and to try and include meat, vegetables, fruits, and milk at every meal. Here is one of the meals he plans to prepare for dinner:

7 oz. baked chicken breast in cream of broccoli soup

1 cup white rice with juices from the broccoli soup as dressing

1 cup of green beans with bacon bits

2 biscuits with butter

½ cup peaches and pears

8 oz. 2%-milk

What foods are high in cholesterol and/or sodium if any? Has Ayvion chosen the right portions and calories for weight loss? If not what should be changed?

Case In Point

NANCY: ADHERING TO A CARDIAC DIET

Nancy is a 62-year-old retired paralegal. The year before she retired she had several episodes of angina in which she thought she was having a heart attack. One of the episodes was so severe, her coworker called EMS. During her hospital visit, the doctor encouraged Nancy to attend a smoking cessation program and to meet with a dietitian to learn about a diet that was low in sodium and cholesterol. Nancy did quit smoking, but found the diet more difficult to adhere to than she imagined.

After she retired, she was attending her grandson's basketball game when she suffered a similar event. This time it was an actual heart attack. Nancy was taken to the hospital and a cardiac catheterization was performed. It was noted that there was a significant amount of blockage. The doctor felt it was necessary to perform surgery immediately. Nancy underwent quadruple bypass.

The doctor requested the hospital dietitian review Nancy's nutritional habits again. When the dietitian asks Nancy about her diet history she admits some changes need to be made. Since Nancy retired she has been able to cook breakfast instead of eating on the run. Her typical breakfast has been sausage or bacon and cheesy eggs. She has never been a coffee drinker so her breakfast caffeine is a diet cola. For lunch her favorite meal is a chicken salad croissant and potato chips. Supper is usually meat and potatoes with gravy. She will include a vegetable with supper, but typically purchases canned vegetables to save money. Once in a while for variety she will bake the vegetables in cheese. Throughout the course of the day her main beverage is typically diet cola.

ASSESSMENT

1. What do you know about Nancy's health?
2. How significant is her health problem?
3. What would the consequences be if Nancy decided to ignore the doctor's advice?
4. What do you know about Nancy's willingness to comply?
5. List all the foods Nancy ate that contained sodium or are usually restricted on a low-sodium diet.
6. List the foods Nancy likes to eat that are high in fat.

DIAGNOSIS

7. Write a diagnostic statement based on Nancy's condition.
8. What does Nancy need to understand about CHF and low-sodium diets?
9. Why does Nancy continue to retain fluid?

PLAN/GOAL

10. What are reasonable, measurable goals for Nancy?

IMPLEMENTATION

11. What are the main topics to teach Nancy about her diet?
12. Modify Nancy's food choices to reflect a low-sodium diet.
13. What food categories can Nancy eat without restrictions?
14. What else does Nancy need in order to control the edema?

EVALUATION/OUTCOME CRITERIA

15. At her 2-week doctor's appointment, what changes can the doctor observe and measure as evidence of the effectiveness of the diet?

THINKING FURTHER

16. Can this disease be cured?
17. Why is managing the disease a constant challenge?

rate this plate

Nancy enjoys preparing meals at home. She is trying to decrease her sodium and fat intake as the registered dietitian instructed. Nancy used a slow-cooker to make the following meal. Rate this plate:

4 oz. beef roast made with cream of mushroom soup and dry onion soup mix

3 oz. cooked potatoes and carrots

1 cup of salad greens with diced tomatoes, cucumbers, cheese, and croutons

2 Tbsp low-fat salad dressing

1 dinner roll with butter

12 oz. diet soda

What changes would you make to her meal, if any? Is she eating according to her sodium restrictions? What do you think about her portion control?

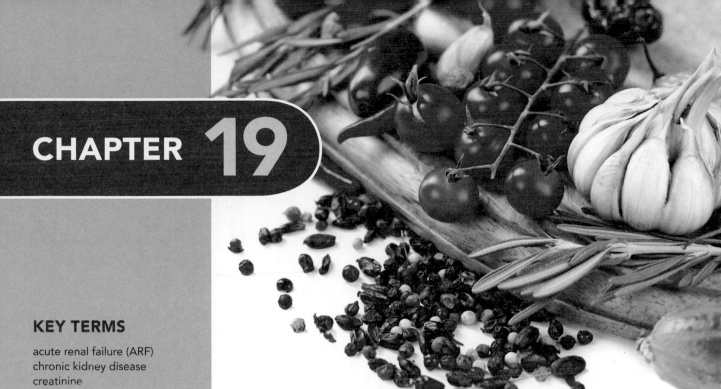

CHAPTER 19

DIET AND RENAL DISEASE

OBJECTIVES

After studying this chapter, you should be able to:

- Describe, in general terms, the work of the kidneys
- Discuss common causes of renal disease
- Explain why protein is restricted for renal clients
- Explain why sodium and water are sometimes restricted for renal clients
- Explain why potassium and phosphorus are sometimes restricted for renal clients

The kidneys are intricate and efficient processing systems that excrete wastes, maintain volume and composition of body fluids, and secrete certain hormones. To accomplish these tasks, they filter the blood, cleansing it of waste products, and recycle other, usable, substances so that the necessary constituents of body fluids are constantly available (Figure 19-1).

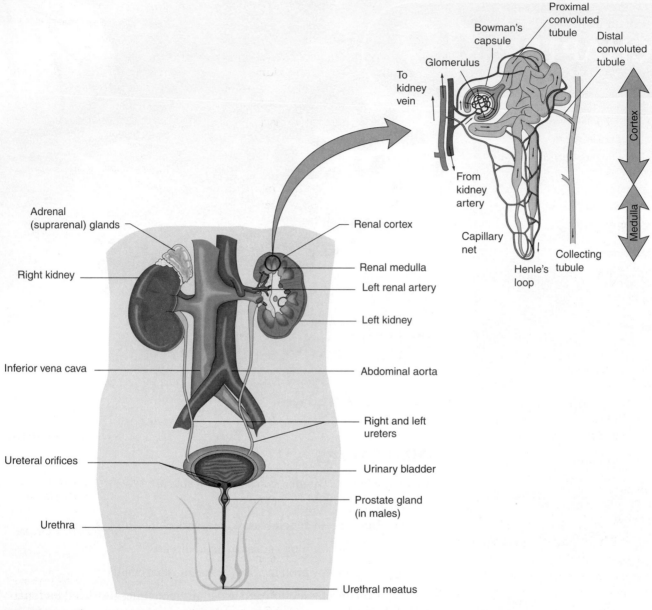

FIGURE 19-1 The urinary system with inset of a nephron.

nephrons
unit of the kidney containing a
glomerulus

glomerulus
filtering unit in the kidneys

ureters
tubes leading from the kidneys to the
bladder

Each kidney contains approximately 1 million working parts called **nephrons**. Each nephron contains a filtering unit, called a **glomerulus**, in which there is a cluster of specialized capillaries (tiny blood vessels connecting veins and arteries). Approximately 180 liters of ultrafiltrate is processed each day. As the filtrate passes through the nephrons, it is concentrated or diluted to meet the body's needs. In this way, the kidneys help maintain both the composition and the volume of body fluids and, consequently, they maintain fluid balance, acid–base balance, and electrolyte balance.

The liquid waste is sent via two tubes called **ureters** from the kidneys to the urinary bladder, from which they are excreted in approximately

1.5 liters of urine per day. These waste materials include end products of protein metabolism (**urea**, **uric acid**, **creatinine**, ammonia, and sulfates), excess water and nutrients, dead renal cells, and toxic substances. When the urinary output is less than 500 ml/day, it is impossible for all the daily wastes to be eliminated. This condition is called **oliguria**. When the kidneys are unable to adequately eliminate nitrogenous waste (end products of protein metabolism), renal failure can result. The recycled materials are reabsorbed (taken back) by the blood. They include amino acids, glucose, minerals, vitamins, and water.

The kidneys synthesize and secrete certain hormones as needed. For example, it is the kidneys that make the final conversion of vitamin D. Active vitamin D promotes the absorption of calcium and the metabolism of calcium and phosphorus. The kidneys indirectly stimulate bone marrow to reproduce red blood cells by producing the hormone erythropoietin.

urea
chief nitrogenous waste product of protein metabolism

uric acid
one of the nitrogenous waste products of protein metabolism

creatinine
an end (waste) product of protein metabolism

oliguria
decreased output of urine to less than 500 ml/day

RENAL DISEASES
Etiology of Renal Disease

Kidney disorders can be initially caused by infection, degenerative changes, diabetes mellitus, high blood pressure, **cysts**, **renal stones**, or trauma (surgery, burns, poisons). When these conditions are severe, renal failure may develop. It may be acute or chronic. **Acute renal failure (ARF)** occurs suddenly and may last a few days or a few weeks. It can be caused by another medical problem such as a serious burn, a crushing injury, or cardiac arrest. It can be expected in some of these situations, so preventive steps should be taken.

cysts
growths

renal stones
kidney stones

acute renal failure (ARF)
suddenly occurring failure of the kidneys

Classification of Renal Disease

Chronic kidney disease develops slowly, causing the number of functioning nephrons to diminish. When renal tissue has been destroyed to a point at which the kidneys are no longer able to filter the blood, excrete wastes, or recycle nutrients as needed, uremia occurs. **Uremia** is a condition in which protein wastes that should normally have been excreted are instead circulating in the blood. Symptoms include nausea, headache, convulsions, and coma. Severe renal failure can result in death unless **dialysis** is begun or a kidney transplant is performed.

Nephritis is a general term referring to the inflammatory diseases of the kidneys. Nephritis can be caused by infection, degenerative processes, or vascular disease.

Glomerulonephritis is an inflammation affecting the capillaries in the glomeruli. It may occur acutely in conjunction with another infection and be self-limiting, or it may lead to serious renal deterioration.

Nephrosclerosis is the hardening of renal arteries. It is caused by arteriosclerosis and hypertension. Although it usually occurs in older people, it sometimes develops in young diabetics.

Polycystic kidney disease is a relatively rare, hereditary disease. Cysts form and press on the kidneys. The kidneys enlarge and lose function.

chronic kidney disease
slow development of kidney failure

uremia
condition in which protein wastes are circulating in the blood

dialysis
mechanical filtration of the blood; used when the kidneys are no longer able to perform normally

nephritis
inflammatory disease of the kidneys

glomerulonephritis
inflammation of the glomeruli of the kidneys

nephrosclerosis
hardening of renal arteries

polycystic kidney disease
rare, hereditary kidney disease causing cysts or growths on the kidneys that can ultimately cause kidney failure in middle age

nephrolithiasis
development of stones in the kidney

cystine
a nonessential amino acid

EXPLORING
THE WEB

Choose one of the renal disorders discussed and thoroughly research the disorder using the Internet. Investigate the causes of the disorder, the presenting signs and symptoms of the disorder, how the disorder is diagnosed, and the treatment choices for the disorder. What role does nutrition play in the prevention, cause, or treatment of the disorder?

Supersize USA

A 23-year-old African American lost the use of his kidneys due to high blood pressure over time. After stabilizing his blood pressure, he began dialysis treatments three times a week and received a renal diet. He also was placed on a kidney transplant list. No matter what your age, you should be checked periodically for high blood pressure, especially if you are obese. A low-sodium, high-potassium diet can help prevent high blood pressure in some people. Prevention is the best way to stay healthy. Start now and improve your health through eating fruits and vegetables and including 30 minutes of exercise per day.

glomerular filtration rate (GFR)
the rate at which the kidneys filter the blood

Although people with this condition have normal kidney function for many years, renal failure may develop near the age of 50.

Nephrolithiasis is a condition in which stones develop in the kidneys. The size of the stones varies from that of a grain of sand to much larger. Some remain at their point of origin, whereas others move. Although the condition is sometimes asymptomatic, symptoms include hematuria (blood in the urine), infection, obstruction, and, if the stones move, intense pain. The stones are classified according to their composition—calcium oxalate, uric acid, **cystine**, calcium phosphate, and magnesium ammonium phosphate (known as struvite). They are associated with metabolic disturbances and immobilization of the client.

SPECIAL CONSIDERATIONS FOR CLIENTS WITH RENAL DISEASES
Dietary Treatment of Renal Disease

Dietary treatment is intended to slow the buildup of waste in the bloodstream. Decreasing waste in the bloodstream will control symptoms of fluid retention, hyperkalemia, and nausea and vomiting. The goal is to reduce the amount of excretory work demanded of the kidneys while helping them maintain fluid, acid–base, and electrolyte balance. While sufficient protein is required to prevent malnutrition and muscle wasting, too much protein can contribute to uremia. Typically, one with chronic renal failure will have protein and sodium, and possibly potassium and phosphorus, restricted.

It is essential that renal clients receive sufficient calories (25–50 calories per kilogram of body weight) unless they are overweight. Energy requirements should be fulfilled by carbohydrates and fat. The fats must be unsaturated to prevent or check hyperlipidemia. If the energy requirement is not met by carbohydrates and fat, ingested protein or body tissue will be metabolized for energy. Either would increase the work of the kidneys because protein increases the amount of nitrogen waste the kidneys must handle. The diet may limit protein to as little as 40 grams for predialysis clients. The specific amount of protein allowed is calculated according to the client's **glomerular filtration rate (GFR)** and weight.

Fluids and sodium may be limited to prevent edema, hypertension, and congestive heart failure. Calcium supplements may be prescribed. In addition, vitamin D may be added and phosphorus limited to prevent osteomalacia (softening of the bones due to excessive loss of calcium). Phosphorus appears to be retained in clients with kidney disorders, and a disproportionately high ratio of phosphorus to calcium tends to increase calcium loss from bones.

Potassium may be restricted in some clients because hyperkalemia tends to occur in **end-stage renal disease (ESRD)**. Excess potassium can cause cardiac arrest. Because of this danger, renal clients should not use salt substitutes or low-sodium milk because the sodium in these products is replaced with potassium. Potassium restriction can be especially difficult. Potassium is particularly high in fruits—one of the few foods someone on a sodium-restricted diet may eat without concern.

Renal clients often have an increased need for vitamins B, C, and D, and supplements are often given. Vitamin A should not be given because the blood level of vitamin A tends to be elevated in uremia. If a client is receiving antibiotics, a vitamin K supplement may be given. Otherwise, supplements of vitamins E and K are not necessary. Iron is commonly prescribed because anemia frequently develops. It is sometimes necessary to increase the amount of simple carbohydrates and unsaturated fats to ensure sufficient calories.

Dialysis

Dialysis is done by either **hemodialysis** or **peritoneal dialysis**. The most common is hemodialysis. Hemodialysis requires permanent access to the bloodstream through a fistula. Fistulas are unusual openings between two organs. They are often created near the wrist and connect an artery and a vein. Hemodialysis is done three times a week for approximately 3–5 hours each visit (Figure 19-2).

Peritoneal dialysis uses the peritoneal cavity as a semipermeable membrane and is less efficient than hemodialysis. Treatments usually last about 10–12 hours a day, three times a week (Figure 19-3). Some clients also use continuous ambulatory peritoneal dialysis (CAPD). The dialysis fluid is exchanged four or five times daily, making this a 24-hour treatment. Clients on CAPD have a more normal lifestyle than do clients on either hemodialysis or

 end-stage renal disease (ESRD)
the stage at which the kidneys have lost most or all of their ability to function

 hemodialysis
cleansing the blood of wastes by circulating the blood through a machine that contains tubing of semipermeable membranes

 peritoneal dialysis
removal of waste products from the blood by injecting the flushing solution into the abdomen and using the client's peritoneum as the semipermeable membrane

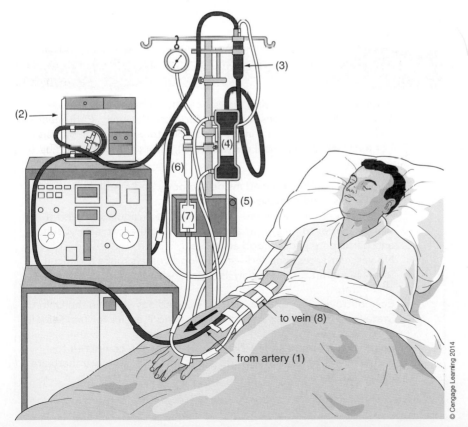

to vein (8)

from artery (1)

© Cengage Learning 2014

FIGURE 19-2 Hemodialysis. (1) Blood leaves the body via an artery. (2) Arterial blood passes through the blood pump. (3) Blood is filtered to remove any clots. (4) Blood passes through the dialyzer. (5) Blood passes into the venous blood line. (6) Blood is filtered to remove any clots. (7) Blood flows through the air detector. (8) Blood returns to the client through the venous blood line.

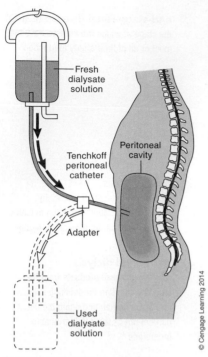

Fresh dialysate solution

Tenchkoff peritoneal catheter

Peritoneal cavity

Adapter

Used dialysate solution

© Cengage Learning 2014

FIGURE 19-3 Peritoneal dialysis.

peritoneal dialysis. Some complications associated with CAPD include peritonitis, hypotension, and weight gain.

Diet During Dialysis

Dialysis clients may need additional protein, but the amount must be carefully controlled to prevent the accumulation of protein waste between treatments.

A client on hemodialysis requires 1.0–1.2 grams of protein per kilogram of body weight to make up for losses during dialysis. A client on peritoneal dialysis will require 1.2–1.5 grams of protein per kilogram of body weight. The protein needs for clients on CAPD are 1.2 grams per kilogram of body weight. Seventy-five percent of this protein should be high biological value (HBV) protein, which is found in eggs, meat, fish, poultry, milk, and cheese.

Potassium is usually restricted for dialysis clients. Healthy people ingest 2,000–6,000 mg per day. The daily intake allowed clients in renal failure is 3,000–4,000 mg. End-stage renal disease further reduces intake allowed to 1,500–2,500 mg per day. The physician will prescribe the milligrams of potassium needed by the client. Table 19-1 lists fruits and vegetables that are low, medium, and high in potassium.

Clients are taught to regulate their intake by making careful choices. Milk is normally restricted to 1/2 cup a day because it is high in potassium and high in methionine, an essential amino acid. A typical renal diet could be written as "80-3-3" which means 80 grams of protein, 3 grams of sodium, and 3 grams of potassium a day. There may be a phosphorus restriction; and

---

SPOTLIGHT *on Life Cycle*

For school-age children, receiving dialysis can be a challenge; however, there are home dialysis options that allow for more flexibility. Peritoneal dialysis (PD), whether through continuous ambulatory peritoneal dialysis (CAPD) or automated peritoneal dialysis (APD), offers many advantages to children:

- Pain free—blood is cleaned inside the body and needles are not required as in hemodialysis.
- Flexible treatment schedule—children are not required to visit a dialysis center to receive treatment, allowing them to attend school and participate in childhood activities.
- No vascular access needed—small blood vessels make it difficult to place a graft for hemodialysis; smaller-sized catheters work well in children.
- Ease of travel—PD supplies can be shipped anywhere in the United States and PD devices are portable, making it easier for families with children receiving treatment to travel together.
- Fewer dietary restrictions—PD is done every day compared to hemodialysis which is done three times a week, therefore there are less restrictions.

(Source: Adapted from DaVita. *Can Children Do Peritoneal Dialysis?* 2012. www.davita.com)

TABLE 19-1 Potassium Content of Selected Fruits and Vegetables

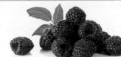

LOW POTASSIUM (<150 MG/SERVING*)	MEDIUM POTASSIUM (150–250 MG/SERVING*)	HIGH POTASSIUM (>250 MG/SERVING*)
Applesauce	Apple juice	Avocado, ½ fruit
Berries: blackberries, blueberries, boysenberries, gooseberries, raspberries, strawberries	Apple, raw, 1 large	Banana, ½ fruit
	Apricots, raw, 2 medium, canned	Dried fruits: figs, apricots, dates, prunes, raisins
Cranberry sauce	Cherries, raw (15) or canned	Kiwifruit
Grape juice	Grapefruit juice	Melons: cantaloupe, ¼ medium; casaba, ¾ cubed; honeydew, ⅛ medium; watermelon, 2 cups, cubed
Grapes, canned or raw	Grapefruit sections	
Lemon or lime, 1 medium	Mango	
Mandarin oranges, canned	Peach, raw, 1 medium	Nectarine, 1 medium
Peaches, canned	Pear, raw, 1 medium	Orange, navel
Pears, canned	Pineapple juice, raw or canned	Orange juice, fresh, frozen, canned
Plums, canned	Pineapple spears	Papaya
Rhubarb	Plums, raw, 2 medium	Prune juice, canned or bottled
	Tangerine	Raisins, seedless
		Tangelo
Bamboo shoots	Asparagus	Artichoke
Bean sprouts	Beets	Beet greens
Beans, green, wax, snap	Brussels sprouts	Dried beans and peas: kidney, lima, garbanzo, navy, and pinto beans; blackeyed peas
Broccoli	Carrots, cooked	
Cabbage	Celery	
Cauliflower	Greens: collard, mustard, kale, dandelion, beet, turnip greens	Potato, ½ cup baked, boiled, or fried
Corn, canned or small ear		Pumpkin
Cucumber	Mixed vegetables	Spinach
Eggplant, cooked	Okra	Sweet potato or yams
Hominy grits, cooked	Peas, green	Tomato, raw or canned
Leek	Peppers	Unsalted tomato juice
Lettuce: cos, romaine, iceberg, leaf, endive, watercress (1 cup shredded)	Summer squash: yellow crookneck, white scallop, zucchini	Winter squash: acorn, butternut, hubbard, spaghetti
Mushrooms		
Onion: green, red, yellow, white		
Peppers, sweet or hot		
Radishes, raw		
Rutabaga		
Summer squash		
Turnips		
Water chestnuts, canned		

*All portions are ½ cup unless otherwise noted.

there is often a need for supplements of water-soluble vitamins, vitamin D, calcium, and iron.

The ability of the kidney to handle sodium and water in ESRD must be assessed often. Usually, the diet contains 3 grams of sodium, which is the equivalent of a no-added-salt diet. Sodium and fluid needs may increase with perspiration, vomiting, fever, and diarrhea. The fluid content of foods, other than liquids, is not counted in fluid restriction. Clients on fluid restriction must be taught to measure their fluid intake and urine output, examine their ankles for edema, and weigh themselves regularly.

Diet After Kidney Transplant

After kidney transplant, there may be a need for extra protein or for the restriction of protein. Carbohydrates and sodium may be restricted. The appropriate amounts of these nutrients will depend largely on the medications given at that time.

Additional calcium and phosphorus may be necessary if there was substantial bone loss before the transplant. There may be an increase in appetite after transplants. Fats and simple carbohydrates may be limited to prevent excessive weight gain.

Dietary Treatment of Renal Stones

Because the causes of renal stones have not been confirmed, treatment of them may vary. In general, however, large amounts of fluid—at least half of it water—are helpful in diluting the urine, as is a well-balanced diet. Once the stones have been analyzed, specific diet modifications may be indicated.

Calcium Oxalate Stones

About 80% of the renal stones formed contain calcium oxalate. Recent studies provide no support for the theory that a diet low in calcium can reduce the risk of calcium oxalate renal stones. In fact, higher dietary calcium intake may decrease the incidence of renal stones for most people. Dietary intake of excessive animal protein has been shown to be a risk factor for stone formation in some clients.

Stones containing oxalate are thought to be partially caused by a diet especially rich in oxalate, which is found in beets, wheat bran, chocolate, tea, rhubarb, strawberries, and spinach (Table 19-2). Evidence also indicates that deficiencies of pyridoxine, thiamine, and magnesium may contribute to the formation of oxalate renal stones.

Uric Acid Stones

purines
end products of nucleoprotein metabolism

When the stones contain uric acid, purine-rich foods are restricted. **Purines** are the end products of nucleoprotein metabolism and are found in all meats, fish, and poultry. Organ meats, anchovies, sardines, meat extracts, excessive alcohol, and broths are especially rich sources of purines. Uric acid stones are usually associated with gout, GI diseases that cause diarrhea, and malignant disease. Medication will prevent gout and other complications by decreasing the formation of uric acid.

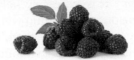

TABLE 19-2 Foods High in Oxalates

FOODS HIGH IN OXALATES

Beets	Soy milk
Black tea and instant tea	Spinach
Chocolate	Sweet potatoes
Dried beans (black, navy, or Great Northern)	Tree nuts (almonds, cashews, hazelnuts)
Peanuts	Wheat bran
Rhubarb	Wheat germ
Soy beans	

© Cengage Learning 2014

In The Media

Kidney Disease Affecting African Americans

African Americans are at an increased risk for kidney disease and failure due to higher rates of diabetes, high blood pressure, and heart disease. African Americans tend to develop kidney failure at an earlier age than white Americans; with the mean age being 56 years. Death rates from high blood pressure and diabetes are on the rise, with diabetes being the leading cause of kidney failure in African Americans. They experience kidney failure about four times more often than white Americans with diabetes. African Americans need to be aware of possible risk factors and visit their doctor regularly to protect against kidney disease.

(Source: Adapted from National Kidney Foundation. Ten Facts About African Americans and Kidney Disease. December 2009. www.kidney.org)

Cystine Stones

Cystine is an amino acid. Cystine stones may form when the cystine concentration in the urine becomes excessive because of a hereditary metabolic disorder. The usual practice is to increase fluids and recommend an alkaline-ash diet.

Struvite Stones

Struvite stones are composed of magnesium ammonium phosphate. They are sometimes called infection stones because they develop following urinary tract infections caused by certain microorganisms. A low-phosphorus diet is often prescribed.

HEALTH AND NUTRITION CONSIDERATIONS

The client with renal disease has a lifelong challenge. Anger and depression are common among these clients. These feelings complicate management of the disease if they contribute to the client's unwillingness to learn about his or her nutritional needs. These complications then add to the client's problems.

It is extremely helpful for the health care professional to develop a trusting relationship with the client. Such a relationship can be established by listening to the client's complaints, needs, and concerns and responding with sincere understanding and sympathy. This approach can help motivate the client to learn how to manage his or her nutritional requirements with assistance from the dietitian.

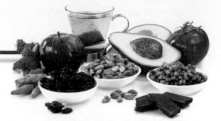

SUMMARY

The kidneys rid the body of liquid wastes; maintain fluid, electrolyte, and acid–base balance; and secrete hormones. When they are damaged by disease or injury, the entire body is affected. Diet therapy for renal disorders can be extremely complex because of the multifaceted nature of the kidneys' functions. Untreated severe kidney disease can result in death unless dialysis or kidney transplant is undertaken.

DISCUSSION TOPICS

1. Discuss the three main tasks of the kidneys.
2. Define nephrons and explain what they do.
3. Discuss some causes of kidney disease.
4. What is nephritis? Glomerulonephritis? Nephrosclerosis?
5. Why is diet therapy for renal disease so complex?
6. Discuss why protein is typically decreased for clients with renal disease.
7. Why are sodium and water sometimes restricted in renal disease?
8. Why is potassium sometimes restricted in renal disease? What is hyperkalemia?
9. Why is phosphorus sometimes restricted in renal disease?
10. Why might calories be restricted in renal disease?
11. What is nephrolithiasis? How is it treated?

SUGGESTED ACTIVITIES

1. Invite a renal educator or dietitian to discuss renal disease with your class.
2. Invite a dialysis client to discuss her or his condition and reactions to dialysis.
3. Using outside sources, prepare a short report on the functions of the circulatory system, the liver, and the kidneys in eliminating nitrogenous waste products from the body.
4. Record your dietary intake for 24 hours. Analyze your choices to see which ones have the highest potassium. (Use Appendix D.)

REVIEW

Multiple choice. Select the *letter* that precedes the best answer.

1. The kidneys maintain the body's
   a. acid–base balance
   b. electrolyte balance
   c. fluid balance
   d. all of these

2. The specialized part within each nephron that actually filters the blood is called the
   a. ureter   c. glomerulus
   b. filter   d. capillary bunch

3. Kidney disorders may be caused by
   a. diabetes   c. burns
   b. infections   d. all of these

4. When renal tissue has been destroyed to a point at which it can no longer filter the blood, which of the following occurs?
   a. nephritis
   b. nephrosclerosis
   c. uremia
   d. nephrolithiasis

5. The general term referring to the inflammatory diseases of the kidneys is
   a. nephritis
   b. nephrosclerosis
   c. uremia
   d. nephrolithiasis

6. The term referring to the hardening of renal arteries is
   a. nephritis
   b. nephrosclerosis
   c. uremia
   d. nephrolithiasis

7. The rare hereditary disease causing cysts to develop on the kidneys is called
   a. nephritis
   b. glomerulonephritis
   c. renal stones
   d. polycystic kidney disease

8. The condition in which stones develop in the kidneys, ureters, or bladder is called
   a. nephritis
   b. nephrolithiasis
   c. polycystic kidney disease
   d. glomerulonephritis

9. Because its nitrogenous wastes contribute to uremia, which nutrient may be restricted in diets of renal clients?
   a. carbohydrate
   b. saturated fat
   c. protein
   d. vitamin A

10. Kidney dialysis
    a. is a means of filtering all protein from the blood
    b. is a means of removing toxic substances from the blood
    c. always requires the client be on a low-protein diet
    d. requires the client to increase his or her sodium intake

11. Sodium and water may be restricted in the diets of renal clients because they
    a. contribute to uremia
    b. increase hypercalcemia
    c. contribute to hyperlipidemia
    d. contribute to fluid retention

12. If osteomalacia occurs in renal clients, which nutrient may be prescribed?
    a. potassium
    b. protein
    c. calcium
    d. phosphorus

13. In a case of hyperkalemia, which nutrient may be restricted?
    a. potassium
    b. protein
    c. calcium
    d. phosphorus

14. Fruits are an especially rich source of
    a. protein
    b. potassium
    c. calcium
    d. phosphorus

15. The vitamins renal clients may have an increased need for are
    a. the water-soluble vitamins
    b. the fat-soluble vitamins
    c. vitamins B, C, and D
    d. vitamins E and A

16. An excess of which nutrient can compound bone loss in renal clients?
    a. phosphorus
    b. carbohydrate
    c. calcium
    d. iron

17. Purine-rich foods include
    a. organ meats and alcohol
    b. dairy foods
    c. vegetables, except corn and lentils
    d. fruits, except cranberries, plums, and prunes

18. An example of nitrogenous waste found in the urine is
    a. ureter
    b. uremia
    c. urea
    d. all of these

19. Which of the following recommendations has been proven to reduce the risk of calcium oxalate stones?
    a. higher whole grain intake
    b. higher dietary calcium intake
    c. increased intake of acetic acid
    d. increased intake of spinach

20. A typical renal diet that could be ordered by the doctor and written by the dietitian is a
    a. 90-2-2 diet
    b. 70-3-2 diet
    c. 80-3-3 diet
    d. 75-3-3 diet

Case In Point

CHARLES: MANAGING DIET AFTER A KIDNEY STONE

Charles is a fourth generation farmer from southern Indiana. He and his wife, Laura, have been married for 42 years. They both were raised on farms and have loved raising their family on a farm as well. At a young age, Charles and his wife learned that to survive as farmers you had to live a very modest lifestyle and let nothing go to waste. Laura is a good cook, and is able to utilize every piece of the farm animals they butcher to provide food for the family. Laura cans the meats, fruits, and vegetables that were grown on the farm so the benefits of the harvest lasts all year long.

Charles is very consistent with his meals. For example, his breakfast always consists of bran flakes with strawberries on top and 2–3 cups of hot tea. As for other meals, he always enjoys a salad along with the main dish. He loves spinach and grew so much of it in the garden that his wife made a spinach salad with beets for supper daily. For dessert, his favorite is rhubarb pie, especially because Laura makes it just like his grandmother's recipe.

One morning, Charles wakes with a sharp, shooting pain in his abdomen. The intense pain radiates completely down his right side. By the time he meets Laura in the kitchen, he is doubled over in pain so severe he can barely move. Laura drives Charles to the emergency room. The doctor assesses Charles and discovers that Charles has a kidney stone. Once Charles is able to pass the urine, the doctor sends it to the lab for analysis. Charles learns that his kidney stone is comprised mainly of calcium oxalate. The doctor informs Charles that these types of stones can be related to a diet that is high in oxalate and animal proteins. The doctor advises Charles and Laura to meet with the hospital dietitian about Charles's diet.

ASSESSMENT

1. What do you know about Charles that put him at risk for kidney stones?
2. What were Charles's symptoms?
3. How will this condition affect Charles for the rest of his life?
4. How significant is this dietary change?

DIAGNOSIS

5. What is the cause of calcium oxalate stones?
6. Complete the following diagnostic statement: Charles's deficient knowledge is related to _____.

PLAN/GOAL

7. What are reasonable, measurable goals for Charles's change in health?

IMPLEMENTATION

8. What changes does Charles need to make in his diet?
9. What would the consequences be if Charles ignored the doctor's advice?
10. Could Charles have another stone?

EVALUATION/OUTCOME CRITERIA

11. How will the doctor know if the plan is effective?

THINKING FURTHER

12. What could someone else learn from Charles's experience?

rate this plate

During his stay at the hospital, Charles spoke with a registered dietitian about his meal planning concerns. The dietitian told Charles that a diet rich in oxalates can lead to the formation of oxalate kidney stones. Charles provided the dietitian with a 24-hour recall of what he typically ate for lunch. Rate this plate:

5 oz. grilled chicken sandwich on whole-grain bun

2 cups fresh spinach salad with strawberries, pecans, and cheese

2 Tbsp light vinaigrette salad dressing

1 medium orange

1 small slice of rhubarb pie

2 cups hot tea

What foods, if any, are high in oxalates? What nutrient deficiencies are common in clients who experience the formation of oxalate kidney stones? What can Charles include in his diet to hopefully prevent the formation of future kidney stones?

Case In Point

LENA: DISCOVERING GLOMERULONEPHRITIS

Lena is a young mother of two boys. She has never considered herself a very healthy person. It seems she is constantly fighting off infections and colds. As far back as she can remember, people have referred to her as "sickly." Even as a child her strong German mother could not understand why Lena was so pale and weak. After having children of her own, her illnesses continued. Every time the boys caught a cold at school or daycare, Lena was sure to end up with it. She had tried to eat healthy and take a regular multivitamin, but still her body just couldn't fight the infections. Recently, Lena has felt especially run down, and she's been experiencing the need to urinate far more often than before. Her urine, too, appears a little darker than usual. Thinking she may be dehydrated, Lena started drinking a lot of water, but this made matters worse.

This morning her urine was a dark orange color and it even looked a little bubbly, like it was foaming. Her stomach ached and she had no appetite.

Lena assumed she had yet another infection and made an appointment with her doctor for later in the day.

The nurse first gathered data for the doctor. She found Lena's blood pressure to be 148/98. She measured her at 5 feet and 7 inches tall and 133 pounds. After examining Lena, the doctor asked her to have some urine and blood work drawn. Upon reviewing the tests, Lena's doctor diagnosed her with glomerulonephritis. He told her that this was an inflammation of the capillaries in the glomeruli of her kidneys. Most likely this had been caused by an infection. He told Lena that it would be necessary for her to start a blood pressure medication as well as a steroid to reduce the inflammation. He wanted her to begin decreasing the sodium, fluid, and protein she consumed. He told her other treatments might become necessary if her kidneys continue to worsen. He referred her to a registered dietitian to be educated regarding the changes necessary in her meal plan.

ASSESSMENT

1. What is the subjective data you have on Lena?
2. What is the objective data you have on Lena?
3. How will this condition affect Lena?

DIAGNOSIS

4. What is the cause of glomerulonephritis?
5. Write a nursing diagnosis for Lena.

PLAN/GOAL

6. What are reasonable, measurable goals for Lena?

IMPLEMENTATION

7. What changes does Lena need to make in her diet?
8. What would the consequences be if Lena did not follow doctor's advice?

EVALUATION/OUTCOME CRITERIA

9. How will the doctor know if the plan is effective?

THINKING FURTHER

10. What are some of the most effective ways to prevent infections?

rate this **plate**

Lena met with a registered dietitian to discuss her concerns about preparing a healthy meal. The dietitian told Lena not to consume more than 48 oz. of fluids per day to help control her blood pressure and lessen the workload on the kidneys. Sodium and potassium intake would be limited to improve blood pressure control and prevent fluid retention. Protein is also restricted to decrease the workload on the kidneys and prevent waste from building up in the blood. Lena's diet should be rich in complex carbohydrates and "good" fats until her body recovers. Rate the plate prepared for dinner.

4 oz. breaded cod fillet

¾ cup brown rice

½ cup broccoli

½ cup fruit salad containing apples, oranges, and grapes

1 cup chocolate ice cream

20 oz. regular soda

Does this meal meet the recommendations advised by the registered dietitian? If not, what can be improved?

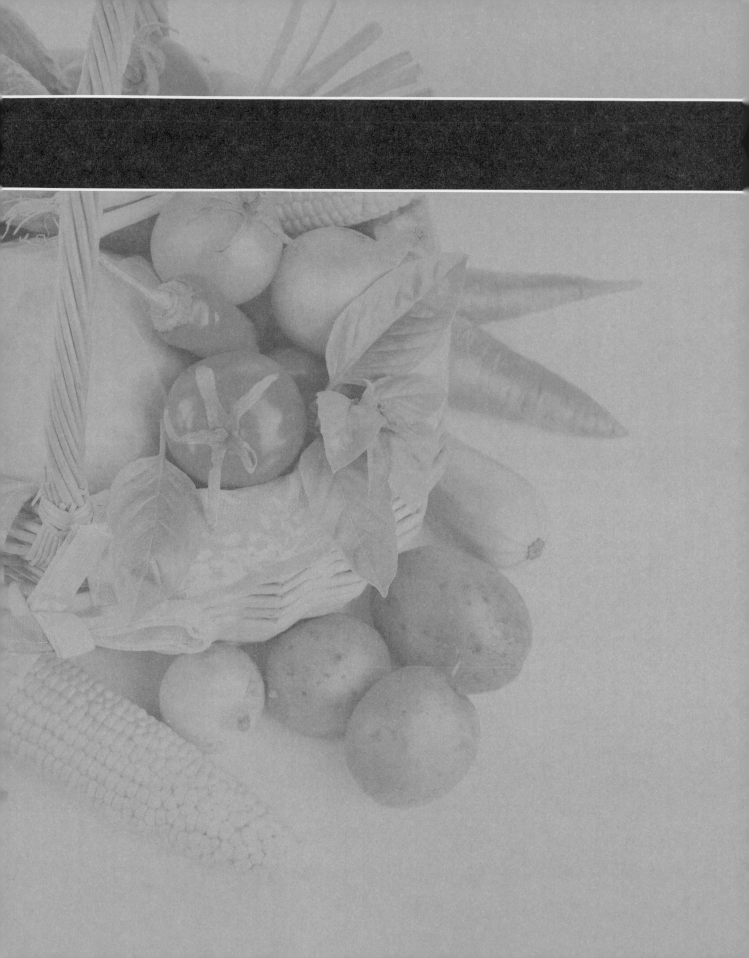

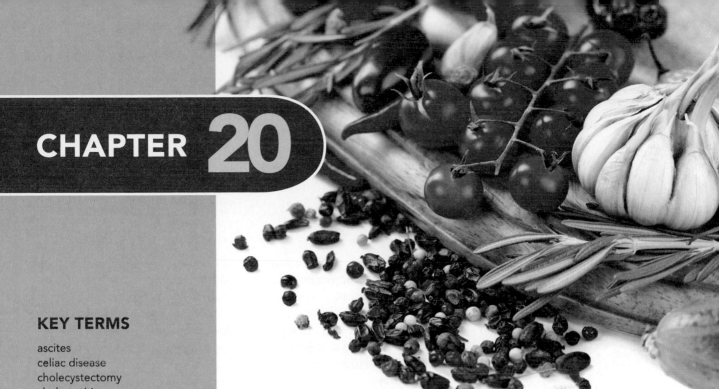

CHAPTER 20

DIET AND GASTROINTESTINAL PROBLEMS

OBJECTIVES

After studying this chapter, you should be able to:

- Explain the uses of diet therapy in gastrointestinal disturbances
- Identify the foods recommended and not recommended in the therapeutic diets discussed
- Adapt normal diets to meet the requirements of clients with these conditions

The gastrointestinal (GI) tract is where digestion and absorption of food occur. The primary organs include the mouth, esophagus, stomach, and small and large intestine. The liver, gallbladder, and pancreas are accessory organs that are also involved in these processes.

Numerous disorders of the gastrointestinal system can make absenteeism from work more prevalent. Some problems are physiologically caused; others can be psychological in origin. It is sometimes difficult to determine the cause(s) of a GI problem. There are numerous treatments and procedures to help identify GI problems and solutions.

DISORDERS OF THE PRIMARY ORGANS
Dyspepsia

dyspepsia
gastrointestinal discomfort of vague origin

Dyspepsia, or indigestion, is a condition of discomfort in the digestive tract that can be physical or psychological in origin. Symptoms include heartburn, bloating, pain, and sometimes regurgitation. If the cause is physical, it can be due to overeating or spicy foods, or it may be a symptom of another problem, such as appendicitis or a kidney, gallbladder, or colon disease or possibly cancer. If the problem is organic in origin, treatment of the underlying cause will be the normal procedure.

Psychological stress can affect stomach secretions and trigger dyspepsia. Treatment should include counseling to help the client:

- Find relief from the underlying stress
- Allow sufficient time to relax and enjoy meals
- Learn to improve eating habits

Esophagitis

esophagitis
inflammation of mucosal lining of the esophagus

gastroesophageal reflux (GER)
backflow of stomach contents into the esophagus

Esophagitis is caused by the irritating effect of acid reflux on the mucosa of the esophagus. Heartburn, regurgitation, and dysphagia (difficulty swallowing) are common symptoms. Acute esophagitis is caused by ingesting an irritating agent, or by **gastroesophageal reflux (GER)**. This can be caused by a hiatal hernia, reduced lower esophageal sphincter (LES) pressure, abdominal pressure, recurrent vomiting, alcohol use, overweight, or smoking. Cancer of the esophagus and silent aspiration may be life-threatening for those with gastroesophageal reflux disease (GERD).

Hiatal Hernia

hiatal hernia
condition wherein part of the stomach protrudes through the diaphragm into the chest cavity

diaphragm
thin membrane or partition

Hiatal hernia is a condition in which a part of the stomach protrudes through the **diaphragm** into the thoracic cavity (Figure 20-1). The hernia prevents the food from moving normally along the digestive tract, although the food does mix somewhat with the gastric juices. Sometimes the food will move back into the esophagus, creating a burning sensation (heartburn), and sometimes food will be regurgitated into the mouth. This condition can be very uncomfortable.

Medical Nutrition Therapy

The symptoms can sometimes be alleviated by serving small, frequent meals (from a well-balanced diet) so that the amount of food in the stomach is never large. Avoid irritants to the esophagus such as carbonated beverages,

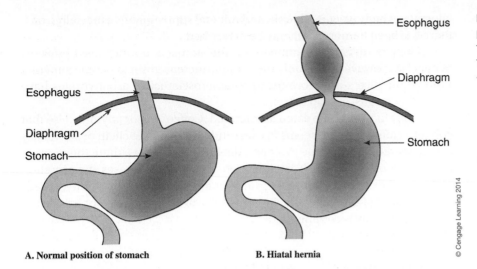

A. Normal position of stomach   B. Hiatal hernia

FIGURE 20-1 A hiatal hernia prevents food from moving through the diaphragm into the thoracic cavity.

chocolate, citrus fruits and juices, tomato products, spicy foods, coffee, pepper, and some herbs. Some foods can cause the lower esophageal sphincter to relax, and these should be avoided. Examples are fatty and fried foods, spicy foods, citrus food, tomato products, onions, chocolate, mint candy, caffeinated beverages, and alcohol. If obesity is present, weight loss may be recommended to reduce pressure on the abdomen. It may also be helpful if clients avoid late-night dinners and lying down for 2–3 hours after eating. When they do lie down, they may be more comfortable sleeping with their heads and upper torso somewhat elevated and wearing loose-fitting clothing. If discomfort cannot be controlled, surgery may be necessary.

Peptic Ulcers

An ulcer is an erosion of the mucous membrane (Figure 20-2). **Peptic ulcers** may occur in the stomach (**gastric ulcer**) or the duodenum (**duodenal ulcer**). The specific cause of ulcers is not clear, but some physicians believe that a number of factors including genetic predisposition, abnormally high secretion of hydrochloric acid by the stomach, stress, excessive use of aspirin or ibuprofen (analgesics), cigarette smoking, and, in some cases, a bacterium called *Helicobacter pylori* may contribute to their development.

A classic symptom is gastric pain, which is sometimes described as burning, and in some cases, hemorrhage is also a symptom. The pain is typically relieved with food or antacids. A hemorrhage usually requires surgery.

Ulcers are generally treated with drugs such as antibiotics and cimetidine. The antibiotics kill the bacteria, and cimetidine inhibits acid secretion in the stomach and thus helps to heal the ulcer. Antacids containing calcium carbonate can also be prescribed to neutralize any excess acid. Stress management may also be beneficial in the treatment of ulcers.

Sufficient low-fat protein should be provided but not in excess because of its ability to stimulate gastric acid secretion. It is recommended that clients receive no less than 0.8 gram of protein per kilogram of body weight. However, if there has been blood loss, protein may be increased to 1–1.5 grams per

peptic ulcers
ulcers of the stomach or duodenum

gastric ulcer
ulcer in the stomach

duodenal ulcer
ulcer occurring in the duodenum

Helicobacter pylori
bacteria that can cause peptic ulcer

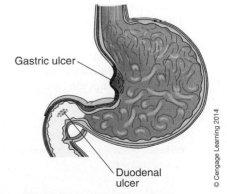

Gastric ulcer

Duodenal ulcer

FIGURE 20-2 Peptic ulcers are erosion of the mucous membrane in the stomach or the duodenum.

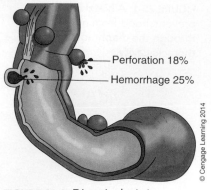

FIGURE 20-3 Diverticulosis is a disorder characterized by little pockets forming in the sides of the large intestine. Rupture of the pockets may result in the need for corrective surgery.

◢ **diverticulosis**
  intestinal disorder characterized by little pockets forming in the sides of the intestines; pockets are called diverticula

◢ **diverticulitis**
  inflammation of the diverticula

◢ **inflammatory bowel diseases (IBDs)**
  chronic condition causing inflammation in the gastrointestinal tract

◢ **ulcerative colitis**
  disease characterized by inflammation and ulceration of the colon, rectum, and sometimes entire large intestine

◢ **Crohn's disease**
  a chronic progressive disorder that causes inflammation, ulcers, and thickening of intestinal walls, sometimes causing obstruction

kilogram of body weight. Vitamin and mineral supplements, especially iron if there has been hemorrhage, may be prescribed.

Since fat delays the emptying of the stomach, an increased intake is beneficial. However, fat is only moderately increased since people suffering from peptic ulcers are more prone to atherosclerosis. Carbohydrates have little effect on gastric acid secretion.

Spicy foods may be eaten as tolerated. Coffee, tea, or anything else that contains caffeine or that seems to cause indigestion in the client or stimulates gastric secretion should be avoided. Alcohol and aspirin irritate the mucous membrane of the stomach, and cigarette smoking decreases the secretion of the pancreas that buffers gastric acid in the duodenum. Currently, a well-balanced diet of three meals a day consisting of foods that do not irritate the client is generally recommended.

Diverticulosis/Diverticulitis

Diverticulosis is an intestinal disorder characterized by little pockets in the sides of the large intestine (colon) (Figure 20-3). When fecal matter collects in these pockets instead of moving on through the colon, bacteria may breed, and inflammation and pain can result, causing **diverticulitis**. If a diverticulum ruptures, surgery may be needed. This condition is thought to be caused by a diet lacking sufficient fiber. A high-fiber diet is commonly recommended for clients with diverticulosis.

Along with antibiotics, diet therapy for diverticulitis may begin with a clear liquid diet, followed by a low-residue diet that allows the bowel to rest and heal. Then a high-fiber diet will be initiated. The bulk provided by the high-fiber diet increases stool volume, reduces the pressure in the colon, and shortens the time the food is in the intestine, giving bacteria less time to grow.

Inflammatory Bowel Disease

Inflammatory bowel diseases (IBDs) are chronic conditions causing inflammation in the gastrointestinal tract. The inflammation causes malabsorption that often leads to malnutrition. The acute phases of these diseases occur at irregular intervals and are followed by periods in which clients are relatively free of symptoms. Neither cause nor cure for these conditions is known.

Two examples are **ulcerative colitis** and **Crohn's disease**. Ulcerative colitis causes inflammation and ulceration of the colon, the rectum, or sometimes the entire large intestine. Crohn's disease, an autoimmune disease, is a chronic progressive disorder that can affect both the small and large intestines. The ulcers can penetrate the entire intestinal wall, and the chronic inflammation can thicken the intestinal wall, causing obstruction.

Both conditions cause bloody diarrhea, cramps, fatigue, nausea, anorexia, malnutrition, and weight loss. Electrolytes, fluids, vitamins, and other minerals are lost in the diarrhea, and the bleeding can cause loss of iron and protein. Clients with Crohn's disease are often thin and may be malnourished due to malabsorption of nutrients. Clients with ulcerative colitis usually experience weight loss related to the severity of the disease.

Treatment may involve anti-inflammatory drugs plus medical nutrition therapy. Usually a low-residue diet is required to avoid irritating the inflamed area and to avoid the danger of obstruction. When tolerated, the diet should include about 100 grams of protein, additional calories, vitamins, and minerals.

In severe cases, **total parenteral nutrition (TPN)** (a process in which nutrients are delivered directly into the superior vena cava; see Chapter 22) may be necessary for a period. As the client begins to regain health, the diet may be increasingly liberalized to suit the client's tastes while maintaining good nutrition.

total parenteral nutrition (TPN)
process of providing all nutrients intravenously

Ileostomy or Colostomy

Clients with severe ulcerative colitis or Crohn's disease frequently require a surgical opening from the body surface to the intestine for the purpose of defecation. The opening that is created is called a **stoma** and is about the size of a nickel. An **ileostomy** (from the ileum to abdomen surface) is required when the entire colon, rectum, and anus must be removed. A **colostomy** (from the colon to abdomen surface) can provide entrance into the colon if the rectum and anus are removed. This can be a temporary or a permanent procedure.

Clients with ileostomies have a greater-than-normal need for salt and water because of excess losses. A vitamin C supplement is recommended and, in some cases, a B_{12} supplement may be needed. Eating a well-balanced individualized diet will prevent a nutritional deficiency for clients with ileostomies and colostomies.

stoma
surgically created opening in the abdominal wall
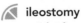
ileostomy
opening from ileum to abdomen surface
colostomy
opening from colon to abdomen surface

Celiac Disease

Celiac disease, also known as **gluten**-sensitive enteropathy or sprue, is a chronic autoimmune disorder caused by intolerance to gluten. Gluten is a protein found in wheat, barley, and rye. Individuals with celiac disease produce antibodies that attack the intestine when they ingest gluten (Figure 20-4).

One third of people carry the genes necessary for celiac disease; however, it appears that unknown environmental factors determine who gets celiac disease or gluten sensitivity and who does not. Symptoms include diarrhea, constipation, weight loss, abdominal cramping and bloating, and malnutrition. Joint pain, anemia, and fatigue are also common findings in individuals who have gluten intolerance, but not all people with celiac disease have symptoms. In children with untreated celiac disease, growth is compromised.

Nearly 1 of 133 Americans suffer from celiac disease according to the latest research from the University of Maryland's Center for Celiac Research. Coming to the forefront is how underdiagnosed gluten intolerance is. In fact, research indicates that celiac disease is twice as common as Crohn's disease, ulcerative colitis, and cystic fibrosis combined.

Specific blood tests, called the "celiac panel," measure immune response to gluten, which must be done prior to the start of a gluten-free diet. A biopsy of the intestine at that stage is also useful for making the diagnosis of

celiac disease
a disorder of the gastrointestinal tract characterized by malabsorption; also called gluten sensitivity

gluten
protein found in grains

FIGURE 20-4 Celiac's damage.

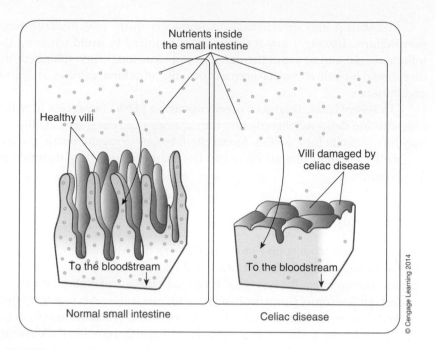

Normal small intestine — Celiac disease

Nutrients inside the small intestine

Healthy villi

Villi damaged by celiac disease

To the bloodstream

To the bloodstream

© Cengage Learning 2014

celiac disease. Some individuals test negative for celiac, but still have some degree of gluten sensitivity. Researchers believe this could be up to 6% of the population. A strict gluten-free diet allows for the intestines to regenerate and heal.

- *Gluten-containing grains to avoid*: barley (including malt extract, beer, and ale), rye, wheat (all types of wheat flour and products made with wheat, bran, germ, starch), spelt, triticale, and farro.

- *Gluten-free grains and starches*: rice, wild rice, millet, amaranth, arrowroot, corn, flax, buckwheat, soy, teff, and flours made from nuts, beans, seeds, potato, tapioca, and sorghum.

Individuals with celiac disease can continue to meet their nutrition needs with naturally gluten-free foods: fruit, vegetables, dairy, eggs, nuts, beans and legumes, oils, butter, margarine, lean meats, and poultry (Table 20-1). When it comes to selecting gluten-free grains, it is recommended that consumers be savvy with choosing the most nutritious high-fiber grains, which include brown rice, wild rice, quinoa, amaranth, buckwheat, gluten-free steel oats, and rice bran. Label reading is important as many gluten-free items sold in stores are made with very refined gluten-free grains with significant added sugars and fats and they may not be fortified. It should be noted that commercially grown oats are contaminated in processing, so individuals must seek out certified gluten-free oats.

At present, if a product contains wheat in any form, it must be stated on the nutrition label. Barley and rye do not have to be listed. Due to increasing incidence of celiac disease, the government is preparing to bring forth regulations for gluten-free food labeling. More and more restaurants are offering gluten-free menu options and are dedicated to preventing cross contamination.

TABLE 20-1 Sample Gluten-Free Menu

BREAKFAST	LUNCH	DINNER
Gluten-free oats	Tuna salad on spinach leaves	Chicken stirfry (gluten-free soy sauce)
Fresh berries	Whole-grain gluten-free crackers with low-fat cheese	Brown rice
Gluten-free bagel with peanut butter	Gluten-free bran muffin	Fruit salad
Milk	Fresh fruit	Milk

SNACKS

Hummus with raw vegetables

Almonds with an apple

© Cengage Learning 2014

In The Media

The Skinny About Gluten-Free Diets

The growing popularity of gluten-free products has led even those without celiac disease to adopt the new diet. Marketing strategies have led people to believe that the gluten-free diet can result in weight loss, improve overall health, and act as a cure for common ailments. However, there is no evidence that replacing a gluten-containing food with a gluten-free food will help someone lose weight. Consuming fewer cakes, cookies, and dinner rolls (products that contain gluten) reduces calorie intake that will lead to weight loss. It is the reduction of calories that yields weight loss, not eliminating gluten from the diet. Gluten-free diets may often be suggested for managing autism, irritable bowel syndrome, and ADHD, but research shows mixed results. The only condition where a totally gluten-free diet is necessary is for celiac sprue disease. Those with gluten sensitivity may benefit from an elimination diet to determine if symptoms can resolve from decreasing gluten intake.

(Source: Adapted from Fontenot, Beth. A Gluten-Free Diet Reality Check. *The Atlantic.* January 3, 2012. http://www.thealtlantic.com)

DISORDERS OF THE ACCESSORY ORGANS
Cirrhosis

The liver is of major importance to, and plays many roles in, metabolism. Except for a few of the fatty acids, all nutrients that are absorbed in the intestines are transported to the liver. The liver dismantles some of these nutrients, stores others, and uses some to synthesize other substances.

The liver determines where amino acids are needed and synthesizes some proteins, enzymes, and urea. It changes the simple sugars to glycogen, provides glucose to body cells, and synthesizes glucose from amino acids, if needed. It converts fats to lipoproteins and synthesizes cholesterol. It stores iron, copper, zinc, and magnesium as well as the fat-soluble vitamins and B vitamins. The liver synthesizes bile and stores it in the gallbladder. It detoxifies many substances such as barbiturates and morphine.

Liver disease may be acute or chronic. Early treatment can usually lead to recovery. **Cirrhosis** is a general term referring to all types of liver disease characterized by cell loss. Alcohol abuse is the most common cause of cirrhosis, but it can also be caused by congenital defects, infections, or other toxic chemicals.

Although the liver does regenerate, the replacement during cirrhosis does not match the loss. In addition to the cell loss during cirrhosis, there is fatty infiltration and **fibrosis**. These developments prevent the liver from functioning normally. Blood flow through the liver is upset, and a form of hypertension, anemia, and hemorrhage in the esophagus can occur. The normal metabolic processes will also be disturbed to such a degree that, in severe cases, death may result.

The dietary treatment of cirrhosis provides at least 25–35 calories or more and 0.8–1.0 gram of protein per kilogram of weight each day, depending on the client's condition. If hepatic coma appears imminent, the lower amount is advocated. Supplements of vitamins and minerals are usually needed. In advanced cirrhosis, 50–60% of the calories should be from carbohydrates.

In some forms of cirrhosis, fat is not tolerated well, so it is restricted. In another form, protein may not be well tolerated, so it is restricted to 35–40 grams a day. Sometimes cirrhosis causes **ascites**. In such a case, sodium and fluids may be restricted. If there is bleeding in the esophagus, fiber can be restricted to prevent irritation of the tissue. Smaller feedings will be better accepted than larger ones. No alcohol is allowed.

Hepatitis

Hepatitis is an inflammation of the liver. It is caused by viruses or toxic agents such as drugs and alcohol. **Necrosis** occurs, and the liver's normal metabolic activities are constricted. Hepatitis may be acute or chronic.

Hepatitis A virus (HAV) is contracted through contaminated drinking water, food, and sewage via a fecal–oral route. Hepatitis B virus (HBV) and hepatitis C virus (HCV) are transmitted through blood, blood products, semen, and saliva. Hepatitis B and C can lead to chronic active hepatitis (CAH), which is diagnosed by liver biopsy. Chronic active hepatitis can lead to liver failure and end-stage liver disease (ESLD).

In mild cases, the cells can be replaced. In severe cases, the damage can be so extensive that the necrosis leads to liver failure and death. There can be bile **stasis** and decreased blood albumin levels. Clients experience nausea, headache, fever, fatigue, tender and enlarged liver, anorexia, and **jaundice**. Weight loss can be pronounced.

Treatment is usually bed rest, plenty of fluids, and medical nutrition therapy. The diet should provide 35–40 calories per kilogram of body weight. Most of the calories should be provided by carbohydrates; there should be moderate amounts of fat and, if the necrosis has not been severe,

---

cirrhosis
generic term for liver disease characterized by cell loss

fibrosis
development of tough, stringy tissue

ascites
abnormal collection of fluid in the abdomen

hepatitis
inflammation of the liver caused by viruses, drugs, or alcohol

necrosis
tissue death due to lack of blood supply

stasis
stoppage or slowing

jaundice
yellow cast of the skin and eyes

up to 70–80 grams of protein for cell regeneration. If the necrosis has been severe and the proteins cannot be properly metabolized, they must be limited to prevent the accumulation of ammonia in the blood. Small frequent meals may be better tolerated for those with liver disease.

Clients with liver disease require a great deal of encouragement because their anorexia and consequent feelings of general malaise can be severe. Their recovery takes patience, rest, and time.

Cholecystitis and Cholelithiasis

The dual function of the gallbladder is the concentration and storage of bile. After bile is formed in the liver, the gallbladder concentrates it to several times its original strength and stores it until needed. Fat in the duodenum triggers the gallbladder to contract and release bile into the common duct for the digestion of fat in the small intestine. If this flow is hindered, there may be pain.

The precise etiology of gallbladder disease is unknown, but heredity factors may be involved. Women develop gallbladder disease more often than men do. Obesity, total parenteral nutrition (TPN), very-low-calorie diets for rapid weight loss, the use of estrogen, and various diseases of the small intestine are frequently associated with gallbladder disease.

Cholecystitis (inflammation) and **cholelithiasis** (gallstones) may inhibit the flow of bile and cause pain. Cholecystitis can cause changes in the gallbladder tissue, which in turn can affect the cholesterol (a constituent of bile), causing it to harden and form stones. It is also thought that chronic overindulgence in fats may contribute to gallstones because the fat stimulates the liver to produce more cholesterol for the bile, which is necessary for the digestion of fat. In addition to pain, which can be severe, there may be indigestion and vomiting, particularly after the ingestion of fatty foods.

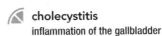

cholecystitis
inflammation of the gallbladder

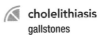

cholelithiasis
gallstones

Treatment may include medication to dissolve the stones and diet therapy. If medication does not succeed, surgery to remove the gallbladder (**cholecystectomy**) may be indicated.

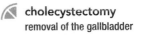

cholecystectomy
removal of the gallbladder

Medical nutrition therapy includes abstinence during the acute phase. This is followed by a clear liquid diet and, gradually, a regular but fat-restricted diet. Amounts of fats allowed run from 40–45 grams per day. In chronic cases, fat may be restricted on a permanent basis. For obese clients, weight loss is recommended in addition to a fat-restricted diet. (For information on fat-restricted diets, see Chapter 18.) Clients with chronic gallbladder conditions may require the water-miscible forms of fat-soluble vitamins.

Pancreatitis

In addition to the hormone insulin, the pancreas produces other hormones and enzymes that are important in the digestion of protein, fats, and carbohydrates. When food reaches the duodenum, the pancreas sends its enzymes to the small intestine to aid in digestion.

Pancreatitis is an inflammation of the pancreas. It may be caused by infections, surgery, alcoholism, biliary tract (includes bile ducts and gallbladder) disease, or certain drugs. It may be acute or chronic.

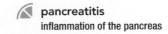

pancreatitis
inflammation of the pancreas

steatorrhea
abnormal amounts of fat in the feces

EXPLORING THE WEB

Choose one of the disorders discussed and thoroughly research it on the Internet. Create a list of the signs and symptoms, the possible causes, and the treatment choices for the disorder. Identify the nutritional needs for a person with this disorder. Can the disorder(s) be controlled through proper nutrition?

Abdominal pain, nausea, and **steatorrhea** are symptoms. Malabsorption (particularly of fat-soluble vitamins) and weight loss occur, and, in cases in which the islets of Langerhans are destroyed, diabetes mellitus may result.

Diet therapy is intended to reduce pancreatic secretions and bile. Just as fat stimulates the gallbladder to secrete bile, protein and hydrochloric acid stimulate the pancreas to secrete its juices and enzymes. During acute pancreatitis, the client is nourished strictly parenterally. Later, when the client can tolerate oral feedings, a liquid diet consisting mainly of carbohydrates is given because, of these three nutrients, carbohydrates have the least stimulatory effect on pancreatic secretions.

As recovery progresses, small, frequent feedings of carbohydrates and protein with little fat or fiber are given. The fat is restricted because of deficiencies of pancreatic lipase. The client is gradually returned to a less-restricted diet as tolerated. Vitamin supplements may be given. Alcohol is forbidden in all cases.

RESIDUE-CONTROLLED DIETS

Fiber is that part of food that is not broken down by digestive enzymes. It is called dietary fiber. Most dietary fiber is found in plant foods. Some is soluble, and some is insoluble (see Chapter 4). Examples of dietary fiber in plants include the outer shells of corn kernels, strings of celery, seeds of strawberries, and the connective tissue of citrus fruits.

Residue is the solid part of feces. Residue is made up of all the undigested and unabsorbed parts of food (including fiber), connective tissue in animal foods, dead cells, and intestinal bacteria and their products. Most of this residue is composed of fiber.

Diets can be adjusted to increase or decrease fiber and residue. The specific names of these diets vary among health care facilities. The specific foods allowed and thus the amount of fiber and residue allowed will depend on the physician's experience and the client's condition.

The High-Fiber Diet

High-fiber diets containing 30 grams or more of dietary fiber are believed to help prevent diverticulosis, constipation, hemorrhoids, and colon cancer. They also are helpful in the treatment of diabetes mellitus (see Chapter 17) and atherosclerosis (see Chapter 18).

It is currently estimated that the normal diet in the United States contains about 15 grams of dietary fiber each day. Recommendations for fiber intake include 38 grams per day for men and 25 grams per day for women, but not to exceed 50 grams per day. The recommended foods for this diet include coarse- and whole-grain breads and cereals, bran, all fruits, vegetables (especially raw), and legumes. Milk, meats, and fats do not contain fiber (Table 20-2). The diet is nutritionally adequate. High-fiber diets must be introduced gradually to prevent the formation of gas and the discomfort that accompanies it. Eight 8-oz glasses of water also must be consumed along with the increased fiber.

TABLE 20-2 Sample Menus for a High-Fiber Diet

BREAKFAST	LUNCH	DINNER
Medium orange	Fresh fruit cup	Baked pork chops
Oatmeal with ½ cup blueberries	Roast beef sandwich on cracked wheat bread	Baked potato
Whole-wheat toast with marmalade	Coleslaw	Fresh broccoli
Coffee	Apple crisp with oat topping	Green salad with oil and vinegar dressing
	Fat-free milk	Whole-grain bread with margarine
	Coffee or tea	Fresh pineapple
		Fat-free milk
		Tea

© Cengage Learning 2014

SPOTLIGHT *on Life Cycle*

Here are some suggestions for helping older adults increase fiber in the diet:

- Eat fresh fruits and vegetables. If the older adult has difficulty chewing raw fruits and vegetables, gently steamed vegetables and soft fruits are appropriate.
- Eat some of the skins of potatoes, apples, pears, and other fruits or vegetables. The outer portion of these foods contains fiber and valuable nutrients.
- Use whole-grain breads and cereals instead of refined white bread and sugary cereals. Instead of meat, add beans (navy, lima, kidney, pinto), all of which are high in fiber and can also be a less expensive source of protein. Beans can also be used in casseroles, soups, stews, and other dishes.
- Try unbuttered air-popped popcorn or the reduced- or low-fat versions of microwave popcorn for a snack. Remind the older adult that dentures and teeth will need special attention during cleaning following a popcorn snack.
- Remember how important it is to increase the water in the diet when the fiber content is increased. At least 8 cups of liquid are needed each day.
- Keep moving; being active helps bowel regularity.

The Low-Residue Diet

The low-residue diet of 5–10 grams of dietary fiber a day is intended to reduce the normal work of the intestines by restricting the amount of dietary fiber and reducing food residue. Low-fiber or residue-restricted diets may be used in cases of severe diarrhea, diverticulitis, ulcerative colitis, and intestinal blockage and in preparation for and immediately after intestinal surgery.

In some facilities, these diets consist of foods that provide no more than 3 grams of fiber a day and that do not increase fecal residue (Tables 20-3 and 20-4). Some foods that do not actually leave residue in the colon are considered "low-residue" foods because they increase stool volume or provide a

Supersize USA

"Baseball games are an American institution. Couldn't wait to eat the hot dogs, peanuts, and nachos and, of course, drink soda to my heart's content! There were nine innings, and then the score was tied at the end of the ninth. I ate my way through all nine and even into the extra innings. Upon leaving the ballpark, I was feeling pain in the upper-right quadrant of my abdomen and straight through to my back. I had had this pain before but never to this extent. What is wrong with me? Did I eat something specifically to cause the pain? What should I eliminate from my diet to prevent future pain?"

You may be having a gallbladder attack. All the foods that have a lot of fat—hot dogs, nachos, peanuts—can cause it. Follow a low-fat diet to prevent future pain.

TABLE 20-3 Foods to Allow and to Avoid on Low-Residue Diets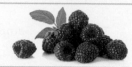

FOODS TO ALLOW	FOODS TO AVOID
Milk, buttermilk (limited to 2 cups daily) if physician allows	Fresh or dried fruits and vegetables
Cottage cheese and some mild cheeses as flavorings in small amounts	Whole-grain breads and cereals
	Legumes, coconut, and marmalade
Butter and margarine	Tough meats
Eggs, except fried	Rich pastries
Tender chicken, fish, ground beef, and ground lamb (meats must be baked, boiled, or broiled)	Milk, unless physician allows
	Meats and fish with tough connective tissue
Soup broth	Potato skin
Cooked, mild-flavored vegetables without coarse fibers; strained fruit juices (except for prune); applesauce; canned fruits including white cherries, peaches, and pears; pureed apricots; ripe bananas	Caffeine
	Popcorn
Refined breads and cereals, white crackers, macaroni, spaghetti, and noodles	
Custard, sherbet, vanilla ice cream; plain gelatin; angel food cake; sponge cake; plain cookies	
Raw vegetables such as lettuce, cucumbers, onions, and zucchini	
Salt, sugar, small amount of spices as permitted by physician	

© Cengage Learning 2014

 TABLE 20-4 Sample Menus for a Low-Residue Diet

BREAKFAST	DINNER	LUNCH OR SUPPER
Strained orange juice	Chicken broth	Tomato juice
Cream of rice cereal with milk and sugar	Ground beef patty	Macaroni and cheese
	Boiled potato, no skin	Green beans
White toast with margarine and jelly	Baked squash	White bread and butter
	Gelatin dessert	Lemon sherbet
Coffee with cream and sugar	Milk	Tea with milk and sugar

© Cengage Learning 2014

laxative effect. Milk and prune juice are examples. Milk increases stool volume, and prune juice acts as a laxative.

HEALTH AND NUTRITION CONSIDERATIONS

Clients with gastrointestinal problems can be frustrated and irritable. Their problems can be psychologically caused; they may fear surgery or cancer; and they may suffer nausea, pain, or both. Some will want to eat foods that are not recommended; others will refuse foods they need.

Health care professionals who show respect and understanding for their clients will have the most success in helping them learn what they should and should not eat, and why.

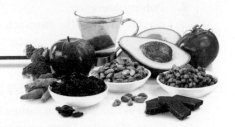

SUMMARY

Disturbances of the gastrointestinal tract require a wide variety of therapeutic diets. Peptic ulcers are treated with drugs, and diet therapy generally involves only the avoidance of alcohol and caffeine. Diverticulosis may be treated with a high-fiber diet, whereas diverticulitis is treated with a gradual progression from clear liquid to the high-fiber diet. Ulcerative colitis may require a low-residue diet combined with high protein and high calories. Cirrhosis requires a substantial, balanced diet, with occasional restrictions of fat, protein, salt, or fluids. Diet therapy for hepatitis may include a full, well-balanced diet, although protein may be restricted, depending upon the client's condition. Cholecystitis and cholelithiasis clients require a fat-restricted diet and, in cases of overweight, a calorie-restricted diet as well. Pancreatitis diet therapy ranges from TPN to an individualized diet as tolerated.

DISCUSSION TOPICS

1. Name the accessory organs in the gastrointestinal system and explain their roles in digestion and metabolism.

2. Discuss dyspepsia. Include its probable causes and the suggested therapy for it.

3. Describe hiatal hernia. Name its symptoms and possible treatment.

4. Define ulcers. Where are they found in the gastrointestinal system, and how are they treated? What substances should not be allowed for a person with an ulcer? Why?

5. Explain the difference between diverticulosis and diverticulitis. How are these conditions treated?

6. Discuss the high-fiber diet. For what conditions might it be used? Compare it with the low-fiber diet. Why is corn on the cob not allowed on the low-fiber diet? Name other foods that are not allowed on the low-fiber diet and tell why they would not be allowed.

7. Discuss ulcerative colitis. What is it? What causes it? How is it treated? How does it differ from other irritable bowel diseases?

SUGGESTED ACTIVITIES

1. Write a report on one or more of the gastrointestinal disturbances included in this chapter and the dietary treatment of them.

2. Adapt the following menu to suit a client on a low-residue diet:
   Orange juice
   Fried egg
   Bacon
   Milk
   Whole-wheat toast with butter and marmalade
   Coffee

3. List 10 of your favorite foods. Circle those foods that would not be allowed on a low-residue diet. Underline the foods that are high in fiber.

4. Using activity 3, replace the low-fiber foods with choices containing high fiber.

REVIEW

Multiple choice. Select the *letter* that precedes the best answer.

1. Dyspepsia
   a. may be an indication of serious gastrointestinal disturbance
   b. is always psychological in origin
   c. cannot be overcome with improved eating habits
   d. is caused by high-fiber foods

2. Hiatal hernia
   a. occurs only in the small intestine
   b. is a typical sign of colon cancer
   c. causes weight loss in all clients
   d. may lead clients to be more comfortable with small, frequent meals

3. Peptic ulcers
    a. can occur in the stomach or the duodenum
    b. cannot be caused by stress
    c. are always treated with aspirin and a low-carbohydrate diet
    d. are usually treated with a low-protein diet

4. Protein foods may be somewhat restricted in cases of peptic ulcers because they
    a. contribute to uremia
    b. contain large amounts of vitamin C
    c. neutralize gastric acid secretions
    d. stimulate gastric acid secretions

5. Diverticulosis
    a. is the inflammation of diverticula
    b. may be initially treated with a clear-liquid diet
    c. may be prevented with a high-fiber diet
    d. occurs in the liver

6. Food residue
    a. is ultimately evacuated in the feces
    b. always involves the small intestine
    c. never leaves the intestines
    d. results from incorrect cooking methods

7. Large amounts of food residue cause
    a. a decrease in fecal matter
    b. an increase in fecal matter
    c. weight gain
    d. diverticulosis

8. Which of the following would be recommended for the high-fiber diet?
    a. pretzels   c. rice pudding
    b. mashed potatoes   d. bran cereal

9. Which of the following would be allowed on a low-residue diet?
    a. fresh oranges   c. macaroni and cheese
    b. corn on the cob   d. fresh fruit cup

10. Ulcerative colitis
    a. affects the small intestine
    b. always requires parenteral feedings
    c. may be treated with a high-residue diet that is also high in calories and protein
    d. may cause malnutrition in clients

11. Which of the following foods would be recommended for an ulcerative colitis client, provided the client tolerates milk?
    a. fresh grapefruit
    b. chicken salad with chopped celery
    c. mashed potatoes with minced onion
    d. bisque tomato soup with crackers

12. The liver
    a. has no role in metabolism
    b. secretes insulin
    c. converts glucose to glycogen
    d. stores water-soluble vitamins

13. Cirrhosis
    a. is a liver disease characterized by cell loss
    b. is always caused by alcoholism
    c. inevitably results in death
    d. occurs only in the large intestine

14. Ascites
    a. is necessary for regeneration of liver cells
    b. is an accumulation of fluid in the abdomen
    c. requires the addition of sodium and water to the diet
    d. is caused by a shortage of iron

15. Hepatitis
    a. only occurs following exposure to HIV
    b. requires clients to follow very-low-carbohydrate diets
    c. is always fatal
    d. may be caused by viruses or toxic agents

16. Gallbladder problems may require
    a. the dietary restriction of dairy products
    b. cholecystectomy
    c. additional fat in the diet
    d. additional protein in the diet

17. Inflammation of the pancreas
    a. is called pancreatitis
    b. is asymptomatic
    c. can require a low-carbohydrate diet
    d. always signifies cancer

18. A client with celiac disease must avoid
    a. soy sauce and brown rice syrup
    b. corn chips and homemade salsa
    c. fruits and vegetables
    d. spinach salad with strawberries and pecans

19. Which IBD appears with a "cobblestoned" appearance in the colon?
    a. diverticulitis   c. Crohn's disease
    b. ulcerative colitis   d. celiac disease

20. Heartburn, regurgitation, and dysphagia are common symptoms of
    a. esophagitis
    b. peptic ulcers
    c. hiatal hernia
    d. duodenal ulcer

Case In Point

Charlotte was diagnosed with type 1 diabetes at the age 8 years. She has been in pretty good control overall. Her most recent A1c was 6.4%. Her doctor seemed very pleased with her control. She also developed thyroid disease in her early 20s. Her endocrinologist told her that people with type 1 diabetes are more at risk for developing other endocrine disorders and he assured her that she did nothing to cause this to happen. Today, at 38 years, Charlotte jokes that she is celebrating her thirtieth anniversary with diabetes. She is otherwise healthy and has not developed any complications as of yet.

This week has been different for Charlotte. She is feeling very run down. She has had several bouts of diarrhea and a chronic stomachache. She loves milk with her breakfast, but barely made it to the bathroom after drinking a glass earlier this week. She is afraid she has an infection or a virus. So many things she eats routinely have made her feel gassy or bloated or given her diarrhea. She stepped on the scale this morning to find that she has lost 10 pounds. Charlotte is only 5 feet 3 inches tall and weighed 115 pounds prior to this last episode, so at 105 pounds she now looks extremely thin. This morning her blood sugar is 258 mg/dl, which is higher than it has been in a long time. She is upset and feels very depressed. She makes an appointment to see her doctor.

After a battery of tests including blood work and an endoscopy of her gastrointestinal tract, her doctor informs Charlotte that she has celiac disease. He explains to her that it is not uncommon in people with type 1 diabetes and other endocrine disorders. He explains that foods containing gluten are causing inflammation and damage to her intestinal tract. She is going to need to begin following a gluten-free meal plan. He refers her to a registered dietitian to provide the education necessary for this new plan.

ASSESSMENT

1. What do you know about Charlotte that puts her at risk for celiac disease?
2. What symptoms did Charlotte have?
3. How will the disease alter her life?
4. How significant is this disease?

DIAGNOSIS

5. Write a diagnostic statement for Charlotte's potential alteration in nutrition.
6. Write a diagnosis for Charlotte's deficient knowledge related to the new diet.

PLAN/GOAL

7. What dietary goals are measurable and appropriate for Charlotte?
8. What education goals are specific and measurable for Charlotte?

IMPLEMENTATION

9. What information about celiac disease does Charlotte need to understand, to make necessary dietary changes?
10. What foods are going to be a problem for Charlotte?

EVALUATION/OUTCOME CRITERIA

11. At her follow-up doctor's appointment, what is her doctor likely to ask to determine if the plan was successful?

THINKING FURTHER

12. Can celiac disease be cured?
13. What medications are typically used to help manage this disease?

rate this plate

Charlotte is overwhelmed by her new diagnosis of gluten sensitivity. As a diabetic, she has learned to control her blood sugar through counting carbohydrates, but following a gluten-free diet seems like a challenge. After receiving education from a registered dietitian, Charlotte feels more confident in preparing a healthy meal. Rate the plate she made for dinner:

2 slices gluten-free pepperoni pizza

1 cup Caesar side salad with croutons

20 oz. iced tea

What types of food contain gluten? Is there anything in this plate that should be eliminated?

Case In Point

Alek is a stockbroker who has been working on Wall Street for nearly 20 years. His career has been high paced and high stress. Despite his demanding career, he has remained quite healthy. Alek is now 43 years old. His only health complaints through the years have been an ulcer and the occasional headache. The ulcer hasn't flared up in quite a while so he was hoping it had resolved. However, Alek has been working late hours and eating take-outs such as pizza, Mexican food, and a spicy oriental chicken from the local restaurants nearby his office. The long, stressful hours have also brought on many headaches. He has been treating these with a few doses of aspirin daily.

Recently while at work, Alek noticed a great amount of burning in his chest and abdomen. Then, throughout the night it became so severe he was sure his ulcer had flared up again. He went to the emergency room for assessment, and was admitted for treatment. Upon discharge, Alek's doctor ordered medications to help treat his ulcer. He also suggested he follow a low-residue diet with no stimulants, spices, or alcohol.

ASSESSMENT

1. What put Alek at risk for his ulcer to bleed?
2. What symptoms did he have?
3. What could have been done to prevent this problem?
4. What impact did this health problem have on Alek?

DIAGNOSIS

5. Write two diagnoses for Alek's problems of diet and lack of knowledge.

PLAN/GOAL

6. What goals would be appropriate for Alek's education and nutrition?

IMPLEMENTATION

7. What does Alek need to learn about his new diet?
8. What does he need to learn about his ulcer and his new medications?
9. What challenges will he face in complying with the diet while at work?
10. Construct a meal that Alek would be likely to find at work.

11. Instead of aspirin, what can Alek use to treat his headaches that will not irritate his ulcer?

EVALUATION/OUTCOME CRITERIA

12. How will Alek's doctor know this plan is effective?

THINKING FURTHER

13. Diet, stress, and medications can contribute to ulcers and prevent them from healing. Can you list some of the other causes and treatments for ulcers?

rate this plate

Following a low-residue diet will allow Alek's ulcer to heal. Rate the plate that Alek ate while working late at the office:

3 Cajun chicken and steak fajitas with onions and peppers

¾ cup Spanish rice

½ cup refried beans

12 oz. caffeine-free lemon-lime soda

How did Alek do with preparing his meal from what was catered in at the office? Can he eat everything? If not, what needs to be changed?

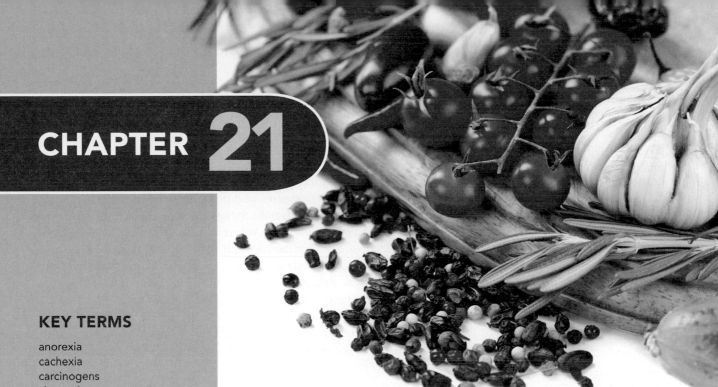

CHAPTER 21

DIET AND CANCER

OBJECTIVES

After studying this chapter, you should be able to:

- Discuss how nutrition can be related to the development or the prevention of cancer
- State the effects of cancer on the nutritional status of the host
- Describe nutritional problems resulting from the medical treatment of cancer
- Describe nutritional therapy for cancer clients

Cancer is the second leading cause of death in the United States. It is a disease characterized by abnormal cell growth and can occur in any organ. In some way the genes lose control of cell growth, and reproduction becomes unstructured and excessive. The developing mass caused by the abnormal growth is called a tumor, or **neoplasm**. Cancer is also called **neoplasia**. Cancerous tumors are **malignant**, affecting the structure and consequently the function of organs. When cancer cells break away from their original site, move through the blood, and spread to a new site, they are said to **metastasize**. The mortality rate for cancer clients is high, but cancer does not always cause death. When it is found early in its development, prompt

389

neoplasm
abnormal growth of new tissue

neoplasia
abnormal development of cells

malignant
life-threatening

metastasize
spread of cancer cells from one organ to another

oncology
the study of cancer

oncologist
doctor specializing in the study of cancer

carcinogens
cancer-causing substances

genetic predisposition
inherited tendency

treatment can eradicate it. **Oncology** is the study of cancer, and a physician who specializes in cancer cases is called an **oncologist**.

THE CAUSES OF CANCER

The precise etiology of cancer is not known, but it is thought that heredity, viruses, environmental **carcinogens**, and possibly emotional stress contribute to its development. Cancer is not inherited, but some families appear to have a **genetic predisposition** for it. When such seems to be the case, environmental carcinogens should be carefully avoided and medical checkups made regularly. Environmental carcinogens include radiation (whether from x-rays, sun, or nuclear wastes), certain chemicals ingested in food or water, some chemicals that touch the skin regularly, and certain substances that are breathed in, such as tobacco smoke and asbestos.

Carcinogens are not known to cause cancer from one or even a few exposures, but after prolonged exposure. For example, skin cancer does not develop after one sunburn.

CLASSIFICATIONS OF CANCER

There are many types of cancer. A classification system was developed based on the type of cell that produced the cancer. The majority of all cancers fall under four headings: carcinomas, sarcomas, lymphomas, and leukemias.

- Carcinomas involve the epithelial cells (cells lining the body). These include the outer layer of the skin, the membranes lining the digestive tract, the bladder, the womb, and any duct or tube that goes through organs in the body.

- Sarcoma is cancer of the soft tissues of the body such as muscle, as well as fat, nerves, tendons, blood and lymph vessels, and any other tissues that support, surround, and protect the organs in the body. Soft tissue sarcomas are uncommon. Sarcomas can also occur in bone rather than soft tissue and primarily in the legs.

- Lymphomas are cancer of the lymphoid tissue. This includes the lymph nodes, bone marrow, spleen, and thymus gland.

- Leukemias develop from the white blood cells and also affect the bone marrow and spleen.

The site where the cancer is located will become part of the diagnosis, such as basal cell carcinoma.

Skin Cancer

Skin cancer is becoming more prevalent. There are three types of skin cancer: basal cell, squamous cell, and melanoma. Basal cell carcinoma is the most common form of skin cancer, affecting the outer skin layer and caused by exposure to sunlight. Those at high risk have fair skin, light hair, and blue, green, or gray eyes and spend considerable leisure time in the sun. Squamous cell carcinoma affects the squamous cells that are in the upper layer of the skin.

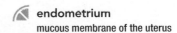

Supersize **USA**

Those who "drive through" do not realize the impact that fast food has on their body. Eating fast food over time can be responsible for considerable weight gain. How would your eating habits and the weight gain put you at risk for cancer?

According to the American Cancer Society, more than 100,000 cases of cancer each year are caused by excess body fat. The American Institute of Cancer Research has directly linked the following cancers to obesity: endometrial, esophageal, pancreatic, breast, and colorectal cancers. To help prevent these cancers, it is recommended that a healthy diet with regular physical activity be adopted.

(Source: Adapted from Sloane, Matt. *Obesity Responsible for 100,000 Cancer Cases Annually*. CNN Medical News. November 5, 2009. www.cnn.com)

Most cases arise from chronic exposure to sunlight, but may also occur where skin has been injured—burns, scars, or long-standing sores. Melanoma is the most serious and deadliest form of skin cancer and originates in the cells that produce the pigment melanin, which colors our skin, hair, and eyes. The majority of melanomas are black or brown, but some melanomas occasionally stop producing pigment and are skin colored, pink, red, or purple. If caught early, melanoma is almost 100% curable; therefore a yearly exam by a dermatologist is recommended for early diagnosis of all skin cancers.

Viral Causes of Cancer

The following viruses have been linked to cancer: Epstein–Barr, hepatitis B, Kaposi sarcoma, herpes virus, retrovirus, and human papilloma virus (HPV). Epstein–Barr virus may cause nasopharyngeal cancer, T-cell lymphoma, Hodgkin's disease, and gastric carcinoma. There is an anticancer vaccine available to prevent hepatitis B and its serious consequences—that is, liver cancer. **Kaposi's sarcoma** is a cancerous tumor of the connective tissue and is often associated with the AIDS virus. More research is being conducted to determine the retroviral cause of cancer. A vaccine is now available to prevent cervical cancer caused by HPV. Cancer research is ongoing in these and other areas.

Kaposi's sarcoma
type of cancer common to individuals with AIDS

RELATIONSHIPS OF FOOD AND CANCER

Although the relationships of food and cancer have not been proved, there appear to be associations between them—both good and bad. Certain substances in foods, for example, are thought to be carcinogenic. Nitrites in cured and smoked foods such as bacon and ham can be changed to nitrosamines (carcinogens) during cooking. Regular ingestion of these foods is associated with cancers of the stomach and esophagus. High-fat diets have been associated with cancers of the uterus, breast, prostate, and colon. The regular, excessive intake of calories is associated with cancers of the gallbladder and **endometrium**. People who smoke and drink alcohol immoderately appear to be at greater risk of cancers of the mouth, pharynx, and esophagus than those who do not.

endometrium
mucous membrane of the uterus

phytochemicals
substances occurring naturally in plant foods

On the positive side, it is thought that diets high in fiber help to protect against colorectal cancer. Diets containing sufficient amounts of vitamin C–rich foods may protect against cancers of the stomach and esophagus. Diets containing sufficient carotene and vitamin A–rich foods may protect against cancers of the lung, bladder, and larynx. **Phytochemicals**, substances that occur naturally in plant foods, are thought to be anticarcinogenic agents. Examples include flavonoids, phenols, and indoles, and fruits and vegetables appear to have an abundance of them. It is advisable to eat 9+ servings of fruits and vegetables each day, including 2½ cups of vegetables and 2 cups of fruit, on a 2,000 calorie diet. Legumes such as soybeans, dried beans, and lentils contain vitamins, minerals, protein, and fiber and may protect against cancer.

Appropriate amounts of protein foods are essential for the maintenance of a healthy immune system. An immune system that has been damaged—possibly through malnutrition—may be a contributing factor in the development of cancer. Excessive protein and fat intake, however, may be a factor in the development of cancer of the colon.

The most important principle is *moderation.* An occasional serving of bacon or buttered popcorn or wine is not likely to cause cancer, but the regular, excessive use of carcinogenic foods may contribute to cancer. Vitamins that are thought to prevent cancer should be ingested in foods that naturally contain them. Excessive intake of vitamin supplements can be harmful. For example, abnormally large amounts of vitamin A can cause bone pain and fragility, hair loss, headaches, and liver and skin problems.

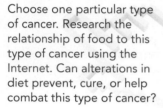

EXPLORING THE WEB

Choose one particular type of cancer. Research the relationship of food to this type of cancer using the Internet. Can alterations in diet prevent, cure, or help combat this type of cancer?

THE EFFECTS OF CANCER

One of the first indications of cancer may be unexplained weight loss because the tumor cells use for their own metabolism and development the nutrients the host has taken in. The host may suffer from weakness, and **anorexia** may occur, which compounds the weight loss. The weight loss includes the loss of muscle tissue and **hypoalbuminemia**, and anemia may develop. The sense of taste and smell may be affected. Some foods may taste different: they may not have much taste, or everything may taste the same. Cancer clients, after chemotherapy, may experience a metallic taste when eating protein foods.

anorexia
a loss of appetite, especially as a result of a disease

hypoalbuminemia
abnormally low amounts of protein in the blood

In The Media

Coffee may Reduce Cancer Risk in Women

A study published in *Cancer Epidemiology, Biomarkers & Prevention* has found a decreased risk of endometrial cancer in women who drank four or more cups of coffee a day. Eight thousand deaths occur every year due to endometrial cancer. Studies indicate that women who drank four or more cups of regular coffee per day lowered their risk of endometrial cancer by 25%. No conclusions have been made about whether caffeine or other ingredients in coffee play a role in decreasing the cancer risk.

(Source: Adapted from Bakalar, Nicholas. Patterns: Coffee May Help Cut Cancer Risk in Women. *The New York Times.* December 12, 2011. www.nytimes.com)

Many clients complain of food tasting too sweet. Radiation to the neck and head can cause damage to the taste buds and could also affect taste and smell, causing loss of appetite and weight loss.

Cancer clients become satiated earlier than normal, possibly because of decreased digestive secretions. Insulin production may be abnormal, and hyperglycemia can delay the stomach's emptying and dull the appetite. Some cancers cause hypercalcemia. If this is chronic, renal stones and impaired kidney function can occur.

The effects of cancer on the host are particularly determined by the location of a tumor. For example, an esophageal or intestinal tumor can cause blockage in the gastrointestinal tract, causing malabsorption. If the cancer is untreated, the continued anorexia and weight loss will create a state of malnutrition, which in turn can lead to **cachexia** and, ultimately, death.

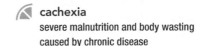

cachexia
severe malnutrition and body wasting caused by chronic disease

THE TREATMENT OF CANCER

Medical treatment of cancer can include surgical removal, radiation, **chemotherapy**, or a combination of these methods. These treatments, unfortunately, have side effects that can further undermine nutritional status. The nutritional effects of surgery in general are discussed in Chapter 22. Cancer surgery, however, can have some additional effects. Surgery on the mouth, for example, might well affect the ability to chew or swallow. Gastric or intestinal **resection** can affect absorption and result in nutritional deficiencies. The removal of the pancreas will result in diabetes mellitus.

Radiation of the head or neck can cause a decrease in salivary secretions, which causes dry mouth (**xerostomia**) and difficulty in swallowing (**dysphagia**). This reduction in saliva also causes tooth decay and sometimes the loss of teeth. Severe weight loss from not eating enough can also result from radiation therapy. Radiation reduces the amount of absorptive tissue in the small intestine. In addition, it can cause bowel obstruction or diarrhea.

Chemotherapy reduces the ability of the small intestine to regenerate absorptive cells, and it can cause hemorrhagic colitis. Both radiation and chemotherapy depress appetite. They may cause nausea, vomiting, and diarrhea leading to fluid and electrolyte imbalances, which can lead to fluid retention. However, when the therapy is completed and a well-balanced diet is resumed, these problems may disappear.

chemotherapy
treatment of diseased tissue with chemicals

resection
reduction

xerostomia
sore, dry mouth caused by a reduction of salivary secretions; may be caused by radiation for treatment of cancer

dysphagia
difficulty in swallowing

NUTRITIONAL CARE OF THE CANCER CLIENT

The nutrients and calorie needs are greater than what they were before the onset of the disease. The cancer causes an increase in the metabolic rate, and the tissue must be rebuilt, and the nutrients lost to cancer must be replaced. Clients who can maintain their weight or minimize its loss increase their chances of responding positively to treatment. Those prescribed a high-protein, high-calorie diet tolerate the side effects of therapy and higher doses of drugs better than those who cannot eat normally. Anorexia can be a major problem despite clients' nutritional needs.

Due to the illness, anorexia can result. It is particularly difficult to combat because cancer clients tend to develop strong food aversions that are
thought to be caused by the effects of chemotherapy. Receiving chemotherapy near mealtime may cause an association between food served and the
nausea caused by the chemotherapy, which can often lead to food aversions.
These aversions result in limited acceptance of food and contribute further to
the client's malnutrition. It is recommended that chemotherapy be withheld
for 2–3 hours before and after meals. The appetite and absorption usually
improve after chemotherapy has been completed. A dietitian, having obtained the likes and dislikes, will create a diet plan containing nutrient- and
calorie-dense foods. Comfort foods should be included liberally.

Diet plans for the cancer client require special attention. A dietitian at
the hospital or oncology center will obtain the client's weight and height to
calculate calorie needs. The dietitian will compile a list of nutrient-rich foods
and comfort foods to encourage nutrient intake and appetite. It is essential
that favorite foods, prepared in familiar ways, be included in the meal plan.
If chewing is a problem, a soft diet may be helpful. If diarrhea is a problem, a
low-residue diet may help (see Chapter 20).

If the client is scheduled to undergo radiation or chemotherapy, these
factors must be included in the diet planning. High-protein, high-calorie
diets may be recommended. Energy demands are high because of the hypermetabolic state often caused by cancer. Calorie needs are individualized, but
30–35 calories per kilogram of body weight may be recommended.

Carbohydrates and fat will be needed to provide this energy and spare
protein for tissue building and the immune system. Clients with good nutritional status will need 1.0–1.2 grams of protein per kilogram of body weight per
day. Malnourished clients may need 1.3–2.0 grams of protein per kilogram of
body weight per day. Vitamins and minerals are essential for metabolism and
tissue maintenance, and they may be supplied in supplemental form. Many
dietary supplements contain levels of antioxidants, such as vitamins C and E,
which are much greater than those recommended for optimal health. During
chemotherapy or radiation, oncologists advise against taking higher doses
of antioxidant supplements. It is best for cancer clients receiving treatment
to avoid dietary supplements that give more than 100% of the Daily Value for
antioxidants, according to the American Cancer Society. Fluids are important
to help the kidneys eliminate the metabolic wastes and the toxins from drugs.

The client's food habits may require change if, before the illness, the person had avoided desserts and high-calorie foods to maintain normal weight.

Sometimes clients may be willing to eat foods that are brought from
home. Some may find cold foods more appealing than hot foods. Meats may
taste bitter so milk, cheese, and eggs may be more appealing. If foods taste
sweeter to the cancer client than to the well person, then foods with citric acid
may be more acceptable.

If the client suffers from dry mouth, salad dressings, gravies, sauces, and
syrups appropriately served on foods can be helpful. Several small meals may
be better tolerated than three large meals. It is preferable to serve nutrient-
dense meals early in the day because the client is less tired and may have a
better appetite at that time. If nausea or pain is a continuous problem, drugs

to control the problem, particularly at mealtimes, may be helpful. Although oral feedings are definitely preferred, enteral or total parenteral nutrition may become necessary if cachexia is extreme. Sometimes an oral diet with a nutritional supplement may be used in conjunction with total parenteral nutrition (see Chapter 22). When appetite is poor, a high-calorie, high-protein liquid supplement may be given. As the client improves, calorie and nutritional content of the diet should be gradually increased.

HEALTH AND NUTRITION CONSIDERATIONS

It is important that the dietitian establish a good relationship with the cancer client as well as encourage and monitor food intake. When appropriate, the dietitian may find it helpful to:

1. Explain why it is important that the client eats.
2. Encourage the client to eat foods he or she enjoys.
3. Recommend that the client avoids eating at the time of day when nausea typically occurs.
4. Refrain from serving foods that give off odors that contribute to nausea.

If the prognosis for the client is not good, nutritional care will not be as important as the client's feelings and immediate comfort.

EXPLORING THE WEB

Search the Internet for the nutritional needs of the chemotherapy client. How do these needs change as the client progresses through therapy? Once therapy is complete, how do nutritional needs change? Plan some sample menus for the chemotherapy client. Check for protein and vitamins that are contraindicated for chemotherapy clients. Check out http://www.cancer.org for more information.

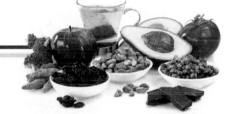

SUMMARY

Cancer is a disease characterized by abnormal cell growth. It can strike any body tissue. Energy needs increase because of the hypermetabolic state and the tumor's needs for energy nutrients. At the same time, anorexia occurs in the client. It causes severe wasting, anemia, and various metabolic problems. Treatment of cancer includes surgery, radiation, and chemotherapy. Improving the client's nutritional state is difficult because of the illness and anorexia. Parenteral or enteral nutrition may be necessary.

DISCUSSION TOPICS

1. Discuss how cancer has affected you, your family, or your friends.
2. Explain why cancer clients lose weight.

3. Why is the anorexia of cancer clients especially difficult to combat? What causes it? Are there any ways it can be prevented?
4. Are supplemental feedings of liquid foods useful in the nutritional rehabilitation of a cancer client? Explain.
5. Discuss enteral and parenteral nutrition in relation to cancer clients.

SUGGESTED ACTIVITIES

1. Invite an oncology nurse to speak to the class.
2. Write an essay about how you might feel if you had just been told that you had a malignant tumor.

3. Plan a day's menus for a cancer client who will eat only the following foods:

Sweetened orange juice	Soda crackers
Bananas	Milkshakes
Applesauce	Eggnog
Cooked pears	Cottage cheese
Puffed rice cereal	Cream of
Rice pudding	chicken soup
White toast with jelly	Poached eggs
	Bouillon

REVIEW

Multiple choice. Select the *letter* that precedes the best answer.

1. Cancer
   a. is characterized by reduced cell growth
   b. growth called a tumor can also be called a neoplasm
   c. inevitably causes death
   d. can metastasize only in clients 50 years and older

2. Carcinogens may include
   a. viruses
   b. certain green vegetables
   c. gluten-containing foods
   d. salmonella

3. Carcinogens
   a. cause cancer after only limited exposure
   b. include some chemical substances
   c. are never found in food or water
   d. are found only in meats and fish

4. Cancer clients
   a. seldom experience weight loss
   b. usually experience an increase in appetite
   c. seldom suffer from anorexia
   d. may suffer from cachexia

5. Radiation and chemotherapy
   a. seldom affect cancer clients' nutritional status
   b. may increase appetite
   c. have no connection to electrolyte imbalance
   d. may create food aversions

6. It is thought that cancer may be caused by
   a. frequent ingestion of smoked meats over a long period
   b. moderate use of alcohol
   c. high-fiber diets
   d. excessive use of vitamin A–rich foods

7. High-fat diets
   a. usually are harmless
   b. have been associated with breast and prostate cancer
   c. provide large amounts of fiber and vitamin C
   d. contribute to the health of the immune system

8. Phytochemicals are
   a. abundantly supplied in fruits and vegetables
   b. widely known carcinogens
   c. most prevalent in carbohydrates and fats
   d. plentifully supplied in proteins

9. It is recommended to cancer clients to take
   a. two multivitamins per day
   b. fish oil and flax seed oil daily
   c. a multivitamin with only 100% of the antioxidants
   d. none of these, as no supplements are required

10. Cachexia
    a. is the result of continued anorexia and weight loss
    b. is inevitable in all cancer clients
    c. occurs only in clients with mouth and throat cancers
    d. does not seem to appear in untreated cancer

Case In Point

KATE: ADJUSTING TO LIFE WITH A COLOSTOMY

Kate turned 50 years old last year. Her family threw a huge party to celebrate. This was a tradition her large, but close-knit Greek family started years ago. Kate always felt they didn't need much of an excuse to celebrate with a party. She went for her routine physical to mark her birthday celebration like she had for many years. Her doctor had told her that now that she was 50, it was time to have a colonoscopy. He explained that it would assess the health of her colon and detect any problems before they could start. He told Kate it was recommended for everyone her age, but he was particularly concerned about Kate because her father had died from colon cancer years ago. Kate had heard so many horror stories about colonoscopies. Several of her friends had the procedure done already and warned Kate about how bad the prep was. She even remembered her parents discussing this when her Dad was so sick. Every time he had a colonoscopy he received more bad news. Kate just wasn't sure she could go through with it. Over the past year, Kate has found numerous excuses as to why she couldn't get the colonoscopy and she kept putting it off.

Lately, Kate hasn't been feeling herself. She has been very tired and her stomach seems to always be cramping up in knots. She has had a lot of diarrhea and is pretty sure that she has a hemorrhoid because she has seen blood in the toilet from time to time. She wishes she felt better, then she could be more excited about the 15 pounds she has lost. Finally, Kate decides to schedule the colonoscopy. The prep was pretty bad, but the procedure was easy. She wakes up remembering nothing about what happened. The doctor meets with Kate after the colonoscopy and informs Kate that they found cancerous tumors in her colon. The doctor explains to Kate that her cancer has only progressed to stage 2, but due to the location of the tumor she will need a colostomy, at least temporarily. Kate's doctor asks her to meet with the nurse educator and dietitian in his practice group following her surgery. The nurse will train Kate on how to change her bag and care for her new colostomy. The dietitian will help Kate find foods that are not irritants to her colon and monitor her weight. He is concerned that because Kate is 5 feet 9 inches tall and currently weighs only 132 pounds, she may be at risk for malnutrition if she continues to lose weight. He asks the dietitian to also work with Kate to find high-protein snacks or supplements that will aid in her healing and prevent further weight loss or wasting.

ASSESSMENT

1. What do you know about Kate?
2. What barriers does she have to balance nutrition?
3. What resources does she have to overcome these barriers?
4. How important is her nutrition to her current health? How about to her future treatments?

DIAGNOSIS

5. Write a diagnosis about potential alteration in nutrition.
6. Write a diagnosis about her deficient knowledge.

PLAN/GOAL

7. What is the immediate goal for Kate's nutrition?
8. What is the long-term goal?

IMPLEMENTATION

9. What does Kate need to learn?
10. List strategies to increase what Kate eats at home.
11. How important is nutrition to her healing?
12. What can a home health care nurse do to enhance Kate's nutrition? What can a dietitian do?

EVALUATION/OUTCOME CRITERIA

13. What can the home health nurse observe and measure as evidence of the success of the plan?

THINKING FURTHER

14. Why is it important to use nutrition to reduce your risk of cancer?

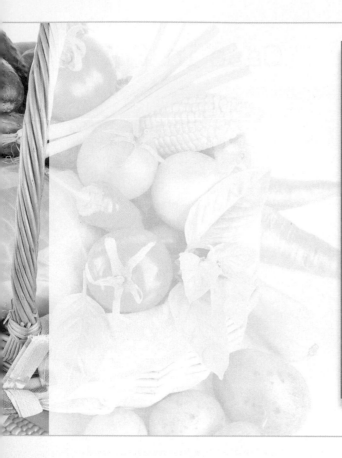

rate this **plate**

The dietitian meets with Kate to discuss protein sources and foods she can include in her diet to help decrease bowel irritation. Everyone's body acts differently to various types of food, so Kate would have to experiment to see what her intestines could tolerate. In order to prevent additional weight loss, the dietitian recommends a protein supplement drink for Kate if she is unable to obtain sufficient protein from her meals and snacks. Rate the plate she plans to eat for lunch, taking into consideration any possible irritants and protein sources:

2 cups spinach salad with mandarin oranges and pecans

3 oz. crispy chicken on top of the salad

¾ cup tomato soup made with water, not milk

½ cup cottage cheese

½ cup sliced peaches

Are there any parts to this meal that may cause Kate some intestinal discomfort? What foods in this meal are rich in protein? Will Kate need to drink the supplement with this meal or does it provide enough protein alone?

Case In Point

DAVE: APPETITE AND WEIGHT LOSS DURING CHEMOTHERAPY

Dave is a 56-year-old Asian man who is currently undergoing chemotherapy. Dave was diagnosed with lymphoma 3 months ago. His initial course of chemotherapy consisted of 10 treatments. Through the first three treatments, Dave experienced a lot of anxiety and fear about how his body would respond to the medications. He had seen people who had undergone chemotherapy and he always thought they appeared very frail and weak. Dave had been trying to maintain as much normalcy in his life as possible while undergoing the chemotherapy. He continued to work as much as he was able. He tried to eat many of his favorite foods to help keep up his strength and prevent a large amount of weight loss. So far, his weight has remained fairly stable.

The oncologist has informed Dave that the treatments will become more difficult each time. He advises him that if he begins losing weight then he will have to prescribe an appetite stimulant for Dave to take during the next few rounds of treatment. He also suggests that Dave meet with a registered dietitian to assess his daily caloric needs.

The dietitian recommends a nutritional supplement for Dave to use between meals if his appetite is poor. She also suggests he weighs himself weekly and notify her if he begins to lose weight. Hopefully, in working with the dietitian, he can avoid having to take one more medication.

ASSESSMENT

1. What has Dave's response to the chemotherapy been so far?
2. What does the doctor suspect will happen to Dave's nutrition during round 4 of chemotherapy?
3. What can the dietitian assess to measure how Dave is eating?

DIAGNOSIS

4. Write a diagnostic statement describing the nutrition problems Dave could have with chemotherapy.

PLAN/GOAL

5. What is the major nutrition goal for Dave?
6. What is the rationale for aggressive proactive nutrition between rounds of chemotherapy?
7. What does Dave need to know related to the nutritional demands of ongoing chemotherapy?

IMPLEMENTATION

8. List four strategies the dietitian can use to encourage Dave to eat.
9. List three strategies that his family can use to help him eat.
10. If Dave eats only 5–10% of his normal food volume, what foods should be a priority? How are fluids important?
11. In preparation for round 5 of chemotherapy, what could Dave do to enhance his nutrition once his appetite returns?

12. How can other cancer clients undergoing chemotherapy and their families help Dave?
13. How can the Internet be of help? Check out the American Cancer Society at http://www.cancer.org.

EVALUATION/OUTCOME CRITERIA

14. How would the doctor evaluate the success of the diet plan?

THINKING FURTHER

15. Why is nutrition so important in the successful treatment of cancer?

rate this plate

Dave has done a good job at eating healthy and maintaining his weight while receiving chemotherapy treatments. Dave will be seeing the dietitian a few times a month to review his food intake and weight status. Using the meal he made for lunch as an example, will Dave be able to maintain his weight? Rate this plate:

- **4 oz. salmon fillet**
- **1 cup mashed potatoes**
- **¾ cup sautéed vegetables including red peppers, broccoli, and zucchini**
- **1 cup romaine salad with dried cranberries and cherries**
- **2 Tbsp light poppy seed dressing**
- **1 toffee nut cookie**

Cancer patients need additional protein because cancer tends to deplete protein stores. Has Dave planned enough protein for this meal? If not, how could he adjust this meal to include more protein?

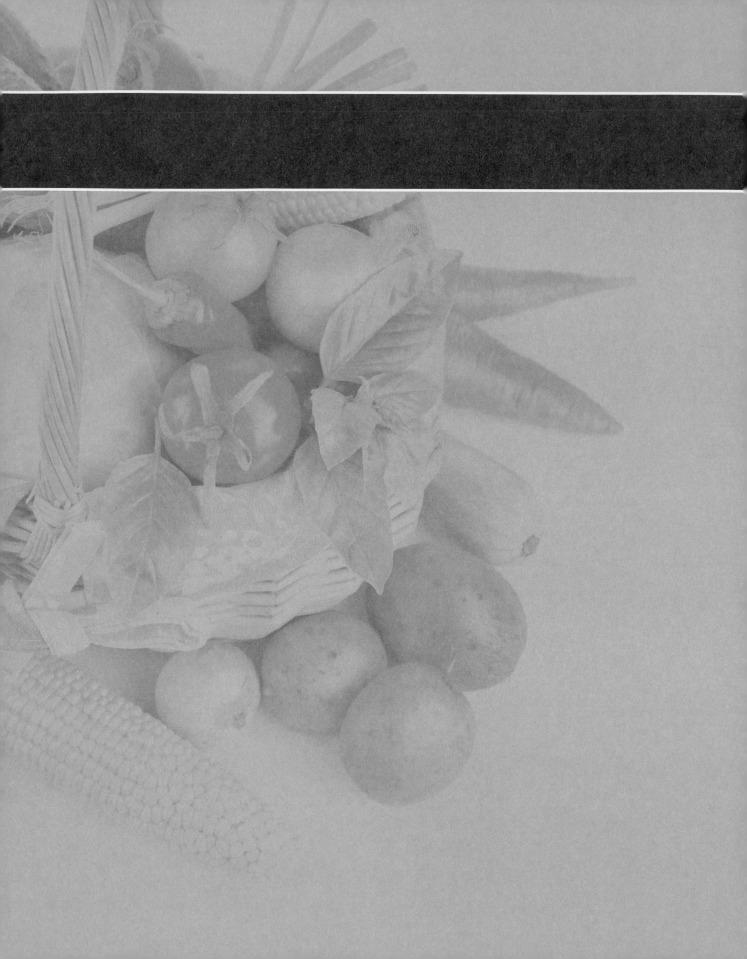

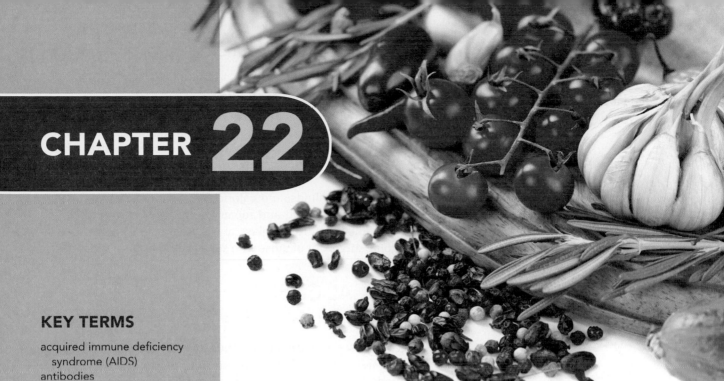

CHAPTER 22

KEY TERMS

acquired immune deficiency
   syndrome (AIDS)
antibodies
aspirated
dumping syndrome
elemental formulas
enteral nutrition
gastrostomy
human immunodeficiency
   virus (HIV)
hydrolyzed formulas
hypermetabolic
hypoalbuminemia
jejunostomy
modular formulas
nasogastric (NG) tube
opportunistic infections
peripheral vein
phlebitis
polymeric formulas
sepsis
thrombosis
thrush
tube feeding (TF)

DIET AND CLIENTS WITH SPECIAL NEEDS

OBJECTIVES

After studying this chapter, you should be able to:

- Describe the body's reactions to stress and relate them to nutrition
- Explain the special dietary needs of surgical and burn clients
- Discuss enteral and parenteral nutrition
- Explain the special dietary needs of clients with fever and infection
- Explain the special dietary needs of AIDS clients

Normally, the human body operates in a state of homeostasis. When the body experiences the trauma of surgery, severe burns, or infections, this balance is upset. The body reacts in an attempt to restore itself to homeostasis.

During its response to physical stress, the body signals the endocrine system, which activates a self-protective, **hypermetabolic** response. This increases energy output. The intensity of the response depends on the severity of the condition.

401

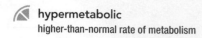

hypermetabolic
higher-than-normal rate of metabolism

Catabolism occurs, causing the rapid breakdown of energy reserves to provide glucose and other substances necessary for the anabolic phase of wound healing and tissue maintenance. Proteins, fats, and minerals are lost in the catabolic phase just when there is an increased need for them to rebuild tissue. When the condition includes hemorrhage and vomiting, these losses are compounded.

Sufficient nutrients, fluids, and calories are required as soon as possible to replace the losses, build and repair tissue, and return the body to homeostasis. Obviously, nutrition plays an important role in the lives of clients undergoing surgery or of those who suffer from burns or infections.

THE SURGICAL CLIENT
Presurgery Nutritional Care

Elective surgery stresses the client prior to the procedure. Prior to surgery, the client's nutritional status should be evaluated and if improvement is needed, it should be undertaken immediately. A good nutritional status before surgery enhances recovery. A nutritional assessment of the client before surgery will be helpful to the dietitian in providing nutrition that will be accepted by the client after surgery, when appetite is poor.

Improvement of nutritional status will usually mean providing extra protein, carbohydrates, vitamins, and minerals. The extra protein is needed for wound healing, tissue building, and blood regeneration. Extra carbohydrates will be converted to glycogen and stored to help provide energy after surgery, when needs are high and when clients may be unable to eat normally. The B vitamins are needed for the increased metabolism, vitamins A and C and zinc for wound healing, vitamin D for the absorption of calcium, and vitamin K for proper clotting of the blood. Iron is necessary for blood building, calcium and phosphorus for bones, and the other minerals for maintenance of acid–base, electrolyte, and fluid balance in the body.

In cases of overweight, improved nutritional status includes weight reduction before surgery whenever possible. Excess fat is a surgical hazard because the extra tissue increases the chances of infection, and fatty tissue tends to retain the anesthetic longer than other tissue.

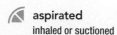

aspirated
inhaled or suctioned

Many physicians order their clients to be NPO (nothing by mouth) after midnight the night before surgery. Withholding food ensures that the stomach contains no food, which could be regurgitated and then **aspirated** into the lungs during surgery. If there is to be gastrointestinal surgery, a low-residue diet may be ordered for a few days before surgery (see Chapter 20), to reduce intestinal residue.

Postsurgery Nutritional Care

The postsurgery diet is intended to provide calories and nutrients in amounts sufficient to fulfill the client's increased metabolic needs and to promote healing and subsequent recovery. In general, during the 24 hours immediately following major surgery, most clients will be given intravenous solutions only. These solutions will contain water, 5–10% dextrose, electrolytes, vitamins, and medications as needed. The maximum calories supplied by intravenous solutions are 400–500 calories per 24-hour period. The estimated daily calorie requirement for adults after surgery is 35–45 calories per kilogram of body weight. A 110-pound individual would require at least 2,000 calories a day. Obviously, until the client can take food, there will be a considerable calorie deficit each day. Body fat will be used to provide energy and to spare body protein, but the calorie intake must be increased to meet energy demands as soon as possible.

Because protein losses following surgery can be significant and because protein is especially needed then to rebuild tissue, control edema, avoid shock, resist infection, and transport fats, a high-protein diet may be recommended. Protein requirements for postsurgical clients can range from 1.5–2.0 g/kg of body weight per day. In addition, extra minerals and vitamins are needed. When peristalsis returns, ice chips may be given; and if they are tolerated, a clear liquid diet can follow. (Peristalsis is evidenced by the presence of bowel sounds.)

Normally in postoperative cases, clients proceed from the clear-liquid diet to the regular diet. Sometimes this change is done directly and sometimes by way of the full-liquid diet, depending on the client and the type of surgery. The average client will be able to take food within 1–4 days after surgery. If the client cannot take food then, parenteral or enteral feeding may be necessary.

Sometimes following gastric surgery, **dumping syndrome** occurs within 15–30 minutes after eating. This is characterized by dizziness, weakness, cramps, vomiting, and diarrhea. It is caused by food moving too quickly from the stomach into the small intestine. It occurs secondary to an increase in insulin, in anticipation of the increase in food, which never comes.

dumping syndrome
nausea and diarrhea caused by food moving too quickly from the stomach to the small intestine

To prevent dumping syndrome, the diet should be high in protein and fat, and carbohydrates should be restricted. Foods should contain little fiber or concentrated sugars and only limited amounts of starch. Complex carbohydrates are gradually reintroduced. Gradual reintroduction is recommended because carbohydrates leave the stomach faster than do proteins and fats. Fluids should be limited to 4 oz at meals, or restricted completely, so as not to fill up the stomach with fluids instead of nutrients. Fluids can be taken 30 minutes after meals. The total daily food intake may be divided and served as several small meals rather than the usual three meals in an attempt to avoid overloading the stomach. Some clients do not tolerate milk well after gastric surgery, so its inclusion in the diet will depend on the client's tolerance.

The food habits of the postoperative client should be closely observed because they will affect recovery. When the client's appetite fails to improve, the physician and the dietitian should be notified, and efforts should be made to offer nutritious foods and supplements (either in liquid or solid form) that the client will ingest. The client should be encouraged to eat slowly to avoid swallowing air, which can cause abdominal distension and pain.

THE CLIENT RECEIVING ENTERAL NUTRITION

The term **enteral nutrition** means the forms of feeding that bring nutrients directly into the digestive tract (Figure 22-1). Oral feeding is the usual method and should be used whenever possible. When clients cannot or will not take food by mouth but their gastrointestinal tract is working, they will be given

enteral nutrition
feeding by tube directly into the client's digestive tract

FIGURE 22-1 Enteral feeding routes.

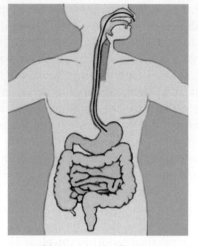

Nasogastric Route

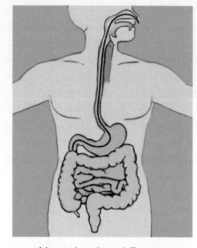

Nasoduodenal Route

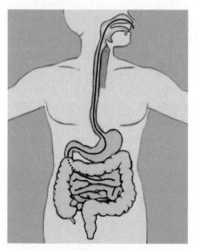

Nasojejunal Route

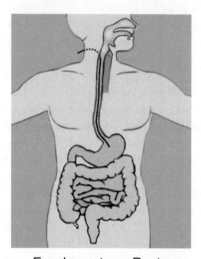

Esophagostomy Route

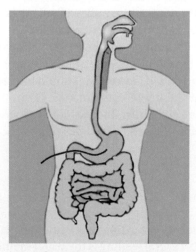

Gastrostomy Route

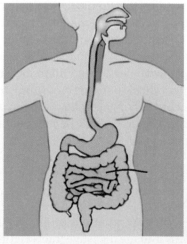

Jejunostomy Route

© Cengage Learning 2014

Supersize USA

Obesity Can Increase Surgery Risks

While obesity is bad for your overall health, it also can pose numerous risks if you are going to have surgery. A recent study from Johns Hopkins University School of Medicine showed increased complications for obese clients after surgery. Being obese increases surgery complications by 18%. Complications include:

- Infection
- Bleeding and blood clots
- Longer surgery time
- Higher amounts of anesthetic drugs
- Longer recovery time

Being of normal weight before surgery poses only a 2% risk for complications. Losing weight before a major surgery can decrease the possible risks as well as lead an individual to feeling better and living longer.

(Source: Adapted from Perry, Arthur. Surgery and Obesity: The Deadly Risks. *The Dr. Oz Show*. July 12, 2011. www.doctoroz.com)

a **tube feeding (TF)**. Sometimes this may be necessary because of unconsciousness, surgery, stroke, severe malnutrition, or extensive burns.

Usually, for periods that do not exceed 6 weeks, tube feeding is administered through a **nasogastric (NG) tube** inserted through the nose and into the stomach or small intestine. When the percutaneous endoscopic gastrostomy (PEG) tube cannot be placed in the nose or when tube feedings will be required for more than 6 weeks, an opening called an ostomy is surgically created into the esophagus (an esophagostomy), the stomach (**gastrostomy**), or the intestine (**jejunostomy**).

The tubes used for these feedings are soft, flexible, and as small as they can be and still allow the feeding to pass through. Although some tubes are weighted to keep them in place in the stomach or intestine, the use of weighted tubes has not been proved to be better than unweighted.

Numerous commercial formulas are available, with varying types and amounts of nutrients. Clients who are able to digest and absorb nutrients can be given **polymeric formulas** (1–2 calories/ml) containing intact proteins, carbohydrates, and fats that require digestion. Clients who have limited ability to digest or absorb nutrients may be given **elemental** or **hydrolyzed formulas** (1 calorie/ml) that contain the products of digestion of proteins, carbohydrates, and fats, and are lactose free. **Modular formulas** (3.8–4.0 calories/ml) can be used as supplements to other formulas or for developing customized formulas for certain clients (such as those with extensive wound-healing needs). The use of modular formulas has been decreasing due to the development of high-protein formulas. Disease-specific formulas have been developed to be used in the acute setting and for a short period of time. Clients admitted to the hospital with renal failure, respiratory failure, or liver failure have been shown to benefit from these specialized formulas.

tube feeding (TF)
feeding by tube directly into the stomach or intestine or via a vein

nasogastric (NG) tube
tube leading from the nose to the stomach for tube feeding

gastrostomy
opening created by the surgeon directly into the stomach for enteral nutrition

jejunostomy
opening created by the surgeon into the intestine for enteral nutrition

polymeric formulas
commercially prepared formulas for tube feedings that contain intact proteins, carbohydrates, and fats that require digestion

elemental formulas
those formulas containing products of digestion of proteins, carbohydrates, and fats; also called hydrolyzed formulas

hydrolyzed formulas
contain products of digestion of proteins, carbohydrates, and fats; also called elemental formulas; used for clients who have difficulty digesting food

modular formulas
made by combining specific nutrients

EXPLORING THE WEB

Search the Web for information on the various types of enteral nutrition formulas discussed in the text. What are the makeups of these formulas? Are any nutrients lacking in these formulas? Is there the potential for side effects of or allergies to these formulas that clients should be aware of and monitored for?

There are three methods for administering tube feedings: continuous, intermittent, and bolus. Intermittent means to only administer tube feeding at night, with solid foods eaten during the day. If there is a food–drug interaction, such as with phenytoin (Dilantin), the TF should be stopped 1 hour before and be restarted 1 hour after administration of the medication via tube.

Daily calorie needs of the client are usually divided into 6 servings per day (not to exceed 400 cc at a time). These feedings are given over a 15-minute time span and followed by 25–60 ml of water, hence the term *bolus.* This method is usually done when a client has a PEG tube, but it could also be done with an NG tube.

Usually the feedings are administered by a pump. This means the feeding is continuous during a 16–24 hour period. Tube feedings need to start slowly, such as 20–25 ml per hour. This rate may be increased by about 25 ml every 4 hours until tolerance has been established and the client is at their goal rate to meet calorie needs. When clients are ready to return to oral feedings, the transfer must be done gradually.

Possible Complications with Enteral Nutrition

The osmolality of a liquid substance indicates the number of particles per kilogram of solution. Solutions with more particles (high osmolality) exert more pressure than solutions with fewer particles. Solutions with high osmolality attract water from nearby fluids that contain lower osmolality. When a formula with high osmolality reaches the intestine, the body may draw fluid from the blood to dilute the formula. This process can cause weakness and diarrhea. However, diarrhea should be attributed to the tube feeding only when all other causes have been ruled out. Liquid medications containing sorbitol or *Clostridium difficile* (C-dif) (the bacterium that causes dysentery) are two possible causes of diarrhea.

Aspiration can occur (some of the formula enters the lung), causing the client to develop pneumonia. The tube may become clogged, or the client may pull the tube out. The placement of the feeding tube should be checked with an x-ray to decrease the possibility of aspiration. Before beginning the tube feeding, the health care provider must administer the flush solution according to the physician's order and raise the head of the bed. If the feeding is continuous, then the head of the bed needs to remain elevated. Some facilities, to verify correct placement of the NG tube in the stomach, will check the gastric pH before each use.

Clients requiring tube feeding may need a great deal of reassurance and support. The health care team should be patient and understanding during the care of tube-fed clients.

THE CLIENT RECEIVING PARENTERAL NUTRITION

Parenteral nutrition is the provision of nutrients intravenously. It is used if the gastrointestinal tract is not functional or if normal feeding is not adequate for the client's needs. It can be used alone or as part of a dietary plan that includes oral or tube feeding as well. When parenteral nutrition is used to provide total nutrition, it is called total parenteral nutrition (TPN) or hyperalimentation.

Nutrient solutions are prescribed by the physician and dietitian and are prepared by a pharmacist. They can be administered via a central vein or, for a period of 2 weeks or less, a **peripheral vein**. Typically, a dextrose/amino acid/fat solution is given. This solution is not combined until just before entry into the vein because the components do not form a stable solution.

Total parenteral nutrition that is required for an extended period is provided via a central vein. A catheter is surgically inserted, under sterile conditions, by a physician or an IV nurse. It is inserted into a subclavian vein or the superior vena cava. The vena cava is used because the high blood flow there facilitates the quick dilution of the highly concentrated TPN solution. Dilution reduces the possibility of **phlebitis** and **thrombosis**.

When parenteral nutrition is no longer necessary, the client must be transferred gradually to an oral diet. Sometimes clients are given tube feeding before oral feeding as they are weaned from TPN.

Possible Complications with Parenteral Nutrition

Infection can occur at the site of the catheter and enter the bloodstream, causing an infection of the blood called **sepsis**. Bacterial or fungal infections can develop in the solution if it is unrefrigerated for over 24 hours. Abnormal electrolyte levels may develop, as can phlebitis or blood clots. Careful monitoring of the client is essential.

THE CLIENT WITH BURNS

In cases of serious burns, the loss of skin surface leads to enormous losses of fluids, electrolytes, and proteins. Water moves from other tissues to the burn site in an effort to compensate for the loss, but this only compounds the problem. This fluid loss can reduce the blood volume and thus blood pressure, as well as urine output.

Fluids and electrolytes are replaced by intravenous therapy immediately to prevent shock. Glucose is not included in these fluids for the first 2–3 days after the burn to avoid hyperglycemia.

The hypermetabolic state after a serious burn continues until the skin is largely healed, so there is an enormous increase in energy needed for the healing process. Calorie requirements are based on weight (size) and the total burned surface, including depth of burns, although most adult calorie needs are calculated at 35–40 kcal/kg per day. Protein needs for adults are as high as 1.5–2.0 g/kg of body weight. Children will need additional protein for healing at 2.5–3.0 g/kg per day. It is reasonable to provide 12–15% of nonprotein calories from fat. A high-protein, high-calorie diet is used. There is an increased need for vitamin C and zinc for healing and B vitamins for the metabolism of the extra nutrients. Vitamin A is important for the immune system and the epithelial tissues. The amino acids arginine and glutamine help increase immune functioning and wound healing. Arginine assists in wound healing

EXPLORING THE WEB

Search the Web for additional information on parenteral nutrition. What types of formulas are used for TPN? Are there nutrients lacking from this form of nutritional support? What possible side effects or allergies should the client be monitored for?

peripheral vein
a vein that is near the surface of the skin

phlebitis
inflammation of a vein

thrombosis
blockage, as a blood clot

sepsis
Infection of the blood

FIGURE 22-2 Adequate nutrition and assistance is essential for clients with severe burns.

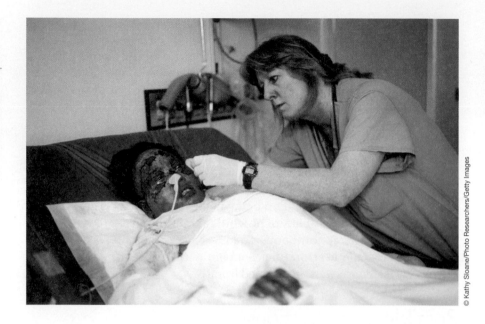

by aiding in collagen formation and nitrogen retention. Some of glutamine's functions are to help prevent bacterial infections, improve immune function, and preserve gut integrity.

Also, it is essential that severely burned clients have sufficient fluids to help the kidneys hold the unusual load of wastes in solution and to replace those lost.

If the client is able to eat, oral feedings are advisable. Liquid commercial formulas may be used at first, and solid food may be added during the second week after the burn. If the client is unable to eat, tube feedings should be started immediately. In some cases, parenteral feeding is required. The foods served should be those the client likes and is willing to eat. To determine this, a registered dietitian must perform an individualized assessment for each burn victim. The best assessment of the adequacy of the nutrients provided is wound healing.

Burn clients need a great deal of encouragement. They are in pain; are worried about disfigurement; and know they face a long, costly, and painful hospital stay with the possibility of surgery.

THE CLIENT WITH INFECTION

Fever typically accompanies an infection. Fevers and infections may be acute or chronic. Fever is a hypermetabolic state in which each degree of fever on the Fahrenheit scale raises the basal metabolic rate (BMR) by 7%. If extra calories are not provided during fever, the body first uses its supply of glycogen, then its stored fat, and finally its own muscle tissue for energy.

Protein intake should be increased because of infections (sepsis) and the amounts required need to be individualized. Protein is needed to replace body tissue and to produce **antibodies** to fight the infection. Minerals are needed to help build and repair body tissue and to maintain acid–base, electrolyte, and fluid balance. Extra calories are needed for the increased metabolic rate. Extra

antibodies
substances produced by the body in reaction to foreign substance; neutralize toxins from foreign bodies

vitamins are also necessary for the increased metabolic rate and to help fight the infection causing the fever. Extra fluid is needed to replace that lost through perspiration, vomiting, or diarrhea, which often accompany infection.

Clients with fever usually have very poor appetites, but they will often accept ice water, fruit juice, and carbonated beverages. Some will accept broth, jello, or popsicles. Usually, the diet during fever and infection progresses from the liquid to the regular diet, with frequent, small meals recommended. It should be high in protein, calories, and vitamins. In some cases, parenteral and enteral feedings are necessary.

High doses of antibiotics or long-term use during infections can lead to oral **thrush**, a yeast infection caused by the *Candida* bacteria. Although the bacteria naturally exist in healthy individuals it can only grow if a client has a compromised immune system. Clients with thrush usually experience decreased appetite due to pain on the tongue during eating. Treatment is not usually needed in oral thrush. Clients can take acidophilus capsules or eat yogurt containing acidophilus to speed recovery.

THE CLIENT WITH AIDS

A virus is a microscopic parasite that invades and lives in or on, and thus infects, another organism, called the host. The virus obtains nourishment from the host and duplicates itself countless times. There are many viruses that infect humans. Some, like those of the common cold, make the host only mildly ill. Others, like the **human immunodeficiency virus (HIV)**, are deadly.

HIV invades the T cells, which are white blood cells that protect the body from infections. When the T cells cannot function normally, the body has no resistance to opportunistic infections. **Opportunistic infections** are caused by other microorganisms that are present but do not affect people who have healthy immune systems.

Persons infected with HIV are said to be HIV positive. HIV infection ultimately leads to **acquired immune deficiency syndrome (AIDS)**, which is incurable and fatal.

HIV can affect anyone exposed to it, regardless of age, sex, or physical condition. HIV infection cannot be cured, but it can be prevented. The virus is not transmitted through casual contact, such as shaking hands. It is transmitted via body fluids, specifically:

- Through sexual contact
- By transfusions of contaminated blood
- By use of contaminated needles during ear piercing, tattooing, acupuncture, or injection of illegal drugs
- By infected mothers to their fetuses during pregnancy or to their infants during lactation

Progression from HIV Infection to AIDS

There are essentially three stages in the progress of AIDS. The first stage begins soon after exposure to HIV, when the body produces antibodies in an

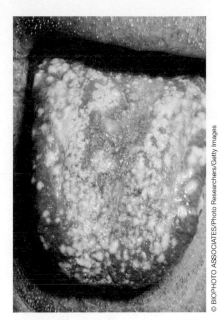

© BIOPHOTO ASSOCIATES/Photo Researchers/Getty Images

FIGURE 22-3 Thrush is very painful.

thrush
a yeast infection of the mucous membrane lining the mouth and tongue

human immunodeficiency virus (HIV)
a virus that weakens the body's immune system and ultimately leads to AIDS

opportunistic infections
caused by microorganisms that are present but that do not normally affect people with healthy immune systems

acquired immune deficiency syndrome (AIDS)
caused by the human immunodeficiency virus (HIV), which weakens the body's immune system, leaving it susceptible to fatal infections

TABLE 22-1　Causes of Nutrient Loss in AIDS Clients
- Anorexia
- Cancer
- Diarrhea
- Increased metabolism due to fever
- Certain medications
- Malabsorption caused by cancer or diarrhea
- Protein energy malnutrition

© Cengage Learning 2014

attempt to destroy the virus. At that time, some people may experience a few days of symptoms resembling mild flu. Others may have no symptoms. At this point and thereafter, the infected person will test positive to HIV and will be among those called HIV positive. Unless tested, the individual will feel normal and will have no idea that he or she is HIV positive for a period ranging from a few months to 10 years.

During this period, the virus is incubating. Viral cells are multiplying in the tonsils, adenoid glands, and spleen, gradually taking over the body's T cells.

Anyone suspecting of exposure to HIV should be tested as soon as possible. An ever-growing number of medications are available that may increase the time the virus needs to multiply and, thus, may prolong the life of the host.

The second stage of HIV is known as the *ARC period. ARC* stands for AIDS-related complex. The body's immune system has by this point grown weaker, and symptoms and opportunistic infections occur. There may be fatigue, skin rashes, headache, night sweats, diarrhea, weight loss, oral lesions or thrush (candidiasis, a fungal infection of the mouth), cough, sore throat, fevers, or shortness of breath (Table 22-1).

The third and end stage of HIV infection is known as AIDS (acquired immune deficiency syndrome). It is manifested by a very low T-cell count, which makes it impossible for the body to fight off infections. Tuberculosis or Kaposi's sarcoma commonly develops at this point. As the T-cell count continues to diminish, other parasites invade and, ultimately, overwhelm the body, causing death.

The Relationship of HIV Infection and Nutrition

A healthful diet is essential for a healthy immune system, which may delay the onset of AIDS. Persons diagnosed as being HIV positive should have a baseline nutrition and diet assessment by a registered dietitian. Unhealthful eating habits can be corrected at an early stage of the disease, and future nutritional needs can be explained.

As the condition progresses, the client begins to experience the physical problems previously listed. Infections increase the metabolic rate and nutrient and calorie needs and, at the same time, decrease the appetite and often the body's ability to absorb nutrients. Medications may further reduce the appetite and cause nausea. When there are oral infections, taste may change, and swallowing can become painful. Anorexia, or loss of appetite, commonly occurs (Table 22-2).

AIDS clients experience serious protein-energy malnutrition (PEM) and, thus, body wasting. This may be referred to as HIV wasting syndrome, which results in **hypoalbuminemia** and weight loss. The immune system is further damaged by insufficient amounts of protein and calories, thus hastening death.

hypoalbuminemia
abnormally low amounts of protein in the blood

Problems Related to Feeding AIDS Clients

Just when an AIDS client most needs a nutrient- and calorie-rich diet, he or she is most apt to refuse it. In some cases, it may be useful to discuss nutritional care with the client. When possible, medications should be given after meals

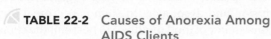

TABLE 22-2 Causes of Anorexia Among AIDS Clients

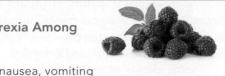

Medications	Cause nausea, vomiting
Oral infections	Diminish saliva, alter taste, cause mouth pain
Altered taste	Changes or exaggerates flavors
Fever	Depresses appetite
Pain	Depresses appetite
Depression	Depresses appetite
Dysphagia	Makes swallowing difficult
Dementia	May cause client to forget to eat

© Cengage Learning 2014

TABLE 22-3 Methods to Improve the Appetite of an AIDS Client

- Give medications *after* meals
- Offer soft food
- Avoid spicy, acidic, and extremely hot or cold foods
- Serve frequent, small meals
- Add sugar and flavorings to liquid supplements
- Take advantage of the "good" days and offer any food the client tolerates
- Talk with the client to help ease concerns about finances, family, and friends

© Cengage Learning 2014

to reduce the chance of nausea. Sores in the mouth or esophagus can make eating painful, and soft foods may be better tolerated than others. Taste can be affected by the disease, so spicy, highly acidic, extremely hot, or extremely cold foods may be rejected. Frequent small meals and, sometimes, liquid supplements may be helpful. Additional sugar and flavoring may increase the acceptability of liquid supplements. Because of the nausea and diarrhea, sufficient fluids are essential. If the client has difficulty swallowing or simply cannot eat, tube feeding may be imperative. If the tube causes pain or if severe diarrhea or malabsorption is present, parenteral nutrition may be necessary.

The client should be helped to eat as much as possible, especially on "good" days (Table 22-3). Clients may suffer from pain and depression, and they may worry about finances and what people think of them. These factors can further diminish their appetites, but positive discussions can help.

In The Media

Treatment Adherence for HIV-Positive Adults

A recent study was conducted on HIV-positive adults to determine the effectiveness of treatment periods on client viral loads, or amount of HIV in the blood. Results indicated that the risk of treatment failure decreases if clients followed their regimens longer than the initial period. Failure of treatment would also become less likely if clients missed less than one dose of medication per week of treatment. Clients taking Sustiva-based and Kaletra-based regimes were tested. Poor compliance to the antiretroviral therapy could lead to higher viral loads, causing a decrease in white blood cells and increased resistance to medications. Results indicated that missing more than one dose per week was associated with higher viral loads and treatment failure. Significant improvement in the treatment failure rates among HIV-positive adults can occur if treatment medications and protocol are followed.

(Source: Adapted from McQueen, Courtney. Early Treatment Adherence Decreases Risk of Treatment Failure in HIV-Positive Adults. *The AIDS Beacon.* 2012. www.aidsbeacon.com)

Neurological impairment usually occurs in varying degrees in AIDS clients and may cause confusion and dysphagia. In such cases, meal trays should be kept simple, the consistency of food modified to best suit the client, and special utensils provided if needed.

Some clients may want to try nontraditional diets, thinking they will help or even cure them. These clients need to be made aware of any potentially harmful effects from such diets. In some cases, the idea of improvement may help the client's appetite.

Those clients who will benefit no further from either medication or nutrition can still be comforted by the health care professional or hospice nurse who shows support, understanding, and respect for them.

HEALTH AND NUTRITION CONSIDERATIONS

Clients who fall within the categories of conditions discussed in this chapter can be a challenge for the health care professional. Surgical clients may seem to make excessive demands due to pain, uncertainty, or anxiety. Clients suffering burns may require extreme patience and the ability of the health care provider to detach emotionally. Clients with fatal infections will require extra time and attention. Clients receiving tube feedings or some medications may suffer from frequent diarrhea and require total client care.

In each of these cases, the health care professional can help herself or himself as well as the client by thinking positively and using therapeutic communication with the client and family.

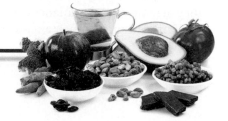

SUMMARY

Surgery, burns, fevers, and infections are traumas that cause the body to respond hypermetabolically. This response creates the need for additional nutrients at the same time that the injury causes a loss of nutrients. Care must be taken to provide extra fluid, proteins, calories, vitamins, minerals, and carbohydrates as needed in these situations. When surgery is elective, nutritional status should be improved before surgery, if necessary. When food cannot be taken orally, enteral or parenteral nutrition may be used.

DISCUSSION TOPICS

1. Describe the body's reaction to trauma and how nutrition is related to it.

2. Why are extra nutrients needed during trauma?

3. When might surgery be elective?

4. In what ways might a diet history of a presurgical client be helpful?

5. Explain why a burn client needs extra protein. What happens when the extra protein is not provided?

6. Why does a surgical client need extra minerals?

7. Why must a client's stomach be empty at the time of surgery?

8. Explain why intravenous dextrose solutions are not sufficient to fulfill nutritional requirements after surgery.

9. Describe dumping syndrome and tell how it may be alleviated.

10. Describe parenteral nutrition. What is it? How is it delivered? What are some dangers related to it?

SUGGESTED ACTIVITIES

1. Ask a certified nutrition support dietitian (CNSD) to visit the class and discuss tube feedings, telling why and when they are used and problems associated with them.

2. Invite a nurse from a local hospital to discuss burns and the nutritional challenges facing clients with burns.

3. If a class member has experienced any of the traumas discussed in this chapter, ask that person to recount it and describe her or his reactions, appetite, and recovery.

4. Role-play a situation in which a client is 5 days' postsurgery and cannot eat and the nurse is trying to convince her to eat.

5. Pretend you are a postsurgical client and are receiving 5–10% dextrose, containing 450 calories per 24 hours. Calculate how much weight you would lose if you remained on the IV for 5 days. Refer to Chapter 16 for assistance.

REVIEW

Multiple choice. Select the *letter* that precedes the best answer.

1. Trauma
   a. can be described as injury
   b. causes a hypometabolic response in the body
   c. usually decreases the body's need for protein
   d. has no relation to nutrition

2. During trauma, there is usually
   a. reduced need for protein and minerals
   b. a hypermetabolic response in the body
   c. only minor changes in nutritional requirements
   d. a decreased need for calories

3. Wound healing, tissue building, and blood regeneration all require
   a. extra fat
   b. extra cholesterol
   c. megadoses of vitamin C
   d. additional protein

4. Intravenous solutions
   a. rarely contain vitamins
   b. usually contain cellulose
   c. are usually given after surgery
   d. provide 2,000 calories per day

5. Protein is needed after major surgery to
   a. provide calories
   b. resist infection
   c. control fat metabolism during trauma
   d. aid in healing

6. It would not be surprising for TPN to be used in the treatment of
   a. a fractured hip
   b. third-degree burns over a large part of the client's body
   c. a broken leg
   d. pancreatitis

7. Dumping syndrome is characterized by
   a. migraine headache
   b. hypertension and tremors
   c. reduced clotting time
   d. dizziness and cramps

8. TPN for more than 2 weeks is given through
   a. a nasogastric tube
   b. a peripheral vein in the ankle
   c. the superior vena cava
   d. an esophagostomy

9. Severely burned clients will need
   a. to replace protein and fluids
   b. extra amounts of glucose the first 2–3 days after the burn
   c. reduced amounts of liquid
   d. a low-protein, low-calorie diet

10. Fever
    a. creates a need for extra calories
    b. clients have enormous appetites
    c. clients experience reduced metabolic rate
    d. clients should be kept on a low-calorie diet

EVALUATION/OUTCOME CRITERIA

17. What criteria would the doctor, physical therapist, and dietitian use to evaluate the effectiveness of the plan?
18. Would weight gain be an effective criterion? If not, why?

THINKING FURTHER

19. How could the lessons from this case be used in other situations?

rate this plate

Along with offering a protein supplement between meals, the dietitian encouraged Betty to include protein sources in her meals and snacks. Increased protein intake will provide her with additional energy and assist in healing her fractures. Rate the plate she ate for breakfast:

½ cup oatmeal

¼ cup blueberries

1 slice whole-wheat toast with butter

4 oz. strawberry yogurt

4 oz. orange juice

Sips of coffee

How many calories and grams of protein did Betty receive from this meal? Was this meal sufficient in calories and protein? What foods can be added to this meal, if any, to increase protein? What can be done to encourage Betty to eat more than 50% of her plate at meal time?

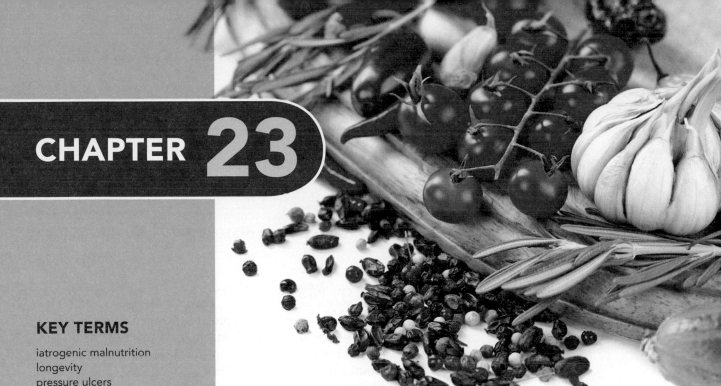

NUTRITIONAL CARE OF CLIENTS

OBJECTIVES

After studying this chapter, you should be able to:

- Describe how illness and surgery can affect the nutrition of clients
- Identify and describe three or more nutrition-related health problems that are common among elderly clients needing long-term care
- Demonstrate correct procedures for feeding a bed-bound client
- Explain the importance of adapting the family's meal to suit the client's nutritional requirements

When clients are unable to feed themselves assistance is required. Each client should have a nutrition assessment to determine the type of feeding best suited for their individual needs. Whether in a hospital, nursing home, at their home, or due to a handicap, clients require extensive help from nurses, nurse's aids, or family. Sufficient time needs to be taken in order for the clients to ingest proper nutrition.

HOSPITALIZED CLIENTS

Illness and surgery can have devastating effects on nutritional status. Fever, nausea, fear, depression, chemotherapy, and radiation can destroy appetite. Vomiting, diarrhea, chemotherapy, radiation, and some medications can reduce or prevent absorption of nutrients. In addition, food is restricted before surgery and some diagnostic tests. Ironically, this reduced nutrient and calorie intake occurs just when requirements are increased. Fluid may also be restricted as most clients are NPO (nothing by mouth) for 12 hours prior to surgery.

Protein Energy Malnutrition

When the increased needs for energy and protein are not met by food intake, the body must use its stores of glycogen and fat. When they have been used, the body breaks down its own protein stores to provide energy. Protein-energy malnutrition, commonly called PEM, can be a problem among hospitalized clients, especially the elderly. It can delay wound healing, contribute to anemia, depress the immune system, and increase susceptibility to infections. Symptoms of PEM include weight loss and dry, pale skin. When malnutrition occurs as a result of hospitalization, it is called **iatrogenic malnutrition**.

 iatrogenic malnutrition
caused by treatment or diagnostic procedures

Improving the Client's Nutritional Status

The importance of improving a client's nutritional status is obvious. Formal nutritional assessments of clients should be made on a regular basis, but all members of the health care team should be alert to signs of malnutrition on a daily basis. The nurse or nursing assistant who sees the client regularly is in the best position to help the client. The nurse will inform the dietitian of decreased intake. The dietitian may implement the following:

1. The client may need information about nutritional needs.
2. The client may need a supplement.
3. The client may want other foods.

If not contraindicated by the client's health condition, it can be helpful to invite friends and relatives to bring the client some of his or her favorite foods.

Serving the Meal

When a meal is served at the bedside, the tray should be lined with a pretty cloth or paper liner. Attractive dishes that fit the tray conveniently without crowding it should be used. The food should be arranged attractively on the plate. Utensils must be arranged conveniently. Water should be served as well as another beverage (unless it is prohibited by the physician). Foods must be served at proper temperatures.

When the client is on complete bed rest, special preparations are required before the meal is served. The client should be given the opportunity

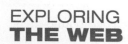

EXPLORING THE WEB

Search the Web for information on nutritional status during acute or chronic illness. Why is appetite affected by illness? For what length of time is it normal to have a decreased appetite when ill? What can be done to improve appetite and maintain nutritional balance when ill?

to use the bedpan and to wash before the meal is served. The client should be helped to a comfortable position, and any unpleasant sights should be removed before the meal is served. Pleasant conversation during the preparations can improve the client's mood considerably. Certain topics of conversation can help stimulate the client's interest in eating. Appropriate remarks on the client's progress, whenever possible, are helpful.

At meal time, the tray should be placed on the bedside table and positioned for easy feeding or if necessary, convenient for someone else to do the feeding. If the client needs help, the napkin should be opened and placed, the bread spread, the meat cut, and the straw offered. The client should be encouraged to eat and be allowed sufficient time.

If the client complains of too much food on the tray, then one might try serving 1–2 dishes at a time. Many older clients find it disturbing to waste food and therefore may benefit from smaller portions at meal times. The physician notes poor intake and may request a calorie and protein count, which is an accurate report of the types and amounts of food eaten.

Feeding the Client Who Requires Assistance

If the client is unable to feed oneself, the person doing the feeding should sit near the side of the bed (Figure 23-1). Small amounts of food should be placed toward the back of the mouth with a slight pressure on the tongue with the spoon or fork. The client must be allowed to help oneself as much as possible. If the client begins to choke, assist in sitting up straight. Do not give food or water while the client is choking. The client's mouth should be wiped as needed. A client diagnosed with dysphagia will require a specialized diet. Depending upon the swallowing abnormality, the client may need pureed foods with either thin or thickened (to a nectar or honey consistency) liquids. A dysphagic client should not use straws.

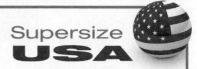

Supersize USA

The elderly have lived through many changes in their lives. One change that might not be easily understood is the supersizing of the dishes they use. Why does a cereal bowl need to hold three or four servings? Plates, cereal-soup bowls, fruit-dessert bowls, and especially serving bowls have all been supersized. Several recent studies have shown that the larger the bowl, the larger the portion one will take. This may be why some elderly complain about "too big of a serving"; it can be overwhelming, causing them to eat very little, or not at all. Having lived through several world wars and the Great Depression, it is distressing for them to know that food will be thrown away. "That is such a waste!" Other elderly clients have adapted to the larger portions and are fighting weight gain and obesity.

Check out some antique dishes and notice the difference in sizes from those you use at home. Measuring portions, rather than eyeballing them, may be wise.

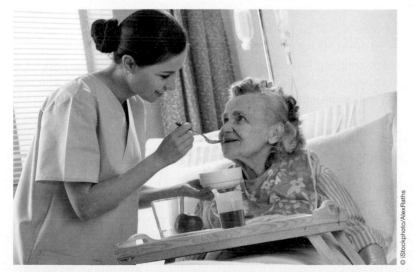

© iStockphoto/AlexRaths

FIGURE 23-1 Some clients require assistance when eating.

In The Media

Four Important Vitamins for Older Brains

Brain scans were performed on elderly test subjects while they conducted mental functioning tests. After ruling out all other factors, researchers concluded that those participants who scored higher on cognitive tests had higher blood levels of the following vitamins:

- Vitamin B
- Vitamin C
- Vitamin D
- Vitamin E

These vitamins are associated with larger brain volume. Omega-3 levels were also found to be linked to higher cognitive functioning. Eating a variety of fresh fruits and vegetables will provide all these nutrients and benefit overall health.

(Source: Adapted from Bakalar, Nicholas. Nutrition: 4 Vitamins that Strengthen Older Brains. *The New York Times.* January 2, 2012. www.nytimes.com)

Feeding the Blind Client

Special care must be taken in serving a meal to a client who is blind. An appetizing description of the meal can help create a desire to eat. To help the client who is blind feed oneself, arrange the food as if the plate were the face of a clock (Figure 23-2). The meat might be put at 6 o'clock, vegetables at 9 o'clock, salad at 12, and bread at 3 o'clock. The person who regularly arranges the meal should remember to use the same pattern for all meals. Plate guards should be placed around the plate to assist with feeding and prevent food from spilling. People who are blind usually feel better when they can help themselves.

longevity
length of life

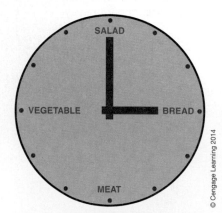

FIGURE 23-2 To a blind client, a plate of food can be pictured as the face of a clock.

© Cengage Learning 2014

LONG-TERM CARE OF THE ELDERLY

Because of increasing **longevity**, the number of elderly people requiring long-term care is increasing. The changes people undergo with age that can affect their nutritional status are discussed in Chapter 15.

Physical Problems of the Institutionalized Elderly

It is estimated that the majority of people 85 and above have at least one chronic disease such as arthritis, osteoporosis, diabetes mellitus, cardiovascular disease, or mental disorder. These conditions affect their attitudes, physical activities, appetites, and, thus, nutritional status. PEM is a major concern for this population.

Anemia can develop if the client has insufficient iron intake. It can contribute to confusion and depression but may go unnoticed because one of its major symptoms, fatigue, may be simply thought to be a characteristic of old age. It is helpful to make sure there is sufficient animal protein and vitamin C (an iron enhancer) in the client's diet.

Pressure ulcers (bedsores) can develop in bedridden clients. The ulcers develop in areas where unrelieved pressure on the skin prevents the blood from bringing nutrients and oxygen and removing wastes. Healing requires treatment of the ulcer, relief of the pressure, a high-calorie diet with sufficient protein, and vitamin C and zinc supplements. Prevention is a must.

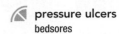
pressure ulcers
bedsores

Constipation can be caused by inadequate fiber, fluid, or exercise; by medication; by reduced peristalsis; or by former abuse of laxatives. It can be relieved by increased fluid, fiber, and exercise (if possible).

Diarrhea can be caused by digestive disorders, medications, viruses, bacteria, and other sources. It will reduce the absorption of nutrients and can contribute to dehydration. An increase of fiber in the diet combined with supplemental vitamins and minerals may be helpful.

The sense of smell declines with age, and the appetite diminishes. A reduced sense of taste can be caused by medications, disease, mineral deficiencies, or xerostomia (dry mouth). The addition of spices, herbs, salt, and sugar (if allowed) can be helpful. Xerostomia can be caused by disease or medications. Drinking water, eating frequent small meals, and chewing sugar-free gums or sucking on hard candies may be helpful. The inadequate amount of saliva in these clients contributes to increased tooth decay.

Dysphagia (difficulty in swallowing) can result from a stroke, closed head trauma, head or neck cancer, surgery, or Alzheimer's and other diseases. A swallow study needs to be done to determine the consistency of diet needed by clients with dysphagia. A swallow study is done by a speech therapist using a video fluoroscope. While being videotaped, the client is given liquids, semiliquids, pureed food, and solid food to determine the consistency of the bolus (food mass) that he or she is able to swallow without aspirating. Many dysphagia clients must have thickened liquids. Dysphagia clients should always be in an upright position with their chin tucked towards their chest when eating. This will prevent aspiration.

FEEDING AT HOME

When a client is discharged from the hospital to go home, the dietitian may be asked to give the client a diet plan. Examples of diet plans include low-sodium, low-cholesterol, and low-residue diets. In the home, the family menu should serve as the basis of the client's meal when possible.

Family meals are easily adapted for the client by omitting or adding certain foods or by varying the method of preparation. For example, the following family menu would need to be adapted for a client needing to limit fat intake:

Fried hamburgers

Mashed potatoes with butter

Buttered carrots

Tossed salad with French dressing

Ice cream with fresh strawberries

Whole milk

EXPLORING THE WEB

Search the Web for information relating to the nutritional status of the elderly. Why does nutritional status decline as one ages? What can be done to prevent the decline of nutritional status among the elderly? Does the American Association of Retired Persons (AARP) offer any guidelines?

Broiling the hamburgers for everyone instead of frying would help limit the fat content. The client's mashed potatoes might be served with little or no butter, and the carrots with only salt and pepper. The client could be served the tossed salad with fat-free dressing and, for dessert, strawberries with low-fat ice cream or whipped topping. Fat-free milk is a simple substitute for whole milk. Enough time should be given to consume the meal. Include the client in meal preparation and dining time if possible.

HEALTH AND NUTRITION CONSIDERATIONS

Bedridden clients are totally dependent on the nursing staff and families for their needs. They are unable to walk, use the bathroom, brush their teeth, or wash their hands without help. The feelings of helplessness they endure are considerable. In addition, they may be embarrassed by their appearance, or by needing a bedpan when only a thin curtain separates them from their roommate's guests.

The needs of many elderly clients in nursing homes are also total. They may be arthritic and unable to walk, some may be incontinent, others may forget their names and how to dress, and they may need to be fed. Each remains an individual. They all need, respond to, and deserve warmth and respect from their caregivers.

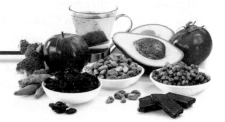

SUMMARY

Illness and surgery can have devastating effects on clients' nutritional status. PEM can be a significant problem. The health care team should work together to improve clients' nutritional status.

Once a client is at home, meals should be adapted from the family's meals. This saves time and expense and allows the client to feel less of a burden and more a part of the family.

A bedridden client should be given the bedpan and then allowed to wash her or his hands before the meal. Clients should be encouraged to feed themselves. However, help should be offered if it is needed. The client who is blind can eat more easily if food is arranged in a set pattern on the plate. Pleasant conversation and cheerfulness on the part of the nurse and/or family can improve the client's appetite. The client's percentage of food eaten should be charted. Elderly clients requiring long-term care may suffer from several nutrition-related health problems that, with proper treatment, can sometimes be relieved.

DISCUSSION TOPICS

1. How do illness and surgery affect one's nutrition?

2. What is iatrogenic malnutrition? How might it develop?

3. In what ways might the nurse help improve the client's nutrition?

4. When might it be unwise to invite a client's friends and family to bring foods to the client? When might it be appropriate? Who would decide?

5. Discuss the importance of proper preparation of the client and room before the meal. What could disturb a client and affect appetite?

6. How may the appearance of the tray affect the client's appetite?

7. Why should the client be encouraged to feed oneself?

8. Why is it important to remove the tray as soon as the client has finished the meal?

9. How can the behavior and attitude of the attending person affect the appetite of the client?

10. Why is anemia so easily overlooked in elderly clients?

11. Discuss how a diminished sense of smell might affect one's appetite.

SUGGESTED ACTIVITIES

1. Have two students participate in the following role-playing situation. The class should evaluate and discuss the "nurse's" tact and skill in dealing with the "client."

   Mrs. Jones is a young, active woman with a family. She is recovering from viral pneumonia. Although she is allowed out of bed, she is not supposed to prepare meals or do housework until her condition improves. Dr. Malcolm has told Ms. Wilson, the nurse, that it is important for Mrs. Jones to regain her lost weight. One day, before her dinner was served, Mrs. Jones complained to Ms. Wilson. She was discouraged about her lack of energy and stated that her family needed her. Ms. Wilson noticed that Mrs. Jones had eaten very little for breakfast and lunch. What should she say to Mrs. Jones?

2. Invite a dietitian to speak to the class on nutrition and the elderly.

3. Invite a nurse who works in a nursing home to talk to the class. Ask the nurse to describe how clients are fed.

4. Visit a local nursing home in groups of two or three. Talk to some of the clients. Write a report on your visit.

REVIEW

Multiple choice. Select the *letter* that precedes the best answer.

1. Surgery
   a. reduces the number of calories normally needed
   b. has only a slight effect on appetite
   c. is always followed by TPN
   d. can temporarily devastate a client's nutritional status

2. Normal absorption of nutrients
   a. is not affected by chemotherapy
   b. is unaffected by diarrhea
   c. can be decreased after surgery
   d. is unaffected by PEM

3. When energy and protein needs are not met by food intake, the body will first use its stores of
   a. fat, and then its glycogen
   b. glycogen, and then its fat
   c. glycogen, and then its protein
   d. protein, and then its glycogen

4. PEM
   a. can delay wound healing
   b. has no relationship to the development of anemia
   c. strengthens the immune system
   d. decreases the risk of infection

5. Surgery may
   a. contribute to the development of PEM
   b. decrease one's calorie requirement
   c. reduce nutritional requirements
   d. increase one's fat requirements

6. Favorite foods brought to hospitalized clients from home
   a. should not be allowed
   b. have no effect on the client's nutritional status
   c. should be approved by the dietitian before being given to the client
   d. are neither helpful nor harmful

7. Iatrogenic malnutrition
   a. is the inevitable result of surgery
   b. can be a result of hospitalization
   c. is commonly caused by low-grade fevers
   d. has no effect on wound healing

8. Dysphagia
   a. means memory loss
   b. is common following bone surgery
   c. can safely be ignored
   d. clients should not be in a supine position when eating

9. Anemia
   a. can result from insufficient fat intake
   b. can contribute to hyperthyroidism
   c. can be helped by the addition of vitamin C and iron
   d. occurs only in males over 50

10. Pressure ulcers
    a. occur only in the stomach
    b. can occur in the duodenum
    c. do not affect bedridden clients
    d. develop in areas where, because of pressure, blood cannot get to the tissue

11. A dietitian is always consulted when
    a. a client is admitted
    b. food intake has decreased
    c. only when a calorie count is ordered
    d. a client gains weight

12. Feeding the client who requires assistance involves
    a. placing small amounts of food toward the back of the tongue
    b. feeding in the supine position
    c. giving sips of fluid between bites
    d. cutting food into bite-size pieces

Case In Point

LOUIS: SUFFERING FROM WEIGHT LOSS AND SKIN BREAKDOWN

Louis is a 79-year-old African American man. He had been married for 47 years until his wife passed away 6 months ago. Since her death, things just haven't been the same for Louis. He finds himself very lonely and at a loss for what to do. He never was a good cook, but now he has no desire to prepare meals at all. He spends most of his days sitting in his recliner watching television. Louis's brother, Lenny, who's also single, has been worried about Louis. He has decided to move in with him, at least temporarily, to help support his brother physically and emotionally.

When Lenny arrives at Louis's house, he notices Louis has lost quite a bit of weight since he last saw him. His skin looks very thin and dry. Lenny begins to prepare meals for Louis. Louis is thankful for the meals, but still has very little appetite. Lenny complies with Louis's request to stay in his recliner for meals.

Louis states his gait has become increasingly unsteady and he prefers to just stay put.

Now that Lenny has been with Louis about a week, he realizes that Louis is even sleeping in his recliner. In fact, Louis really only gets up when he needs to use the bathroom. Lenny decides he needs to assist his brother in getting a shower and a little activity. While assisting Louis, his brother notices a large pressure ulcer on his tailbone. Lenny is very concerned and decides to take Louis to the doctor. Louis's doctor determines he needs to have surgery to clean and repair the ulcer, and then Louis must keep off his tailbone for several weeks. Louis is also instructed to increase his protein intake, to assist in wound healing. Louis's doctor asks the two men to meet with a dietitian to review a meal plan that would facilitate wound healing and help Louis regain some of the weight he has lost over the past several months.

ASSESSMENT
1. What do you know about Louis and his nutrition?
2. Did he eat a balanced diet?
3. What barriers were there to his healing?
4. What foods are priorities for healing?
5. How significant is nutrition to this problem?

DIAGNOSIS
6. Write at least two diagnoses that apply to Louis's problem.

PLAN/GOAL
7. What is the priority goal for Louis?

IMPLEMENTATION

8. What does the dietitian need to know about Louis to help?
9. What is the dietitian likely to recommend?
10. How could vitamin supplements help?
11. Who else can help?
12. What strategies could be helpful to get Louis to eat?
13. What could a home health nurse do?
14. What does Louis need to do to help himself?
15. If Louis is unable to eat enough food to maintain his weight, what alternatives does the doctor have?

EVALUATION/OUTCOME CRITERIA

16. What needs to happen for Louis to avoid having a feeding tube?
17. What criteria will the doctor use to determine if the plan is effective?

THINKING FURTHER

18. How are Louis's needs similar to those of any other surgical client?
19. What are the most serious consequences if Louis is unable to heal, even with tube feedings?

rate this **plate**

Lenny made the following meal for Louis. Rate this plate on protein quality:

6 oz. baked meatloaf

1 medium baked potato with shredded cheese and butter

¾ cup mixed vegetables

1 dinner roll with butter

4 oz. custard cup

How many grams of protein are in this meal? Is it enough to support the healing of Louis's ulcer?

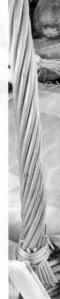

Case In Point

DUMISANI: ADJUSTING TO LIFE IN ASSISTED LIVING

Dumisani's wife passed away 5 years ago. He is 82 years old and has had an increasingly difficult time caring for himself. He and his wife had been together for so long; he is lost without her. When they were just 18 years old, the couple traveled from their native Egypt to the United States to start a new life together. Living without her is difficult. After much discussion with his son, he felt it was in his best interest to move to an assisted living nursing home. In his new home, his meals are prepared for him and the nursing staff monitors his medications. Dumisani has settled into his new home and has even enjoyed the company of many of the others who live there. He has been able to be more active and social than he has been in many years. He has been attending bingo games and playing cards with some other men who live in the facility. Dumisani developed an upper respiratory infection 3 weeks ago and was on a 10-day course of antibiotics. Before completing the course of antibiotics, he began noticing he was having frequent loose stools. He assumed this was a side effect of the medication and was not concerned. However, it has been a week since he finished the medication and he is still having loose stools every time he uses the bathroom. His appetite has decreased of the past few days. His nurse took his temperature today and noticed he had a fever of 102 degrees. Dumisani is somewhat disoriented this morning with his surroundings. His nurse decides to contact the physician to notify him of the change in status.

ASSESSMENT

1. What has happened to Dumisani?
2. What data do you have to support your findings?
3. What conditions will occur if Dumisani's diarrhea and temperature are not treated?
4. Because of his age, what do you know about Dumisani's total body water content?

DIAGNOSIS

5. Complete the following nursing diagnosis statement: Dumisani's deficient fluid volume is related to _____ and fever as evidenced by his behavior of _____.

PLAN/GOAL

6. What is your immediate concern for Dumisani?
7. What is your concern for the next 24 hours?

IMPLEMENTATION

8. What fluid would be most helpful to Dumisani and why?
9. How much fluid should he have?
10. What else should be done to treat Dumisani?
11. What should Dumisani do the next time he starts to have diarrhea?

EVALUATION/OUTCOME CRITERIA

12. What changes will you expect to see if your plan is effective?

THINKING FURTHER

13. At what point could Dumisani have avoided this problem?
14. How could you use this lesson in your future experiences as a nurse?

rate this **plate**

Chronic diarrhea can lead to dehydration so it is important for Dumisani to be drinking fluids regularly. It is also important to replenish lost electrolytes and sodium. Rate this plate that Dumisani received for lunch:

1 cup chicken noodle soup

1 small baked potato with butter

½ cup fruited orange gelatin

½ cup chocolate pudding

8 oz. apple juice

Use Appendix D to list the water and sodium content of these foods. Will this meal provide Dumisani with adequate fluids?

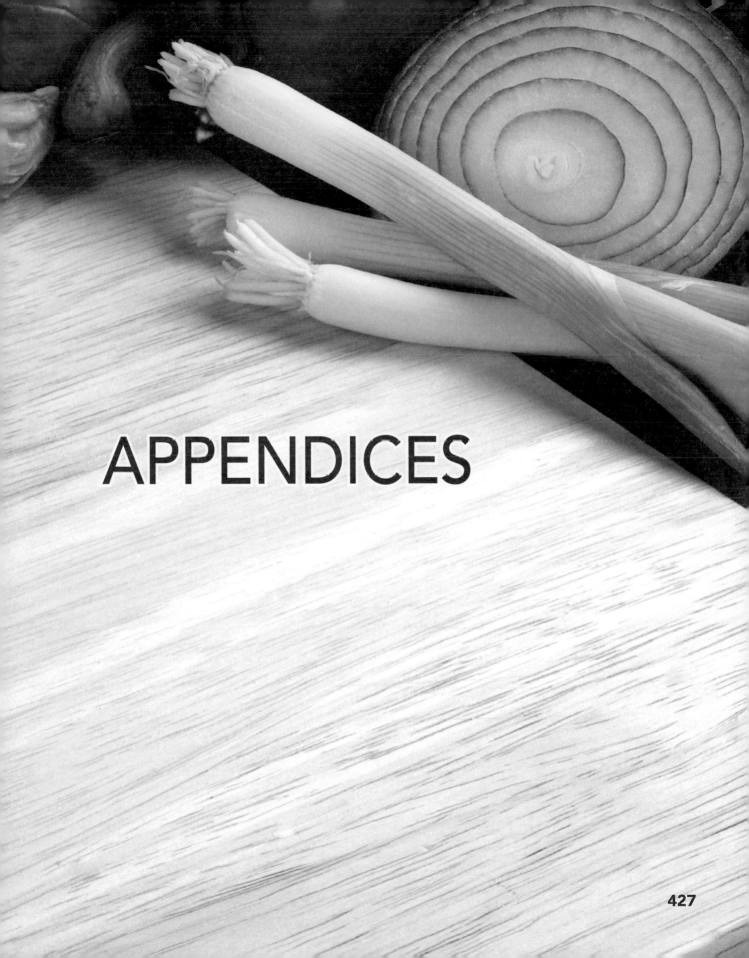

APPENDICES

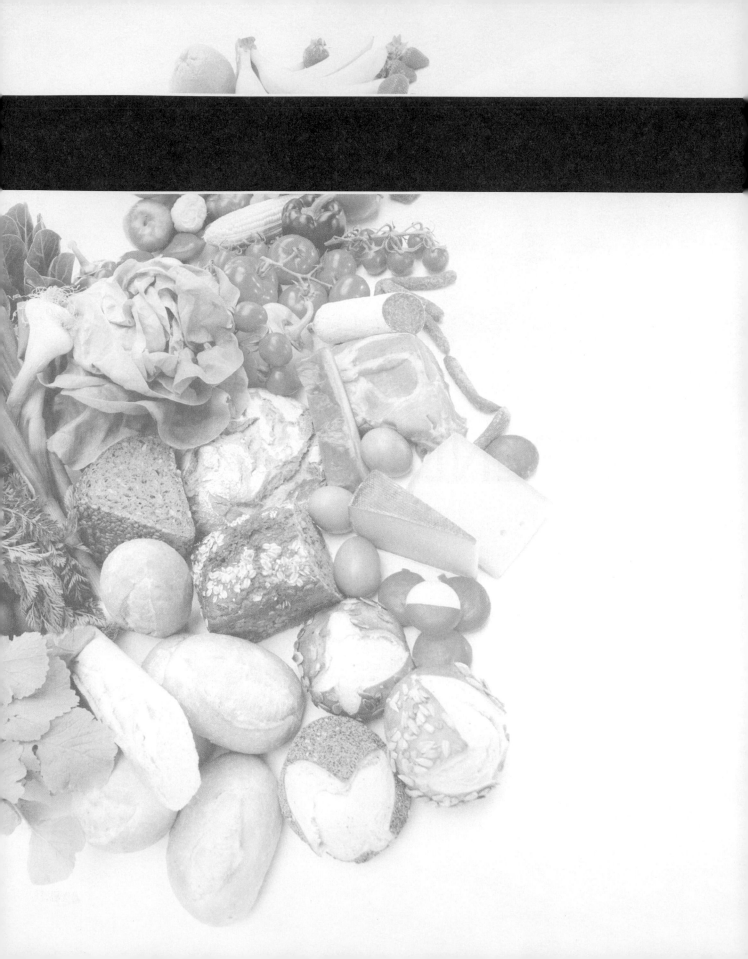

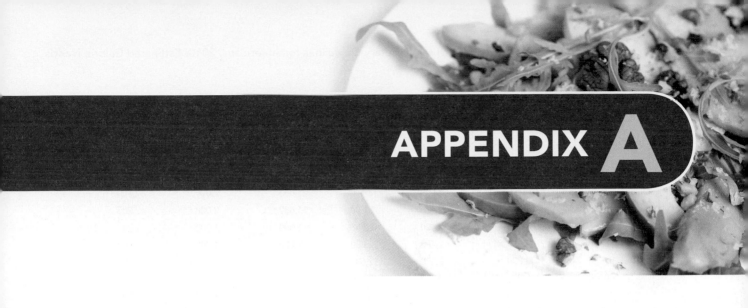

DIETARY GUIDELINES FOR AMERICANS, 2010: ESTIMATED CALORIE NEEDS PER DAY BY AGE, GENDER, AND PHYSICAL ACTIVITY LEVEL[a]

Reprinted from *Dietary Guidelines for Americans, 2010* (7th ed.), by the U.S. Department of Health and Human Services and U.S. Department of Agriculture, 2010, Washington, DC: U.S. Government Printing Office.

Gender/ activity level[b]	Male/ Sedentary	Male/ Moderately active	Male/ Active	Female[c]/ Sedentary	Female[c]/ Moderately active	Female[c]/ Active
Age (years)						
2	1,000	1,000	1,000	1,000	1,000	1,000
3	1,200	1,400	1,400	1,000	1,200	1,400
4	1,200	1,400	1,600	1,200	1,400	1,400
5	1,200	1,400	1,600	1,200	1,400	1,600
6	1,400	1,600	1,800	1,200	1,400	1,600
7	1,400	1,600	1,800	1,200	1,600	1,800
8	1,400	1,600	2,000	1,400	1,600	1,800
9	1,600	1,800	2,000	1,400	1,600	1,800
10	1,600	1,800	2,200	1,400	1,800	2,000
11	1,800	2,000	2,200	1,600	1,800	2,000
12	1,800	2,200	2,400	1,600	2,000	2,200
13	2,000	2,200	2,600	1,600	2,000	2,200
14	2,000	2,400	2,800	1,800	2,000	2,400
15	2,200	2,600	3,000	1,800	2,000	2,400
16	2,400	2,800	3,200	1,800	2,000	2,400
17	2,400	2,800	3,200	1,800	2,000	2,400
18	2,400	2,800	3,200	1,800	2,000	2,400
19–20	2,600	2,800	3,000	2,000	2,200	2,400
21–25	2,400	2,800	3,000	2,000	2,200	2,400
26–30	2,400	2,600	3,000	1,800	2,000	2,400
31–35	2,400	2,600	3,000	1,800	2,000	2,200
36–40	2,400	2,600	2,800	1,800	2,000	2,200

(continues)

(continued)

Gender/ activity level[b]	Male/ Sedentary	Male/ Moderately active	Male/ Active	Female[c]/ Sedentary	Female[c]/ Moderately active	Female[c]/ Active
Age (years)						
41–45	2,200	2,600	2,800	1,800	2,000	2,200
46–50	2,200	2,400	2,800	1,800	2,000	2,200
51–55	2,200	2,400	2,800	1,600	1,800	2,200
56–60	2,200	2,400	2,600	1,600	1,800	2,200
61–65	2,000	2,400	2,600	1,600	1,800	2,000
66–70	2,000	2,200	2,600	1,600	1,800	2,000
71–75	2,000	2,200	2,600	1,600	1,800	2,000
76+	2,000	2,200	2,400	1,600	1,800	2,000

Estimated amounts of calories needed to maintain calorie balance for various gender and age groups at three different levels of physical activity. The estimates are rounded to the nearest 200 calories. An individual's calorie needs may be higher or lower than these average estimates.

[a]Based on Estimated Energy Requirements (EER) equations, using reference heights (average) and reference weights (healthy) for each age-gender group. For children and adolescents, reference height and weight vary. For adults, the reference man is 5 feet 10 inches tall and weighs 154 pounds. The reference woman is 5 feet 4 inches tall and weighs 126 pounds. EER equations are from the Institute of Medicine. Dietary Reference Intakes for Energy, Carbohydrate, Fiber, Fat, Fatty Acids, Cholesterol, Protein, and Amino Acids. Washington (DC): The National Academies Press; 2002.

[b]Sedentary means a lifestyle that includes only the light physical activity associated with typical day-to-day life. Moderately active means a lifestyle that includes physical activity equivalent to walking about 1.5 to 3 miles per day at 3 to 4 miles per hour, in addition to the light physical activity associated with typical day-to-day life. Active means a lifestyle that includes physical activity equivalent to walking more than 3 miles per day at 3 to 4 miles per hour, in addition to the light physical activity associated with typical day-to-day life.

[c]Estimates for females do not include women who are pregnant or breastfeeding.

Source: Britten P, Marcoe K, Yamini S, Davis C. Development of food intake patterns for the MyPyramid Food Guidance System. *J Nutr Educ Behav* 2006;38(6 Suppl):S78–S92.

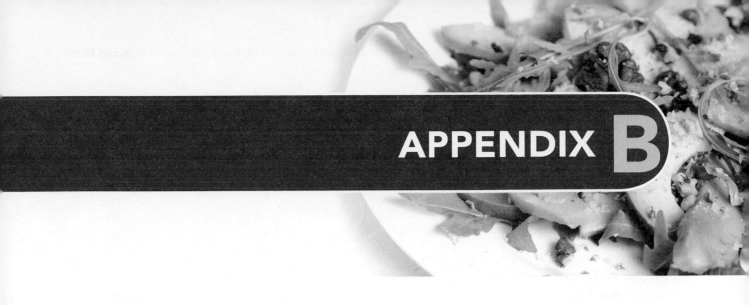

APPENDIX B

DIETARY GUIDELINES FOR AMERICANS, 2010: FOOD SOURCES OF SELECTED NUTRIENTS

Reprinted from *Dietary Guidelines for Americans, 2010* (7th ed.), by the U.S. Department of Health and Human Services and U.S. Department of Agriculture, 2010, Washington, DC: U.S. Government Printing Office.

Appendix B-1

Selected food sources ranked by amounts of potassium and calories per standard food portion.

Food	Standard portion size	Calories in standard portion[a]	Potassium in standard portion (mg)[a]
Potato, baked, flesh and skin	1 small potato	128	738
Prune juice, canned	1 cup	182	707
Carrot juice, canned	1 cup	94	689
Tomato paste	¼ cup	54	664
Beet greens, cooked	½ cup	19	654
White beans, canned	½ cup	149	595
Tomato juice, canned	1 cup	41	556
Plain yogurt, nonfat or low-fat	8 ounces	127–143	531–579
Tomato puree	½ cup	48	549
Sweet potato, baked in skin	1 medium	103	542
Clams, canned	3 ounces	126	534
Orange juice, fresh	1 cup	112	496
Halibut, cooked	3 ounces	119	490
Soybeans, green, cooked	½ cup	127	485
Tuna, yellowfin, cooked	3 ounces	118	484
Lima beans, cooked	½ cup	108	478
Soybeans, mature, cooked	½ cup	149	443
Rockfish, Pacific, cooked	3 ounces	103	442
Cod, Pacific, cooked	3 ounces	89	439
Evaporated milk, nonfat	½ cup	100	425
Low-fat (1%) or reduced-fat (2%) chocolate milk	1 cup	158–190	422–425
Bananas	1 medium	105	422

(continues)

(continued)

Food	Standard portion size	Calories in standard portion[a]	Potassium in standard portion (mg)[a]
Spinach, cooked	½ cup	21–25	370–419
Tomato sauce	½ cup	29	405
Peaches, dried, uncooked	¼ cup	96	398
Prunes, stewed	½ cup	133	398
Skim milk (nonfat)	1 cup	83	382
Rainbow trout, cooked	3 ounces	128	381
Apricots, dried, uncooked	¼ cup	78	378
Pinto beans, cooked	½ cup	122	373
Pork loin, center rib, lean, roasted	3 ounces	190	371
Low-fat milk or buttermilk (1%)	1 cup	98–102	366–370
Lentils, cooked	½ cup	115	365
Plantains, cooked	½ cup	89	358
Kidney beans, cooked	½ cup	112	358

[a]Source: U.S. Department of Agriculture, Agricultural Research Service, Nutrient Data Laboratory. 2009. USDA National Nutrient Database for Standard Reference, Release 22. Available at: http://www.ars.usda.gov/ba/bhnrc/ndl.

Appendix B-2
Selected food sources ranked by amounts of dietary fiber and calories per standard food portion.

Food	Standard portion size	Calories in standard portion[a]	Dietary fiber in standard portion (g)[a]
Beans (navy, pinto, black, kidney, white, great northern, lima), cooked	½ cup	104–149	6.2–9.6
Bran ready-to-eat cereal (100%)	⅓ cup (about 1 ounce)	81	9.1
Split peas, lentils, chickpeas, or cowpeas, cooked	½ cup	108–134	5.6–8.1
Artichoke, cooked	½ cup hearts	45	7.2
Pear	1 medium	103	5.5
Soybeans, mature, cooked	½ cup	149	5.2
Plain rye wafer crackers	2 wafers	73	5.0
Bran ready-to-eat cereals (various)	⅓–¾ cup (about 1 ounce)	88–91	2.6–5.0
Asian pear	1 small	51	4.4
Green peas, cooked	½ cup	59–67	3.5–4.4
Whole-wheat English muffin	1 muffin	134	4.4
Bulgur, cooked	½ cup	76	4.1
Mixed vegetables, cooked	½ cup	59	4.0
Raspberries	½ cup	32	4.0
Sweet potato, baked in skin	1 medium	103	3.8
Blackberries	½ cup	31	3.8
Soybeans, green, cooked	½ cup	127	3.8
Prunes, stewed	½ cup	133	3.8
Shredded wheat ready-to-eat cereal	½ cup (about 1 ounce)	95–100	2.7–3.8
Figs, dried	¼ cup	93	3.7

(continues)

(continued)

Food	Standard portion size	Calories in standard portion[a]	Dietary fiber in standard portion (g)[a]
Apple, with skin	1 small	77	3.6
Pumpkin, canned	½ cup	42	3.6
Greens (spinach, collards, turnip greens), cooked	½ cup	14–32	2.5–3.5
Almonds	1 ounce	163	3.5
Sauerkraut, canned	½ cup	22	3.4
Whole wheat spaghetti, cooked	½ cup	87	3.1
Banana	1 medium	105	3.1
Orange	1 medium	62	3.1
Guava	1 fruit	37	3.0
Potato, baked, with skin	1 small	128	3.0
Oat bran muffin	1 small	178	3.0
Pearled barley, cooked	½ cup	97	3.0
Dates	¼ cup	104	2.9
Winter squash, cooked	½ cup	38	2.9
Parsnips, cooked	½ cup	55	2.8
Tomato paste	¼ cup	54	2.7
Broccoli, cooked	½ cup	26–27	2.6–2.8
Okra, cooked from frozen	½ cup	26	2.6

[a]Source: U.S. Department of Agriculture, Agricultural Research Service, Nutrient Data Laboratory. 2009. USDA National Nutrient Database for Standard Reference, Release 22. Available at: http://www.ars.usda.gov/ba/bhnrc/ndl.

Appendix B-3
Selected food sources ranked by amounts of calcium and calories per standard food portion.

Food	Standard portion size	Calories in standard portion[a]	Calcium in standard portion[a] (mg)
Fortified ready-to-eat cereals (various)	¾–1 cup (about 1 ounce)	100–210	250–1,000
Orange juice, calcium fortified	1 cup	117	500
Plain yogurt, nonfat	8 ounces	127	452
Romano cheese	1½ ounces	165	452
Pasteurized process Swiss cheese	2 ounces	189	438
Evaporated milk, nonfat	½ cup	100	371
Tofu, regular, prepared with calcium sulfate	½ cup	94	434
Plain yogurt, low-fat	8 ounces	143	415
Fruit yogurt, low-fat	8 ounces	232	345
Ricotta cheese, part skim	½ cup	171	337
Swiss cheese	1½ ounces	162	336
Sardines, canned in oil, drained	3 ounces	177	325
Pasteurized process American cheese food	2 ounces	187	323
Provolone cheese	1½ ounces	149	321
Mozzarella cheese, part-skim	1½ ounces	128	311
Cheddar cheese	1½ ounces	171	307

(continues)

(continued)

Food	Standard portion size	Calories in standard portion[a]	Calcium in standard portion[a] (mg)
Low-fat milk (1%)	1 cup	102	305
Muenster cheese	1½ ounces	156	305
Skim milk (nonfat)	1 cup	83	299
Soymilk, original and vanilla, with added calcium	1 cup	104	299
Reduced fat milk (2%)	1 cup	122	293
Low-fat chocolate milk (1%)	1 cup	158	290
Low-fat buttermilk (1%)	1 cup	98	284
Rice milk, with added calcium	1 cup	113	283
Whole chocolate milk	1 cup	208	280
Whole milk	1 cup	149	276
Plain yogurt, whole milk	8 ounces	138	275
Reduced fat chocolate milk (2%)	1 cup	190	272
Ricotta cheese, whole milk	½ cup	216	257
Tofu, firm, prepared with calcium sulfate and magnesium choloride	½ cup	88	253

[a]Source: U.S. Department of Agriculture, Agricultural Research Service, Nutrient Data Laboratory. 2009. USDA National Nutrient Database for Standard Reference, Release 22. Available at: http://www.ars.usda.gov/ba/bhnrc/ndl.

Appendix B-4

Selected food sources ranked by amounts of vitamin D and calories per standard food portion.

Food	Standard portion size	Calories in standard portion[a]	Vitamin D in standard portion[a,b] (mcg)
Salmon, sockeye, cooked	3 ounces	184	19.8
Salmon, smoked	3 ounces	99	14.5
Salmon, canned	3 ounces	118	11.6
Rockfish, cooked	3 ounces	103	6.5
Tuna, light, canned in oil, drained	3 ounces	168	5.7
Orange juice[c]	1 cup	118	3.4
Sardine, canned in oil, drained	3 ounces	177	4.1
Tuna, light, canned in water, drained	3 ounces	99	3.8
Whole milk[c]	1 cup	149	3.2
Whole chocolate milk[c]	1 cup	208	3.2
Reduced fat chocolate milk (2%)[c]	1 cup	190	3.0
Milk (nonfat, 1% and 2%)[c]	1 cup	83–122	2.9
Low-fat chocolate milk (1%)[c]	1 cup	158	2.8
Soymilk[c]	1 cup	104	2.7
Evaporated milk, nonfat[c]	½ cup	100	2.6
Flatfish (flounder and sole), cooked	3 ounces	99	2.5
Fortified ready-to-eat cereals (various)[c]	¾–1¼ cup (about 1 ounce)	92–190	0.9–2.5
Rice drink[c]	1 cup	113	2.4

(continues)

(continued)

Food	Standard portion size	Calories in standard portion[a]	Vitamin D in standard portion[a,b] (mcg)
Herring, pickled	3 ounces	223	2.4
Pork, cooked (various cuts)	3 ounces	153–337	0.6–2.2
Cod, cooked	3 ounces	89	1.0
Beef liver, cooked	3 ounces	149	1.0
Cured ham	3 ounces	133–207	0.6–0.8
Egg, hard-boiled	1 large	78	0.7
Shiitake mushrooms	½ cup	41	0.6
Canadian bacon	2 slices (about 1½ ounces)	87	0.5

[a]Source: U.S. Department of Agriculture, Agricultural Research Service, Nutrient Data Laboratory. 2009. USDA National Nutrient Database for Standard Reference, Release 22. Available at: http://www.ars.usda.gov/ba/bhnrc/ndl.

[b]1 mcg of vitamin D is equivalent to 40 IU.

[c]Vitamin D fortified.

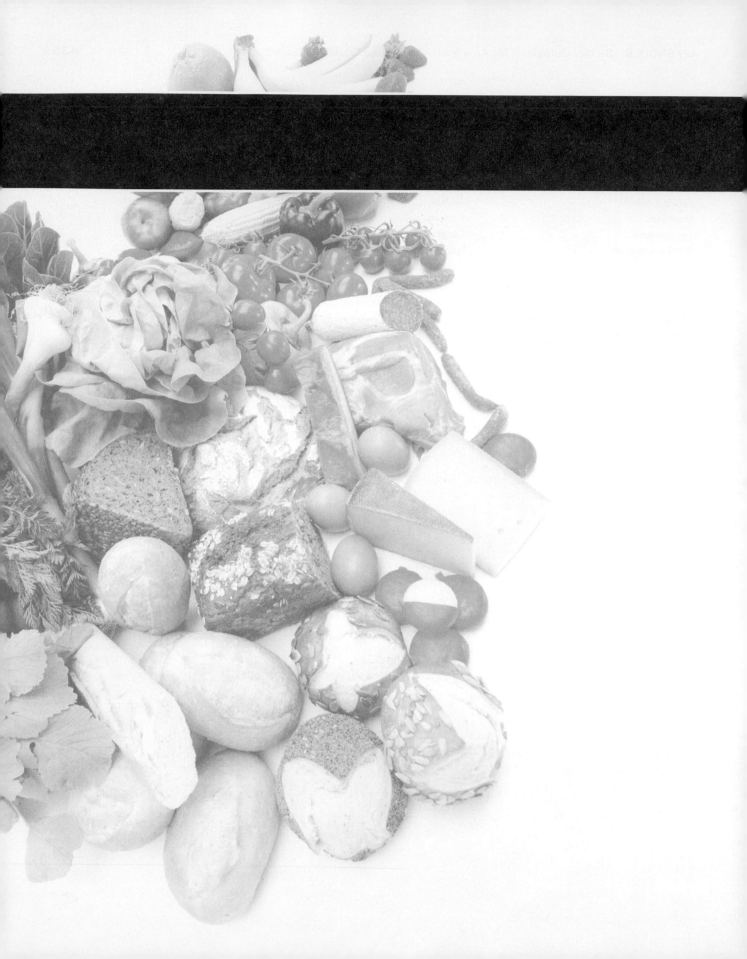

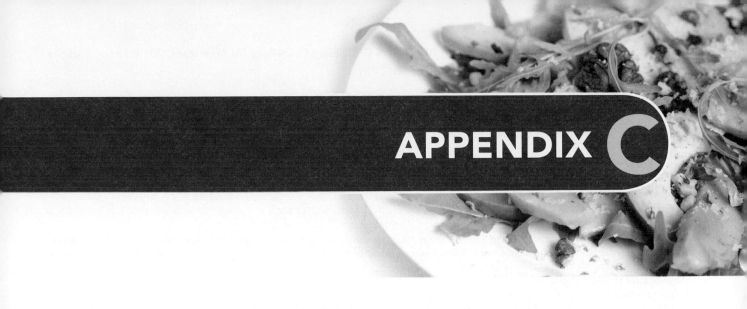

APPENDIX C

DIETARY GUIDELINES FOR AMERICANS, 2010: EATING PATTERNS

Reprinted from *Dietary Guidelines for Americans, 2010* (7th ed.), by the U.S. Department of Health and Human Services and U.S. Department of Agriculture, 2010, Washington, DC: U.S. Government Printing Office.

Appendix C-1

The DASH Eating Plan at Specific Calorie Levels
The DASH Eating Plan is based on various calorie levels. The number of daily servings in a food group varies depending on caloric needs[a] (see Appendix A to determine caloric needs). This chart can aid in planning menus and food selection in restaurants and grocery stores.

Food group[b]	1,200 calories	1,400 calories	1,600 calories	1,800 calories	2,000 calories	2,600 calories	3,100 calories	Serving sizes
Grains	4–5	5–6	6	6	6–8	10–11	12–13	1 slice bread; 1 oz dry cereal[c]; ½ cup cooked rice, pasta, or cereal[c]
Vegetables	3–4	3–4	3–4	4–5	4–5	5–6	6	1 cup raw leafy vegetable; ½ cup cut-up raw or cooked vegetable; ½ cup vegetable juice
Fruits	3–4	4	4	4–5	4–5	5–6	6	1 medium fruit; ¼ cup dried fruit; ½ cup fresh, frozen, or canned fruit; ½ cup fruit juice
Fat-free or low-fat milk and milk products	2–3	2–3	2–3	2–3	2–3	3	3–4	1 cup milk or yogurt; 1½ oz cheese
Lean meats, poultry, and fish	3 or less	3–4 or less	3–4 or less	6 or less	6 or less	6 or less	6–9	1 oz cooked meats, poultry, or fish; 1 egg
Nuts, seeds, and legumes	3 per week	3 per week	3–4 per week	4 per week	4–5 per week	1	1	⅓ cup or 1½ oz nuts; 2 Tbsp peanut butter; 2 Tbsp or ½ oz seeds; ½ cup cooked legumes (dried beans, peas)
Fats and oils	1	1	2	2–3	2–3	3	4	1 tsp soft margarine; 1 tsp vegetable oil; 1 Tbsp mayonnaise; 1 Tbsp salad dressing

(continues)

(continued)

Food group[b]	1,200 calories	1,400 calories	1,600 calories	1,800 calories	2,000 calories	2,600 calories	3,100 calories	Serving sizes
Sweets and added sugars	3 or less per week	3 or less per week	3 or less per week	5 or less per week	5 or less per week	< 2	< 2	1 Tbsp sugar; 1 Tbsp jelly or jam; ½ cup sorbet, gelatin dessert; 1 cup lemonade
Maximum sodium limit[d]	2,300 mg/day	2,300 mg/day	2,300 mg/day	2,300 mg/day	2,300 mg/day	2,300 mg/day	2,300 mg/day	

[a]The DASH eating patterns from 1,200 to 1,800 calories meet the nutritional needs of children 4 to 8 years old. Patterns from 1,600 to 3,100 calories meet the nutritional needs of children 9 years and older and adults. See Appendix A for estimated calorie needs per day by age, gender, and physical activity level.

[b]Significance to DASH Eating Plan, selection notes, and examples of foods in each food group.

• Grains: Major sources of energy and fiber. Whole grains are recommended for most grain servings as a good source of fiber and nutrients. Examples: Whole-wheat bread and rolls; whole-wheat pasta, English muffin, pita bread, bagel, cereals; grits, oatmeal, brown rice; unsalted pretzels and popcorn.

• Vegetables: Rich sources of potassium, magnesium, and fiber. Examples: Broccoli, carrots, collards, green beans, green peas, kale, lima beans, potatoes, spinach, squash, sweet potatoes, tomatoes.

• Fruits: Important sources of potassium, magnesium, and fiber. Examples: Apples, apricots, bananas, dates, grapes, oranges, grape-fruit, grapefruit juice, mangoes, melons, peaches, pineapples, raisins, strawberries, tangerines.

• Fat-free or low-fat milk and milk products: Major sources of calcium and protein. Examples: Fat-free milk or buttermilk; fat-free, low-fat, or reduced-fat cheese; fat-free/low-fat regular or frozen yogurt.

• Lean meats, poultry, and fish: Rich sources of protein and magnesium. Select only lean; trim away visible fats; broil, roast, or poach; remove skin from poultry. Since eggs are high in cholesterol, limit egg yolk intake to no more than four per week; two egg whites have the same protein content as 1 oz meat.

• Nuts, seeds, and legumes: Rich sources of energy, magnesium, protein, and fiber. Examples: Almonds, filberts, mixed nuts, peanuts, walnuts, sunflower seeds, peanut butter, kidney beans, lentils, split peas.

• Fats and oils: DASH study had 27 percent of calories as fat, including fat in or added to foods. Fat content changes serving amount for fats and oils. For example, 1 Tbsp regular salad dressing = one serving; 2 Tbsp low-fat dressing = one serving; 1 Tbsp fat-free dressing = zero servings. Examples: Soft margarine, vegetable oil (canola, corn, olive, safflower), low-fat mayonnaise, light salad dressing.

• Sweets and added sugars: Sweets should be low in fat. Examples: Fruit-flavored gelatin, fruit punch, hard candy, jelly, maple syrup, sorbet and ices, sugar.

[c]Serving sizes vary between ½ cup and 1¼ cups, depending on cereal type. Check product's Nutrition Facts label.

[d]The DASH Eating Plan consists of patterns with a sodium limit of 2,300 mg and 1,500 mg per day.

Source: U.S. Department of Agriculture and U.S. Department of Health and Human Services. Dietary Guidelines for Americans, 2010. 7th Edition, Washington, DC: U.S. Government Printing Office, December 2010

Appendix C-2
USDA Food Patterns

The suggested amounts of food to consume from the basic food groups, subgroups, and oils to meet recommended nutrient intakes at 12 different calorie levels. Nutrient and energy contributions from each group are calculated according to the nutrient-dense forms of foods in each group (e.g., lean meats and fat-free milk).
For each food group or subgroup,[a] recommended average daily intake amounts[b] at all calorie levels. Recommended intakes from vegetable and protein foods subgroups are per week. For more information and tools for application, go to MyPyramid.gov.

Calorie level of pattern[c]	1,000	1,200	1,400	1,600	1,800	2,000	2,200	2,400	2,600	2,800	3,000	3,200
Fruits	1 c	1 c	1½ c	1½ c	1½ c	2 c	2 c	2 c	2 c	2½ c	2½ c	2½ c
Vegetables[d]	1 c	1½ c	1½ c	2 c	2½ c	2½ c	3 c	3 c	3½ c	3½ c	4 c	4 c
Dark-green vegetables	½ c/wk	1 c/wk	1 c/wk	1½ c/wk	1½ c/wk	1½ c/wk	2 c/wk	2 c/wk	2½ c/wk	2½ c/wk	2½ c/wk	2½ c/wk
Red and orange vegetables	2½ c/wk	3 c/wk	3 c/wk	4 c/wk	5½ c/wk	5½ c/wk	6 c/wk	6 c/wk	7 c/wk	7 c/wk	7½ c/wk	7½ c/wk

(continues)

(continued)

Beans and peas (legumes)	½ c/wk	½ c/wk	½ c/wk	1 c/wk	1½ c/wk	1½ c/wk	2 c/wk	2 c/wk	2½ c/wk	2½ c/wk	3 c/wk	3 c/wk
Starchy vegetables	2 c/wk	3½ c/wk	3½ c/wk	4 c/wk	5 c/wk	5 c/wk	6 c/wk	6 c/wk	7 c/wk	7 c/wk	8 c/wk	8 c/wk
Other vegetables	1½ c/wk	2½ c/wk	2½ c/wk	3½ c/wk	4 c/wk	4 c/wk	5 c/wk	5 c/wk	5½ c/wk	5½ c/wk	7 c/wk	7 c/wk
Grains[e]	3 oz-eq	4 oz-eq	5 oz-eq	5 oz-eq	6 oz-eq	6 oz-eq	7 oz-eq	8 oz-eq	9 oz-eq	10 oz-eq	10 oz-eq	10 oz-eq
Whole grains	1½ oz-eq	2 oz-eq	2½ oz-eq	3 oz-eq	3 oz-eq	3 oz-eq	3½ oz-eq	4 oz-eq	4½ oz-eq	5 oz-eq	5 oz-eq	5 oz-eq
Enriched grains	1½ oz-eq	2 oz-eq	2½ oz-eq	2 oz-eq	3 oz-eq	3 oz-eq	3½ oz-eq	4 oz-eq	4½ oz-eq	5 oz-eq	5 oz-eq	5 oz-eq
Protein foods[d]	2 oz-eq	3 oz-eq	4 oz-eq	5 oz-eq	5 oz-eq	5½ oz-eq	6 oz-eq	6½ oz-eq	6½ oz-eq	7 oz-eq	7 oz-eq	7 oz-eq
Seafood	3 oz/wk	5 oz/wk	6 oz/wk	8 oz/wk	8 oz/wk	8 oz/wk	9 oz/wk	10 oz/wk	10 oz/wk	11 oz/wk	11 oz/wk	11 oz/wk
Meat, poultry, eggs	10 oz/wk	14 oz/wk	19 oz/wk	24 oz/wk	24 oz/wk	26 oz/wk	29 oz/wk	31 oz/wk	31 oz/wk	34 oz/wk	34 oz/wk	34 oz/wk
Nuts, seeds, soy products	1 oz/wk	2 oz/wk	3 oz/wk	4 oz/wk	4 oz/wk	4 oz/wk	4 oz/wk	5 oz/wk	5 oz/wk	5 oz/wk	5 oz/wk	5 oz/wk
Dairy[f]	2 c	2½ c	2½ c	3 c	3 c	3 c	3 c	3 c	3 c	3 c	3 c	3 c
Oils[g]	15 g	17 g	17 g	22 g	24 g	27 g	29 g	31 g	34 g	36 g	44 g	51 g
Maximum SoFAS[h] **limit, calories (% of calories)**	137 (14%)	121 (10%)	121 (9%)	121 (8%)	161 (9%)	258 (13%)	266 (12%)	330 (14%)	362 (14%)	395 (14%)	459 (15%)	596 (19%)

[a]All foods are assumed to be in nutrient-dense forms, lean or low-fat, and prepared without added fats, sugars, or salt. Solid fats and added sugars may be included up to the daily maximum limit identified in the table. Food items in each group and subgroup are:

- Fruits: All fresh, frozen, canned, and dried fruits and fruit juices: for example, oranges and orange juice, apples and apple juice, bananas, grapes, melons, berries, raisins.
- Vegetables
  - Dark green vegetables: All fresh, frozen, and canned dark-green leafy vegetables and broccoli, cooked or raw: for example, broccoli; spinach; romaine; collard, turnip, and mustard greens.
  - Red and orange vegetables: All fresh, frozen, and canned red and orange vegetables, cooked or raw: for example, tomatoes, red peppers, carrots, sweet potatoes, winter squash, and pumpkin.
  - Beans and peas (legumes): All cooked beans and peas: for example, kidney beans, lentils, chickpeas, and pinto beans. Does not include green beans or green peas. (See additional comment under protein foods group.)
  - Starchy vegetables: All fresh, frozen, and canned starchy vegetables: for example, white potatoes, corn, green peas.
  - Other vegetables: All fresh, frozen, and canned other vegetables, cooked or raw: for example, iceberg lettuce, green beans, and onions.
- Grains
  - Whole grains: All whole-grain products and whole grains used as ingredients: for example, whole-wheat bread, whole-grain cereals and crackers, oatmeal, and brown rice.
  - Enriched grains: All enriched refined-grain products and enriched refined grains used as ingredients: for example, white breads, enriched grain cereals and crackers, enriched pasta, white rice.
  - Protein foods: All meat, poultry, seafood, eggs, nuts, seeds, and processed soy products. Meat and poultry should be lean or low-fat and nuts should be unsalted. Beans and peas are considered part of this group as well as the vegetable group, but should be counted in one group only.
  - Dairy: All milks, including lactose-free and lactose-reduced products and fortified soy beverages, yogurts, frozen yogurts, dairy desserts, and cheeses. Most choices should be fat-free or low-fat. Cream, sour cream, and cream cheese are not included due to their low calcium content.

[b]Food group amounts are shown in cup (c) or ounce-equivalents (oz-eq). Oils are shown in grams (g). Quantity equivalents for each food group are:

- Grains, 1 ounce-equivalent is: 1 ounce slice bread; 1 ounce uncooked pasta or rice; ½ cup cooked rice, pasta, or cereal; 1 tortilla (6″ diameter); 1 pancake (5″ diameter); 1 ounce ready-to-eat cereal (about 1 cup cereal flakes).
- Vegetables and fruits, 1 cup equivalent is: 1 cup raw or cooked vegetable or fruit; ½ cup dried vegetable or fruit; 1 cup vegetable or fruit juice; 2 cups leafy salad greens.
- Protein foods, 1 ounce-equivalent is: 1 ounce lean meat, poultry, seafood; 1 egg; 1 Tbsp peanut butter; ½ ounce nuts or seeds. Also, ¼ cup cooked beans or peas may also be counted as 1 ounce-equivalent.
- Dairy, 1 cup equivalent is: 1 cup milk, fortified soy beverage, or yogurt; 1½ ounces natural cheese (e.g., cheddar); 2 ounces of processed cheese (e.g., American).

(continues)

(continued)

[c]See Appendix A for estimated calorie needs per day by age, gender, and physical activity level. Food intake patterns at 1,000, 1,200, and 1,400 calories meet the nutritional needs of children ages 2 to 8 years. Patterns from 1,600 to 3,200 calories meet the nutritional needs of children ages 9 years and older and adults. If a child ages 4 to 8 years needs more calories and, therefore, is following a pattern at 1,600 calories or more, the recommended amount from the dairy group can be 2½ cups per day. Children ages 9 years and older and adults should not use the 1,000, 1,200, or 1,400 calorie patterns.

[d]Vegetable and protein foods subgroup amounts are shown in this table as weekly amounts, because it would be difficult for consumers to select foods from all subgroups daily.

[e]Whole-grain subgroup amounts shown in this table are minimums. More whole grains up to all of the grains recommended may be selected, with offsetting decreases in the amounts of enriched refined grains.

[f]The amount of dairy foods in the 1,200 and 1,400 calorie patterns have increased to reflect new RDAs for calcium that are higher than previous recommendations for children ages 4 to 8 years.

[g]Oils and soft margarines include vegetable, nut, and fish oils and soft vegetable oil table spreads that have no *trans* fats.

[h]SoFAS are calories from solid fats and added sugars. The limit for SoFAS is the remaining amount of calories in each food pattern after selecting the specified amounts in each food group in nutrient-dense forms (forms that are fat-free or low-fat and with no added sugars). The number of SoFAS is lower in the 1,200, 1,400, and 1,600 calorie patterns than in the 1,000 calorie pattern. The nutrient goals for the 1,200 to 1,600 calorie patterns are higher and require that more calories be used for nutrient-dense foods from the food groups.

Source: U.S. Department of Agriculture and U.S. Department of Health and Human Services. Dietary Guidelines for Americans, 2010. 7th Edition, Washington, DC: U.S. Government Printing Office, December 2010

Appendix C-3
Lacto-ovo vegetarian adaptation of the USDA food patterns.
For each food group or subgroup,[a] recommended average daily intake amounts[b] at all calorie levels. Recommended intakes from vegetable and protein foods subgroups are per week. For more information and tools for application, go to MyPyramid.gov.

Calorie level of pattern[c]	1,000	1,200	1,400	1,600	1,800	2,000	2,200	2,400	2,600	2,800	3,000	3,200
Fruits	1 c	1 c	1½ c	1½ c	1½ c	2 c	2 c	2 c	2 c	2½ c	2½ c	2½ c
Vegetables[d]	1 c	1½ c	1½ c	2 c	2½ c	2½ c	3 c	3 c	3½ c	3½ c	4 c	4 c
Dark green vegetables	½ c/wk	1 c/wk	1 c/wk	1½ c/wk	1½ c/wk	1½ c/wk	2 c/wk	2 c/wk	2½ c/wk	2½ c/wk	2½ c/wk	2½ c/wk
Red and orange vegetables	2½ c/wk	3 c/wk	3 c/wk	4 c/wk	5½ c/wk	5½ c/wk	6 c/wk	6 c/wk	7 c/wk	7 c/wk	7½ c/wk	7½ c/wk
Beans and peas (legumes)	½ c/wk	½ c/wk	½ c/wk	1 c/wk	1½ c/wk	1½ c/wk	2 c/wk	2 c/wk	2½ c/wk	2½ c/wk	3 c/wk	3 c/wk
Starchy vegetables	2 c/wk	3½ c/wk	3½ c/wk	4 c/wk	5 c/wk	5 c/wk	6 c/wk	6 c/wk	7 c/wk	7 c/wk	8 c/wk	8 c/wk
Other vegetables	1½ c/wk	2½ c/wk	2½ c/wk	3½ c/wk	4 c/wk	4 c/wk	5 c/wk	5 c/wk	5½ c/wk	5½ c/wk	7 c/wk	7 c/wk
Grains[e]	3 oz-eq	4 oz-eq	5 oz-eq	5 oz-eq	6 oz-eq	6 oz-eq	7 oz-eq	8 oz-eq	9 oz-eq	10 oz-eq	10 oz-eq	10 oz-eq
Whole grains	1½ oz-eq	2 oz-eq	2½ oz-eq	3 oz-eq	3 oz-eq	3 oz-eq	3½ oz-eq	4 oz-eq	4½ oz-eq	5 oz-eq	5 oz-eq	5 oz-eq
Refined grains	1½ oz-eq	2 oz-eq	2½ oz-eq	2 oz-eq	3 oz-eq	3 oz-eq	3½ oz-eq	4 oz-eq	4½ oz-eq	5 oz-eq	5 oz-eq	5 oz-eq
Protein foods[d]	2 oz-eq	3 oz-eq	4 oz-eq	5 oz-eq	5 oz-eq	5½ oz-eq	6 oz-eq	6½ oz-eq	6½ oz-eq	7 oz-eq	7 oz-eq	7 oz-eq
Eggs	1 oz-eq/wk	2 oz-eq/wk	3 oz-eq/wk	4 oz-eq/wk	4 oz-eq/wk	4 oz-eq/wk	4 oz-eq/wk	5 oz-eq/wk	5 oz-eq/wk	5 oz-eq/wk	5 oz-eq/wk	5 oz-eq/wk
Beans and peas[f]	3½ oz-eq/wk	5 oz-eq/wk	7 oz-eq/wk	9 oz-eq/wk	9 oz-eq/wk	10 oz-eq/wk	10 oz-eq/wk	11 oz-eq/wk	11 oz-eq/wk	12 oz-eq/wk	12 oz-eq/wk	12 oz-eq/wk
Soy products	4 oz-eq/wk	6 oz-eq/wk	8 oz-eq/wk	11 oz-eq/wk	11 oz-eq/wk	12 oz-eq/wk	13 oz-eq/wk	14 oz-eq/wk	14 oz-eq/wk	15 oz-eq/wk	15 oz-eq/wk	15 oz-eq/wk
Nuts and seeds	5 oz-eq/wk	7 oz-eq/wk	10 oz-eq/wk	12 oz-eq/wk	12 oz-eq/wk	13 oz-eq/wk	15 oz-eq/wk	16 oz-eq/wk	16 oz-eq/wk	17 oz-eq/wk	17 oz-eq/wk	17 oz-eq/wk
Dairy[g]	2 c	2½ c	2½ c	3 c	3 c	3 c	3 c	3 c	3 c	3 c	3 c	3 c
Oils[h]	12 g	13 g	12 g	15 g	17 g	19 g	21 g	22 g	25 g	26 g	34 g	41 g
Maximum SoFAS[i] **limit, calories (% total calories)**	137 (14%)	121 (10%)	121 (9%)	121 (8%)	161 (9%)	258 (13%)	266 (12%)	330 (14%)	362 (14%)	395 (14%)	459 (15%)	596 (19%)

(continues)

a,b,c,d,e See Appendix C-2, notes a through e.

f Total recommended beans and peas amounts would be the sum of amounts recommended in the vegetable and the protein foods groups. An ounce-equivalent of beans and peas in the protein foods group is ¼ cup, cooked. For example, in the 2,000 calorie pattern, total weekly beans and peas recommendation is (10 oz-eq/4) + 1½ cups = about 4 cups, cooked.

g,h,i See Appendix C-2, notes f, g, and h.

Source: U.S. Department of Agriculture and U.S. Department of Health and Human Services. Dietary Guidelines for Americans, 2010. 7th Edition, Washington, DC: U.S. Government Printing Office, December 2010

Appendix C-4

Vegan adaptation of the USDA food patterns.
For each food group or subgroup,[a] recommended average daily intake amounts[b] at all calorie levels. Recommended intakes from vegetable and protein foods subgroups are per week. For more information and tools for application, go to MyPyramid.gov.

Calorie level of pattern[c]	1,000	1,200	1,400	1,600	1,800	2,000	2,200	2,400	2,600	2,800	3,000	3,200
Fruits	1 c	1 c	1½ c	1½ c	1½ c	2 c	2 c	2 c	2 c	2½ c	2½ c	2½ c
Vegetables[d]	1 c	1½ c	1½ c	2 c	2½ c	2½ c	3 c	3 c	3½ c	3½ c	4 c	4 c
Dark green vegetables	½ c/wk	1 c/wk	1 c/wk	1½ c/wk	1½ c/wk	1½ c/wk	2 c/wk	2 c/wk	2½ c/wk	2½ c/wk	2½ c/wk	2½ c/wk
Red and orange vegetables	2½ c/wk	3 c/wk	3 c/wk	4 c/wk	5½ c/wk	5½ c/wk	6 c/wk	6 c/wk	7 c/wk	7 c/wk	7½ c/wk	7½ c/wk
Beans and peas (legumes)	½ c/wk	½ c/wk	½ c/wk	1 c/wk	1½ c/wk	1½ c/wk	2 c/wk	2 c/wk	2½ c/wk	2½ c/wk	3 c/wk	3 c/wk
Starchy vegetables	2 c/wk	3½ c/wk	3½ c/wk	4 c/wk	5 c/wk	5 c/wk	6 c/wk	6 c/wk	7 c/wk	7 c/wk	8 c/wk	8 c/wk
Other vegetables	1½ c/wk	2½ c/wk	2½ c/wk	3½ c/wk	4 c/wk	4 c/wk	5 c/wk	5 c/wk	5½ c/wk	5½ c/wk	7 c/wk	7 c/wk
Grains[e]	3 oz-eq	4 oz-eq	5 oz-eq	5 oz-eq	6 oz-eq	6 oz-eq	7 oz-eq	8 oz-eq	9 oz-eq	10 oz-eq	10 oz-eq	10 oz-eq
Whole grains	1½ oz-eq	2 oz-eq	2½ oz-eq	3 oz-eq	3 oz-eq	3 oz-eq	3½ oz-eq	4 oz-eq	4½ oz-eq	5 oz-eq	5 oz-eq	5 oz-eq
Refined grains	1½ oz-eq	2 oz-eq	2½ oz-eq	2 oz-eq	3 oz-eq	3 oz-eq	3½ oz-eq	4 oz-eq	4½ oz-eq	5 oz-eq	5 oz-eq	5 oz-eq
Protein foods[d]	2 oz-eq	3 oz-eq	4 oz-eq	5 oz-eq	5 oz-eq	5½ oz-eq	6 oz-eq	6½ oz-eq	6½ oz-eq	7 oz-eq	7 oz-eq	7 oz-eq
Beans and peas[f]	5 oz-eq/wk	7 oz-eq/wk	10 oz-eq/wk	12 oz-eq/wk	12 oz-eq/wk	13 oz-eq/wk	15 oz-eq/wk	16 oz-eq/wk	16 oz-eq/wk	17 oz-eq/wk	17 oz-eq/wk	17 oz-eq/wk
Soy products	4 oz-eq/wk	5 oz-eq/wk	7 oz-eq/wk	9 oz-eq/wk	9 oz-eq/wk	10 oz-eq/wk	11 oz-eq/wk	11 oz-eq/wk	11 oz-eq/wk	12 oz-eq/wk	12 oz-eq/wk	12 oz-eq/wk
Nuts and seeds	6 oz-eq/wk	8 oz-eq/wk	11 oz-eq/wk	14 oz-eq/wk	14 oz-eq/wk	15 oz-eq/wk	17 oz-eq/wk	18 oz-eq/wk	18 oz-eq/wk	20 oz-eq/wk	20 oz-eq/wk	20 oz-eq/wk
Dairy (vegan)[g]	2 c	2½ c	2½ c	3 c	3 c	3 c	3 c	3 c	3 c	3 c	3 c	3 c
Oils[h]	12 g	12 g	11 g	14 g	16 g	18 g	20 g	21 g	24 g	25 g	33 g	40 g
Maximum SoFAS[i] limit, calories (% total calories)	137 (14%)	121 (10%)	121 (9%)	121 (8%)	161 (9%)	258 (13%)	266 (12%)	330 (14%)	362 (14%)	395 (14%)	459 (15%)	596 (19%)

a,b,c,d,e See Appendix C-2, notes a through e.

f Total recommended beans and peas amounts would be the sum of amounts recommended in the vegetable and the protein foods groups. An ounce-equivalent of beans and peas in the protein foods group is ¼ cup, cooked. For example, in the 2,000 calorie pattern, total weekly beans and peas recommendation is (13 oz-eq/4) + 1½ cups = about 5 cups, cooked.

g The vegan "dairy group" is composed of calcium-fortified beverages and foods from plant sources. For analysis purposes the following products were included: calcium-fortified soy beverage, calcium-fortified rice milk, tofu made with calcium-sulfate, and calcium-fortified soy yogurt. The amounts in the 1,200 and 1,400 calorie patterns have increased to reflect new RDAs for calcium that are higher than previous recommendations for children ages 4 to 8 years.

h,i See Appendix C-2, notes g and h.

Source: U.S. Department of Agriculture and U.S. Department of Health and Human Services. Dietary Guidelines for Americans, 2010. 7th Edition, Washington, DC: U.S. Government Printing Office, December 2010

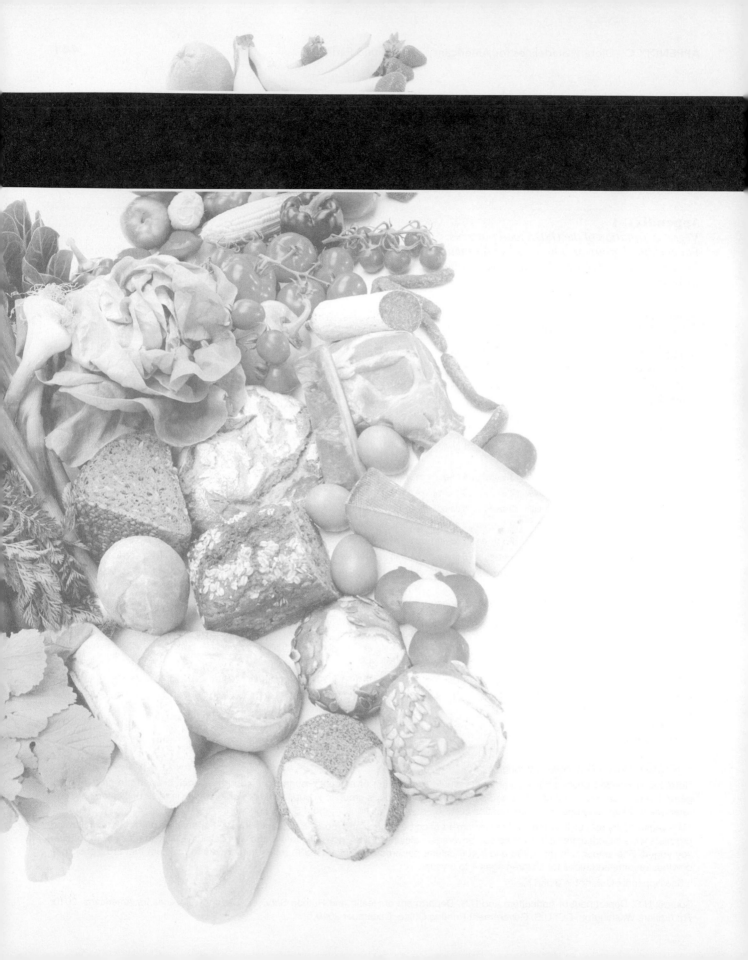

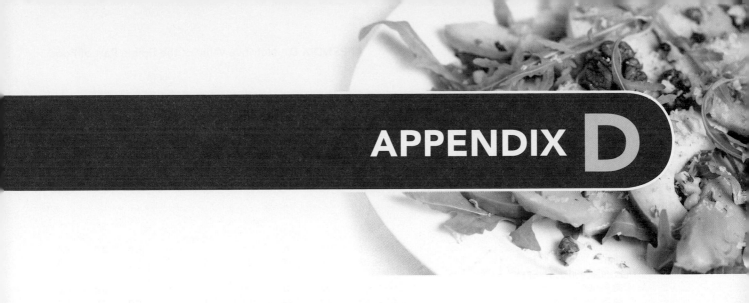

APPENDIX D

NUTRITIVE VALUE OF THE EDIBLE PART OF FOOD

Reprinted from "Nutritive value of foods" by S. E. Gebhardt and R. G. Thomas, 2002, U.S. Department of Agriculture, Agricultural Research, *Home and Garden Bulletin, 72,* 14–89.

Food No.	Food Description	Measure of Edible Portion	Weight (g)	Water (%)	Calories (kcal)	Protein (g)	Total Fat (g)	Fatty Acids Satu-rated (g)	Fatty Acids Mono-unsatu-rated (g)	Fatty Acids Poly-unsatu-rated (g)
BEVERAGES										
	ALCOHOLIC									
	BEER									
1	REGULAR	12 FL OZ	355	92	146	1	0	0.0	0.0	0.0
2	LIGHT	12 FL OZ	354	95	99	1	0	0.0	0.0	0.0
	GIN, RUM, VODKA, WHISKEY									
3	80 PROOF	1.5 FL OZ	42	67	97	0	0	0.0	0.0	0.0
4	86 PROOF	1.5 FL OZ	42	64	105	0	0	0.0	0.0	0.0
5	90 PROOF	1.5 FL OZ	42	62	110	0	0	0.0	0.0	0.0
6	LIQUEUR, COFFEE, 53 PROOF	1.5 FL OZ	52	31	175	TR	TR	0.1	TR	0.1
	MIXED DRINKS, PREPARED FROM RECIPE									
7	DAIQUIRI	2 FL OZ	60	70	112	TR	TR	TR	TR	TR
8	PINA COLADA	4.5 FL OZ	141	65	262	1	3	1.2	0.2	0.5
	WINE									
	DESSERT									
9	DRY	3.5 FL OZ	103	80	130	TR	0	0.0	0.0	0.0
10	SWEET	3.5 FL OZ	103	73	158	TR	0	0.0	0.0	0.0
	TABLE									
11	RED	3.5 FL OZ	103	89	74	TR	0	0.0	0.0	0.0
12	WHITE	3.5 FL OZ	103	90	70	TR	0	0.0	0.0	0.0
	CARBONATED*									
13	CLUB SODA	12 FL OZ	355	100	0	0	0	0.0	0.0	0.0
14	COLA TYPE	12 FL OZ	370	89	152	0	0	0.0	0.0	0.0
	DIET, SWEETENED WITH ASPARTAME									
15	COLA	12 FL OZ	355	100	4	TR	0	0.0	0.0	0.0
16	OTHER THAN COLA OR PEPPER TYPE	12 FL OZ	355	100	0	TR	0	0.0	0.0	0.0
17	GINGER ALE	12 FL OZ	366	91	124	0	0	0.0	0.0	0.0
18	GRAPE	12 FL OZ	372	89	160	0	0	0.0	0.0	0.0
19	LEMON LIME	12 FL OZ	368	90	147	0	0	0.0	0.0	0.0
20	ORANGE	12 FL OZ	372	88	179	0	0	0.0	0.0	0.0
21	PEPPER TYPE	12 FL OZ	368	89	151	0	TR	0.3	0.0	0.0
22	ROOT BEER	12 FL OZ	370	89	152	0	0	0.0	0.0	0.0
	CHOCOLATE-FLAVORED BEVERAGE MIX									
23	POWDER	2–3 HEAPING TSP	22	1	75	1	1	0.4	0.2	TR
24	PREPARED WITH MILK	1 CUP	266	81	226	9	9	5.5	2.6	0.3
	COCOA									
	POWDER CONTAINING NONFAT DRY MILK									
25	POWDER	3 HEAPING TSP	28	2	102	3	1	0.7	0.4	TR
26	PREPARED (6 OZ WATER PLUS 1 OZ POWDER)	1 SERVING	206	86	103	3	1	0.7	0.4	TR
	POWDER CONTAINING NONFAT DRY MILK AND ASPARTAME									
27	POWDER	1/2-OZ ENVELOPE	5	3	48	4	TR	0.3	0.1	TR
28	PREPARED (6 OZ WATER PLUS 1 ENVELOPE MIX)	1 SERVING	192	92	48	4	TR	0.3	0.1	TR
	COFFEE									
29	BREWED	6 FL OZ	178	99	4	TR	0	TR	0.0	TR
30	ESPRESSO	2 FL OZ	60	98	5	TR	TR	0.1	0.0	0.1
31	INSTANT, PREPARED (1 ROUNDED TSP POWDER PLUS 6 FL OZ WATER)	6 FL OZ	179	99	4	TR	0	TR	0.0	TR

*Mineral content varies depending on water source.

Cholesterol (mg)	Carbohydrate (g)	Total Dietary Fiber (g)	Calcium (mg)	Iron (mg)	Potassium (mg)	Sodium (mg)	Vitamin A		Thiamine (mg)	Riboflavin (mg)	Niacin (mg)	Ascorbic Acid (mg)	Food No.
							(IU)	(RE)					
0	13	0.7	18	0.1	89	18	0	0	0.02	0.09	1.6	0	1
0	5	0.0	18	0.1	64	11	0	0	0.03	0.11	1.4	0	2
0	0	0.0	0	TR	1	TR	0	0	TR	TR	TR	0	3
0	TR	0.0	0	TR	1	TR	0	0	TR	TR	TR	0	4
0	0	0.0	0	TR	1	TR	0	0	TR	TR	TR	0	5
0	24	0.0	1	TR	16	4	0	0	TR	0.01	0.1	0	6
0	4	0.0	2	0.1	13	3	2	0	0.01	TR	TR	1	7
0	40	0.8	11	0.3	100	8	3	0	0.04	0.02	0.2	7	8
0	4	0.0	8	0.2	95	9	0	0	0.02	0.02	0.2	0	9
0	12	0.0	8	0.2	95	9	0	0	0.02	0.02	0.2	0	10
0	2	0.0	8	0.4	115	5	0	0	0.01	0.03	0.1	0	11
0	1	0.0	9	0.3	82	5	0	0	TR	0.01	0.1	0	12
0	0	0.0	18	TR	7	75	0	0	0.00	0.00	0.0	0	13
0	38	0.0	11	0.1	4	15	0	0	0.00	0.00	0.0	0	14
0	TR	0.0	14	0.1	0	21	0	0	0.02	0.08	0.0	0	15
0	0	0.0	14	0.1	7	21	0	0	0.00	0.00	0.0	0	16
0	32	0.0	11	0.7	4	26	0	0	0.00	0.00	0.0	0	17
0	42	0.0	11	0.3	4	56	0	0	0.00	0.00	0.0	0	18
0	38	0.0	7	0.3	4	40	0	0	0.00	0.00	0.1	0	19
0	46	0.0	19	0.2	7	45	0	0	0.00	0.00	0.0	0	20
0	38	0.0	11	0.1	4	37	0	0	0.00	0.00	0.0	0	21
0	39	0.0	19	0.2	4	48	0	0	0.00	0.00	0.0	0	22
0	20	1.3	8	0.7	128	45	4	TR	0.01	0.03	0.1	TR	23
32	31	1.3	301	0.8	497	165	311	77	0.10	0.43	0.3	2	24
1	22	0.3	92	0.3	202	143	4	1	0.03	0.16	0.2	1	25
2	22	2.5	97	0.4	202	148	4	0	0.03	0.16	0.2	TR	26
1	9	0.4	86	0.7	405	168	5	1	0.04	0.21	0.2	0	27
2	8	0.4	90	0.7	405	173	4	0	0.04	0.21	0.2	0	28
0	1	0.0	4	0.1	96	4	0	0	0.00	0.00	0.4	0	29
0	1	0.0	1	0.1	69	8	0	0	TR	0.11	3.1	TR	30
0	1	0.0	5	0.1	64	5	0	0	0.00	TR	0.5	0	31

Food No.	Food Description	Measure of Edible Portion	Weight (g)	Water (%)	Calories (kcal)	Protein (g)	Total Fat (g)	Fatty Acids Saturated (g)	Monounsaturated (g)	Polyunsaturated (g)
BEVERAGES (CONTINUED)										
	FRUIT DRINKS, NONCARBONATED, CANNED OR BOTTLED, WITH ADDED ASCORBIC ACID									
32	CRANBERRY JUICE COCKTAIL	8 FL OZ	253	86	144	0	TR	TR	TR	0.1
33	FRUIT PUNCH DRINK	8 FL OZ	248	88	117	0	0	TR	TR	TR
34	GRAPE DRINK	8 FL OZ	250	88	113	0	0	TR	0.0	TR
35	PINEAPPLE GRAPEFRUIT JUICE DRINK	8 FL OZ	250	88	118	1	TR	TR	TR	0.1
36	PINEAPPLE ORANGE JUICE DRINK	8 FL OZ	250	87	125	3	0	0.0	0.0	0.0
	LEMONADE									
37	FROZEN CONCENTRATE, PREPARED	8 FL OZ	248	89	99	TR	0	TR	TR	TR
	POWDER, PREPARED WITH WATER									
38	REGULAR	8 FL OZ	266	89	112	0	0	TR	TR	TR
39	LOW CALORIE, SWEETENED WITH ASPARTAME	8 FL OZ	237	99	5	0	0	0.0	0.0	0.0
	MALTED MILK, WITH ADDED NUTRIENTS									
	CHOCOLATE									
40	POWDER	3 HEAPING TSP	21	3	75	1	1	0.4	0.2	0.1
41	PREPARED	1 CUP	265	81	225	9	9	5.5	2.6	0.4
	NATURAL									
42	POWDER	4–5 HEAPING TSP	21	3	80	2	1	0.3	0.2	0.1
43	PREPARED	1 CUP	265	81	231	10	9	5.4	2.5	0.4
	MILK AND MILK BEVERAGES. SEE DAIRY PRODUCTS.									
44	RICE BEVERAGE, CANNED (RICE DREAM)	1 CUP	245	89	120	TR	2	0.2	1.3	0.3
	SOY MILK. SEE LEGUMES, NUTS, AND SEEDS.									
	TEA									
	BREWED									
45	BLACK	6 FL OZ	178	100	2	0	0	TR	TR	TR
	HERB									
46	CHAMOMILE	6 FL OZ	178	100	2	0	0	TR	TR	TR
47	OTHER THAN CHAMOMILE	6 FL OZ	178	100	2	0	0	TR	TR	TR
	INSTANT, POWDER, PREPARED									
48	UNSWEETENED	8 FL OZ	237	100	2	0	0	0.0	0.0	0.0
49	SWEETENED, LEMON FLAVOR	8 FL OZ	259	91	88	TR	0	TR	TR	TR
50	SWEETENED WITH SACCHARIN, LEMON FLAVOR	8 FL OZ	237	99	5	0	0	0.0	0.0	TR
51	WATER, TAP	8 FL OZ	237	100	0	0	0	0.0	0.0	0.0
DAIRY PRODUCTS										
	BUTTER. SEE FATS AND OILS.									
	CHEESE									
	NATURAL									
52	BLUE	1 OZ	28	42	100	6	8	5.3	2.2	0.2
53	CAMEMBERT (3 WEDGES PER 4-OZ CONTAINER)	1 WEDGE	38	52	114	8	9	5.8	2.7	0.3
	CHEDDAR									
54	CUT PIECES	1 OZ	28	37	114	7	9	6.0	2.7	0.3
55		1 CUBIC IN.	17	37	68	4	6	3.6	1.6	0.2
56	SHREDDED	1 CUP	113	37	455	28	37	23.8	10.6	1.1

Cholesterol (mg)	Carbo-hydrate (g)	Total Dietary Fiber (g)	Calcium (mg)	Iron (mg)	Potassium (mg)	Sodium (mg)	Vitamin A		Thiamine (mg)	Ribo-flavin (mg)	Niacin (mg)	Ascorbic Acid (mg)	Food No.
							(IU)	(RE)					
0	36	0.3	8	0.4	46	5	10	0	0.02	0.02	0.1	90	32
0	30	0.2	20	0.5	62	55	35	2	0.05	0.06	0.1	73	33
0	29	0.0	8	0.4	13	15	3	0	0.01	0.01	0.1	85	34
0	29	0.3	18	0.8	153	35	88	10	0.08	0.04	0.7	115	35
0	30	0.3	13	0.7	115	8	1,328	133	0.08	0.05	0.5	56	36
0	26	0.2	7	0.4	37	7	52	5	0.01	0.05	TR	10	37
0	29	0.0	29	0.1	3	19	0	0	0.00	TR	0.0	34	38
0	1	0.0	50	0.1	0	7	0	0	0.00	0.00	0.0	6	39
1	18	0.2	93	3.6	251	125	2,751	824	0.64	0.86	10.7	32	40
34	29	0.3	384	3.8	620	244	3,058	901	0.73	1.26	10.9	34	41
4	17	0.1	79	3.5	203	85	2,222	668	0.62	0.75	10.2	27	42
34	28	0.0	371	3.6	572	204	2,531	742	0.71	1.14	10.4	29	43
0	25	0.0	20	0.2	69	86	5	0	0.08	0.01	1.9	1	44
0	1	0.0	0	TR	66	5	0	0	0.00	0.02	0.0	0	45
0	TR	0.0	4	0.1	16	2	36	4	0.02	0.01	0.0	0	46
0	TR	0.0	4	0.1	16	2	0	0	0.02	0.01	0.0	0	47
0	TR	0.0	5	TR	47	7	0	0	0.00	TR	0.1	0	48
0	22	0.0	5	0.1	49	8	0	0	0.00	0.05	0.1	0	49
0	1	0.0	5	0.1	40	24	0	0	0.00	0.01	0.1	0	50
0	0	0.0	5	TR	0	7	0	0	0.00	0.00	0.0	0	51
21	1	0.0	150	0.1	73	396	204	65	0.01	0.11	0.3	0	52
27	TR	0.0	147	0.1	71	320	351	96	0.01	0.19	0.2	0	53
30	TR	0.0	204	0.2	28	176	300	79	0.01	0.11	TR	0	54
18	TR	0.0	123	0.1	17	105	180	47	TR	0.06	TR	0	55
119	1	0.0	815	0.8	111	701	1,197	314	0.03	0.42	0.1	0	56

Food No.	Food Description	Measure of Edible Portion	Weight (g)	Water (%)	Calories (kcal)	Protein (g)	Total Fat (g)	Fatty Acids Satu- rated (g)	Mono- unsatu- rated (g)	Poly- unsatu- rated (g)
DAIRY PRODUCTS (CONTINUED)										
	CHEESE (CONTINUED)									
	NATURAL (CONTINUED)									
	COTTAGE									
	CREAMED (4% FAT)									
57	LARGE CURD	1 CUP	225	79	233	28	10	6.4	2.9	0.3
58	SMALL CURD	1 CUP	210	79	217	26	9	6.0	2.7	0.3
59	WITH FRUIT	1 CUP	226	72	279	22	8	4.9	2.2	0.2
60	LOW FAT (2%)	1 CUP	226	79	203	31	4	2.8	1.2	0.1
61	LOW FAT (1%)	1 CUP	226	82	164	28	2	1.5	0.7	0.1
62	UNCREAMED (DRY CURD, LESS THAN 1/2% FAT)	1 CUP	145	80	123	25	1	0.4	0.2	TR
	CREAM									
63	REGULAR	1 OZ	28	54	99	2	10	6.2	2.8	0.4
64		1 TBSP	15	54	51	1	5	3.2	1.4	0.2
65	LOW FAT	1 TBSP	15	64	35	2	3	1.7	0.7	0.1
66	FAT FREE	1 TBSP	16	76	15	2	TR	0.1	0.1	TR
67	FETA	1 OZ	28	55	75	4	6	4.2	1.3	0.2
68	LOW FAT, CHEDDAR OR COLBY	1 OZ	28	63	49	7	2	1.2	0.6	0.1
	MOZZARELLA, MADE WITH									
69	WHOLE MILK	1 OZ	28	54	80	6	6	3.7	1.9	0.2
70	PART SKIM MILK (LOW MOISTURE)	1 OZ	28	49	79	8	5	3.1	1.4	0.1
71	MUENSTER	1 OZ	28	42	104	7	9	5.4	2.5	0.2
72	NEUFCHATEL	1 OZ	28	62	74	3	7	4.2	1.9	0.2
73	PARMESAN, GRATED	1 CUP	100	18	456	42	30	19.1	8.7	0.7
74		1 TBSP	5	18	23	2	2	1.0	0.4	TR
75		1 OZ	28	18	129	12	9	5.4	2.5	0.2
76	PROVOLONE	1 OZ	28	41	100	7	8	4.8	2.1	0.2
	RICOTTA, MADE WITH									
77	WHOLE MILK	1 CUP	246	72	428	28	32	20.4	8.9	0.9
78	PART SKIM MILK	1 CUP	246	74	340	28	19	12.1	5.7	0.6
79	SWISS	1 OZ	28	37	107	8	8	5.0	2.1	0.3
	PASTEURIZED PROCESS CHEESE									
	AMERICAN									
80	REGULAR	1 OZ	28	39	106	6	9	5.6	2.5	0.3
81	FAT FREE	1 SLICE	21	57	31	5	TR	0.1	TR	TR
82	SWISS	1 OZ	28	42	95	7	7	4.5	2.0	0.2
83	PASTEURIZED PROCESS CHEESE FOOD, AMERICAN	1 OZ	28	43	93	6	7	4.4	2.0	0.2
84	PASTEURIZED PROCESS CHEESE SPREAD, AMERICAN	1 OZ	28	48	82	5	6	3.8	1.8	0.2
	CREAM, SWEET									
85	HALF AND HALF (CREAM AND MILK)	1 CUP	242	81	315	7	28	17.3	8.0	1.0
86		1 TBSP	15	81	20	TR	2	1.1	0.5	0.1
87	LIGHT, COFFEE, OR TABLE	1 CUP	240	74	469	6	46	28.8	13.4	1.7
88		1 TBSP	15	74	29	TR	3	1.8	0.8	0.1
	WHIPPING, UNWHIPPED (VOLUME ABOUT DOUBLE WHEN WHIPPED)									
89	LIGHT	1 CUP	239	64	699	5	74	46.2	21.7	2.1
90		1 TBSP	15	64	44	TR	5	2.9	1.4	0.1
91	HEAVY	1 CUP	238	58	821	5	88	54.8	25.4	3.3
92		1 TBSP	15	58	52	TR	6	3.5	1.6	0.2

Cholesterol (mg)	Carbo-hydrate (g)	Total Dietary Fiber (g)	Calcium (mg)	Iron (mg)	Potassium (mg)	Sodium (mg)	Vitamin A (IU)	Vitamin A (RE)	Thiamine (mg)	Ribo-flavin (mg)	Niacin (mg)	Ascorbic Acid (mg)	Food No.
34	6	0.0	135	0.3	190	911	367	108	0.05	0.37	0.3	0	57
31	6	0.0	126	0.3	177	850	342	101	0.04	0.34	0.3	0	58
25	30	0.0	108	0.2	151	915	278	81	0.04	0.29	0.2	0	59
19	8	0.0	155	0.4	217	918	158	45	0.05	0.42	0.3	0	60
10	6	0.0	138	0.3	193	918	84	25	0.05	0.37	0.3	0	61
10	3	0.0	46	0.3	47	19	44	12	0.04	0.21	0.2	0	62
31	1	0.0	23	0.3	34	84	405	108	TR	0.06	TR	0	63
16	TR	0.0	12	0.2	17	43	207	55	TR	0.03	TR	0	64
8	1	0.0	17	0.3	25	44	108	33	TR	0.04	TR	0	65
1	1	0.0	29	TR	25	85	145	44	0.01	0.03	TR	0	66
25	1	0.0	140	0.2	18	316	127	36	0.04	0.24	0.3	0	67
6	1	0.0	118	0.1	19	174	66	18	TR	0.06	TR	0	68
22	1	0.0	147	0.1	19	106	225	68	TR	0.07	TR	0	69
15	1	0.0	207	0.1	27	150	199	54	0.01	0.10	TR	0	70
27	TR	0.0	203	0.1	38	178	318	90	TR	0.09	TR	0	71
22	1	0.0	21	0.1	32	113	321	85	TR	0.06	TR	0	72
79	4	0.0	1,376	1.0	107	1,862	701	173	0.05	0.39	0.3	0	73
4	TR	0.0	69	TR	5	93	35	9	TR	0.02	TR	0	74
22	1	0.0	390	0.3	30	528	199	49	0.01	0.11	0.1	0	75
20	1	0.0	214	0.1	39	248	231	75	0.01	0.09	TR	0	76
124	7	0.0	509	0.9	257	207	1,205	330	0.03	0.48	0.3	0	77
76	13	0.0	669	1.1	308	307	1,063	278	0.05	0.46	0.2	0	78
26	1	0.0	272	TR	31	74	240	72	0.01	0.10	TR	0	79
27	TR	0.0	174	0.1	46	406	343	82	0.01	0.10	TR	0	80
2	3	0.0	145	0.1	60	321	308	92	0.01	0.10	TR	0	81
24	1	0.0	219	0.2	61	388	229	65	TR	0.08	TR	0	82
18	2	0.0	163	0.2	79	337	259	62	0.01	0.13	TR	0	83
16	2	0.0	159	0.1	69	381	223	54	0.01	0.12	TR	0	84
89	10	0.0	254	0.2	314	98	1,050	259	0.08	0.36	0.2	2	85
6	1	0.0	16	TR	19	6	65	16	0.01	0.02	TR	TR	86
159	9	0.0	231	0.1	292	95	1,519	437	0.08	0.36	0.1	2	87
10	1	0.0	14	TR	18	6	95	27	TR	0.02	TR	TR	88
265	7	0.0	166	0.1	231	82	2,694	705	0.06	0.30	0.1	1	89
17	TR	0.0	10	TR	15	5	169	44	TR	0.02	TR	TR	90
326	7	0.0	154	0.1	179	89	3,499	1,002	0.05	0.26	0.1	1	91
21	TR	0.0	10	TR	11	6	221	63	TR	0.02	TR	TR	92

Food No.	Food Description	Measure of Edible Portion	Weight (g)	Water (%)	Calories (kcal)	Protein (g)	Total Fat (g)	Fatty Acids Saturated (g)	Fatty Acids Mono-unsaturated (g)	Fatty Acids Poly-unsaturated (g)
DAIRY PRODUCTS (CONTINUED)										
93	WHIPPED TOPPING (PRESSURIZED)	1 CUP	60	61	154	2	13	8.3	3.9	0.5
94		1 TBSP	3	61	8	TR	1	0.4	0.2	TR
	CREAM, SOUR									
95	REGULAR	1 CUP	230	71	493	7	48.0	30.0	13.9	1.8
96		1 TBSP	12	71	26	TR	3	1.6	0.7	0.1
97	REDUCED FAT	1 TBSP	15	80	20	TR	2	1.1	0.5	0.1
98	FAT FREE	1 TBSP	16	81	12	TR	0	0.0	0.0	0.0
	CREAM PRODUCT, IMITATION (MADE WITH VEGETABLE FAT)*									
	SWEET									
	CREAMER									
99	LIQUID (FROZEN)	1 TBSP	15	77	20	TR	1	0.3	1.1	TR
100	POWDERED	1 TSP	2	2	11	TR	1	0.7	TR	TR
	WHIPPED TOPPING									
101	FROZEN	1 CUP	75	50	239	1	19	16.3	1.2	0.4
102		1 TBSP	4	50	13	TR	1	0.9	0.1	TR
103	POWDERED, PREPARED WITH WHOLE MILK	1 CUP	80	67	151	3	10	8.5	0.7	0.2
104		1 TBSP	4	67	8	TR	TR	0.4	TR	TR
105	PRESSURIZED	1 CUP	70	60	184	1	16	13.0	2.0	1.3
106		1 TBSP	4	60	11	TR	1	0.8	0.1	TR
107	SOUR DRESSING (FILLED CREAM TYPE, NONBUTTERFAT)	1 CUP	235	75	417	8	39	31.2	4.6	1.1
108		1 TBSP	12	75	21	TR	2	1.6	0.2	0.1
	FROZEN DESSERT									
	FROZEN YOGURT, SOFT SERVE									
109	CHOCOLATE	1/2 CUP	72	64	115	3	4	2.6	1.3	0.2
110	VANILLA	1/2 CUP	72	65	114	3	4	2.5	1.1	0.2
	ICE CREAM									
	REGULAR									
111	CHOCOLATE	1/2 CUP	66	56	143	3	7	4.5	2.1	0.3
112	VANILLA	1/2 CUP	66	61	133	2	7	4.5	2.1	0.3
113	LIGHT (50% REDUCED FAT), VANILLA	1/2 CUP	66	68	92	3	3	1.7	0.8	0.1
114	PREMIUM LOW FAT, CHOCOLATE	1/2 CUP	72	61	113	3	2	1.0	0.6	0.1
115	RICH, VANILLA	1/2 CUP	74	57	178	3	12	7.4	3.4	0.4
116	SOFT SERVE, FRENCH VANILLA.	1/2 CUP	86	60	185	4	11	6.4	3.0	0.4
117	SHERBET, ORANGE	1/2 CUP	74	66	102	1	1	0.9	0.4	0.1
	MILK									
	FLUID, NO MILK SOLIDS ADDED									
118	WHOLE (3.3% FAT)	1 CUP	244	88	150	8	8	5.1	2.4	0.3
119	REDUCED FAT (2%)	1 CUP	244	89	121	8	5	2.9	1.4	0.2
120	LOW FAT (1%)	1 CUP	244	90	102	8	3	1.6	0.7	0.1
121	NONFAT (SKIM)	1 CUP	245	91	86	8	TR	0.3	0.1	TR
122	BUTTERMILK	1 CUP	245	90	99	8	2	1.3	0.6	0.1
	CANNED									
123	CONDENSED, SWEETENED	1 CUP	306	27	982	24	27	16.8	7.4	1.0
	EVAPORATED									
124	WHOLE MILK	1 CUP	252	74	339	17	19	11.6	5.9	0.6
125	SKIM MILK	1 CUP	256	79	199	19	1	0.3	0.2	TR
	DRIED									
126	BUTTERMILK	1 CUP	120	3	464	41	7	4.3	2.0	0.3

*The vitamin A values listed for imitation sweet cream products are mostly from beta-carotene added for coloring.

Cholesterol (mg)	Carbo-hydrate (g)	Total Dietary Fiber (g)	Calcium (mg)	Iron (mg)	Potassium (mg)	Sodium (mg)	Vitamin A (IU)	Vitamin A (RE)	Thiamine (mg)	Ribo-flavin (mg)	Niacin (mg)	Ascorbic Acid (mg)	Food No.
46	7	0.0	61	TR	88	78	506	124	0.02	0.04	TR	0	93
2	TR	0.0	3	TR	4	4	25	6	TR	TR	TR	0	94
102	10	0.0	268	0.1	331	123	1,817	449	0.08	0.34	0.2	2	95
5	1	0.0	14	TR	17	6	95	23	TR	0.02	TR	TR	96
6	1	0.0	16	TR	19	6	68	17	0.01	0.02	TR	TR	97
1	2	0.0	20	0.0	21	23	100	13	0.01	0.02	TR	0	98
0	2	0.0	1	TR	29	12	13*	1*	0.00	0.00	0.0	0	99
0	1	0.0	TR	TR	16	4	4	TR	0.00	TR	0.0	0	100
0	17	0.0	5	0.1	14	19	646*	65*	0.00	0.00	0.0	0	101
0	1	0.0	TR	TR	1	1	34*	3*	0.00	0.00	0.0	0	102
8	13	0.0	72	TR	121	53	289*	39*	0.02	0.09	TR	1	103
TR	1	0.0	4	TR	6	3	14*	2*	TR	TR	TR	TR	104
0	11	0.0	4	TR	13	43	331*	33*	0.00	0.00	0.0	0	105
0	1	0.0	TR	TR	1	2	19*	2*	0.00	0.00	0.0	0	106
13	11	0.0	266	0.1	380	113	24	5	0.09	0.38	0.2	2	107
1	1	0.0	14	TR	19	6	1	TR	TR	0.02	TR	TR	108
4	18	1.6	106	0.9	188	71	115	31	0.03	0.15	0.2	TR	109
1	17	0.0	103	0.2	152	63	153	41	0.03	0.16	0.2	1	110
22	19	0.8	72	0.6	164	50	275	79	0.03	0.13	0.1	TR	111
29	16	0.0	84	0.1	131	53	270	77	0.03	0.16	0.1	TR	112
9	15	0.0	92	0.1	139	56	109	31	0.04	0.17	0.1	1	113
7	22	0.7	107	0.4	179	50	163	47	0.02	0.13	0.1	1	114
45	17	0.0	87	TR	118	41	476	136	0.03	0.12	0.1	1	115
78	19	0.0	113	0.2	152	52	464	132	0.04	0.16	0.1	1	116
4	22	0.0	40	0.1	71	34	56	10	0.02	0.06	TR	2	117
33	11	0.0	291	0.1	370	120	307	76	0.09	0.40	0.2	2	118
18	12	0.0	297	0.1	377	122	500	139	0.10	0.40	0.2	2	119
10	12	0.0	300	0.1	381	123	500	144	0.10	0.41	0.2	2	120
4	12	0.0	302	0.1	406	126	500	149	0.09	0.34	0.2	2	121
9	12	0.0	285	0.1	371	257	81	20	0.08	0.38	0.1	2	122
104	166	0.0	868	0.6	1,136	389	1,004	248	0.28	1.27	0.6	8	123
74	25	0.0	657	0.5	764	267	612	136	0.12	0.80	0.5	5	124
9	29	0.0	741	0.7	849	294	1,004	300	0.12	0.79	0.4	3	125
83	59	0.0	1,421	0.4	1,910	621	262	65	0.47	1.89	1.1	7	126

Food No.	Food Description	Measure of Edible Portion	Weight (g)	Water (%)	Calories (kcal)	Protein (g)	Total Fat (g)	Fatty Acids Satu-rated (g)	Mono-unsatu-rated (g)	Poly-unsatu-rated (g)
DAIRY PRODUCTS (CONTINUED)										
127	NONFAT, INSTANT, WITH ADDED VITAMIN A	1 CUP	68	4	244	24	TR	0.3	0.1	TR
	MILK BEVERAGE									
	CHOCOLATE MILK (COMMERCIAL)									
128	WHOLE	1 CUP	250	82	208	8	8	5.3	2.5	0.3
129	REDUCED FAT (2%)	1 CUP	250	84	179	8	5	3.1	1.5	0.2
130	LOW FAT (1%)	1 CUP	250	85	158	8	3	1.5	0.8	0.1
131	EGGNOG (COMMERCIAL)	1 CUP	254	74	342	10	19	11.3	5.7	0.9
	MILK SHAKE, THICK									
132	CHOCOLATE	10.6 FL OZ	300	72	356	9	8	5.0	2.3	0.3
133	VANILLA	11 FL OZ	313	74	350	12	9	5.9	2.7	0.4
	SHERBET. SEE DAIRY PRODUCTS, FROZEN DESSERT									
	YOGURT									
	WITH ADDED MILK SOLIDS									
	MADE WITH LOW FAT MILK									
134	FRUIT FLAVORED	8-OZ CONTAINER	227	74	231	10	2	1.6	0.7	0.1
135	PLAIN	8-OZ CONTAINER	227	85	144	12	4	2.3	1.0	0.1
	MADE WITH NONFAT MILK									
136	FRUIT FLAVORED	8-OZ CONTAINER	227	75	213	10	TR	0.3	0.1	TR
137	PLAIN	8-OZ CONTAINER	227	85	127	13	TR	0.3	0.1	TR
	WITHOUT ADDED MILK SOLIDS									
138	MADE WITH WHOLE MILK, PLAIN	8-OZ CONTAINER	227	88	139	8	7	4.8	2.0	0.2
139	MADE WITH NON-FAT MILK, LOW-CALORIE SWEETENER, VANILLA OR LEMON FLAVOR	8-OZ CONTAINER	227	87	98	9	TR	0.3	0.1	TR
EGGS										
	EGG									
	RAW									
140	WHOLE	1 MEDIUM	44	75	66	5	4	1.4	1.7	0.6
141		1 LARGE	50	75	75	6	5	1.6	1.9	0.7
142		1 EXTRA LARGE	58	75	86	7	6	1.8	2.2	0.8
143	WHITE	1 LARGE	33	88	17	4	0	0.0	0.0	0.0
144	YOLK	1 LARGE	17	49	59	3	5	1.6	1.9	0.7
	COOKED, WHOLE									
145	FRIED, IN MARGARINE, WITH SALT	1 LARGE	46	69	92	6	7	1.9	2.7	1.3
146	HARD COOKED, SHELL REMOVED	1 LARGE	50	75	78	6	5	1.6	2.0	0.7
147		1 CUP, CHOPPED	136	75	211	17	14	4.4	5.5	1.9
148	POACHED, WITH SALT	1 LARGE	50	75	75	6	5	1.5	1.9	0.7
149	SCRAMBLED, IN MARGARINE, WITH WHOLE MILK, SALT	1 LARGE	61	73	101	7	7	2.2	2.9	1.3
150	EGG SUBSTITUTE, LIQUID	1/4 CUP	63	83	53	8	2	0.4	0.6	1.0
FATS AND OILS										
	BUTTER (4 STICKS PER LB)									
151	SALTED	1 STICK	113	16	813	1	92	57.3	26.6	3.4
152		1 TBSP	14	16	102	TR	12	7.2	3.3	0.4
153		1 TSP	5	16	36	TR	4	2.5	1.2	0.2
154	UNSALTED	1 STICK	113	18	813	1	92	57.3	26.6	3.4

Cholesterol (mg)	Carbo-hydrate (g)	Total Dietary Fiber (g)	Calcium (mg)	Iron (mg)	Potassium (mg)	Sodium (mg)	Vitamin A (IU)	Vitamin A (RE)	Thiamine (mg)	Ribo-flavin (mg)	Niacin (mg)	Ascorbic Acid (mg)	Food No.
12	35	0.0	837	0.2	1,160	373	1,612	483	0.28	1.19	0.6	4	127
31	26	2.0	280	0.6	417	149	303	73	0.09	0.41	0.3	2	128
17	26	1.3	284	0.6	422	151	500	143	0.09	0.41	0.3	2	129
7	26	1.3	287	0.6	426	152	500	148	0.10	0.42	0.3	2	130
149	34	0.0	330	0.5	420	138	894	203	0.09	0.48	0.3	4	131
32	63	0.9	396	0.9	672	333	258	63	0.14	0.67	0.4	0	132
37	56	0.0	457	0.3	572	299	357	88	0.09	0.61	0.5	0	133
10	43	0.0	345	0.2	442	133	104	25	0.08	0.40	0.2	1	134
14	16	0.0	415	0.2	531	159	150	36	0.10	0.49	0.3	2	135
5	43	0.0	345	0.2	440	132	16	5	0.09	0.41	0.2	2	136
4	17	0.0	452	0.2	579	174	16	5	0.11	0.53	0.3	2	137
29	11	0.0	274	0.1	351	105	279	68	0.07	0.32	0.2	1	138
5	17	0.0	325	0.3	402	134	0	0	0.08	0.37	0.2	2	139
187	1	0.0	22	0.6	53	55	279	84	0.03	0.22	TR	0	140
213	1	0.0	25	0.7	61	63	318	96	0.03	0.25	TR	0	141
247	1	0.0	28	0.8	70	73	368	111	0.04	0.29	TR	0	142
0	TR	0.0	2	TR	48	55	0	0	TR	0.15	TR	0	143
213	TR	0.0	23	0.6	16	7	323	97	0.03	0.11	TR	0	144
211	1	0.0	25	0.7	61	162	394	114	0.03	0.24	TR	0	145
212	1	0.0	25	0.6	63	62	280	84	0.03	0.26	TR	0	146
577	2	0.0	68	1.6	171	169	762	228	0.09	0.70	0.1	0	147
212	1	0.0	25	0.7	60	140	316	95	0.02	0.22	TR	0	148
215	1	0.0	43	0.7	84	171	416	119	0.03	0.27	TR	TR	149
1	TR	0.0	33	1.3	208	112	1,361	136	0.07	0.19	0.1	0	150
248	TR	0.0	27	0.2	29	937	3,468	855	0.01	0.04	TR	0	151
31	TR	0.0	3	TR	4	117	434	107	TR	TR	TR	0	152
11	TR	0.0	1	TR	1	41	153	38	TR	TR	TR	0	153
248	TR	0.0	27	0.2	29	12	3,468	855	0.01	0.04	TR	0	154

Food No.	Food Description	Measure of Edible Portion	Weight (g)	Water (%)	Calories (kcal)	Protein (g)	Total Fat (g)	Fatty Acids Saturated (g)	Mono-unsaturated (g)	Poly-unsaturated (g)
FATS AND OILS (CONTINUED)										
155	LARD	1 CUP	205	0	1,849	0	205	80.4	92.5	23.0
156		1 TBSP	13	0	115	0	13	5.0	5.8	1.4
	MARGARINE, VITAMIN A–FORTIFIED, SALT ADDED									
	REGULAR (ABOUT 80% FAT)									
157	HARD (4 STICKS PER LB)	1 STICK	113	16	815	1	91	17.9	40.6	28.8
158		1 TBSP	14	16	101	TR	11	2.2	5.0	3.6
159		1 TSP	5	16	34	TR	4	0.7	1.7	1.2
160	SOFT	1 CUP	227	16	1,626	2	183	31.3	64.7	78.5
161		1 TSP	5	16	34	TR	4	0.6	1.3	1.6
	SPREAD (ABOUT 60% FAT)									
162	HARD (4 STICKS PER LB)	1 STICK	115	37	621	1	70	16.2	29.9	20.8
163		1 TBSP	14	37	76	TR	9	2.0	3.6	2.5
164		1 TSP	5	37	26	TR	3	0.7	1.2	0.9
165	SOFT	1 CUP	229	37	1,236	1	139	29.3	72.1	31.6
166		1 TSP	5	37	26	TR	3	0.6	1.5	0.7
167	SPREAD (ABOUT 40% FAT)	1 CUP	232	58	801	1	90	17.9	36.4	32.0
168		1 TSP	5	58	17	TR	2	0.4	0.8	0.7
169	MARGARINE BUTTER BLEND	1 STICK	113	16	811	1	91	32.1	37.0	18.0
170		1 TBSP	14	16	102	TR	11	4.0	4.7	2.3
	OILS, SALAD OR COOKING									
171	CANOLA	1 CUP	218	0	1,927	0	218	15.5	128.4	64.5
172		1 TBSP	14	0	124	0	14	1.0	8.2	4.1
173	CORN	1 CUP	218	0	1,927	0	218	27.7	52.8	128.0
174		1 TBSP	14	0	120	0	14	1.7	3.3	8.0
175	OLIVE	1 CUP	216	0	1,909	0	216	29.2	159.2	18.1
176		1 TBSP	14	0	119	0	14	1.8	9.9	1.1
177	PEANUT	1 CUP	216	0	1,909	0	216	36.5	99.8	69.1
178		1 TBSP	14	0	119	0	14	2.3	6.2	4.3
179	SAFFLOWER, HIGH OLEIC	1 CUP	218	0	1,927	0	218	13.5	162.7	31.3
180		1 TBSP	14	0	120	0	14	0.8	10.2	2.0
181	SESAME	1 CUP	218	0	1,927	0	218	31.0	86.5	90.9
182		1 TBSP	14	0	120	0	14	1.9	5.4	5.7
183	SOYBEAN, HYDROGENATED	1 CUP	218	0	1,927	0	218	32.5	93.7	82.0
184		1 TBSP	14	0	120	0	14	2.0	5.8	5.1
185	SOYBEAN, HYDROGENATED AND COTTONSEED OIL BLEND	1 CUP	218	0	1,927	0	218	39.2	64.3	104.9
186		1 TBSP	14	0	120	0	14	2.4	4.0	6.5
187	SUNFLOWER	1 CUP	218	0	1,927	0	218	22.5	42.5	143.2
188		1 TBSP	14	0	120	0	14	1.4	2.7	8.9
	SALAD DRESSINGS									
	COMMERCIAL									
	BLUE CHEESE									
189	REGULAR	1 TBSP	15	32	77	1	8	1.5	1.9	4.3
190	LOW CALORIE	1 TBSP	15	80	15	1	1	0.4	0.3	0.4
	CAESAR									
191	REGULAR	1 TBSP	15	34	78	TR	8	1.3	2.0	4.8
192	LOW CALORIE	1 TBSP	15	73	17	TR	1	0.1	0.2	0.4
	FRENCH									
193	REGULAR	1 TBSP	16	38	67	TR	6	1.5	1.2	3.4
194	LOW CALORIE	1 TBSP	16	69	22	TR	1	0.1	0.2	0.6

Cholesterol (mg)	Carbo-hydrate (g)	Total Dietary Fiber (g)	Calcium (mg)	Iron (mg)	Potassium (mg)	Sodium (mg)	Vitamin A (IU)	Vitamin A (RE)	Thiamine (mg)	Ribo-flavin (mg)	Niacin (mg)	Ascorbic Acid (mg)	Food No.
195	0	0.0	TR	0.0	TR	TR	0	0	0.00	0.00	0.0	0	155
12	0	0.0	TR	0.0	TR	TR	0	0	0.00	0.00	0.0	0	156
0	1	0.0	34	0.1	48	1,070	4,050	906	0.01	0.04	TR	TR	157
0	TR	0.0	4	TR	6	132	500	112	TR	0.01	TR	TR	158
0	TR	0.0	1	TR	2	44	168	38	TR	TR	TR	TR	159
0	1	0.0	60	0.0	86	2,449	8,106	1,814	0.02	0.07	TR	TR	160
0	TR	0.0	1	0.0	2	51	168	38	TR	TR	TR	TR	161
0	0	0.0	24	0.0	34	1,143	4,107	919	0.01	0.03	TR	TR	162
0	0	0.0	3	0.0	4	139	500	112	TR	TR	TR	TR	163
0	0	0.0	1	0.0	1	48	171	38	TR	TR	TR	TR	164
0	0	0.0	48	0.0	68	2,276	8,178	1,830	0.02	0.06	TR	TR	165
0	0	0.0	1	0.0	1	48	171	38	TR	TR	TR	TR	166
0	1	0.0	41	0.0	50	2,226	8,285	1,854	0.01	0.05	TR	TR	167
0	TR	0.0	1	0.0	1	46	171	38	TR	TR	TR	TR	168
99	1	0.0	32	0.1	41	1,014	4,035	903	0.01	0.04	TR	TR	169
12	TR	0.0	4	TR	5	127	507	113	TR	TR	TR	TR	170
0	0	0.0	0	0.0	0	0	0	0	0.00	0.00	0.0	0	171
0	0	0.0	0	0.0	0	0	0	0	0.00	0.00	0.0	0	172
0	0	0.0	0	0.0	0	0	0	0	0.00	0.00	0.0	0	173
0	0	0.0	0	0.0	0	0	0	0	0.00	0.00	0.0	0	174
0	0	0.0	TR	0.8	0	TR	0	0	0.00	0.00	0.0	0	175
0	0	0.0	TR	0.1	0	TR	0	0	0.00	0.00	0.0	0	176
0	0	0.0	TR	0.1	TR	TR	0	0	0.00	0.00	0.0	0	177
0	0	0.0	TR	TR	TR	TR	0	0	0.00	0.00	0.0	0	178
0	0	0.0	0	0.0	0	0	0	0	0.00	0.00	0.0	0	179
0	0	0.0	0	0.0	0	0	0	0	0.00	0.00	0.0	0	180
0	0	0.0	0	0.0	0	0	0	0	0.00	0.00	0.0	0	181
0	0	0.0	0	0.0	0	0	0	0	0.00	0.00	0.0	0	182
0	0	0.0	0	0.0	0	0	0	0	0.00	0.00	0.0	0	183
0	0	0.0	0	0.0	0	0	0	0	0.00	0.00	0.0	0	184
0	0	0.0	0	0.0	0	0	0	0	0.00	0.00	0.0	0	185
0	0	0.0	0	0.0	0	0	0	0	0.00	0.00	0.0	0	186
0	0	0.0	0	0.0	0	0	0	0	0.00	0.00	0.0	0	187
0	0	0.0	0	0.0	0	0	0	0	0.00	0.00	0.0	0	188
3	1	0.0	12	TR	6	167	32	10	TR	0.02	TR	TR	189
TR	TR	0.0	14	0.1	1	184	2	TR	TR	0.02	TR	TR	190
TR	TR	TR	4	TR	4	158	3	TR	TR	TR	TR	0	191
TR	3	TR	4	TR	4	162	3	TR	TR	TR	TR	0	192
0	3	0.0	2	0.1	12	214	203	20	TR	TR	TR	0	193
0	4	0.0	2	0.1	13	128	212	21	0.00	0.00	0.0	0	194

Food No.	Food Description	Measure of Edible Portion	Weight (g)	Water (%)	Calories (kcal)	Protein (g)	Total Fat (g)	Fatty Acids Saturated (g)	Fatty Acids Mono-unsaturated (g)	Fatty Acids Poly-unsaturated (g)
FATS AND OILS (CONTINUED)										
	ITALIAN									
195	REGULAR	1 TBSP	15	38	69	TR	7	1.0	1.6	4.1
196	LOW CALORIE	1 TBSP	15	82	16	TR	1	0.2	0.3	0.9
	MAYONNAISE									
197	REGULAR	1 TBSP	14	15	99	TR	11	1.6	3.1	5.7
198	LIGHT, CHOLESTEROL FREE	1 TBSP	15	56	49	TR	5	0.7	1.1	2.8
199	FAT FREE	1 TBSP	16	84	12	0	TR	0.1	0.1	0.2
	RUSSIAN									
200	REGULAR	1 TBSP	15	35	76	TR	8	1.1	1.8	4.5
201	LOW CALORIE	1 TBSP	16	65	23	TR	1	0.1	0.1	0.4
	THOUSAND ISLAND									
202	REGULAR	1 TBSP	16	46	59	TR	6	0.9	1.3	3.1
203	LOW CALORIE	1 TBSP	15	69	24	TR	2	0.2	0.4	0.9
	PREPARED FROM HOME RECIPE									
204	COOKED, MADE WITH MARGARINE	1 TBSP	16	69	25	1	2	0.5	0.6	0.3
205	FRENCH	1 TBSP	14	24	88	TR	10	1.8	2.9	4.7
206	VINEGAR AND OIL	1 TBSP	16	47	70	0	8	1.4	2.3	3.8
207	SHORTENING (HYDROGENATED SOYBEAN AND COTTON-SEED OILS)	1 CUP	205	0	1,812	0	205	51.3	91.2	53.5
208		1 TBSP	13	0	113	0	13	3.2	5.7	3.3
FISH AND SHELLFISH										
209	CATFISH, BREADED, FRIED	3 OZ	85	59	195	15	11	2.8	4.8	2.8
	CLAM									
210	RAW, MEAT ONLY	3 OZ	85	82	63	11	1	0.1	0.1	0.2
211		1 MEDIUM	15	82	11	2	TR	TR	TR	TR
212	BREADED, FRIED	3/4 CUP	115	29	451	13	26	6.6	11.4	6.8
213	CANNED, DRAINED SOLIDS	3 OZ	85	64	126	22	2	0.2	0.1	0.5
214		1 CUP	160	64	237	41	3	0.3	0.3	0.9
	COD									
215	BAKED OR BROILED	3 OZ	85	76	89	20	1	0.1	0.1	0.3
216		1 FILLET	90	76	95	21	1	0.1	0.1	0.3
217	CANNED, SOLIDS AND LIQUID	3 OZ	85	76	89	19	1	0.1	0.1	0.2
	CRAB									
	ALASKA KING									
218	STEAMED	1 LEG	134	78	130	26	2	0.2	0.2	0.7
219		3 OZ	85	78	82	16	1	0.1	0.2	0.5
220	IMITATION, FROM SURIMI	3 OZ	85	74	87	10	1	0.2	0.2	0.6
	BLUE									
221	STEAMED	3 OZ	85	77	87	17	2	0.2	0.2	0.6
222	CANNED CRABMEAT	1 CUP	135	76	134	28	2	0.3	0.3	0.6
223	CRAB CAKE, WITH EGG, ONION, FRIED IN MARGARINE	1 CAKE	60	71	93	12	5	0.9	1.7	1.4
224	FISH FILLET, BATTERED OR BREADED, FRIED	1 FILLET	91	54	211	13	11	2.6	2.3	5.7
225	FISH STICK AND PORTION, BREADED, FROZEN, REHEATED	1 STICK (4″ × 1″ × 1/2″)	28	46	76	4	3	0.9	1.4	0.9
226		1 PORTION (4″ × 2″ × 1/2″)	57	46	155	9	7	1.8	2.9	1.8
227	FLOUNDER OR SOLE, BAKED OR BROILED	3 OZ	85	73	99	21	1	0.3	0.2	0.5
228		1 FILLET	127	73	149	31	2	0.5	0.3	0.8

Cholesterol (mg)	Carbo-hydrate (g)	Total Dietary Fiber (g)	Calcium (mg)	Iron (mg)	Potassium (mg)	Sodium (mg)	Vitamin A (IU)	(RE)	Thiamine (mg)	Ribo-flavin (mg)	Niacin (mg)	Ascorbic Acid (mg)	Food No.
0	1	0.0	1	TR	2	116	11	4	TR	TR	TR	0	195
1	1	TR	TR	TR	2	118	0	0	0.00	0.00	0.0	0	196
8	TR	0.0	2	0.1	5	78	39	12	0.00	0.00	TR	0	197
0	1	0.0	0	0.0	10	107	18	2	0.00	0.00	0.0	0	198
0	2	0.6	0	0.0	15	190	0	0	0.00	0.00	0.0	0	199
3	2	0.0	3	0.1	24	133	106	32	0.01	0.01	0.1	1	200
1	4	TR	3	0.1	26	141	9	3	TR	TR	TR	1	201
4	2	0.0	2	0.1	18	109	50	15	TR	TR	TR	0	202
2	2	0.2	2	0.1	17	153	49	15	TR	TR	TR	0	203
9	2	0.0	13	0.1	19	117	66	20	0.01	0.02	TR	TR	204
0	TR	0.0	1	TR	3	92	72	22	TR	TR	TR	TR	205
0	TR	0.0	0	0.0	1	TR	0	0	0.00	0.00	0.0	0	206
0	0	0.0	0	0.0	0	0	0	0	0.00	0.00	0.0	0	207
0	0	0.0	0	0.0	0	0	0	0	0.00	0.00	0.0	0	200
69	7	0.6	37	1.2	289	238	24	7	0.06	0.11	1.9	0	209
29	2	0.0	39	11.9	267	48	255	77	0.07	0.18	1.5	11	210
5	TR	0.0	7	2.0	46	8	44	13	0.01	0.03	0.3	2	211
87	39	0.3	21	3.0	266	834	122	37	0.21	0.26	2.9	0	212
57	4	0.0	78	23.8	534	95	485	145	0.13	0.36	2.9	19	213
107	8	0.0	147	44.7	1,005	179	912	274	0.24	0.68	5.4	35	214
40	0	0.0	8	0.3	439	77	27	9	0.02	0.04	2.1	3	215
42	0	0.0	8	0.3	465	82	29	9	0.02	0.05	2.2	3	216
47	0	0.0	18	0.4	449	185	39	12	0.07	0.07	2.1	1	217
71	0	0.0	79	1.0	351	1,436	39	12	0.07	0.07	1.8	10	218
45	0	0.0	50	0.6	223	911	25	8	0.05	0.05	1.1	6	219
17	9	0.0	11	0.3	77	715	56	17	0.03	0.02	0.2	0	220
85	0	0.0	88	0.8	275	237	5	2	0.09	0.04	2.8	3	221
120	0	0.0	136	1.1	505	450	7	3	0.11	0.11	1.8	4	222
90	TR	0.0	63	0.6	194	198	151	49	0.05	0.05	1.7	2	223
31	15	0.5	16	1.9	291	484	35	11	0.10	0.10	1.9	0	224
31	7	0.0	6	0.2	73	163	30	9	0.04	0.05	0.6	0	225
64	14	0.0	11	0.4	149	332	60	18	0.07	0.10	1.2	0	226
58	0	0.0	15	0.3	292	89	32	9	0.07	0.10	1.9	0	227
86	0	0.0	23	0.4	437	133	48	14	0.10	0.14	2.8	0	228

Food No.	Food Description	Measure of Edible Portion	Weight (g)	Water (%)	Calories (kcal)	Protein (g)	Total Fat (g)	Fatty Acids Satu- rated (g)	Mono- unsatu- rated (g)	Poly- unsatu- rated (g)
FISH AND SHELLFISH (CONTINUED)										
229	HADDOCK, BAKED OR BROILED	3 OZ	85	74	95	21	1	0.1	0.1	0.3
230		1 FILLET	150	74	168	36	1	0.3	0.2	0.5
231	HALIBUT, BAKED OR BROILED	3 OZ	85	72	119	23	2	0.4	0.8	0.8
232		1/2 FILLET	159	72	223	42	5	0.7	1.5	1.5
233	HERRING, PICKLED	3 OZ	85	55	223	12	15	2.0	10.2	1.4
234	LOBSTER, STEAMED	3 OZ	85	76	83	17	1	0.1	0.1	0.1
235	OCEAN PERCH, BAKED OR BROILED	3 OZ	85	73	103	20	2	0.3	0.7	0.5
236		1 FILLET	50	73	61	12	1	0.2	0.4	0.3
	OYSTER									
237	RAW, MEAT ONLY	1 CUP	248	85	169	17	6	1.9	0.8	2.4
238		6 MEDIUM	84	85	57	6	2	0.6	0.3	0.8
239	BREADED, FRIED	3 OZ	85	65	167	7	11	2.7	4.0	2.8
240	POLLOCK, BAKED OR BROILED	3 OZ	85	74	96	20	1	0.2	0.1	0.4
241		1 FILLET	60	74	68	14	1	0.1	0.1	0.3
242	ROCKFISH, BAKED OR BROILED	3 OZ	85	73	103	20	2	0.4	0.4	0.5
243		1 FILLET	149	73	180	36	3	0.7	0.7	0.9
244	ROUGHY, ORANGE, BAKED OR BROILED	3 OZ	85	69	76	16	1	TR	0.5	TR
	SALMON									
245	BAKED OR BROILED (RED)	3 OZ	85	62	184	23	9	1.6	4.5	2.0
246		1/2 FILLET	155	62	335	42	17	3.0	8.2	3.7
247	CANNED (PINK), SOLIDS AND LIQUID (INCLUDES BONES)	3 OZ	85	69	118	17	5	1.3	1.5	1.7
248	SMOKED (CHINOOK)	3 OZ	85	72	99	16	4	0.8	1.7	0.8
249	SARDINE, ATLANTIC, CANNED IN OIL, DRAINED SOLIDS (INCLUDES BONES)	3 OZ	85	60	177	21	10	1.3	3.3	4.4
	SCALLOP, COOKED									
250	BREADED, FRIED	6 LARGE	93	58	200	17	10	2.5	4.2	2.7
251	STEAMED	3 OZ	85	73	95	20	1	0.1	0.1	0.4
	SHRIMP									
252	BREADED, FRIED	3 OZ	85	53	206	18	10	1.8	3.2	4.3
253		6 LARGE	45	53	109	10	6	0.9	1.7	2.3
254	CANNED, DRAINED SOLIDS	3 OZ	85	73	102	20	2	0.3	0.2	0.6
255	SWORDFISH, BAKED OR BROILED	3 OZ	85	69	132	22	4	1.2	1.7	1.0
256		1 PIECE	106	69	164	27	5	1.5	2.1	1.3
257	TROUT, BAKED OR BROILED	3 OZ	85	68	144	21	6	1.8	1.8	2.0
258		1 FILLET	71	68	120	17	5	1.5	1.5	1.7
	TUNA									
259	BAKED OR BROILED	3 OZ	85	63	118	25	1	0.3	0.2	0.3
	CANNED, DRAINED SOLIDS									
260	OIL PACK, CHUNK LIGHT	3 OZ	85	60	168	25	7	1.3	2.5	2.5
261	WATER PACK, CHUNK LIGHT	3 OZ	85	75	99	22	1	0.2	0.1	0.3
262	WATER PACK, SOLID WHITE	3 OZ	85	73	109	20	3	0.7	0.7	0.9
263	TUNA SALAD: LIGHT TUNA IN OIL, PICKLE RELISH, MAYO-TYPE SALAD DRESSING	1 CUP	205	63	383	33	19	3.2	5.9	8.5
FRUITS AND FRUIT JUICES										
	APPLES									
	RAW									
264	UNPEELED, 2 3/4″ DIA (ABOUT 3 PER LB)	1 APPLE	138	84	81	TR	TR	0.1	TR	0.1

Cholesterol (mg)	Carbo-hydrate (g)	Total Dietary Fiber (g)	Calcium (mg)	Iron (mg)	Potassium (mg)	Sodium (mg)	Vitamin A (IU)	(RE)	Thiamine (mg)	Ribo-flavin (mg)	Niacin (mg)	Ascorbic Acid (mg)	Food No.
63	0	0.0	36	1.1	339	74	54	16	0.03	0.04	3.9	0	229
111	0	0.0	63	2.0	599	131	95	29	0.06	0.07	6.9	0	230
35	0	0.0	51	0.9	490	59	152	46	0.06	0.08	6.1	0	231
65	0	0.0	95	1.7	916	110	285	86	0.11	0.14	11.3	0	232
11	8	0.0	65	1.0	59	740	732	219	0.03	0.12	2.8	0	233
61	1	0.0	52	0.3	299	323	74	22	0.01	0.06	0.9	0	234
46	0	0.0	116	1.0	298	82	39	12	0.11	0.11	2.1	1	235
27	0	0.0	69	0.6	175	48	23	7	0.07	0.07	1.2	TR	236
131	10	0.0	112	16.5	387	523	248	74	0.25	0.24	3.4	9	237
45	3	0.0	38	5.6	131	177	84	25	0.08	0.08	1.2	3	238
69	10	0.2	53	5.9	207	354	257	77	0.13	0.17	1.4	3	239
82	0	0.0	5	0.2	329	99	65	20	0.06	0.06	1.4	0	240
58	0	0.0	4	0.2	232	70	46	14	0.04	0.05	1.0	0	241
37	0	0.0	10	0.5	442	65	186	56	0.04	0.07	3.3	0	242
66	0	0.0	18	0.8	775	115	326	98	0.07	0.13	5.8	0	243
22	0	0.0	32	0.2	327	69	69	20	0.10	0.16	3.1	0	244
74	0	0.0	6	0.5	319	56	178	54	0.18	0.15	5.7	0	245
135	0	0.0	11	0.9	581	102	324	98	0.33	0.27	10.3	0	246
47	0	0.0	181	0.7	277	471	47	14	0.02	0.16	5.6	0	247
20	0	0.0	9	0.7	149	666	75	22	0.02	0.09	4.0	0	248
121	0	0.0	325	2.5	337	429	190	57	0.07	0.19	4.5	0	249
57	9	0.2	39	0.8	310	432	70	20	0.04	0.10	1.4	2	250
45	3	0.0	98	2.6	405	225	85	26	0.00	0.06	1.1	0	251
150	10	0.3	57	1.1	191	292	161	48	0.11	0.12	2.6	1	252
80	5	0.2	30	0.6	101	155	85	25	0.06	0.06	1.4	1	253
147	1	0.0	50	2.3	179	144	51	15	0.02	0.03	2.3	2	254
43	0	0.0	5	0.9	314	98	116	35	0.04	0.10	10.0	1	255
53	0	0.0	6	1.1	391	122	145	43	0.05	0.12	12.5	1	256
58	0	0.0	73	0.3	375	36	244	73	0.20	0.07	7.5	3	257
48	0	0.0	61	0.2	313	30	204	61	0.17	0.06	6.2	2	258
49	0	0.0	18	0.8	484	40	58	17	0.43	0.05	10.1	1	259
15	0	0.0	11	1.2	176	301	66	20	0.03	0.10	10.5	0	260
26	0	0.0	9	1.3	201	287	48	14	0.03	0.06	11.3	0	261
36	0	0.0	12	0.8	201	320	16	5	0.01	0.04	4.9	0	262
27	19	0.0	35	2.1	365	824	199	55	0.06	0.14	13.7	5	263
0	21	3.7	10	0.2	159	0	73	7	0.02	0.02	0.1	8	264

Food No.	Food Description	Measure of Edible Portion	Weight (g)	Water (%)	Calories (kcal)	Protein (g)	Total Fat (g)	Fatty Acids Saturated (g)	Monounsaturated (g)	Polyunsaturated (g)
FRUITS AND FRUIT JUICES (CONTINUED)										
265	PEELED, SLICED	1 CUP	110	84	63	TR	TR	0.1	TR	0.1
266	DRIED (SODIUM BISULFITE USED TO PRESERVE COLOR)	5 RINGS	32	32	78	TR	TR	TR	TR	TR
267	APPLE JUICE, BOTTLED OR CANNED	1 CUP	248	88	117	TR	TR	TR	TR	0.1
268	APPLE PIE FILLING, CANNED	1/8 OF 21-OZ CAN	74	73	75	TR	TR	TR	0.0	TR
	APPLESAUCE, CANNED									
269	SWEETENED	1 CUP	255	80	194	TR	TR	0.1	TR	0.1
270	UNSWEETENED	1 CUP	244	88	105	TR	TR	TR	TR	TR
	APRICOTS									
271	RAW, WITHOUT PITS (ABOUT 12 PER LB WITH PITS)	1 APRICOT	35	86	17	TR	TR	TR	0.1	TR
	CANNED, HALVES, FRUIT AND LIQUID									
272	HEAVY SYRUP PACK	1 CUP	258	78	214	1	TR	TR	0.1	TR
273	JUICE PACK	1 CUP	244	87	117	2	TR	TR	TR	TR
274	DRIED, SULFURED	10 HALVES	35	31	83	1	TR	TR	0.1	TR
275	APRICOT NECTAR, CANNED, WITH ADDED ASCORBIC ACID	1 CUP	251	85	141	1	TR	TR	0.1	TR
	ASIAN PEAR, RAW									
276	2 1/4" HIGH × 2 1/2" DIA	1 PEAR	122	88	51	1	TR	TR	0.1	0.1
277	3 3/8" HIGH × 3" DIA	1 PEAR	275	88	116	1	1	TR	0.1	0.2
	AVOCADOS, RAW, WITHOUT SKIN AND SEED									
278	CALIFORNIA (ABOUT 1/5 WHOLE)	1 OZ	28	73	50	1	5	0.7	3.2	0.6
279	FLORIDA (ABOUT 1/10 WHOLE)	1 OZ	28	80	32	TR	3	0.5	1.4	0.4
	BANANAS, RAW									
280	WHOLE, MEDIUM (7" TO 7 7/8" LONG)	1 BANANA	118	74	109	1	1	0.2	TR	0.1
281	SLICED	1 CUP	150	74	138	2	1	0.3	0.1	0.1
282	BLACKBERRIES, RAW	1 CUP	144	86	75	1	1	TR	0.1	0.3
	BLUEBERRIES									
283	RAW	1 CUP	145	85	81	1	1	TR	0.1	0.2
284	FROZEN, SWEETENED, THAWED	1 CUP	230	77	186	1	TR	TR	TR	0.1
	CANTALOUPE. SEE MELONS.									
	CARAMBOLA (STARFRUIT), RAW									
285	WHOLE (3 5/8" LONG)	1 FRUIT	91	91	30	TR	TR	TR	TR	0.2
286	SLICED	1 CUP	108	91	36	1	TR	TR	TR	0.2
	CHERRIES									
287	SOUR, RED, PITTED, CANNED, WATER PACK	1 CUP	244	90	88	2	TR	0.1	0.1	0.1
288	SWEET, RAW, WITHOUT PITS AND STEMS	10 CHERRIES	68	81	49	1	1	0.1	0.2	0.2
289	CHERRY PIE FILLING, CANNED	1/5 OF 21-OZ CAN	74	71	85	TR	TR	TR	TR	TR
290	CRANBERRIES, DRIED, SWEETENED	1/4 CUP	28	12	92	TR	TR	TR	TR	0.1
291	CRANBERRY SAUCE, SWEETENED, CANNED (ABOUT 8 SLICES PER CAN)	1 SLICE	57	61	86	TR	TR	TR	TR	TR
	DATES, WITHOUT PITS									
292	WHOLE	5 DATES	42	23	116	1	TR	0.1	0.1	TR
293	CHOPPED	1 CUP	178	23	490	4	1	0.3	0.3	0.1
294	FIGS, DRIED	2 FIGS	38	28	97	1	TR	0.1	0.1	0.2
	FRUIT COCKTAIL, CANNED, FRUIT AND LIQUID									

Cholesterol (mg)	Carbo-hydrate (g)	Total Dietary Fiber (g)	Calcium (mg)	Iron (mg)	Potassium (mg)	Sodium (mg)	Vitamin A (IU)	Vitamin A (RE)	Thiamine (mg)	Ribo-flavin (mg)	Niacin (mg)	Ascorbic Acid (mg)	Food No.
0	16	2.1	4	0.1	124	0	48	4	0.02	0.01	0.1	4	265
0	21	2.8	4	0.4	144	28	0	0	0.00	0.05	0.3	1	266
0	29	0.2	17	0.9	295	7	2	0	0.05	0.04	0.2	2	267
0	19	0.7	3	0.2	33	33	10	1	0.01	0.01	TR	1	268
0	51	3.1	10	0.9	156	8	28	3	0.03	0.07	0.5	4	269
0	28	2.9	7	0.3	183	5	71	7	0.03	0.06	0.5	3	270
0	4	0.8	5	0.2	104	TR	914	91	0.01	0.01	0.2	4	271
0	55	4.1	23	0.8	361	10	3,173	317	0.05	0.06	1.0	8	272
0	30	3.9	29	0.7	403	10	4,126	412	0.04	0.05	0.8	12	273
0	22	3.2	16	1.6	482	4	2,534	253	TR	0.05	1.0	1	274
0	36	1.5	18	1.0	286	8	3,303	331	0.02	0.04	0.7	137	275
0	13	4.4	5	0.0	148	0	0	0	0.01	0.01	0.3	5	276
0	29	9.9	11	0.0	333	0	0	0	0.02	0.03	0.6	10	277
0	2	1.4	3	0.3	180	3	174	17	0.03	0.03	0.5	2	278
0	3	1.5	3	0.2	138	1	174	17	0.03	0.03	0.5	2	279
0	28	2.8	7	0.4	467	1	96	9	0.05	0.12	0.6	11	280
0	35	3.6	9	0.5	594	2	122	12	0.07	0.15	0.8	14	281
0	18	7.6	46	0.8	282	0	238	23	0.04	0.06	0.6	30	282
0	20	3.9	9	0.2	129	9	145	15	0.07	0.07	0.5	19	283
0	50	4.8	14	0.9	138	2	101	9	0.05	0.12	0.6	2	284
0	7	2.5	4	0.2	148	2	449	45	0.03	0.02	0.4	19	285
0	8	2.9	4	0.3	176	2	532	53	0.03	0.03	0.4	23	286
0	22	2.7	27	3.3	239	17	1,840	183	0.04	0.10	0.4	5	287
0	11	1.6	10	0.3	152	0	146	14	0.03	0.04	0.3	5	288
0	21	0.4	8	0.2	78	13	152	16	0.02	0.01	0.1	3	289
0	24	2.5	5	0.1	24	1	0	0	0.01	0.03	TR	TR	290
0	22	0.6	2	0.1	15	17	11	1	0.01	0.01	0.1	1	291
0	31	3.2	13	0.5	274	1	21	2	0.04	0.04	0.9	0	292
0	131	13.4	57	2.0	1,161	5	89	9	0.16	0.18	3.9	0	293
0	25	4.6	55	0.8	271	4	51	5	0.03	0.03	0.3	TR	294

Food No.	Food Description	Measure of Edible Portion	Weight (g)	Water (%)	Calories (kcal)	Protein (g)	Total Fat (g)	Fatty Acids Saturated (g)	Mono-unsaturated (g)	Poly-unsaturated (g)
FRUITS AND FRUIT JUICES (CONTINUED)										
295	HEAVY SYRUP PACK	1 CUP	248	80	181	1	TR	TR	TR	0.1
296	JUICE PACK	1 CUP	237	87	109	1	TR	TR	TR	TR
	GRAPEFRUIT									
	RAW, WITHOUT PEEL, MEMBRANE									
	AND SEEDS (3 3/4″ DIA)									
297	PINK OR RED	1/2 GRAPEFRUIT	123	91	37	1	TR	TR	TR	TR
298	WHITE	1/2 GRAPEFRUIT	118	90	39	1	TR	TR	TR	TR
299	CANNED, SECTIONS WITH LIGHT SYRUP	1 CUP	254	84	152	1	TR	TR	TR	0.1
	GRAPEFRUIT JUICE									
	RAW									
300	PINK	1 CUP	247	90	96	1	TR	TR	TR	0.1
301	WHITE	1 CUP	247	90	96	1	TR	TR	TR	0.1
	CANNED									
302	UNSWEETENED	1 CUP	247	90	94	1	TR	TR	TR	0.1
303	SWEETENED	1 CUP	250	87	115	1	TR	TR	TR	0.1
	FROZEN CONCENTRATE,									
	UNSWEETENED									
304	UNDILUTED	6-FL-OZ CAN	207	62	302	4	1	0.1	0.1	0.2
305	DILUTED WITH 3 PARTS									
	WATER BY VOLUME	1 CUP	247	89	101	1	TR	TR	TR	0.1
306	GRAPES, SEEDLESS, RAW	10 GRAPES	50	81	36	TR	TR	0.1	TR	0.1
307		1 CUP	160	81	114	1	1	0.3	TR	0.3
	GRAPE JUICE									
308	CANNED OR BOTTLED	1 CUP	253	84	154	1	TR	0.1	TR	0.1
	FROZEN CONCENTRATE, SWEETENED,									
	WITH ADDED VITAMIN C									
309	UNDILUTED	6-FL-OZ CAN	216	54	387	1	1	0.2	TR	0.2
310	DILUTED WITH 3 PARTS WATER BY									
	VOLUME	1 CUP	250	87	128	TR	TR	0.1	TR	0.1
311	KIWI FRUIT, RAW, WITHOUT SKIN									
	(ABOUT 5 PER LB WITH SKIN)	1 MEDIUM	76	83	46	1	TR	TR	TR	0.2
312	LEMONS, RAW, WITHOUT PEEL									
	(2 1/8″ DIA WITH PEEL)	1 LEMON	58	89	17	1	TR	TR	TR	0.1
	LEMON JUICE									
313	RAW (FROM 2 1/8″ DIA LEMON)	JUICE OF								
		1 LEMON	47	91	12	TR	0	0.0	0.0	0.0
314	CANNED OR BOTTLED, UNSWEETENED	1 CUP	244	92	51	1	1	0.1	TR	0.2
315		1 TBSP	15	92	3	TR	TR	TR	TR	TR
	LIME JUICE									
316	RAW (FROM 2″ DIA LIME)	JUICE OF								
		1 LIME	38	90	10	TR	TR	TR	TR	TR
317	CANNED, UNSWEETENED	1 CUP	246	93	52	1	1	0.1	0.1	0.2
318		1 TBSP	15	93	3	TR	TR	TR	TR	TR
	MANGOS, RAW, WITHOUT SKIN AND SEED									
	(ABOUT 1 1/2 PER LB WITH SKIN AND SEED)									
319	WHOLE	1 MANGO	207	82	135	1	1	0.1	0.2	0.1
320	SLICED	1 CUP	165	82	107	1	TR	0.1	0.2	0.1
	MELONS, RAW, WITHOUT RIND AND									
	CAVITY CONTENTS									

*Sodium benzoate and sodium bisulfite added as preservatives.

Cholesterol (mg)	Carbo-hydrate (g)	Total Dietary Fiber (g)	Calcium (mg)	Iron (mg)	Potassium (mg)	Sodium (mg)	Vitamin A		Thiamine (mg)	Ribo-flavin (mg)	Niacin (mg)	Ascorbic Acid (mg)	Food No.
							(IU)	(RE)					
0	47	2.5	15	0.7	218	15	508	50	0.04	0.05	0.9	5	295
0	28	2.4	19	0.5	225	9	723	73	0.03	0.04	1.0	6	296
0	9	1.4	14	0.1	159	0	319	32	0.04	0.02	0.2	47	297
0	10	1.3	14	0.1	175	0	12	1	0.04	0.02	0.3	39	298
0	39	1.0	36	1.0	328	5	0	0	0.10	0.05	0.6	54	299
0	23	0.2	22	0.5	400	2	1,087	109	0.10	0.05	0.5	94	300
0	23	0.2	22	0.5	400	2	25	2	0.10	0.05	0.5	94	301
0	22	0.2	17	0.5	378	2	17	2	0.10	0.05	0.6	72	302
0	28	0.3	20	0.9	405	5	0	0	0.10	0.06	0.8	67	303
0	72	0.8	56	1.0	1,002	6	64	6	0.30	0.16	1.6	248	304
0	24	0.2	20	0.3	336	2	22	2	0.10	0.05	0.5	83	305
0	9	0.5	6	0.1	93	1	37	4	0.05	0.03	0.2	5	306
0	28	1.6	18	0.4	296	3	117	11	0.15	0.09	0.5	17	307
0	38	0.3	23	0.6	334	8	20	3	0.07	0.09	0.7	TR	308
0	96	0.6	28	0.8	160	15	58	6	0.11	0.20	0.9	179	309
0	32	0.3	10	0.3	53	5	20	3	0.04	0.07	0.3	60	310
0	11	2.6	20	0.3	252	4	133	14	0.02	0.04	0.4	74	311
0	5	1.6	15	0.3	80	1	17	2	0.02	0.01	0.1	31	312
0	4	0.2	3	TR	58	TR	9	1	0.01	TR	TR	22	313
0	16	1.0	27	0.3	249	51*	37	5	0.10	0.02	0.5	61	314
0	1	0.1	2	TR	16	3*	2	TR	0.01	TR	TR	4	315
0	3	0.2	3	TR	41	TR	4	TR	0.01	TR	TR	11	316
0	16	1.0	30	0.6	185	39*	39	5	0.08	0.01	0.4	16	317
0	1	0.1	2	TR	11	2*	2	TR	TR	TR	TR	1	318
0	35	3.7	21	0.3	323	4	8,061	805	0.12	0.12	1.2	57	319
0	28	3.0	17	0.2	257	3	6,425	642	0.10	0.09	1.0	46	320

Food No.	Food Description	Measure of Edible Portion	Weight (g)	Water (%)	Calories (kcal)	Protein (g)	Total Fat (g)	Fatty Acids Satu-rated (g)	Mono-unsatu-rated (g)	Poly-unsatu-rated (g)
FRUITS AND FRUIT JUICES (CONTINUED)										
	CANTALOUPE (5″ DIA)									
321	WEDGE	1/8 MELON	69	90	24	1	TR	TR	TR	0.1
322	CUBES	1 CUP	160	90	56	1	TR	0.1	TR	0.2
	HONEYDEW (6″–7″ DIA)									
323	WEDGE	1/8 MELON	160	90	56	1	TR	TR	TR	0.1
324	DICED (ABOUT 20 PIECES PER CUP)	1 CUP	170	90	60	1	TR	TR	TR	0.1
325	MIXED FRUIT, FROZEN, SWEETENED, THAWED (PEACH, CHERRY, RASPBERRY, GRAPE, AND BOYSENBERRY)	1 CUP	250	74	245	4	TR	0.1	0.1	0.2
326	NECTARINES, RAW (2 1/2″ DIA)	1 NECTARINE	136	86	67	1	1	0.1	0.2	0.3
	ORANGES, RAW									
327	WHOLE, WITHOUT PEEL AND SEEDS (2 5/8″ DIA)	1 ORANGE	131	87	62	1	TR	TR	TR	TR
328	SECTIONS WITHOUT MEMBRANES	1 CUP	180	87	85	2	TR	TR	TR	TR
	ORANGE JUICE									
329	RAW, ALL VARIETIES	1 CUP	248	88	112	2	TR	0.1	0.1	0.1
330		JUICE FROM 1 ORANGE	86	88	39	1	TR	TR	TR	TR
331	CANNED, UNSWEETENED	1 CUP	249	89	105	1	TR	TR	0.1	0.1
332	CHILLED (REFRIGERATOR CASE)	1 CUP	249	88	110	2	1	0.1	0.1	0.2
	FROZEN CONCENTRATE									
333	UNDILUTED	6-FL-OZ CAN	213	58	339	5	TR	0.1	0.1	0.1
334	DILUTED WITH 3 PARTS WATER BY VOLUME	1 CUP	249	88	112	2	TR	TR	TR	TR
	PAPAYAS, RAW									
335	1/2″ CUBES	1 CUP	140	89	55	1	TR	0.1	0.1	TR
336	WHOLE (5 1/8″ LONG × 3″ DIA)	1 PAPAYA	304	89	119	2	TR	0.1	0.1	0.1
	PEACHES									
	RAW									
337	WHOLE, 2 1/2″ DIA, PITTED (ABOUT 4 PER LB)	1 PEACH	98	88	42	1	TR	TR	TR	TR
338	SLICED	1 CUP	170	88	73	1	TR	TR	0.1	0.1
	CANNED, FRUIT AND LIQUID									
339	HEAVY SYRUP PACK	1 CUP	262	79	194	1	TR	TR	0.1	0.1
340		1 HALF	98	79	73	TR	TR	TR	TR	TR
341	JUICE PACK	1 CUP	248	87	109	2	TR	TR	TR	TR
342		1 HALF	98	87	43	1	TR	TR	TR	TR
343	DRIED, SULFURED	3 HALVES	39	32	93	1	TR	TR	0.1	0.1
344	FROZEN, SLICED, SWEETENED, WITH ADDED ASCORBIC ACID, THAWED	1 CUP	250	75	235	2	TR	TR	0.1	0.2
	PEARS									
345	RAW, WITH SKIN, CORED, 2 1/2″ DIA	1 PEAR	166	84	98	1	1	TR	0.1	0.2
	CANNED, FRUIT AND LIQUID									
346	HEAVY SYRUP PACK	1 CUP	266	80	197	1	TR	TR	0.1	0.1
347		1 HALF	76	80	56	TR	TR	TR	TR	TR
348	JUICE PACK	1 CUP	248	86	124	1	TR	TR	TR	TR
349		1 HALF	76	86	38	TR	TR	TR	TR	TR
	PINEAPPLE									
350	RAW, DICED	1 CUP	155	87	76	1	1	TR	0.1	0.2

Cholesterol (mg)	Carbo-hydrate (g)	Total Dietary Fiber (g)	Calcium (mg)	Iron (mg)	Potassium (mg)	Sodium (mg)	Vitamin A		Thiamine (mg)	Ribo-flavin (mg)	Niacin (mg)	Ascorbic Acid (mg)	Food No.
							(IU)	(RE)					
0	6	0.6	8	0.1	213	6	2,225	222	0.02	0.01	0.4	29	321
0	13	1.3	18	0.3	494	14	5,158	515	0.06	0.03	0.9	68	322
0	15	1.0	10	0.1	434	16	64	6	0.12	0.03	1.0	40	323
0	16	1.0	10	0.1	461	17	68	7	0.13	0.03	1.0	42	324
0	61	4.8	18	0.7	328	8	805	80	0.04	0.09	1.0	188	325
0	16	2.2	7	0.2	288	0	1,001	101	0.02	0.06	1.3	7	326
0	15	3.1	52	0.1	237	0	269	28	0.11	0.05	0.4	70	327
0	21	4.3	72	0.2	326	0	369	38	0.16	0.07	0.5	96	328
0	26	0.5	27	0.5	496	2	496	50	0.22	0.07	1.0	124	329
0	9	0.2	9	0.2	172	1	172	17	0.08	0.03	0.3	43	330
0	25	0.5	20	1.1	436	5	436	45	0.15	0.07	0.8	86	331
0	25	0.5	25	0.4	473	2	194	20	0.28	0.05	0.7	82	332
0	81	1.7	68	0.7	1,436	6	588	60	0.60	0.14	1.5	294	333
0	27	0.5	22	0.2	473	2	194	20	0.20	0.04	0.5	97	334
0	14	2.5	34	0.1	360	4	398	39	0.04	0.04	0.5	87	335
0	30	5.5	73	0.3	781	9	863	85	0.08	0.10	1.0	188	336
0	11	2.0	5	0.1	193	0	524	53	0.02	0.04	1.0	6	337
0	19	3.4	9	0.2	335	0	910	92	0.03	0.07	1.7	11	338
0	52	3.4	8	0.7	241	16	870	86	0.03	0.06	1.6	7	339
0	20	1.3	3	0.3	90	6	325	32	0.01	0.02	0.6	3	340
0	29	3.2	15	0.7	317	10	945	94	0.02	0.04	1.4	9	341
0	11	1.3	6	0.3	125	4	373	37	0.01	0.02	0.6	4	342
0	24	3.2	11	1.6	388	3	844	84	TR	0.08	1.7	2	343
0	60	4.5	8	0.9	325	15	710	70	0.03	0.09	1.6	236	344
0	25	4.0	18	0.4	208	0	33	3	0.03	0.07	0.2	7	345
0	51	4.3	13	0.6	173	13	0	0	0.03	0.06	0.6	3	346
0	15	1.2	4	0.2	49	4	0	0	0.01	0.02	0.2	1	347
0	32	4.0	22	0.7	238	10	15	2	0.03	0.03	0.5	4	348
0	10	1.2	7	0.2	73	3	5	1	0.01	0.01	0.2	1	349
0	19	1.9	11	0.6	175	2	36	3	0.14	0.06	0.7	24	350

Food No.	Food Description	Measure of Edible Portion	Weight (g)	Water (%)	Calories (kcal)	Protein (g)	Total Fat (g)	Fatty Acids Satu- rated (g)	Mono- unsatu- rated (g)	Poly- unsatu- rated (g)
FRUITS AND FRUIT JUICES (CONTINUED)										
	CANNED, FRUIT AND LIQUID									
	HEAVY SYRUP PACK									
351	CRUSHED, SLICED, OR CHUNKS	1 CUP	254	79	198	1	TR	TR	TR	0.1
352	SLICES (3″ DIA)	1 SLICE	49	79	38	TR	TR	TR	TR	TR
	JUICE PACK									
353	CRUSHED, SLICED, OR CHUNKS	1 CUP	249	84	149	1	TR	TR	TR	0.1
354	SLICE (3″ DIA)	1 SLICE	47	84	28	TR	TR	TR	TR	TR
355	PINEAPPLE JUICE, UNSWEETENED, CANNED	1 CUP	250	86	140	1	TR	TR	TR	0.1
	PLANTAIN, WITHOUT PEEL									
356	RAW	1 MEDIUM	179	65	218	2	1	0.3	0.1	0.1
357	COOKED, SLICES	1 CUP	154	67	179	1	TR	0.1	TR	0.1
	PLUMS									
358	RAW (2 1/8″ DIA)	1 PLUM	66	85	36	1	TR	TR	0.3	0.1
	CANNED, PURPLE, FRUIT AND LIQUID									
359	HEAVY SYRUP PACK	1 CUP	258	76	230	1	TR	TR	0.2	0.1
360		1 PLUM	46	76	41	TR	TR	TR	TR	TR
361	JUICE PACK	1 CUP	252	84	146	1	TR	TR	TR	TR
362		1 PLUM	46	84	27	TR	TR	TR	TR	TR
	PRUNES, DRIED, PITTED									
363	UNCOOKED	5 PRUNES	42	32	100	1	TR	TR	0.1	TR
364	STEWED, UNSWEETENED,									
	FRUIT AND LIQUID	1 CUP	248	70	265	3	1	TR	0.4	0.1
365	PRUNE JUICE, CANNED OR BOTTLED	1 CUP	256	81	182	2	TR	TR	0.1	TR
	RAISINS, SEEDLESS									
366	CUP, NOT PACKED	1 CUP	145	15	435	5	1	0.2	TR	0.2
367	PACKET, 1/2 OZ (1 1/2 TBSP)	1 PACKET	14	15	42	TR	TR	TR	TR	TR
	RASPBERRIES									
368	RAW	1 CUP	123	87	60	1	1	TR	0.1	0.4
369	FROZEN, SWEETENED, THAWED	1 CUP	250	73	258	2	TR	TR	TR	0.2
370	RHUBARB, FROZEN, COOKED, WITH SUGAR	1 CUP	240	68	278	1	TR	TR	TR	0.1
	STRAWBERRIES									
	RAW, CAPPED									
371	LARGE (1 1/8″ DIA)	1 STRAWBERRY	18	92	5	TR	TR	TR	TR	TR
372	MEDIUM (1 1/4″ DIA)	1 STRAWBERRY	12	92	4	TR	TR	TR	TR	TR
373	SLICED	1 CUP	166	92	50	1	1	TR	0.1	0.3
374	FROZEN, SWEETENED,									
	SLICED, THAWED	1 CUP	255	73	245	1	TR	TR	TR	0.2
	TANGERINES									
375	RAW, WITHOUT PEEL AND SEEDS									
	(2 3/8″ DIA)	1 TANGERINE	84	88	37	1	TR	TR	TR	TR
376	CANNED (MANDARIN ORANGES),									
	LIGHT SYRUP, FRUIT AND LIQUID	1 CUP	252	83	154	1	TR	TR	TR	0.1
377	TANGERINE JUICE, CANNED, SWEETENED	1 CUP	249	87	125	1	TR	TR	TR	0.1
	WATERMELON, RAW (15″ LONG × 7 1/2″ DIA)									
378	WEDGE (ABOUT 1/16 OF MELON)	1 WEDGE	286	92	92	2	1	0.1	0.3	0.4
379	DICED	1 CUP	152	92	49	1	1	0.1	0.2	0.2
GRAIN PRODUCTS										
	BAGELS, ENRICHED									
380	PLAIN	3 1/2″ BAGEL	71	33	195	7	1	0.2	0.1	0.5
381		4″ BAGEL	89	33	245	9	1	0.2	0.1	0.6

Cholesterol (mg)	Carbo-hydrate (g)	Total Dietary Fiber (g)	Calcium (mg)	Iron (mg)	Potassium (mg)	Sodium (mg)	Vitamin A		Thiamine (mg)	Ribo-flavin (mg)	Niacin (mg)	Ascorbic Acid (mg)	Food No.
							(IU)	(RE)					
0	51	2.0	36	1.0	264	3	36	3	0.23	0.06	0.7	19	351
0	10	0.4	7	0.2	51	TR	7	TR	0.04	0.01	0.1	4	352
0	39	2.0	35	0.7	304	2	95	10	0.24	0.05	0.7	24	353
0	7	0.4	7	0.1	57	TR	18	2	0.04	0.01	0.1	4	354
0	34	0.5	43	0.7	335	3	13	0	0.14	0.06	0.6	27	355
0	57	4.1	5	1.1	893	7	2,017	202	0.09	0.10	1.2	33	356
0	48	3.5	3	0.9	716	8	1,400	140	0.07	0.08	1.2	17	357
0	9	1.0	3	0.1	114	0	213	21	0.03	0.06	0.3	6	358
0	60	2.6	23	2.2	235	49	668	67	0.04	0.10	0.8	1	359
0	11	0.5	4	0.4	42	9	119	12	0.01	0.02	0.1	TR	360
0	38	2.6	26	0.9	388	3	2,543	255	0.06	0.15	1.2	7	361
0	7	0.5	5	0.2	71	TR	464	46	0.01	0.03	0.2	1	362
0	26	3.0	21	1.0	313	2	835	84	0.03	0.07	0.8	1	363
0	70	16.4	57	2.8	828	5	759	77	0.06	0.25	1.8	7	364
0	45	2.6	31	3.0	707	10	8	0	0.04	0.18	2.0	10	365
0	115	5.8	71	3.0	1,089	17	12	1	0.23	0.13	1.2	5	366
0	11	0.6	7	0.3	105	2	1	TR	0.02	0.01	0.1	TR	367
0	14	8.4	27	0.7	187	0	160	16	0.04	0.11	1.1	31	368
0	65	11.0	38	1.6	285	3	150	15	0.05	0.11	0.6	41	369
0	76	4.8	318	0.6	200	2	100	17	0.04	0.09	0.5	0	370
0	1	0.4	3	0.1	30	TR	5	1	TR	0.01	TR	10	371
0	1	0.3	2	TR	20	TR	3	TR	TR	0.01	TR	7	372
0	12	3.8	23	0.6	276	2	45	5	0.03	0.11	0.4	94	373
0	66	4.8	28	1.5	250	8	61	5	0.04	0.13	1.0	106	374
0	9	1.9	12	0.1	132	1	773	77	0.09	0.02	0.1	26	375
0	41	1.8	18	0.9	197	15	2,117	212	0.13	0.11	1.1	50	376
0	30	0.5	45	0.5	443	2	1,046	105	0.15	0.05	0.2	55	377
0	21	1.4	23	0.5	332	6	1,047	106	0.23	0.06	0.6	27	378
0	11	0.8	12	0.3	176	3	556	56	0.12	0.03	0.3	15	379
0	38	1.6	53	2.5	72	379	0	0	0.38	0.22	3.2	0	380
0	48	2.0	66	3.2	90	475	0	0	0.48	0.28	4.1	0	381

Food No.	Food Description	Measure of Edible Portion	Weight (g)	Water (%)	Calories (kcal)	Protein (g)	Total Fat (g)	Fatty Acids Saturated (g)	Mono-unsaturated (g)	Poly-unsaturated (g)
GRAIN PRODUCTS (CONTINUED)										
382	CINNAMON RAISIN	3 1/2″ BAGEL	71	32	195	7	1	0.2	0.1	0.5
383		4″ BAGEL	89	32	244	9	2	0.2	0.2	0.6
384	EGG	3 1/2″ BAGEL	71	33	197	8	1	0.3	0.3	0.5
385		4″ BAGEL	89	33	247	9	2	0.4	0.4	0.6
386	BANANA BREAD, PREPARED FROM RECIPE, WITH MARGARINE	1 SLICE	60	29	196	3	6	1.3	2.7	1.9
	BARLEY, PEARLED									
387	UNCOOKED	1 CUP	200	10	704	20	2	0.5	0.3	1.1
388	COOKED	1 CUP	157	69	193	4	1	0.1	0.1	0.3
	BISCUITS, PLAIN OR BUTTERMILK, ENRICHED									
389	PREPARED FROM RECIPE, WITH 2% MILK	2 1/2″ BISCUIT	60	29	212	4	10	2.6	4.2	2.5
390		4″ BISCUIT	101	29	358	7	16	4.4	7.0	4.2
	REFRIGERATED DOUGH, BAKED									
391	REGULAR	2 1/2″ BISCUIT	27	28	93	2	4	1.0	2.2	0.5
392	LOWER FAT	2 1/4″ BISCUIT	21	28	63	2	1	0.3	0.6	0.2
	BREADS, ENRICHED									
393	CRACKED WHEAT	1 SLICE	25	36	65	2	1	0.2	0.5	0.2
394	EGG BREAD (CHALLAH)	1/2″ SLICE	40	35	115	4	2	0.6	0.9	0.4
395	FRENCH OR VIENNA (INCLUDES SOURDOUGH)	1/2 SLICE	25	34	69	2	1	0.2	0.3	0.2
396	INDIAN FRY (NAVAJO) BREAD	5″ BREAD	90	27	296	6	9	2.1	3.6	2.3
397		10 1/2″ BREAD	160	27	526	11	15	3.7	6.4	4.1
398	ITALIAN	1 SLICE	20	36	54	2	1	0.2	0.3	0.2
	MIXED GRAIN									
399	UNTOASTED	1 SLICE	26	38	65	3	1	0.2	0.4	0.2
400	TOASTED	1 SLICE	24	32	65	3	1	0.2	0.4	0.2
	OATMEAL									
401	UNTOASTED	1 SLICE	27	37	73	2	1	0.2	0.4	0.5
402	TOASTED	1 SLICE	25	31	73	2	1	0.2	0.4	0.5
403	PITA	4 PITA	28	32	77	3	TR	TR	TR	0.1
404		6 1/2″ PITA	60	32	165	5	1	0.1	0.1	0.3
	PUMPERNICKEL									
405	UNTOASTED	1 SLICE	32	38	80	3	1	0.1	0.3	0.4
406	TOASTED	1 SLICE	29	32	80	3	1	0.1	0.3	0.4
	RAISIN									
407	UNTOASTED	1 SLICE	26	34	71	2	1	0.3	0.6	0.2
408	TOASTED	1 SLICE	24	28	71	2	1	0.3	0.6	0.2
	RYE									
409	UNTOASTED	1 SLICE	32	37	83	3	1	0.2	0.4	0.3
410	TOASTED	1 SLICE	24	31	68	2	1	0.2	0.3	0.2
411	RYE, REDUCED CALORIE	1 SLICE	23	46	47	2	1	0.1	0.2	0.2
	WHEAT									
412	UNTOASTED	1 SLICE	25	37	65	2	1	0.2	0.4	0.2
413	TOASTED	1 SLICE	23	32	65	2	1	0.2	0.4	0.2
414	WHEAT, REDUCED CALORIE	1 SLICE	23	43	46	2	1	0.1	0.1	0.2
	WHITE									
415	UNTOASTED	1 SLICE	25	37	67	2	1	0.1	0.2	0.5
416	TOASTED	1 SLICE	22	30	64	2	1	0.1	0.2	0.5
417	SOFT CRUMBS	1 CUP	45	37	120	4	2	0.2	0.3	0.9
418	WHITE, REDUCED CALORIE	1 SLICE	23	43	48	2	1	0.1	0.2	0.1

Cholesterol (mg)	Carbo-hydrate (g)	Total Dietary Fiber (g)	Calcium (mg)	Iron (mg)	Potassium (mg)	Sodium (mg)	Vitamin A (IU)	Vitamin A (RE)	Thiamine (mg)	Ribo-flavin (mg)	Niacin (mg)	Ascorbic Acid (mg)	Food No.
0	39	1.6	13	2.7	105	229	52	0	0.27	0.20	2.2	TR	382
0	49	2.0	17	3.4	132	287	65	0	0.34	0.25	2.7	1	383
17	38	1.6	9	2.8	48	359	77	23	0.38	0.17	2.4	TR	384
21	47	2.0	12	3.5	61	449	97	29	0.48	0.21	3.1	1	385
26	33	0.7	13	0.8	80	181	278	72	0.10	0.12	0.9	1	386
0	155	31.2	58	5.0	560	18	44	4	0.38	0.23	9.2	0	387
0	44	6.0	17	2.1	146	5	11	2	0.13	0.10	3.2	0	388
2	27	0.9	141	1.7	73	348	49	14	0.21	0.19	1.8	TR	389
3	45	1.5	237	2.9	122	586	83	23	0.36	0.31	3.0	TR	390
0	13	0.4	5	0.7	42	325	0	0	0.09	0.06	0.8	0	391
0	12	0.4	4	0.6	39	305	0	0	0.09	0.05	0.7	0	392
0	12	1.4	11	0.7	44	135	0	0	0.09	0.06	0.9	0	393
20	19	0.9	37	1.2	46	197	30	9	0.18	0.17	1.9	0	394
0	13	0.8	19	0.6	28	152	0	0	0.13	0.08	1.2	0	395
0	48	1.6	210	3.2	67	626	0	0	0.39	0.27	3.3	0	396
0	05	2.9	373	5.0	110	1,112	0	0	0.69	0.49	5.8	0	397
0	10	0.5	16	0.6	22	117	0	0	0.09	0.06	0.9	0	398
0	12	1.7	24	0.9	53	127	0	0	0.11	0.09	1.1	TR	399
0	12	1.6	24	0.9	53	127	0	0	0.08	0.08	1.0	TR	400
0	13	1.1	18	0.7	38	162	4	1	0.11	0.06	0.8	0	401
0	13	1.1	18	0.7	39	163	4	1	0.09	0.06	0.8	TR	402
0	16	0.6	24	0.7	34	150	0	0	0.17	0.09	1.3	0	403
0	33	1.3	52	1.6	72	322	0	0	0.36	0.20	2.8	0	404
0	15	2.1	22	0.9	67	215	0	0	0.10	0.10	1.0	0	405
0	15	2.1	21	0.9	66	214	0	0	0.08	0.09	0.9	0	406
0	14	1.1	17	0.8	59	101	0	0	0.09	0.10	0.9	TR	407
0	14	1.1	17	0.8	59	102	TR	0	0.07	0.09	0.8	TR	408
0	15	1.9	23	0.9	53	211	2	TR	0.14	0.11	1.2	TR	409
0	13	1.5	19	0.7	44	174	1	0	0.09	0.08	0.9	TR	410
0	9	2.8	17	0.7	23	93	1	0	0.08	0.06	0.6	TR	411
0	12	1.1	26	0.8	50	133	0	0	0.10	0.07	1.0	0	412
0	12	1.2	26	0.8	50	132	0	0	0.08	0.06	0.9	0	413
0	10	2.8	18	0.7	28	118	0	0	0.10	0.07	0.9	TR	414
TR	12	0.6	27	0.8	30	135	0	0	0.12	0.09	1.0	0	415
TR	12	0.6	26	0.7	29	130	0	0	0.09	0.07	0.9	0	416
TR	22	1.0	49	1.4	54	242	0	0	0.21	0.15	1.8	0	417
0	10	2.2	22	0.7	17	104	1	TR	0.09	0.07	0.8	TR	418

Food No.	Food Description	Measure of Edible Portion	Weight (g)	Water (%)	Calories (kcal)	Protein (g)	Total Fat (g)	Fatty Acids Saturated (g)	Monounsaturated (g)	Polyunsaturated (g)
GRAIN PRODUCTS (CONTINUED)										
	BREAD, WHOLE WHEAT									
419	UNTOASTED	1 SLICE	28	38	69	3	1	0.3	0.5	0.3
420	TOASTED	1 SLICE	25	30	69	3	1	0.3	0.5	0.3
	BREAD CRUMBS, DRY, GRATED									
421	PLAIN, ENRICHED	1 CUP	108	6	427	14	6	1.3	2.6	1.2
422		1 OZ	28	6	112	4	2	0.3	0.7	0.3
423	SEASONED, UNENRICHED	1 CUP	120	6	440	17	3	0.9	1.2	0.8
	BREAD CRUMBS, SOFT. SEE WHITE BREAD.									
424	BREAD STUFFING, PREPARED									
	FROM DRY MIX	1/2 CUP	100	65	178	3	9	1.7	3.8	2.6
425	BREAKFAST BAR, CEREAL									
	CRUST WITH FRUIT FILLING, FAT FREE	1 BAR	37	14	121	2	TR	TR	TR	0.1
	BREAKFAST CEREALS									
	HOT TYPE, COOKED									
	CORN (HOMINY) GRITS									
	REGULAR OR QUICK, ENRICHED									
426	WHITE	1 CUP	242	85	145	3	TR	0.1	0.1	0.2
427	YELLOW	1 CUP	242	85	145	3	TR	0.1	0.1	0.2
428	INSTANT, PLAIN	1 PACKET	137	82	89	2	TR	TR	TR	0.1
	CREAM OF WHEAT									
429	REGULAR	1 CUP	251	87	133	4	1	0.1	0.1	0.3
430	QUICK	1 CUP	239	87	129	4	TR	0.1	0.1	0.3
431	MIX'N EAT, PLAIN	1 PACKET	142	82	102	3	TR	TR	TR	0.2
432	MALT O MEAL	1 CUP	240	88	122	4	TR	0.1	0.1	TR
	OATMEAL									
433	REGULAR, QUICK OR INSTANT, PLAIN,									
	NONFORTIFIED	1 CUP	234	85	145	6	2	0.4	0.7	0.9
434	INSTANT, FORTIFIED, PLAIN	1 PACKET	177	86	104	4	2	0.3	0.6	0.7
	QUAKER INSTANT									
435	APPLES AND CINNAMON	1 PACKET	149	79	125	3	1	0.3	0.5	0.6
436	MAPLE AND BROWN									
	SUGAR	1 PACKET	155	75	153	4	2	0.4	0.6	0.7
437	WHEATENA	1 CUP	243	85	136	5	1	0.2	0.2	0.6
	READY TO EAT									
438	ALL BRAN	1/2 CUP	30	3	79	4	1	0.2	0.2	0.5
439	APPLE CINNAMON CHEERIOS	3/4 CUP	30	3	118	2	2	0.3	0.6	0.2
440	APPLE JACKS	1 CUP	30	3	116	1	TR	0.1	0.1	0.2
441	BASIC 4	1 CUP	55	7	201	4	3	0.4	1.0	1.1
442	BERRY BERRY KIX	3/4 CUP	30	2	120	1	1	0.2	0.5	0.1
443	CAP'N CRUNCH	3/4 CUP	27	2	107	1	1	0.4	0.3	0.2
444	CAP'N CRUNCH'S CRUNCHBERRIES	3/4 CUP	26	2	104	1	1	0.3	0.3	0.2
445	CAP'N CRUNCH'S PEANUT BUTTER									
	CRUNCH	3/4 CUP	27	2	112	2	2	0.5	0.8	0.5
446	CHEERIOS	1 CUP	30	3	110	3	2	0.4	0.6	0.2
	CHEX									
447	CORN	1 CUP	30	3	113	2	TR	0.1	0.1	0.2
448	HONEY NUT	3/4 CUP	30	2	117	2	1	0.1	0.4	0.2
449	MULTI BRAN	1 CUP	49	3	165	4	1	0.2	0.3	0.5
450	RICE	1 1/4 CUP	31	3	117	2	TR	TR	TR	TR
451	WHEAT	1 CUP	30	3	104	3	1	0.1	0.1	0.3
452	CINNAMON LIFE	1 CUP	50	4	190	4	2	0.3	0.6	0.8

Cholesterol (mg)	Carbo-hydrate (g)	Total Dietary Fiber (g)	Calcium (mg)	Iron (mg)	Potassium (mg)	Sodium (mg)	Vitamin A (IU)	Vitamin A (RE)	Thiamine (mg)	Ribo-flavin (mg)	Niacin (mg)	Ascorbic Acid (mg)	Food No.
0	13	1.9	20	0.9	71	148	0	0	0.10	0.06	1.1	0	419
0	13	1.9	20	0.9	71	148	0	0	0.08	0.05	1.0	0	420
0	78	2.6	245	6.6	239	931	1	0	0.83	0.47	7.4	0	421
0	21	0.7	64	1.7	63	244	TR	0	0.22	0.12	1.9	0	422
1	84	5.0	119	3.8	324	3,180	16	4	0.19	0.20	3.3	TR	423
0	22	2.9	32	1.1	74	543	313	81	0.14	0.11	1.5	0	424
TR	28	0.8	49	4.5	92	203	1,249	125	1.01	0.42	5.0	1	425
0	31	0.5	0	1.5	53	0	0	0	0.24	0.15	2.0	0	426
0	31	0.5	0	1.5	53	0	145	15	0.24	0.15	2.0	0	427
0	21	1.2	8	8.2	38	289	0	0	0.15	0.08	1.4	0	428
0	28	1.8	50	10.3	43	3	0	0	0.25	0.00	1.5	0	429
0	27	1.2	50	10.3	45	139	0	0	0.24	0.00	1.4	0	430
0	21	0.4	20	8.1	38	241	1,252	376	0.43	0.28	5.0	0	431
0	26	1.0	5	9.6	31	2	0	0	0.48	0.24	5.8	0	432
0	25	4.0	19	1.6	131	2	37	5	0.26	0.05	0.3	0	433
0	18	3.0	163	6.3	99	285	1,510	453	0.53	0.28	5.5	0	434
0	26	2.5	104	3.9	106	121	1,019	306	0.30	0.35	4.1	TR	435
0	31	2.6	105	3.9	112	234	1,008	302	0.30	0.34	4.0	0	436
0	29	6.6	10	1.4	187	5	0	0	0.02	0.05	1.3	0	437
0	23	9.7	106	4.5	342	61	750	225	0.39	0.42	5.0	15	438
0	25	1.6	35	4.5	60	150	750	225	0.38	0.43	5.0	15	439
0	27	0.6	3	4.5	32	134	750	225	0.39	0.42	5.0	15	440
0	42	3.4	310	4.5	162	323	1,250	375	0.37	0.42	5.0	15	441
0	26	0.2	66	4.5	24	185	750	225	0.38	0.43	5.0	15	442
0	23	0.9	5	4.5	35	208	36	4	0.38	0.42	5.0	0	443
0	22	0.6	7	4.5	37	190	33	5	0.37	0.42	5.0	TR	444
0	22	0.8	3	4.5	62	204	37	4	0.38	0.42	5.0	0	445
0	23	2.6	55	8.1	89	284	1,250	375	0.38	0.43	5.0	15	446
0	26	0.5	100	9.0	32	289	0	0	0.38	0.00	5.0	6	447
0	26	0.4	102	9.0	27	224	0	0	0.38	0.44	5.0	6	448
0	41	6.4	95	13.7	191	325	0	0	0.32	0.00	4.4	5	449
0	27	0.3	104	9.0	36	291	0	0	0.38	0.02	5.0	6	450
0	24	3.3	60	9.0	116	269	0	0	0.23	0.04	3.0	4	451
0	40	3.0	135	7.5	113	220	16	2	0.63	0.71	8.4	TR	452

Food No.	Food Description	Measure of Edible Portion	Weight (g)	Water (%)	Calories (kcal)	Protein (g)	Total Fat (g)	Fatty Acids Satu- rated (g)	Mono- unsatu- rated (g)	Poly- unsatu- rated (g)
GRAIN PRODUCTS (CONTINUED)										
453	CINNAMON TOAST CRUNCH	3/4 CUP	30	2	124	2	3	0.5	0.9	0.5
454	COCOA KRISPIES	3/4 CUP	31	2	120	2	1	0.6	0.1	0.1
455	COCOA PUFFS	1 CUP	30	2	119	1	1	0.2	0.3	TR
	CORN FLAKES									
456	GENERAL MILLS, TOTAL	1 1/3 CUP	30	3	112	2	TR	0.2	0.1	TR
457	KELLOGG'S	1 CUP	28	3	102	2	TR	0.1	TR	0.1
458	CORN POPS	1 CUP	31	3	118	1	TR	0.1	0.1	TR
459	CRISPIX	1 CUP	29	3	108	2	TR	0.1	0.1	0.1
460	COMPLETE WHEAT BRAN FLAKES	3/4 CUP	29	4	95	3	1	0.1	0.1	0.4
461	FROOT LOOPS	1 CUP	30	2	117	1	1	0.4	0.2	0.3
462	FROSTED FLAKES	3/4 CUP	31	3	119	1	TR	0.1	TR	0.1
	FROSTED MINI WHEATS									
463	REGULAR	1 CUP	51	5	173	5	1	0.2	0.1	0.6
464	BITE SIZE	1 CUP	55	5	187	5	1	0.2	0.2	0.6
465	GOLDEN GRAHAMS	3/4 CUP	30	3	116	2	1	0.2	0.3	0.2
466	HONEY FROSTED WHEATIES	3/4 CUP	30	3	110	2	TR	0.1	TR	TR
467	HONEY NUT CHEERIOS	1 CUP	30	2	115	3	1	0.2	0.5	0.2
468	HONEY NUT CLUSTERS	1 CUP	55	3	213	5	3	0.4	1.8	0.4
469	KIX	1 1/3 CUP	30	2	114	2	1	0.2	0.1	TR
470	LIFE	3/4 CUP	32	4	121	3	1	0.2	0.4	0.6
471	LUCKY CHARMS	1 CUP	30	2	116	2	1	0.2	0.4	0.2
472	NATURE VALLEY GRANOLA	3/4 CUP	55	4	248	6	10	1.3	6.5	1.9
	100% NATURAL CEREAL									
473	WITH OATS, HONEY, AND RAISINS	1/2 CUP	51	4	218	5	7	3.2	3.2	0.8
474	WITH RAISINS, LOW FAT	1/2 CUP	50	4	195	4	3	0.8	1.3	0.5
475	PRODUCT 19	1 CUP	30	3	110	3	TR	TR	0.2	0.2
476	PUFFED RICE	1 CUP	14	3	56	1	TR	TR	TR	TR
477	PUFFED WHEAT	1 CUP	12	3	44	2	TR	TR	TR	TR
	RAISIN BRAN									
478	GENERAL MILLS, TOTAL	1 CUP	55	9	178	4	1	0.2	0.2	0.2
479	KELLOGG'S	1 CUP	61	8	186	6	1	0.0	0.2	0.8
480	RAISIN NUT BRAN	1 CUP	55	5	209	5	4	0.7	1.9	0.5
481	REESE'S PEANUT BUTTER PUFFS	3/4 CUP	30	2	129	3	3	0.6	1.4	0.6
482	RICE KRISPIES	1 1/4 CUP	33	3	124	2	TR	0.1	0.1	0.2
483	RICE KRISPIES TREATS CEREAL	3/4 CUP	30	4	120	1	2	0.4	1.0	0.2
484	SHREDDED WHEAT	2 BISCUITS	46	4	156	5	1	0.1	NA	NA
485	SMACKS	3/4 CUP	27	3	103	2	1	0.3	0.1	0.2
486	SPECIAL K	1 CUP	31	3	115	6	TR	0.0	0.0	0.2
487	QUAKER TOASTED OATMEAL, HONEY NUT	1 CUP	49	3	191	5	3	0.5	1.2	0.7
488	TOTAL, WHOLE GRAIN	3/4 CUP	30	3	105	3	1	0.2	0.1	0.1
489	TRIX	1 CUP	30	2	122	1	2	0.4	0.9	0.3
490	WHEATIES	1 CUP	30	3	110	3	1	0.2	0.2	0.2
	BROWNIES, WITHOUT ICING COMMERCIALLY PREPARED									
491	REGULAR, LARGE (2 3/4″ SQ × 7/8″)	1 BROWNIE	56	14	227	3	9	2.4	5.0	1.3

Cholesterol (mg)	Carbo-hydrate (g)	Total Dietary Fiber (g)	Calcium (mg)	Iron (mg)	Potassium (mg)	Sodium (mg)	Vitamin A (IU)	Vitamin A (RE)	Thiamine (mg)	Ribo-flavin (mg)	Niacin (mg)	Ascorbic Acid (mg)	Food No.
0	24	1.5	42	4.5	44	210	750	225	0.38	0.43	5.0	15	453
0	27	0.4	4	1.8	60	210	750	225	0.37	0.43	5.0	15	454
0	27	0.2	33	4.5	52	181	0	0	0.38	0.43	5.0	15	455
0	26	0.8	237	18.0	34	203	1,250	375	1.50	1.70	20.1	60	456
0	24	0.8	1	8.7	25	298	700	210	0.36	0.39	4.7	14	457
0	28	0.4	2	1.9	23	123	775	233	0.40	0.43	5.2	16	458
0	25	0.6	3	1.8	35	240	750	225	0.38	0.44	5.0	15	459
0	23	4.6	14	8.1	175	226	1,208	363	0.38	0.44	5.0	15	460
0	26	0.6	3	4.2	32	141	703	211	0.39	0.42	5.0	14	461
0	28	0.6	1	4.5	20	200	750	225	0.37	0.43	5.0	15	462
0	42	5.5	18	14.3	170	2	0	0	0.36	0.41	5.0	0	463
0	45	5.9	0	15.4	186	2	0	0	0.33	0.39	4.7	0	464
0	26	0.9	14	4.5	53	275	750	225	0.38	0.43	5.0	15	465
0	26	1.5	8	4.5	56	211	750	225	0.38	0.43	5.0	15	466
0	24	1.6	20	4.5	85	259	750	225	0.38	0.43	5.0	15	467
0	43	4.2	72	4.5	171	239	0	0	0.37	0.42	5.0	9	468
0	26	0.8	44	8.1	41	263	1,250	375	0.38	0.43	5.0	15	469
0	25	2.0	98	9.0	79	174	12	1	0.40	0.45	5.3	0	470
0	25	1.2	32	4.5	54	203	750	225	0.38	0.43	5.0	15	471
0	36	3.5	41	1.7	183	89	0	0	0.17	0.06	0.6	0	472
1	36	3.7	39	1.7	214	11	4	1	0.14	0.09	0.8	TR	473
1	40	3.0	30	1.3	169	129	9	1	0.15	0.06	0.9	TR	474
0	25	1.0	3	18.0	41	216	750	225	1.50	1.71	20.0	60	475
0	13	0.2	1	4.4	16	TR	0	0	0.36	0.25	4.9	0	476
0	10	0.5	3	3.8	42	TR	0	0	0.31	0.22	4.2	0	477
0	43	5.0	238	18.0	287	240	1,250	375	1.50	1.70	20.0	0	478
0	47	8.2	35	5.0	437	354	832	250	0.43	0.49	5.6	0	479
0	41	5.1	74	4.5	218	246	0	0	0.37	0.42	5.0	0	480
0	23	0.4	21	4.5	62	177	750	225	0.38	0.43	5.0	15	481
0	29	0.4	3	2.0	42	354	825	248	0.43	0.46	5.5	17	482
0	26	0.3	2	1.8	19	190	750	225	0.39	0.42	5.0	15	483
0	38	5.3	20	1.4	196	3	0	NA	0.12	0.05	2.6	0	484
0	24	0.9	3	1.8	42	51	750	225	0.38	0.43	5.0	15	485
0	22	1.0	5	8.7	55	250	750	225	0.53	0.59	7.0	15	486
TR	39	3.3	27	4.5	185	166	500	150	0.37	0.42	5.0	6	487
0	24	2.6	258	18.0	97	199	1,250	375	1.50	1.70	20.1	60	488
0	26	0.7	32	4.5	18	197	750	225	0.38	0.43	5.0	15	489
0	24	2.1	55	8.1	104	222	750	225	0.38	0.43	5.0	15	490
10	36	1.2	16	1.3	83	175	39	3	0.14	0.12	1.0	0	491

Food No.	Food Description	Measure of Edible Portion	Weight (g)	Water (%)	Calories (kcal)	Protein (g)	Total Fat (g)	Fatty Acids Saturated (g)	Mono-unsaturated (g)	Poly-unsaturated (g)
GRAIN PRODUCTS (CONTINUED)										
492	FAT FREE, 2″ SQ	1 BROWNIE	28	12	89	1	TR	0.2	0.1	TR
493	PREPARED FROM DRY MIX, REDUCED CALORIE, 2″ SQ	1 BROWNIE	22	13	84	1	2	1.1	1.0	0.2
494	BUCKWHEAT FLOUR, WHOLE GROAT	1 CUP	120	11	402	15	4	0.8	1.1	1.1
495	BUCKWHEAT GROATS, ROASTED (KASHA), COOKED	1 CUP	168	76	155	6	1	0.2	0.3	0.3
	BULGUR									
496	UNCOOKED	1 CUP	140	9	479	17	2	0.3	0.2	0.8
497	COOKED	1 CUP	182	78	151	6	TR	0.1	0.1	0.2
	CAKES, PREPARED FROM DRY MIX									
498	ANGELFOOD (1/12 OF 10″ DIA)	1 PIECE	50	33	129	3	TR	TR	TR	0.1
499	YELLOW, LIGHT, WITH WATER, EGG WHITES, NO FROSTING (1/12 OF 9″ DIA)	1 PIECE	69	37	181	3	2	1.1	0.9	0.2
	CAKES, PREPARED FROM RECIPE									
500	CHOCOLATE, WITHOUT FROSTING (1/12 OF 9″ DIA)	1 PIECE	95	24	340	5	14	5.2	5.7	2.6
501	GINGERBREAD (1/9 OF 8″ SQUARE)	1 PIECE	74	28	263	3	12	3.1	5.3	3.1
502	PINEAPPLE UPSIDE DOWN (1/9 OF 8″ SQUARE)	1 PIECE	115	32	367	4	14	3.4	6.0	3.8
503	SHORTCAKE, BISCUIT TYPE (ABOUT 3″ DIA)	1 SHORTCAKE	65	28	225	4	9	2.5	3.9	2.4
504	SPONGE (1/12 OF 16-OZ CAKE)	1 PIECE	63	29	187	5	3	0.8	1.0	0.4
	WHITE									
505	WITH COCONUT FROSTING (1/12 OF 9″ DIA)	1 PIECE	112	21	399	5	12	4.4	4.1	2.4
506	WITHOUT FROSTING (1/12 OF 9″ DIA)	1 PIECE	74	23	264	4	9	2.4	3.9	2.3
	CAKES, COMMERCIALLY PREPARED									
507	ANGELFOOD (1/12 OF 12-OZ CAKE)	1 PIECE	28	33	72	2	TR	TR	TR	0.1
508	BOSTON CREAM (1/6 OF PIE)	1 PIECE	92	45	232	2	8	2.2	4.2	0.9
509	CHOCOLATE WITH CHOCOLATE FROSTING (1/8 OF 18-OZ CAKE)	1 PIECE	64	23	235	3	10	3.1	5.6	1.2
510	COFFEECAKE, CRUMB (1/9 OF 20-OZ CAKE)	1 PIECE	63	22	263	4	15	3.7	8.2	2.0
511	FRUITCAKE	1 PIECE	43	25	139	1	4	0.5	1.8	1.4
	POUND									
512	BUTTER (1/12 OF 12-OZ CAKE)	1 PIECE	28	25	109	2	6	3.2	1.7	0.3
513	FAT FREE (3 1/4″ × 2 3/4″ × 5/8″ SLICE)	1 SLICE	28	31	79	2	TR	0.1	TR	0.1
	SNACK CAKES									
514	CHOCOLATE, CREAM FILLED, WITH FROSTING	1 CUPCAKE	50	20	188	2	7	1.4	2.8	2.6
515	CHOCOLATE, WITH FROSTING, LOW FAT	1 CUPCAKE	43	23	131	2	2	0.5	0.8	0.2
516	SPONGE, CREAM FILLED	1 CAKE	43	20	155	1	5	1.1	1.7	1.4
517	SPONGE, INDIVIDUAL SHORTCAKE	1 SHORTCAKE	30	30	87	2	1	0.2	0.3	0.1
	YELLOW									
518	WITH CHOCOLATE FROSTING	1 PIECE	64	22	243	2	11	3.0	6.1	1.4
519	WITH VANILLA FROSTING	1 PIECE	64	22	239	2	9	1.5	3.9	3.3
520	CHEESECAKE (1/6 OF 17-OZ CAKE)	1 PIECE	80	46	257	4	18	7.9	6.9	1.3
521	CHEESE FLAVOR PUFFS OR TWISTS	1 OZ	28	2	157	2	10	1.9	5.7	1.3
522	CHEX MIX	1 OZ (ABOUT 2/3 CUP)	28	4	120	3	5	1.6	NA	NA
	COOKIES									
523	BUTTER, COMMERCIALLY PREPARED CHOCOLATE CHIP, MEDIUM (2 1/4″–2 1/2″ DIA)	1 COOKIE	5	5	23	TR	1	0.6	0.3	TR

Cholesterol (mg)	Carbo-hydrate (g)	Total Dietary Fiber (g)	Calcium (mg)	Iron (mg)	Potassium (mg)	Sodium (mg)	Vitamin A (IU)	Vitamin A (RE)	Thiamine (mg)	Ribo-flavin (mg)	Niacin (mg)	Ascorbic Acid (mg)	Food No.
0	22	1.0	17	0.7	89	90	1	TR	0.03	0.04	0.3	TR	492
0	16	0.8	3	0.3	69	21	0	0	0.02	0.03	0.2	0	493
0	85	12.0	49	4.9	692	13	0	0	0.50	0.23	7.4	0	494
0	33	4.5	12	1.3	148	7	0	0	0.07	0.07	1.6	0	495
0	106	25.6	49	3.4	574	24	0	0	0.32	0.16	7.2	0	496
0	34	8.2	18	1.7	124	9	0	0	0.10	0.05	1.8	0	497
0	29	0.1	42	0.1	68	255	0	0	0.05	0.10	0.1	0	498
0	37	0.6	69	0.6	41	279	6	1	0.06	0.12	0.6	0	499
55	51	1.5	57	1.5	133	299	133	38	0.13	0.20	1.1	TR	500
24	36	0.7	63	2.1	325	242	36	10	0.14	0.12	1.3	TR	501
25	58	0.9	138	1.7	129	367	291	75	0.18	0.18	1.4	1	502
2	32	0.8	133	1.7	69	329	47	12	0.20	0.18	1.7	TR	503
107	36	0.4	26	1.0	89	144	163	49	0.10	0.19	0.8	0	504
1	71	1.1	101	1.3	111	318	43	12	0.14	0.21	1.2	TR	505
1	42	0.6	96	1.1	70	242	41	12	0.14	0.18	1.1	TR	506
0	16	0.4	39	0.1	26	210	0	0	0.03	0.14	0.2	0	507
34	39	1.3	21	0.3	36	132	74	21	0.38	0.25	0.2	TR	508
27	35	1.8	28	1.4	128	214	54	16	0.02	0.09	0.4	TR	509
20	29	1.3	34	1.2	77	221	70	21	0.13	0.14	1.1	TR	510
2	26	1.6	14	0.9	66	116	9	2	0.02	0.04	0.3	TR	511
62	14	0.1	10	0.4	33	111	170	44	0.04	0.06	0.4	0	512
0	17	0.3	12	0.6	31	95	27	8	0.04	0.08	0.2	0	513
9	30	0.4	37	1.7	61	213	9	3	0.11	0.15	1.2	0	514
0	29	1.8	15	0.7	96	178	0	0	0.02	0.06	0.3	0	515
7	27	0.2	19	0.5	37	155	7	2	0.07	0.06	0.5	TR	516
31	18	0.2	21	0.8	30	73	46	14	0.07	0.08	0.6	0	517
35	35	1.2	24	1.3	114	216	70	21	0.08	0.10	0.8	0	518
35	38	0.2	40	0.7	34	220	40	12	0.06	0.04	0.3	0	519
44	20	0.3	41	0.5	72	166	438	117	0.02	0.15	0.2	TR	520
1	15	0.3	16	0.7	47	298	75	10	0.07	0.10	0.9	TR	521
0	18	1.6	10	7.0	76	288	41	4	0.44	0.14	4.8	13	522
6	3	TR	1	0.1	6	18	34	8	0.02	0.02	0.2	0	523

GRAIN PRODUCTS (CONTINUED)

Food No.	Food Description	Measure of Edible Portion	Weight (g)	Water (%)	Calories (kcal)	Protein (g)	Total Fat (g)	Fatty Acids Saturated (g)	Fatty Acids Mono-unsaturated (g)	Fatty Acids Poly-unsaturated (g)
	COMMERCIALLY PREPARED									
524	REGULAR	1 COOKIE	10	4	48	1	2	0.7	1.2	0.2
525	REDUCED FAT	1 COOKIE	10	4	45	1	2	0.4	0.6	0.5
526	FROM REFRIGERATED DOUGH (SPOONED FROM ROLL)	1 COOKIE	26	3	128	1	6	2.0	2.9	0.6
527	PREPARED FROM RECIPE, WITH MARGARINE	1 COOKIE	16	6	78	1	5	1.3	1.7	1.3
528	DEVIL'S FOOD, COMMERCIALLY PREPARED, FAT FREE	1 COOKIE	16	18	49	1	TR	0.1	TR	TR
529	FIG BAR	1 COOKIE	16	17	56	1	1	0.2	0.5	0.4
	MOLASSES									
530	MEDIUM	1 COOKIE	15	6	65	1	2	0.5	1.1	0.3
531	LARGE (3 1/2"–4" DIA)	1 COOKIE	32	6	138	2	4	1.0	2.3	0.6
	OATMEAL									
	COMMERCIALLY PREPARED, WITH OR WITHOUT RAISINS									
532	REGULAR, LARGE	1 COOKIE	25	6	113	2	5	1.1	2.5	0.6
533	SOFT TYPE	1 COOKIE	15	11	61	1	2	0.5	1.2	0.3
534	FAT FREE	1 COOKIE	11	13	36	1	TR	TR	TR	0.1
535	PREPARED FROM RECIPE, WITH RAISINS (2 5/8" DIA)	1 COOKIE	15	6	65	1	2	0.5	1.0	0.8
	PEANUT BUTTER									
536	COMMERCIALLY PREPARED	1 COOKIE	15	6	72	1	4	0.7	1.9	0.8
537	PREPARED FROM RECIPE, WITH MARGARINE (3" DIA)	1 COOKIE	20	6	95	2	5	0.9	2.2	1.4
	SANDWICH TYPE, WITH CREAM FILLING									
538	CHOCOLATE COOKIE	1 COOKIE	10	2	47	TR	2	0.4	0.9	0.7
	VANILLA COOKIE									
539	OVAL	1 COOKIE	15	2	72	1	3	0.4	1.3	1.1
540	ROUND	1 COOKIE	10	2	48	TR	2	0.3	0.8	0.8
	SHORTBREAD, COMMERCIALLY PREPARED									
541	PLAIN (1 5/8" SQ)	1 COOKIE	8	4	40	TR	2	0.5	1.1	0.3
	PECAN									
542	REGULAR (2" DIA)	1 COOKIE	14	3	76	1	5	1.1	2.6	0.6
543	REDUCED FAT	1 COOKIE	16	5	73	1	3	0.6	1.6	0.4
	SUGAR									
544	COMMERCIALLY PREPARED	1 COOKIE	15	5	72	1	3	0.8	1.8	0.4
545	FROM REFRIGERATED DOUGH	1 COOKIE	15	5	73	1	3	0.9	2.0	0.4
546	PREPARED FROM RECIPE, WITH MARGARINE (3" DIA)	1 COOKIE	14	9	66	1	3	0.7	1.4	1.0
547	VANILLA WAFER, LOWER FAT, MEDIUM SIZE	1 COOKIE	4	5	18	TR	1	0.2	0.3	0.2
	CORN CHIPS									
548	PLAIN	1 OZ	28	1	153	2	9	1.3	2.7	4.7
549	BARBECUE FLAVOR	1 OZ	28	1	148	2	9	1.3	2.7	4.6
	CORNBREAD									
550	PREPARED FROM MIX, PIECE 3 3/4" × 2 1/2" × 3/4"	1 PIECE	60	32	188	4	6	1.6	3.1	0.7
551	PREPARED FROM RECIPE, WITH 2% MILK, PIECE 2 1/2" SQ × 1 1/2"	1 PIECE	65	39	173	4	5	1.0	1.2	2.1
	CORNMEAL, YELLOW, DRY FORM									
552	WHOLE GRAIN	1 CUP	122	10	442	10	4	0.6	1.2	2.0

Cholesterol (mg)	Carbo-hydrate (g)	Total Dietary Fiber (g)	Calcium (mg)	Iron (mg)	Potassium (mg)	Sodium (mg)	Vitamin A (IU)	Vitamin A (RE)	Thiamine (mg)	Ribo-flavin (mg)	Niacin (mg)	Ascorbic Acid (mg)	Food No.
0	7	0.3	3	0.3	14	32	TR	0	0.02	0.03	0.3	0	524
0	7	0.4	2	0.3	12	38	TR	0	0.03	0.03	0.3	0	525
7	18	0.4	7	0.7	52	60	15	4	0.04	0.05	0.5	0	526
5	9	0.4	6	0.4	36	58	102	26	0.03	0.03	0.2	TR	527
0	12	0.3	5	0.4	18	28	TR	NA	0.01	0.03	0.2	TR	528
0	11	0.7	10	0.5	33	56	5	1	0.03	0.03	0.3	TR	529
0	11	0.1	11	1.0	52	69	0	0	0.05	0.04	0.5	0	530
0	24	0.3	24	2.1	111	147	0	0	0.11	0.08	1.0	0	531
0	17	0.7	9	0.6	36	96	5	1	0.07	0.06	0.6	TR	532
1	10	0.4	14	0.4	20	52	5	1	0.03	0.03	0.3	TR	533
0	9	0.8	4	0.2	23	33	0	0	0.02	0.03	0.1	0	534
5	10	0.5	15	0.4	36	81	96	25	0.04	0.02	0.2	TR	535
TR	9	0.3	5	0.4	25	62	1	TR	0.03	0.03	0.6	0	536
6	12	0.4	8	0.4	46	104	120	31	0.04	0.04	0.7	TR	537
0	7	0.3	3	0.4	18	60	TR	0	0.01	0.02	0.2	0	538
0	11	0.2	4	0.3	14	52	0	0	0.04	0.04	0.4	0	539
0	7	0.2	3	0.2	9	35	0	0	0.03	0.02	0.3	0	540
2	5	0.1	3	0.2	8	36	7	1	0.03	0.03	0.3	0	541
5	8	0.3	4	0.3	10	39	TR	TR	0.04	0.03	0.3	0	542
0	11	0.2	8	0.5	15	55	1	TR	0.05	0.03	0.4	TR	543
8	10	0.1	3	0.3	9	54	14	4	0.03	0.03	0.4	TR	544
5	10	0.1	14	0.3	24	70	6	2	0.03	0.02	0.4	0	545
4	8	0.2	10	0.3	11	69	135	35	0.04	0.04	0.3	TR	546
2	3	0.1	2	0.1	4	12	1	TR	0.01	0.01	0.1	0	547
0	16	1.4	36	0.4	40	179	27	3	0.01	0.04	0.3	0	548
0	16	1.5	37	0.4	67	216	173	17	0.02	0.06	0.5	TR	549
37	29	1.4	44	1.1	77	467	123	26	0.15	0.16	1.2	TR	550
26	28	1.9	162	1.6	96	428	180	35	0.19	0.19	1.5	TR	551
0	94	8.9	7	4.2	350	43	572	57	0.47	0.25	4.4	0	552

Food No.	Food Description	Measure of Edible Portion	Weight (g)	Water (%)	Calories (kcal)	Protein (g)	Total Fat (g)	Fatty Acids Satu- rated (g)	Mono- unsatu- rated (g)	Poly- unsatu- rated (g)
GRAIN PRODUCTS (CONTINUED)										
553	DEGERMED, ENRICHED	1 CUP	138	12	505	12	2	0.3	0.6	1.0
554	SELF-RISING, DEGERMED, ENRICHED	1 CUP	138	10	490	12	2	0.3	0.6	1.0
555	CORNSTARCH	1 TBSP	8	8	30	TR	TR	TR	TR	TR
	COUSCOUS									
556	UNCOOKED	1 CUP	173	9	650	22	1	0.2	0.2	0.4
557	COOKED	1 CUP	157	73	176	6	TR	TR	TR	0.1
	CRACKERS									
558	CHEESE, 1″ SQ	10 CRACKERS	10	3	50	1	3	0.9	1.2	0.2
	GRAHAM, PLAIN									
559	2 1/2″ SQ	2 SQUARES	14	4	59	1	1	0.2	0.6	0.5
560	CRUSHED	1 CUP	84	4	355	6	8	1.3	3.4	3.2
561	MELBA TOAST, PLAIN	4 PIECES	20	5	78	2	1	0.1	0.2	0.3
562	RYE WAFER, WHOLE GRAIN, PLAIN	1 WAFER	11	5	37	1	TR	TR	TR	TR
	SALTINE									
563	SQUARE	4 CRACKERS	12	4	52	1	1	0.4	0.8	0.2
564	OYSTER TYPE	1 CUP	45	4	195	4	5	1.3	2.9	0.8
	SANDWICH TYPE									
565	WHEAT WITH CHEESE	1 SANDWICH	7	4	33	1	1	0.4	0.8	0.2
566	CHEESE WITH PEANUT BUTTER	1 SANDWICH	7	4	34	1	2	0.4	0.8	0.3
	STANDARD SNACK TYPE									
567	BITE SIZE	1 CUP	62	4	311	5	16	2.3	6.6	5.9
568	ROUND	4 CRACKERS	12	4	60	1	3	0.5	1.3	1.1
569	WHEAT, THIN SQUARE	4 CRACKERS	8	3	38	1	2	0.4	0.9	0.2
570	WHOLE WHEAT	4 CRACKERS	16	3	71	1	3	0.5	0.9	1.1
571	CROISSANT, BUTTER	1 CROISSANT	57	23	231	5	12	6.6	3.1	0.6
572	CROUTONS, SEASONED	1 CUP	40	4	186	4	7	2.1	3.8	0.9
	DANISH PASTRY, ENRICHED									
573	CHEESE FILLED	1 DANISH	71	31	266	6	16	4.8	8.0	1.8
574	FRUIT FILLED	1 DANISH	71	27	263	4	13	3.5	7.1	1.7
	DOUGHNUTS									
575	CAKE TYPE	1 HOLE	14	21	59	1	3	0.5	1.3	1.1
576		1 MEDIUM	47	21	198	2	11	1.7	4.4	3.7
577	YEAST LEAVENED, GLAZED	1 HOLE	13	25	52	1	3	0.8	1.7	0.4
578		1 MEDIUM	60	25	242	4	14	3.5	7.7	1.7
579	ECLAIR, PREPARED FROM RECIPE, 5″ × 2″ × 1 3/4″	1 ECLAIR	100	52	262	6	16	4.1	6.5	3.9
	ENGLISH MUFFIN, PLAIN, ENRICHED									
580	UNTOASTED	1 MUFFIN	57	42	134	4	1	0.1	0.2	0.5
581	TOASTED	1 MUFFIN	52	37	133	4	1	0.1	0.2	0.5
	FRENCH TOAST									
582	PREPARED FROM RECIPE, WITH 2% MILK, FRIED IN MARGARINE	1 SLICE	65	55	149	5	7	1.8	2.9	1.7
583	FROZEN, READY TO HEAT	1 SLICE	59	53	126	4	4	0.9	1.2	0.7
	GRANOLA BAR									
584	HARD, PLAIN	1 BAR	28	4	134	3	6	0.7	1.2	3.4
	SOFT, UNCOATED									
585	CHOCOLATE CHIP	1 BAR	28	5	119	2	5	2.9	1.0	0.6
586	RAISIN	1 BAR	28	6	127	2	5	2.7	0.8	0.9
587	SOFT, CHOCOLATE-COATED, PEANUT BUTTER	1 BAR	28	3	144	3	9	4.8	1.9	0.5
588	MACARONI (ELBOWS), ENRICHED, COOKED	1 CUP	140	66	197	7	1	0.1	0.1	0.4

Cholesterol (mg)	Carbo-hydrate (g)	Total Dietary Fiber (g)	Calcium (mg)	Iron (mg)	Potassium (mg)	Sodium (mg)	Vitamin A (IU)	Vitamin A (RE)	Thiamine (mg)	Ribo-flavin (mg)	Niacin (mg)	Ascorbic Acid (mg)	Food No.
0	107	10.2	7	5.7	224	4	570	57	0.99	0.56	6.9	0	553
0	103	9.8	483	6.5	235	1,860	570	57	0.94	0.53	6.3	0	554
0	7	0.1	TR	TR	TR	1	0	0	0.00	0.00	0.0	0	555
0	134	8.7	42	1.9	287	17	0	0	0.28	0.13	6.0	0	556
0	36	2.2	13	0.6	91	8	0	0	0.10	0.04	1.5	0	557
1	6	0.2	15	0.5	15	100	16	3	0.06	0.04	0.5	0	558
0	11	0.4	3	0.5	19	85	0	0	0.03	0.04	0.6	0	559
0	65	2.4	20	3.1	113	508	0	0	0.19	0.26	3.5	0	560
0	15	1.3	19	0.7	40	166	0	0	0.08	0.05	0.8	0	561
0	9	2.5	4	0.7	54	87	1	0	0.05	0.03	0.2	TR	562
0	9	0.4	14	0.6	15	156	0	0	0.07	0.06	0.6	0	563
0	32	1.4	54	2.4	58	586	0	0	0.25	0.21	2.4	0	564
TR	4	0.1	18	0.2	30	98	5	1	0.03	0.05	0.3	TR	565
TR	4	0.2	6	0.2	17	69	22	2	0.03	0.02	0.5	TR	566
0	38	1.0	74	2.2	82	525	0	0	0.25	0.21	2.5	0	567
0	7	0.2	14	0.4	16	102	0	0	0.05	0.04	0.5	0	568
0	5	0.4	4	0.4	15	64	0	0	0.04	0.03	0.4	0	569
0	11	1.7	8	0.5	48	105	0	0	0.03	0.02	0.7	0	570
38	26	1.5	21	1.2	67	424	424	106	0.22	0.14	1.2	TR	571
3	25	2.0	38	1.1	72	495	16	4	0.20	0.17	1.9	0	572
11	26	0.7	25	1.1	70	320	104	32	0.13	0.18	1.4	TR	573
81	34	1.3	33	1.3	59	251	53	16	0.19	0.16	1.4	3	574
5	7	0.2	6	0.3	18	76	8	2	0.03	0.03	0.3	TR	575
17	23	0.7	21	0.9	60	257	27	8	0.10	0.11	0.9	TR	576
1	6	0.2	6	0.3	14	44	2	1	0.05	0.03	0.4	TR	577
4	27	0.7	26	1.2	65	205	8	2	0.22	0.13	1.7	TR	578
127	24	0.6	63	1.2	117	337	718	191	0.12	0.27	0.8	TR	579
0	26	1.5	99	1.4	75	264	0	0	0.25	0.16	2.2	0	580
0	26	1.5	98	1.4	74	262	0	0	0.20	0.14	2.0	TR	581
75	16	0.7	65	1.1	87	311	315	86	0.13	0.21	1.1	TR	582
48	19	0.7	63	1.3	79	292	110	32	0.16	0.22	1.6	TR	583
0	18	1.5	17	0.8	95	83	43	4	0.07	0.03	0.4	TR	584
TR	20	1.4	26	0.7	96	77	12	1	0.06	0.04	0.3	0	585
TR	19	1.2	29	0.7	103	80	0	0	0.07	0.05	0.3	0	586
3	15	0.8	31	0.4	96	55	37	10	0.03	0.06	0.9	TR	587
0	40	1.8	10	2.0	43	1	0	0	0.29	0.14	2.3	0	588

Food No.	Food Description	Measure of Edible Portion	Weight (g)	Water (%)	Calories (kcal)	Protein (g)	Total Fat (g)	Fatty Acids Satu-rated (g)	Fatty Acids Mono-unsatu-rated (g)	Fatty Acids Poly-unsatu-rated (g)
GRAIN PRODUCTS (CONTINUED)										
589	MATZO, PLAIN	1 MATZO	28	4	112	3	TR	0.1	TR	0.2
	MUFFINS									
	BLUEBERRY									
590	COMMERCIALLY PREPARED (2 3/4″ DIA × 2″)	1 MUFFIN	57	38	158	3	4	0.8	1.1	1.4
591	PREPARED FROM MIX (2 1/4″ DIA × 1 3/4″)	1 MUFFIN	50	36	150	3	4	0.7	1.8	1.5
592	PREPARED FROM RECIPE, WITH 2% MILK	1 MUFFIN	57	40	162	4	6	1.2	1.5	3.1
593	BRAN WITH RAISINS, TOASTER TYPE, TOASTED	1 MUFFIN	34	27	106	2	3	0.5	0.8	1.7
	CORN									
594	COMMERCIALLY PREPARED (2 1/2″ DIA × 2 1/4″)	1 MUFFIN	57	33	174	3	5	0.8	1.2	1.8
595	PREPARED FROM MIX (2 1/4″ DIA × 1 1/2″)	1 MUFFIN	50	31	161	4	5	1.4	2.6	0.6
596	OAT BRAN, COMMERCIALLY PREPARED (2 1/2″ DIA × 2 1/4″)	1 MUFFIN	57	35	154	4	4	0.6	1.0	2.4
597	NOODLES, CHOW MEIN, CANNED	1 CUP	45	1	237	4	14	2.0	3.5	7.8
	NOODLES (EGG NOODLES), ENRICHED, COOKED									
598	REGULAR	1 CUP	160	69	213	8	2	0.5	0.7	0.7
599	SPINACH	1 CUP	160	69	211	8	3	0.6	0.8	0.6
600	NUTRI GRAIN CEREAL BAR, FRUIT FILLED	1 BAR	37	15	136	2	3	0.6	1.9	0.3
	OAT BRAN									
601	UNCOOKED	1 CUP	94	7	231	16	7	1.2	2.2	2.6
602	COOKED	1 CUP	219	84	88	7	2	0.4	0.6	0.7
603	ORIENTAL SNACK MIX	1 OZ (ABOUT 1/4 CUP)	28	3	156	5	7	1.1	2.8	3.0
	PANCAKES, PLAIN (4″ DIA)									
604	FROZEN, READY TO HEAT	1 PANCAKE	36	45	82	2	1	0.3	0.4	0.3
605	PREPARED FROM COMPLETE MIX	1 PANCAKE	38	53	74	2	1	0.2	0.3	0.3
606	PREPARED FROM INCOMPLETE MIX, WITH 2% MILK, EGG, AND OIL	1 PANCAKE	38	53	83	3	3	0.8	0.8	1.1
	PIE CRUST, BAKED									
	STANDARD TYPE									
607	FROM RECIPE	1 PIE SHELL	180	10	949	12	62	15.5	27.3	16.4
608	FROM FROZEN	1 PIE SHELL	126	11	648	6	41	13.3	19.8	5.1
609	GRAHAM CRACKER	1 PIE SHELL	239	4	1,181	10	60	12.4	27.2	16.5
	PIES									
	COMMERCIALLY PREPARED (1/6 OF 8″ DIA)									
610	APPLE	1 PIECE	117	52	277	2	13	4.4	5.1	2.6
611	BLUEBERRY	1 PIECE	117	53	271	2	12	2.0	5.0	4.1
612	CHERRY	1 PIECE	117	46	304	2	13	3.0	6.8	2.4
613	CHOCOLATE CREAM	1 PIECE	113	44	344	3	22	5.6	12.6	2.7
614	COCONUT CUSTARD	1 PIECE	104	49	270	6	14	6.1	5.7	1.2
615	LEMON MERINGUE	1 PIECE	113	42	303	2	10	2.0	3.0	4.1
616	PECAN	1 PIECE	113	19	452	5	21	4.0	12.1	3.6
617	PUMPKIN	1 PIECE	109	58	229	4	10	1.9	4.4	3.4
	PREPARED FROM RECIPE (1/8 OF 9″ DIA)									
618	APPLE	1 PIECE	155	47	411	4	19	4.7	8.4	5.2
619	BLUEBERRY	1 PIECE	147	51	360	4	17	4.3	7.5	4.5
620	CHERRY	1 PIECE	180	46	486	5	22	5.4	9.6	5.8
621	LEMON MERINGUE	1 PIECE	127	43	362	5	16	4.0	7.1	4.2

Cholesterol (mg)	Carbo-hydrate (g)	Total Dietary Fiber (g)	Calcium (mg)	Iron (mg)	Potassium (mg)	Sodium (mg)	Vitamin A (IU)	Vitamin A (RE)	Thiamine (mg)	Ribo-flavin (mg)	Niacin (mg)	Ascorbic Acid (mg)	Food No.
0	24	0.9	4	0.9	32	1	0	0	0.11	0.08	1.1	0	589
17	27	1.5	32	0.9	70	255	19	5	0.08	0.07	0.6	1	590
23	24	0.6	13	0.6	39	219	39	11	0.07	0.16	1.1	1	591
21	23	1.1	108	1.3	70	251	80	22	0.16	0.16	1.3	1	592
3	19	2.8	13	1.0	60	179	58	16	0.07	0.10	0.8	0	593
15	29	1.9	42	1.6	39	297	119	21	0.16	0.19	1.2	0	594
31	25	1.2	38	1.0	66	398	105	23	0.12	0.14	1.1	TR	595
0	28	2.6	36	2.4	289	224	0	0	0.15	0.05	0.2	0	596
0	26	1.8	9	2.1	54	198	38	4	0.26	0.19	2.7	0	597
53	40	1.8	19	2.5	45	11	32	10	0.30	0.13	2.4	0	598
53	39	3.7	30	1.7	59	19	165	22	0.39	0.20	2.4	0	599
0	27	0.8	15	1.8	73	110	750	227	0.37	0.41	5.0	0	600
0	62	14.5	55	5.1	532	4	0	0	1.10	0.21	0.9	0	601
0	25	5.7	22	1.9	201	2	0	0	0.35	0.07	0.3	0	602
0	15	3.7	15	0.7	93	117	1	0	0.09	0.04	0.9	TR	603
3	16	0.6	22	1.3	26	183	36	10	0.14	0.17	1.4	TR	604
5	14	0.5	48	0.6	67	239	12	3	0.08	0.08	0.7	TR	605
27	11	0.7	82	0.5	76	192	95	27	0.08	0.12	0.5	TR	606
0	86	3.0	18	5.2	121	976	0	0	0.70	0.50	6.0	0	607
0	62	1.3	26	2.8	139	815	0	0	0.35	0.48	3.1	0	608
0	156	3.6	50	5.2	210	1,365	1,876	483	0.25	0.42	5.1	0	609
0	40	1.9	13	0.5	76	311	145	35	0.03	0.03	0.3	4	610
0	41	1.2	9	0.4	59	380	164	40	0.01	0.04	0.4	3	611
0	47	0.9	14	0.6	95	288	329	63	0.03	0.03	0.2	1	612
6	38	2.3	41	1.2	144	154	0	0	0.04	0.12	0.8	0	613
36	31	1.9	84	0.8	182	348	114	28	0.09	0.15	0.4	1	614
51	53	1.4	63	0.7	101	165	198	59	0.07	0.24	0.7	4	615
36	65	4.0	19	1.2	84	479	198	53	0.10	0.14	0.3	1	616
22	30	2.9	65	0.9	168	307	3,743	405	0.06	0.17	0.2	1	617
0	58	3.6	11	1.7	122	327	90	19	0.23	0.17	1.9	3	618
0	49	3.6	10	1.8	74	272	62	6	0.22	0.19	1.8	1	619
0	69	3.5	18	3.3	139	344	736	86	0.27	0.23	2.3	2	620
67	50	0.7	15	1.3	83	307	203	56	0.15	0.20	1.2	4	621

Food No.	Food Description	Measure of Edible Portion	Weight (g)	Water (%)	Calories (kcal)	Protein (g)	Total Fat (g)	Fatty Acids Satu-rated (g)	Mono-unsatu-rated (g)	Poly-unsatu-rated (g)
GRAIN PRODUCTS (CONTINUED)										
622	PECAN	1 PIECE	122	20	503	6	27	4.9	13.6	7.0
623	PUMPKIN	1 PIECE	155	59	316	7	14	4.9	5.7	2.8
624	FRIED, CHERRY	1 PIE	128	38	404	4	21	3.1	9.5	6.9
	POPCORN									
625	AIR POPPED, UNSALTED	1 CUP	8	4	31	1	TR	TR	0.1	0.2
626	OIL POPPED, SALTED	1 CUP	11	3	55	1	3	0.5	0.9	1.5
	CARAMEL-COATED									
627	WITH PEANUTS	1 CUP	42	3	168	3	3	0.4	1.1	1.4
628	WITHOUT PEANUTS	1 CUP	35	3	152	1	5	1.3	1.0	1.6
629	CHEESE FLAVOR	1 CUP	11	3	58	1	4	0.7	1.1	1.7
630	POPCORN CAKE	1 CAKE	10	5	38	1	TR	TR	0.1	0.1
	PRETZELS, MADE WITH ENRICHED FLOUR									
631	STICK, 2 1/4″ LONG	10 PRETZELS	3	3	11	TR	TR	TR	TR	TR
632	TWISTED, REGULAR	10 PRETZELS	60	3	229	5	2	0.5	0.8	0.7
633	TWISTED, DUTCH, 2 3/4″ × 2 5/8″	1 PRETZEL	16	3	61	1	1	0.1	0.2	0.2
	RICE									
634	BROWN, LONG GRAIN, COOKED	1 CUP	195	73	216	5	2	0.4	0.6	0.6
	WHITE, LONG GRAIN, ENRICHED									
	REGULAR									
635	RAW	1 CUP	185	12	675	13	1	0.3	0.4	0.3
636	COOKED	1 CUP	158	68	205	4	TR	0.1	0.1	0.1
637	INSTANT, PREPARED	1 CUP	165	76	162	3	TR	0.1	0.1	0.1
	PARBOILED									
638	RAW	1 CUP	185	10	686	13	1	0.3	0.3	0.3
639	COOKED	1 CUP	175	72	200	4	TR	0.1	0.1	0.1
640	WILD, COOKED	1 CUP	164	74	166	7	1	0.1	0.1	0.3
641	RICE CAKE, BROWN RICE, PLAIN	1 CAKE	9	6	35	1	TR	0.1	0.1	0.1
642	RICE KRISPIES TREAT SQUARES	1 BAR	22	6	91	1	2	0.3	0.6	1.1
	ROLLS									
643	DINNER	1 ROLL	28	32	84	2	2	0.5	1.0	0.3
644	HAMBURGER OR HOTDOG	1 ROLL	43	34	123	4	2	0.5	0.4	1.1
645	HARD, KAISER	1 ROLL	57	31	167	6	2	0.3	0.6	1.0
	SPAGHETTI, COOKED									
646	ENRICHED	1 CUP	140	66	197	7	1	0.1	0.1	0.4
647	WHOLE WHEAT	1 CUP	140	67	174	7	1	0.1	0.1	0.3
	SWEET ROLLS, CINNAMON									
648	COMMERCIAL, WITH RAISINS	1 ROLL	60	25	223	4	10	1.8	2.9	4.5
649	REFRIGERATED DOUGH, BAKED, WITH FROSTING	1 ROLL	30	23	109	2	4	1.0	2.2	0.5
650	TACO SHELL, BAKED	1 MEDIUM	13	6	62	1	3	0.4	1.2	1.1
651	TAPIOCA, PEARL, DRY	1 CUP	152	11	544	TR	TR	TR	TR	TR
	TOASTER PASTRIES									
652	BROWN SUGAR CINNAMON	1 PASTRY	50	11	206	3	7	1.8	4.0	0.9
653	CHOCOLATE WITH FROSTING	1 PASTRY	52	13	201	3	5	1.0	2.7	1.1
654	FRUIT FILLED	1 PASTRY	52	12	204	2	5	0.8	2.2	2.0
655	LOW FAT	1 PASTRY	52	12	193	2	3	0.7	1.7	0.5
	TORTILLA CHIPS									
	PLAIN									
656	REGULAR	1 OZ	28	2	142	2	7	1.4	4.4	1.0
657	LOW FAT, BAKED	10 CHIPS	14	2	54	2	1	0.1	0.2	0.4
	NACHO FLAVOR									
658	REGULAR	1 OZ	28	2	141	2	7	1.4	4.3	1.0
659	LIGHT, REDUCED FAT	1 OZ	28	1	126	2	4	0.8	2.5	0.6

Cholesterol (mg)	Carbo-hydrate (g)	Total Dietary Fiber (g)	Calcium (mg)	Iron (mg)	Potassium (mg)	Sodium (mg)	Vitamin A (IU)	(RE)	Thiamine (mg)	Ribo-flavin (mg)	Niacin (mg)	Ascorbic Acid (mg)	Food No.
106	64	2.2	39	1.8	162	320	410	109	0.23	0.22	1.0	TR	622
65	41	2.9	146	2.0	288	349	11,833	1,212	0.14	0.31	1.2	3	623
0	55	3.3	28	1.6	83	479	220	22	0.18	0.14	1.8	2	624
0	6	1.2	1	0.2	24	TR	16	2	0.02	0.02	0.2	0	625
0	6	1.1	1	0.3	25	97	17	2	0.01	0.01	0.2	TR	626
0	34	1.6	28	1.6	149	124	27	3	0.02	0.05	0.8	0	627
2	28	1.8	15	0.6	38	73	18	4	0.02	0.02	0.8	0	628
1	6	1.1	12	0.2	29	98	27	5	0.01	0.03	0.2	TR	629
0	8	0.3	1	0.2	33	29	7	1	0.01	0.02	0.6	0	630
0	2	0.1	1	0.1	4	51	0	0	0.01	0.02	0.2	0	631
0	48	1.9	22	2.6	88	1,029	0	0	0.28	0.37	3.2	0	632
0	13	0.5	6	0.7	23	274	0	0	0.07	0.10	0.8	0	633
0	45	3.5	20	0.8	84	10	0	0	0.19	0.05	3.0	0	634
0	148	2.4	52	8.0	213	9	0	0	1.07	0.09	7.8	0	635
0	45	0.6	16	1.9	55	2	0	0	0.26	0.02	2.3	0	636
0	35	1.0	13	1.0	7	5	0	0	0.12	0.08	1.5	0	637
0	151	3.1	111	6.6	222	9	0	0	1.10	0.13	6.7	0	638
0	43	0.7	33	2.0	65	5	0	0	0.44	0.03	2.5	0	639
0	35	3.0	5	1.0	166	5	0	0	0.09	0.14	2.1	0	640
0	7	0.4	1	0.1	26	29	4	TR	0.01	0.01	0.7	0	641
0	18	0.1	1	0.5	9	77	200	60	0.15	0.18	2.0	0	642
TR	14	0.8	33	0.9	37	146	0	0	0.14	0.09	1.1	TR	643
0	22	1.2	60	1.4	61	241	0	0	0.21	0.13	1.7	TR	644
0	30	1.3	54	1.9	62	310	0	0	0.27	0.19	2.4	0	645
0	40	2.4	10	2.0	43	1	0	0	0.29	0.14	2.3	0	646
0	37	6.3	21	1.5	62	4	0	0	0.15	0.06	1.0	0	647
40	31	1.4	43	1.0	67	230	129	38	0.19	0.16	1.4	1	648
0	17	0.6	10	0.8	19	250	1	0	0.12	0.07	1.1	TR	649
0	8	1.0	21	0.3	24	49	0	0	0.03	0.01	0.2	0	650
0	135	1.4	30	2.4	17	2	0	0	0.01	0.00	0.0	0	651
0	34	0.5	17	2.0	57	212	493	112	0.19	0.29	2.3	TR	652
0	37	0.6	20	1.8	82	203	500	NA	0.16	0.16	2.0	0	653
0	37	1.1	14	1.8	58	218	501	2	0.15	0.19	2.0	TR	654
0	40	0.8	23	1.8	34	131	494	49	0.15	0.29	2.0	2	655
0	18	1.8	44	0.4	56	150	56	6	0.02	0.05	0.4	0	656
0	11	0.7	22	0.2	37	57	52	6	0.03	0.04	0.1	TR	657
1	18	1.5	42	0.4	61	201	105	12	0.04	0.05	0.4	1	658
1	20	1.4	45	0.5	77	284	108	12	0.06	0.08	0.1	TR	659

Food No.	Food Description	Measure of Edible Portion	Weight (g)	Water (%)	Calories (kcal)	Protein (g)	Total Fat (g)	Fatty Acids Satu-rated (g)	Fatty Acids Mono-unsatu-rated (g)	Fatty Acids Poly-unsatu-rated (g)
GRAIN PRODUCTS (CONTINUED)										
	TORTILLAS, READY TO COOK (ABOUT 6″ DIA)									
660	CORN	1 TORTILLA	26	44	58	1	1	0.1	0.2	0.3
661	FLOUR	1 TORTILLA	32	27	104	3	2	0.6	1.2	0.3
	WAFFLES, PLAIN									
662	PREPARED FROM RECIPE, 7″ DIA	1 WAFFLE	75	42	218	6	11	2.1	2.6	5.1
663	FROZEN, TOASTED, 4″ DIA	1 WAFFLE	33	42	87	2	3	0.5	1.1	0.9
664	LOW FAT, 4″ DIA	1 WAFFLE	35	43	83	2	1	0.3	0.4	0.4
	WHEAT FLOURS									
	ALL PURPOSE, ENRICHED									
665	SIFTED, SPOONED	1 CUP	115	12	419	12	1	0.2	0.1	0.5
666	UNSIFTED, SPOONED	1 CUP	125	12	455	13	1	0.2	0.1	0.5
667	BREAD, ENRICHED	1 CUP	137	13	495	16	2	0.3	0.2	1.0
668	CAKE OR PASTRY FLOUR, ENRICHED, UNSIFTED, SPOONED	1 CUP	137	13	496	11	1	0.2	0.1	0.5
669	SELF-RISING, ENRICHED, UNSIFTED, SPOONED	1 CUP	125	11	443	12	1	0.2	0.1	0.5
670	WHOLE WHEAT, FROM HARD WHEATS, STIRRED, SPOONED	1 CUP	120	10	407	16	2	0.4	0.3	0.9
671	WHEAT GERM, TOASTED, PLAIN	1 TBSP	7	6	27	2	1	0.1	0.1	0.5
LEGUMES, NUTS, AND SEEDS										
	ALMONDS, SHELLED									
672	SLICED	1 CUP	95	5	549	20	48	3.7	30.5	11.6
673	WHOLE	1 OZ (24 NUTS)	28	5	164	6	14	1.1	9.1	3.5
	BEANS, DRY									
	COOKED									
674	BLACK	1 CUP	172	66	227	15	1	0.2	0.1	0.4
675	GREAT NORTHERN	1 CUP	177	69	209	15	1	0.2	TR	0.3
676	KIDNEY, RED	1 CUP	177	67	225	15	1	0.1	0.1	0.5
677	LIMA, LARGE	1 CUP	188	70	216	15	1	0.2	0.1	0.3
678	PEA (NAVY)	1 CUP	182	63	258	16	1	0.3	0.1	0.4
679	PINTO	1 CUP	171	64	234	14	1	0.2	0.2	0.3
	CANNED, SOLIDS AND LIQUID									
	BAKED BEANS									
680	PLAIN OR VEGETARIAN	1 CUP	254	73	236	12	1	0.3	0.1	0.5
681	WITH FRANKFURTERS	1 CUP	259	69	368	17	17	6.1	7.3	2.2
682	WITH PORK IN TOMATO SAUCE	1 CUP	253	73	248	13	3	1.0	1.1	0.3
683	WITH PORK IN SWEET SAUCE	1 CUP	253	71	281	13	4	1.4	1.6	0.5
684	KIDNEY, RED	1 CUP	256	77	218	13	1	0.1	0.1	0.5
685	LIMA, LARGE	1 CUP	241	77	190	12	TR	0.1	TR	0.2
686	WHITE	1 CUP	262	70	307	19	1	0.2	0.1	0.3
	BLACK-EYED PEAS, DRY									
687	COOKED	1 CUP	172	70	200	13	1	0.2	0.1	0.4
688	CANNED, SOLIDS AND LIQUID	1 CUP	240	80	185	11	1	0.3	0.1	0.6
689	BRAZIL NUTS, SHELLED	1 OZ (6–8 NUTS)	28	3	186	4	19	4.6	6.5	6.8
690	CAROB FLOUR	1 CUP	103	4	229	5	1	0.1	0.2	0.2
	CASHEWS, SALTED									
691	DRY ROASTED	1 OZ	28	2	163	4	13	2.6	7.7	2.2
692	OIL ROASTED	1 CUP	130	4	749	21	63	12.4	36.9	10.6
693		1 OZ (18 NUTS)	28	4	163	5	14	2.7	8.1	2.3
694	CHESTNUTS, EUROPEAN, ROASTED, SHELLED	1 CUP	143	40	350	5	3	0.6	1.1	1.2
	CHICKPEAS, DRY									

Cholesterol (mg)	Carbo-hydrate (g)	Total Dietary Fiber (g)	Calcium (mg)	Iron (mg)	Potassium (mg)	Sodium (mg)	Vitamin A		Thiamine (mg)	Ribo-flavin (mg)	Niacin (mg)	Ascorbic Acid (mg)	Food No.
							(IU)	(RE)					
0	12	1.4	46	0.4	40	42	0	0	0.03	0.02	0.4	0	660
0	18	1.1	40	1.1	42	153	0	0	0.17	0.09	1.1	0	661
52	25	0.7	191	1.7	119	383	171	49	0.20	0.26	1.6	TR	662
8	13	0.8	77	1.5	42	260	400	120	0.13	0.16	1.5	0	663
9	15	0.4	20	1.9	50	155	506	NA	0.31	0.26	2.6	0	664
0	88	3.1	17	5.3	123	2	0	0	0.90	0.57	6.8	0	665
0	95	3.4	19	5.8	134	3	0	0	0.98	0.62	7.4	0	666
0	99	3.3	21	6.0	137	3	0	0	1.11	0.70	10.3	0	667
0	107	2.3	19	10.0	144	3	0	0	1.22	0.59	9.3	0	668
0	93	3.4	423	5.8	155	1,588	0	0	0.84	0.52	7.3	0	669
0	87	14.6	41	4.7	486	6	0	0	0.54	0.26	7.6	0	670
0	3	0.9	3	0.6	66	TR	0	0	0.12	0.06	0.4	TR	671
0	19	11.2	236	4.1	692	1	10	1	0.23	0.77	3.7	0	672
0	6	3.3	70	1.2	206	TR	3	TR	0.07	0.23	1.1	0	673
0	41	15.0	40	3.6	611	2	10	2	0.42	0.10	0.9	0	674
0	37	12.4	120	3.8	692	4	2	0	0.28	0.10	1.2	2	675
0	40	13.1	50	5.2	713	4	0	0	0.28	0.10	1.0	2	676
0	39	13.2	32	4.5	955	4	0	0	0.30	0.10	0.8	0	677
0	48	11.6	127	4.5	670	2	4	0	0.37	0.11	1.0	2	678
0	44	14.7	82	4.5	800	3	3	0	0.32	0.16	0.7	4	679
0	52	12.7	127	0.7	752	1,008	434	43	0.39	0.15	1.1	8	680
16	40	17.9	124	4.5	609	1,114	399	39	0.15	0.15	2.3	6	681
18	49	12.1	142	8.3	759	1,113	314	30	0.13	0.12	1.3	8	682
18	53	13.2	154	4.2	673	850	288	28	0.12	0.15	0.9	8	683
0	40	16.4	61	3.2	658	873	0	0	0.27	0.23	1.2	3	684
0	36	11.6	51	4.4	530	810	0	0	0.13	0.08	0.6	0	685
0	57	12.6	191	7.8	1,189	13	0	0	0.25	0.10	0.3	0	686
0	36	11.2	41	4.3	478	7	26	3	0.35	0.09	0.9	1	687
0	33	7.9	48	2.3	413	718	31	2	0.18	0.18	0.8	6	688
0	4	1.5	50	1.0	170	1	0	0	0.28	0.03	0.5	TR	689
0	92	41.0	358	3.0	852	36	14	1	0.05	0.47	2.0	TR	690
0	9	0.9	13	1.7	160	181	0	0	0.06	0.06	0.4	0	691
0	37	4.9	53	5.3	689	814	0	0	0.55	0.23	2.3	0	692
0	8	1.1	12	1.2	150	177	0	0	0.12	0.05	0.5	0	693
0	76	7.3	41	1.3	847	3	34	3	0.35	0.25	1.9	37	694

Food No.	Food Description	Measure of Edible Portion	Weight (g)	Water (%)	Calories (kcal)	Protein (g)	Total Fat (g)	Fatty Acids Saturated (g)	Fatty Acids Monounsaturated (g)	Fatty Acids Polyunsaturated (g)
LEGUMES, NUTS, AND SEEDS (CONTINUED)										
695	COOKED	1 CUP	164	60	269	15	4	0.4	1.0	1.9
696	CANNED, SOLIDS AND LIQUID	1 CUP	240	70	286	12	3	0.3	0.6	1.2
	COCONUT									
	RAW									
697	PIECE, ABOUT 2″ × 2″ × 1/2″	1 PIECE	45	47	159	1	15	13.4	0.6	0.2
698	SHREDDED, NOT PACKED	1 CUP	80	47	283	3	27	23.8	1.1	0.3
699	DRIED, SWEETENED, SHREDDED	1 CUP	93	13	466	3	33	29.3	1.4	0.4
700	HAZELNUTS (FILBERTS), CHOPPED	1 CUP	115	5	722	17	70	5.1	52.5	9.1
701		1 OZ	28	5	178	4	17	1.3	12.9	2.2
702	HUMMUS, COMMERCIAL	1 TBSP	14	67	23	1	1	0.2	0.6	0.5
703	LENTILS, DRY, COOKED	1 CUP	198	70	230	18	1	0.1	0.1	0.3
704	MACADAMIA NUTS, DRY ROASTED, SALTED	1 CUP	134	2	959	10	102	16.0	79.4	2.0
705		1 OZ (10–12 NUTS)	28	2	203	2	22	3.4	16.8	0.4
	MIXED NUTS, WITH PEANUTS, SALTED									
706	DRY ROASTED	1 OZ	28	2	168	5	15	2.0	8.9	3.1
707	OIL ROASTED	1 OZ	28	2	175	5	16	2.5	9.0	3.8
	PEANUTS									
	DRY ROASTED									
708	SALTED	1 OZ (ABOUT 28)	28	2	166	7	14	2.0	7.0	4.4
709	UNSALTED	1 CUP	146	2	854	35	73	10.1	36.0	22.9
710		1 OZ (ABOUT 28)	28	2	166	7	14	2	7.0	4.4
711	OIL ROASTED, SALTED	1 CUP	144	2	837	38	71	9.9	35.2	22.4
712		1 OZ	28	2	165	7	14	1.9	6.9	4.4
	PEANUT BUTTER									
	REGULAR									
713	SMOOTH STYLE	1 TBSP	16	1	95	4	8	1.7	3.9	2.2
714	CHUNK STYLE	1 TBSP	16	1	94	4	8	1.5	3.8	2.3
715	REDUCED FAT, SMOOTH	1 TBSP	18	1	94	5	6	1.3	2.9	1.8
716	PEAS, SPLIT, DRY, COOKED	1 CUP	196	69	231	16	1	0.1	0.2	0.3
717	PECANS, HALVES	1 CUP	108	4	746	10	78	6.7	44.0	23.3
718		1 OZ (20 HALVES)	28	4	196	3	20	1.8	11.6	6.1
719	PINE NUTS (PIGNOLIA), SHELLED	1 OZ	28	7	160	7	14	2.2	5.4	6.1
720		1 TBSP	9	7	49	2	4	0.7	1.6	1.8
721	PISTACHIO NUTS, DRY ROASTED, WITH SALT, SHELLED	1 OZ (47 NUTS)	28	2	161	6	13	1.6	6.8	3.9
722	PUMPKIN AND SQUASH KERNELS, ROASTED, WITH SALT	1 OZ (142 SEEDS)	28	7	148	9	12	2.3	3.7	5.4
723	REFRIED BEANS, CANNED	1 CUP	252	76	237	14	3	1.2	1.4	0.4
724	SESAME SEEDS	1 TBSP	8	5	47	2	4	0.6	1.7	1.9
725	SOYBEANS, DRY, COOKED	1 CUP	172	63	298	29	15	2.2	3.4	8.7
	SOY PRODUCTS									
726	MISO	1 CUP	275	41	567	32	17	2.4	3.7	9.4
727	SOY MILK	1 CUP	245	93	81	7	5	0.5	0.8	2.0
	TOFU									
728	FIRM	1/4 BLOCK	81	84	62	7	4	0.5	0.8	2.0
729	SOFT, PIECE 2 1/2″ × 2 3/4″ × 1″	1 PIECE	120	87	73	8	4	0.6	1.0	2.5
730	SUNFLOWER SEED KERNELS, DRY ROASTED, WITH SALT	1/4 CUP	32	1	186	6	16	1.7	3.0	10.5

Cholesterol (mg)	Carbo-hydrate (g)	Total Dietary Fiber (g)	Calcium (mg)	Iron (mg)	Potassium (mg)	Sodium (mg)	Vitamin A (IU)	Vitamin A (RE)	Thiamine (mg)	Ribo-flavin (mg)	Niacin (mg)	Ascorbic Acid (mg)	Food No.
0	45	12.5	80	4.7	477	11	44	5	0.19	0.10	0.9	2	695
0	54	10.6	77	3.2	413	718	58	5	0.07	0.08	0.3	9	696
0	7	4.1	6	1.1	160	9	0	0	0.03	0.01	0.2	1	697
0	12	7.2	11	1.9	285	16	0	0	0.05	0.02	0.4	3	698
0	44	4.2	14	1.8	313	244	0	0	0.03	0.02	0.4	1	699
0	19	11.2	131	5.4	782	0	46	5	0.74	0.13	2.1	7	700
0	5	2.7	32	1.3	193	0	11	1	0.18	0.03	0.5	2	701
0	2	0.8	5	0.3	32	53	4	TR	0.03	0.01	0.1	0	702
0	40	15.6	38	6.6	731	4	16	2	0.33	0.14	2.1	3	703
0	17	10.7	94	3.6	486	355	0	0	0.95	0.12	3.0	1	704
0	4	2.3	20	0.8	103	75	0	0	0.20	0.02	0.6	TR	705
0	7	2.6	20	1.0	169	190	4	TR	0.06	0.06	1.3	TR	706
0	6	2.6	31	0.9	165	185	5	1	0.14	0.06	1.4	TR	707
0	6	2.3	15	0.6	187	230	0	0	0.12	0.03	3.8	0	708
0	31	11.7	79	3.3	961	9	0	0	0.64	0.14	19.7	0	709
0	6	2.3	15	0.6	187	2	0	0	0.12	0.03	3.8	0	710
0	27	13.2	127	2.6	982	624	0	0	0.36	0.16	20.6	0	711
0	5	2.6	25	0.5	193	123	0	0	0.07	0.03	4.0	0	712
0	3	0.9	6	0.3	107	75	0	0	0.01	0.02	2.1	0	713
0	3	1.1	7	0.3	120	78	0	0	0.02	0.02	2.2	0	714
0	6	0.9	6	0.3	120	97	0	0	0.05	0.01	2.6	0	715
0	41	16.3	27	2.5	710	4	14	2	0.37	0.11	1.7	1	716
0	15	10.4	76	2.7	443	0	83	9	0.71	0.14	1.3	1	717
0	4	2.7	20	0.7	116	0	22	2	0.19	0.04	0.3	TR	718
0	4	1.3	7	2.6	170	1	8	1	0.23	0.05	1.0	1	719
0	1	0.4	2	0.8	52	TR	2	TR	0.07	0.02	0.3	TR	720
0	8	2.9	31	1.2	293	121	151	15	0.24	0.04	0.4	1	721
0	4	1.1	12	4.2	229	163	108	11	0.06	0.09	0.5	1	722
20	39	13.4	88	4.2	673	753	0	0	0.07	0.04	0.8	15	723
0	1	0.9	10	0.6	33	3	5	1	0.06	0.01	0.4	0	724
0	17	10.3	175	8.8	886	2	15	2	0.27	0.49	0.7	3	725
0	77	14.9	182	7.5	451	10,029	239	25	0.27	0.69	2.4	0	726
0	4	3.2	10	1.4	345	29	78	7	0.39	0.17	0.4	0	727
0	2	0.3	131	1.2	143	6	6	1	0.08	0.08	TR	TR	728
0	2	0.2	133	1.3	144	10	8	1	0.06	0.04	0.6	TR	729
0	8	2.9	22	1.2	272	250	0	0	0.03	0.08	2.3	TR	730

Food No.	Food Description	Measure of Edible Portion	Weight (g)	Water (%)	Calories (kcal)	Protein (g)	Total Fat (g)	Fatty Acids Saturated (g)	Mono-unsaturated (g)	Poly-unsaturated (g)
LEGUMES, NUTS, AND SEEDS (CONTINUED)										
731		1 OZ	28	1	165	5	14	1.5	2.7	9.3
732	TAHINI	1 TBSP	15	3	89	3	8	1.1	3.0	3.5
733	WALNUTS, ENGLISH	1 CUP, CHOPPED	120	4	785	18	78	7.4	10.7	56.6
734		1 OZ (14 HALVES)	28	4	185	4	18	1.7	2.5	13.4
MEAT AND MEAT PRODUCTS										
	BEEF, COOKED									
	CUTS BRAISED, SIMMERED, OR POT ROASTED									
	RELATIVELY FAT, SUCH AS CHUCK BLADE, PIECE, 2 1/2″ × 2 1/2″ × 3/4″									
735	LEAN AND FAT	3 OZ	85	47	293	23	22	8.7	9.4	0.8
736	LEAN ONLY	3 OZ	85	55	213	26	11	4.3	4.8	0.4
	RELATIVELY LEAN, SUCH AS BOTTOM ROUND, PIECE, 4 1/8″ × 2 1/4″ × 1/2″									
737	LEAN AND FAT	3 OZ	85	52	234	24	14	5.4	6.2	0.5
738	LEAN ONLY	3 OZ	85	58	178	27	7	2.4	3.1	0.3
	GROUND BEEF, BROILED									
739	83% LEAN	3 OZ	85	57	218	22	14	5.5	6.1	0.5
740	79% LEAN	3 OZ	85	56	231	21	16	6.2	6.9	0.6
741	73% LEAN	3 OZ	85	54	246	20	18	6.9	7.7	0.7
742	LIVER, FRIED, SLICE, 6 1/2″ × 2 3/8″ × 3/8″	3 OZ	85	56	184	23	7	2.3	1.4	1.5
	ROAST, OVEN COOKED, NO LIQUID ADDED									
	RELATIVELY FAT, SUCH AS RIB, 2 PIECES, 4 1/8″ × 2 1/4″ × 1/4″									
743	LEAN AND FAT	3 OZ	85	47	304	19	25	9.9	10.6	0.9
744	LEAN ONLY	3 OZ	85	59	195	23	11	4.2	4.5	0.3
	RELATIVELY LEAN, SUCH AS EYE OF ROUND, 2 PIECES, 2 1/2″ × 2 1/2″ × 3/8″									
745	LEAN AND FAT	3 OZ	85	59	195	23	11	4.2	4.7	0.4
746	LEAN ONLY	3 OZ	85	65	143	25	4	1.5	1.8	0.1
	STEAK, SIRLOIN, BROILED, PIECE, 2 1/2″ × 2 1/2″ × 3/4″									
747	LEAN AND FAT	3 OZ	85	57	219	24	13	5.2	5.6	0.5
748	LEAN ONLY	3 OZ	85	62	166	26	6	2.4	2.6	0.2
749	BEEF, CANNED, CORNED	3 OZ	85	58	213	23	13	5.3	5.1	0.5
750	BEEF, DRIED, CHIPPED	1 OZ	28	57	47	8	1	0.5	0.5	0.1
	LAMB, COOKED									
	CHOPS									
	ARM, BRAISED									
751	LEAN AND FAT	3 OZ	85	44	294	26	20	8.4	8.7	1.5
752	LEAN ONLY	3 OZ	85	49	237	30	12	4.3	5.2	0.8
	LOIN, BROILED									
753	LEAN AND FAT	3 OZ	85	52	269	21	20	8.4	8.2	1.4
754	LEAN ONLY	3 OZ	85	61	184	25	8	3.0	3.6	0.5
	LEG, ROASTED, 2 PIECES, 4 1/8″ × 2 1/4″ × 1/4″									
755	LEAN AND FAT	3 OZ	85	57	219	22	14	5.9	5.9	1.0
756	LEAN ONLY	3 OZ	85	64	162	24	7	2.3	2.9	0.4
	RIB, ROASTED, 3 PIECES, 2 1/2″ × 2 1/2″ × 1/4″									
757	LEAN AND FAT	3 OZ	85	48	305	18	25	10.9	10.6	1.8
758	LEAN ONLY	3 OZ	85	60	197	22	11	4.0	5.0	0.7

Cholesterol (mg)	Carbo-hydrate (g)	Total Dietary Fiber (g)	Calcium (mg)	Iron (mg)	Potassium (mg)	Sodium (mg)	Vitamin A (IU)	(RE)	Thiamine (mg)	Ribo-flavin (mg)	Niacin (mg)	Ascorbic Acid (mg)	Food No.
0	7	2.6	20	1.1	241	221	0	0	0.03	0.07	2.0	TR	731
0	3	1.4	64	1.3	62	17	10	1	0.18	0.07	0.8	0	732
0	16	8.0	125	3.5	529	2	49	5	0.41	0.18	2.3	2	733
0	4	1.9	29	0.8	125	1	12	1	0.10	0.04	0.5	TR	734
88	0	0.0	11	2.6	196	54	0	0	0.06	0.20	2.1	0	735
90	0	0.0	11	3.1	224	60	0	0	0.07	0.24	2.3	0	736
82	0	0.0	5	2.7	240	43	0	0	0.06	0.20	3.2	0	737
82	0	0.0	4	2.9	262	43	0	0	0.06	0.22	3.5	0	738
71	0	0.0	6	2.0	266	60	0	0	0.05	0.23	4.2	0	739
74	0	0.0	9	1.8	256	65	0	0	0.04	0.18	4.4	0	740
77	0	0.0	9	2.1	248	71	0	0	0.03	0.16	4.9	0	741
410	7	0.0	9	5.3	309	90	30,689	9,120	0.18	3.52	12.3	20	742
71	0	0.0	9	2.0	256	54	0	0	0.06	0.14	2.9	0	743
68	0	0.0	9	2.4	318	61	0	0	0.07	0.18	3.5	0	744
61	0	0.0	5	1.6	308	50	0	0	0.07	0.14	3.0	0	745
59	0	0.0	4	1.7	336	53	0	0	0.08	0.14	3.2	0	746
77	0	0.0	9	2.6	311	54	0	0	0.09	0.23	3.3	0	747
76	0	0.0	9	2.9	343	56	0	0	0.11	0.25	3.6	0	748
73	0	0.0	10	1.8	116	855	0	0	0.02	0.12	2.1	0	749
12	TR	0.0	2	1.3	126	984	0	0	0.02	0.06	1.5	0	750
102	0	0.0	21	2.0	260	61	0	0	0.06	0.21	5.7	0	751
103	0	0.0	22	2.3	287	65	0	0	0.06	0.23	5.4	0	752
85	0	0.0	17	1.5	278	65	0	0	0.09	0.21	6.0	0	753
81	0	0.0	16	1.7	320	71	0	0	0.09	0.24	5.8	0	754
79	0	0.0	9	1.7	266	56	0	0	0.09	0.23	5.6	0	755
76	0	0.0	7	1.8	287	58	0	0	0.09	0.25	5.4	0	756
82	0	0.0	19	1.4	230	62	0	0	0.08	0.18	5.7	0	757
75	0	0.0	18	1.5	268	69	0	0	0.08	0.20	5.2	0	758

Food No.	Food Description	Measure of Edible Portion	Weight (g)	Water (%)	Calories (kcal)	Protein (g)	Total Fat (g)	Fatty Acids Saturated (g)	Fatty Acids Mono-unsaturated (g)	Fatty Acids Poly-unsaturated (g)
MEAT AND MEAT PRODUCTS (CONTINUED)										
	PORK, CURED, COOKED									
	BACON									
759	REGULAR	3 MEDIUM SLICES	19	13	109	6	9	3.3	4.5	1.1
760	CANADIAN STYLE (6 SLICES PER 6-OZ PKG)	2 SLICES	47	62	86	11	4	1.3	1.9	0.4
	HAM, LIGHT CURE, ROASTED, 2 PIECES, 4 1/8″ × 2 1/4″ × 1/4″									
761	LEAN AND FAT	3 OZ	85	58	207	18	14	5.1	6.7	1.5
762	LEAN ONLY	3 OZ	85	66	133	21	5	1.6	2.2	0.5
763	HAM, CANNED, ROASTED, 2 PIECES, 4 1/8″ × 21/4″ × 1/4″	3 OZ	85	67	142	18	7	2.4	3.5	0.8
	PORK, FRESH, COOKED									
	CHOP, LOIN (CUT 3 PER LB WITH BONE)									
	BROILED									
764	LEAN AND FAT	3 OZ	85	58	204	24	11	4.1	5.0	0.8
765	LEAN ONLY	3 OZ	85	61	172	26	7	2.5	3.1	0.5
	PAN FRIED									
766	LEAN AND FAT	3 OZ	85	53	235	25	14	5.1	6.0	1.6
767	LEAN ONLY	3 OZ	85	57	197	27	9	3.1	3.8	1.1
	HAM (LEG), ROASTED, PIECE, 2 1/2″ × 2 1/2″ × 3/4″									
768	LEAN AND FAT	3 OZ	85	55	232	23	15	5.5	6.7	1.4
769	LEAN ONLY	3 OZ	85	61	179	25	8	2.8	3.8	0.7
	RIB ROAST, PIECE, 2 1/2″ × 2 1/2″ × 3/4″									
770	LEAN AND FAT	3 OZ	85	56	217	23	13	5.0	5.9	1.1
771	LEAN ONLY	3 OZ	85	59	190	24	9	3.7	4.5	0.7
	RIBS, LEAN AND FAT, COOKED									
772	BACKRIBS, ROASTED	3 OZ	85	45	315	21	25	9.3	11.4	2.0
773	COUNTRY STYLE, BRAISED	3 OZ	85	54	252	20	18	6.8	7.9	1.6
774	SPARERIBS, BRAISED	3 OZ	85	40	337	25	26	9.5	11.5	2.3
	SHOULDER CUT, BRAISED, 3 PIECES, 2 1/2″ × 2 1/2″ × 1/4″									
775	LEAN AND FAT	3 OZ	85	48	280	24	20	7.2	8.8	1.9
776	LEAN ONLY	3 OZ	85	54	211	27	10	3.5	4.9	1.0
	SAUSAGES AND LUNCHEON MEATS									
777	BOLOGNA, BEEF AND PORK (8 SLICES PER 8-OZ PKG)	2 SLICES	57	54	180	7	16	6.1	7.6	1.4
778	BRAUNSCHWEIGER (6 SLICES PER 6-OZ PKG)	2 SLICES	57	48	205	8	18	6.2	8.5	2.1
779	BROWN AND SERVE, COOKED, LINK, 4″ × 7/8″ RAW	2 LINKS	26	45	103	4	9	3.4	4.5	1.0
	CANNED, MINCED LUNCHEON MEAT									
780	PORK, HAM, AND CHICKEN, REDUCED SODIUM (7 SLICES PER 7-OZ CAN)	2 SLICES	57	56	172	7	15	5.1	7.1	1.5
781	PORK WITH HAM (12 SLICES PER 12-OZ CAN)	2 SLICES	57	52	188	8	17	5.7	7.7	1.2
782	PORK AND CHICKEN (12 SLICES PER 12-OZ CAN)	2 SLICES	57	64	117	9	8	2.7	3.8	0.8
783	CHOPPED HAM (8 SLICES PER 6-OZ PKG)	2 SLICES	21	64	48	4	4	1.2	1.7	0.4
	COOKED HAM (8 SLICES PER 8-OZ PKG)									
784	REGULAR	2 SLICES	57	65	104	10	6	1.9	2.8	0.7
785	EXTRA LEAN	2 SLICES	57	71	75	11	3	0.9	1.3	0.3
	FRANKFURTER (10 PER 1-LB PKG), HEATED									

Cholesterol (mg)	Carbo-hydrate (g)	Total Dietary Fiber (g)	Calcium (mg)	Iron (mg)	Potassium (mg)	Sodium (mg)	Vitamin A (IU)	Vitamin A (RE)	Thiamine (mg)	Ribo-flavin (mg)	Niacin (mg)	Ascorbic Acid (mg)	Food No.
16	TR	0.0	2	0.3	92	303	0	0	0.13	0.05	1.4	0	759
27	1	0.0	5	0.4	181	719	0	0	0.38	0.09	3.2	0	760
53	0	0.0	6	0.7	243	1,009	0	0	0.51	0.19	3.8	0	761
47	0	0.0	6	0.8	269	1,128	0	0	0.58	0.22	4.3	0	762
35	TR	0.0	6	0.9	298	908	0	0	0.82	0.21	4.3	0	763
70	0	0.0	28	0.7	304	49	8	3	0.91	0.24	4.5	TR	764
70	0	0.0	26	0.7	319	51	7	2	0.98	0.26	4.7	TR	765
78	0	0.0	23	0.8	361	68	7	2	0.97	0.26	4.8	1	766
78	0	0.0	20	0.8	382	73	7	2	1.06	0.28	5.1	1	767
80	0	0.0	12	0.9	299	51	9	3	0.54	0.27	3.9	TR	768
00	0	0.0	6	1.0	317	54	8	3	0.59	0.30	4.2	TR	769
62	0	0.0	24	0.8	358	39	5	2	0.62	0.26	5.2	TR	770
60	0	0.0	22	0.8	371	40	5	2	0.64	0.27	5.5	TR	771
100	0	0.0	38	1.2	268	86	8	3	0.36	0.17	3.0	TR	772
74	0	0.0	25	1.0	279	50	7	2	0.43	0.22	3.3	1	773
103	0	0.0	40	1.6	272	79	9	3	0.35	0.32	4.7	0	774
93	0	0.0	15	1.4	314	75	8	3	0.46	0.26	4.4	TR	775
97	0	0.0	7	1.7	344	87	7	2	0.51	0.31	5.0	TR	776
31	2	0.0	7	0.9	103	581	0	0	0.10	0.08	1.5	0	777
89	2	0.0	5	5.3	113	652	8,009	2,405	0.14	0.87	4.8	0	778
18	1	0.0	3	0.3	49	209	0	0	0.09	0.04	0.9	0	779
43	1	0.0	0	0.4	321	539	0	0	0.15	0.10	1.8	18	780
40	1	0.0	0	0.4	233	758	0	0	0.18	0.10	2.0	0	781
43	1	0.0	0	0.7	352	539	0	0	0.10	0.12	2.0	18	782
11	0	0.0	1	0.2	67	288	0	0	0.13	0.04	0.8	0	783
32	2	0.0	4	0.6	189	751	0	0	0.49	0.14	3.0	0	784
27	1	0.0	4	0.4	200	815	0	0	0.53	0.13	2.8	0	785

Food No.	Food Description	Measure of Edible Portion	Weight (g)	Water (%)	Calories (kcal)	Protein (g)	Total Fat (g)	Fatty Acids Saturated (g)	Mono-unsaturated (g)	Poly-unsaturated (g)
MEAT AND MEAT PRODUCTS (CONTINUED)										
786	BEEF AND PORK	1 FRANK	45	54	144	5	13	4.8	6.2	1.2
787	BEEF	1 FRANK	45	55	142	5	13	5.4	6.1	0.6
	PORK SAUSAGE, FRESH, COOKED									
788	LINK (4″ × 7/8″ RAW)	2 LINKS	26	45	96	5	8	2.8	3.6	1.0
789	PATTY (3 7/8″ × 1/4″ RAW)	1 PATTY	27	45	100	5	8	2.9	3.8	1.0
	SALAMI, BEEF AND PORK									
790	COOKED TYPE (8 SLICES PER 8-OZ PKG)	2 SLICES	57	60	143	8	11	4.6	5.2	1.2
791	DRY TYPE, SLICE, 3 1/8″ × 1/16″	2 SLICES	20	35	84	5	7	2.4	3.4	0.6
792	SANDWICH SPREAD (PORK, BEEF)	1 TBSP	15	60	35	1	3	0.9	1.1	0.4
793	VIENNA SAUSAGE (7 PER 4-OZ CAN)	1 SAUSAGE	16	60	45	2	4	1.5	2.0	0.3
	VEAL, LEAN AND FAT, COOKED									
794	CUTLET, BRAISED, 4 1/8″ × 2 1/4″ × 1/2″	3 OZ	85	55	179	31	5	2.2	2.0	0.4
795	RIB, ROASTED, 2 PIECES, 4 1/8″ × 2 1/4″ × 1/4″	3 OZ	85	60	194	20	12	4.6	4.6	0.8
MIXED DISHES AND FAST FOODS										
	MIXED DISHES									
796	BEEF MACARONI, FROZEN, HEALTHY CHOICE	1 PACKAGE	240	78	211	14	2	0.7	1.2	0.3
797	BEEF STEW, CANNED	1 CUP	232	82	218	11	12	5.2	5.5	0.5
798	CHICKEN POT PIE, FROZEN	1 SMALL PIE	217	60	484	13	29	9.7	12.5	4.5
799	CHILI CON CARNE WITH BEANS, CANNED	1 CUP	222	74	255	20	8	2.1	2.2	1.4
800	MACARONI AND CHEESE, CANNED, MADE WITH CORN OIL	1 CUP	252	82	199	8	6	3.0	NA	1.3
801	MEATLESS BURGER CRUMBLES, MORNINGSTAR FARMS	1 CUP	110	60	231	22	13	3.3	4.6	4.9
802	MEATLESS BURGER PATTY, FROZEN, MORNINGSTAR FARMS	1 PATTY	85	71	91	14	1	0.1	0.3	0.2
803	PASTA WITH MEATBALLS IN TOMATO SAUCE, CANNED	1 CUP	252	78	260	11	10	4.0	4.2	0.6
804	SPAGHETTI BOLOGNESE (MEAT SAUCE), FROZEN, HEALTHY CHOICE	1 PACKAGE	283	78	255	14	3	1.0	0.9	0.9
805	SPAGHETTI IN TOMATO SAUCE WITH CHEESE, CANNED	1 CUP	252	80	192	6	2	0.7	0.3	0.3
806	SPINACH SOUFFLE, HOME-PREPARED	1 CUP	136	74	219	11	18	7.1	6.8	3.1
807	TORTELLINI, PASTA WITH CHEESE FILLING, FROZEN	3/4 CUP (YIELDS 1 CUP COOKED)	81	31	249	11	6	2.9	1.7	0.4
	FAST FOODS									
	BREAKFAST ITEMS									
808	BISCUIT WITH EGG AND SAUSAGE	1 BISCUIT	180	43	581	19	39	15.0	16.4	4.4
809	CROISSANT WITH EGG, CHEESE, BACON	1 CROISSANT	129	44	413	16	28	15.4	9.2	1.8
	DANISH PASTRY									
810	CHEESE FILLED	1 PASTRY	91	34	353	6	25	5.1	15.6	2.4
811	FRUIT FILLED	1 PASTRY	94	29	335	5	16	3.3	10.1	1.6
812	ENGLISH MUFFIN WITH EGG, CHEESE, CANADIAN BACON	1 MUFFIN	137	57	289	17	13	4.7	4.7	1.6
813	FRENCH TOAST WITH BUTTER	2 SLICES	135	51	356	10	19	7.7	7.1	2.4
814	FRENCH TOAST STICKS	5 STICKS	141	30	513	8	29	4.7	12.6	9.9
815	HASHED BROWN POTATOES	1/2 CUP	72	60	151	2	9	4.3	3.9	0.5
816	PANCAKES WITH BUTTER, SYRUP	2 PANCAKES	232	50	520	8	14	5.9	5.3	2.0

Cholesterol (mg)	Carbo-hydrate (g)	Total Dietary Fiber (g)	Calcium (mg)	Iron (mg)	Potassium (mg)	Sodium (mg)	Vitamin A (IU)	Vitamin A (RE)	Thiamine (mg)	Ribo-flavin (mg)	Niacin (mg)	Ascorbic Acid (mg)	Food No.
23	1	0.0	5	0.5	75	504	0	0	0.09	0.05	1.2	0	786
27	1	0.0	9	0.6	75	462	0	0	0.02	0.05	1.1	0	787
22	TR	0.0	8	0.3	94	336	0	0	0.19	0.07	1.2	1	788
22	TR	0.0	9	0.3	97	349	0	0	0.20	0.07	1.2	1	789
37	1	0.0	7	1.5	113	607	0	0	0.14	0.21	2.0	0	790
16	1	0.0	2	0.3	76	372	0	0	0.12	0.06	1.0	0	791
6	2	TR	2	0.1	17	152	13	1	0.03	0.02	0.3	0	792
8	TR	0.0	2	0.1	16	152	0	0	0.01	0.02	0.3	0	793
114	0	0.0	7	1.1	326	57	0	0	0.05	0.30	9.0	0	794
94	0	0.0	9	0.8	251	78	0	0	0.04	0.23	5.9	0	795
14	33	4.6	46	2.7	365	444	514	50	0.28	0.16	3.1	58	796
37	16	3.5	28	1.6	404	947	3,860	494	0.17	0.14	2.9	10	797
41	43	1.7	33	2.1	256	857	2,285	343	0.25	0.36	4.1	2	798
24	24	8.2	67	3.3	608	1,032	884	93	0.15	0.15	2.1	1	799
8	29	3.0	113	2.0	123	1,058	713	NA	0.28	0.25	2.5	0	800
0	7	5.1	79	6.4	178	476	0	0	9.92	0.35	3.0	0	801
0	8	4.3	87	2.9	434	383	0	0	0.26	0.55	4.1	0	802
20	31	6.8	28	2.3	416	1,053	920	93	0.19	0.16	3.3	8	803
17	43	5.1	51	3.5	408	473	492	48	0.35	3.77	0.5	15	804
8	39	7.8	40	2.8	305	963	932	58	0.35	0.28	4.5	10	805
184	3	NA	230	1.3	201	763	3,461	675	0.09	0.30	0.5	3	806
34	38	1.5	123	1.2	72	279	50	13	0.25	0.25	2.2	0	807
302	41	0.9	155	4.0	320	1,141	635	164	0.50	0.45	3.6	0	808
215	24	NA	151	2.2	201	889	472	120	0.35	0.34	2.2	2	809
20	29	NA	70	1.8	116	319	155	43	0.26	0.21	2.5	3	810
19	45	NA	22	1.4	110	333	86	24	0.29	0.21	1.8	2	811
234	27	1.5	151	2.4	199	729	586	156	0.49	0.45	3.3	2	812
116	36	NA	73	1.9	177	513	473	146	0.58	0.50	3.9	TR	813
75	58	2.7	78	3.0	127	499	45	13	0.23	0.25	3.0	0	814
9	16	NA	7	0.5	267	290	18	3	0.08	0.01	1.1	5	815
58	91	NA	128	2.6	251	1,104	281	70	0.39	0.56	3.4	3	816

Food No.	Food Description	Measure of Edible Portion	Weight (g)	Water (%)	Calories (kcal)	Protein (g)	Total Fat (g)	Fatty Acids Satu-rated (g)	Mono-unsatu-rated (g)	Poly-unsatu-rated (g)
MIXED DISHES AND FAST FOODS (CONTINUED)										
	BURRITO									
817	WITH BEANS AND CHEESE	1 BURRITO	93	54	189	8	6	3.4	1.2	0.9
818	WITH BEANS AND MEAT	1 BURRITO	116	52	255	11	9	4.2	3.5	0.6
	CHEESEBURGER									
	REGULAR SIZE, WITH CONDIMENTS									
819	DOUBLE PATTY WITH MAYO-TYPE DRESSING, VEGETABLES	1 SANDWICH	166	51	417	21	21	8.7	7.8	2.7
820	SINGLE PATTY	1 SANDWICH	113	48	295	16	14	6.3	5.3	1.1
	REGULAR SIZE, PLAIN									
821	DOUBLE PATTY	1 SANDWICH	155	42	457	28	28	13.0	11.0	1.9
822	DOUBLE PATTY WITH 3-PIECE BUN	1 SANDWICH	160	43	461	22	22	9.5	8.3	1.8
823	SINGLE PATTY	1 SANDWICH	102	37	319	15	15	6.5	5.8	1.5
	LARGE, WITH CONDIMENTS									
824	SINGLE PATTY WITH MAYO-TYPE DRESSING, VEGETABLES	1 SANDWICH	219	53	563	28	33	15.0	12.6	2.0
825	SINGLE PATTY WITH BACON	1 SANDWICH	195	44	608	32	37	16.2	14.5	2.7
826	CHICKEN FILLET (BREADED AND FRIED) SANDWICH, PLAIN	1 SANDWICH	182	47	515	24	29	8.5	10.4	8.4
	CHICKEN, FRIED. SEE POULTRY AND POULTRY PRODUCTS.									
827	CHICKEN PIECES, BONELESS, BREADED AND FRIED, PLAIN	6 PIECES	106	47	319	18	21	4.7	10.5	4.6
828	CHILI CON CARNE	1 CUP	253	77	256	25	8	3.4	3.4	0.5
829	CHIMICHANGA WITH BEEF	1 CHIMICHANGA	174	51	425	20	20	8.5	8.1	1.1
830	COLESLAW	3/4 CUP	99	74	147	1	11	1.6	2.4	6.4
	DESSERTS									
831	ICE MILK, SOFT, VANILLA, IN CONE	1 CONE	103	65	164	4	6	3.5	1.8	0.4
832	PIE, FRIED, WITH FRUIT FILLING (5″ X 3 3/4″)	1 PIE	128	38	404	4	21	3.1	9.5	6.9
833	SUNDAE, HOT FUDGE	1 SUNDAE	158	60	284	6	9	5.0	2.3	0.8
834	ENCHILADA WITH CHEESE	1 ENCHILADA	163	63	319	10	19	10.6	6.3	0.8
835	FISH SANDWICH, WITH TARTAR SAUCE AND CHEESE	1 SANDWICH	183	45	523	21	29	8.1	8.9	9.4
836	FRENCH FRIES	1 SMALL	85	35	291	4	16	3.3	9.0	2.7
837		1 MEDIUM	134	35	458	6	25	5.2	14.3	4.2
838		1 LARGE	169	35	578	7	31	6.5	18.0	5.3
839	FRIJOLES (REFRIED BEANS, CHILI SAUCE, CHEESE)	1 CUP	167	69	225	11	8	4.1	2.6	0.7
	HAMBURGER									
	REGULAR SIZE, WITH CONDIMENTS									
840	DOUBLE PATTY	1 SANDWICH	215	51	576	32	32	12.0	14.1	2.8
841	SINGLE PATTY	1 SANDWICH	106	45	272	12	10	3.6	3.4	1.0
	LARGE, WITH CONDIMENTS, MAYO-TYPE DRESSING, AND VEGETABLES									
842	DOUBLE PATTY	1 SANDWICH	226	54	540	34	27	10.5	10.3	2.8
843	SINGLE PATTY	1 SANDWICH	218	56	512	26	27	10.4	11.4	2.2
	HOT DOG									
844	PLAIN	1 SANDWICH	98	54	242	10	15	5.1	6.9	1.7
845	WITH CHILI	1 SANDWICH	114	48	296	14	13	4.9	6.6	1.2
846	WITH CORN FLOUR COATING (CORNDOG)	1 CORNDOG	175	47	460	17	19	5.2	9.1	3.5
847	HUSH PUPPIES	5 PIECES	78	32	257	5	12	2.7	7.8	0.4

Cholesterol (mg)	Carbo-hydrate (g)	Total Dietary Fiber (g)	Calcium (mg)	Iron (mg)	Potassium (mg)	Sodium (mg)	Vitamin A (IU)	Vitamin A (RE)	Thiamine (mg)	Ribo-flavin (mg)	Niacin (mg)	Ascorbic Acid (mg)	Food No.
14	27	NA	107	1.1	248	583	625	119	0.11	0.35	1.8	1	817
24	33	NA	53	2.5	329	670	319	32	0.27	0.42	2.7	1	818
60	35	NA	171	3.4	335	1,051	398	65	0.35	0.28	8.1	2	819
37	27	NA	111	2.4	223	616	462	94	0.25	0.23	3.7	2	820
110	22	NA	233	3.4	308	636	332	79	0.25	0.37	6.0	0	821
80	44	NA	224	3.7	285	891	277	66	0.34	0.38	6.0	0	822
50	32	NA	141	2.4	164	500	153	37	0.40	0.40	3.7	0	823
88	38	NA	206	4.7	445	1,108	613	129	0.39	0.46	7.4	8	824
111	37	NA	162	4.7	332	1,043	406	80	0.31	0.41	6.6	2	825
60	39	NA	60	4.7	353	957	100	31	0.33	0.24	6.8	9	826
61	15	0.0	14	0.9	305	513	0	0	0.12	0.16	7.5	0	827
134	22	NA	68	5.2	691	1,007	1,662	167	0.13	1.14	2.5	2	828
9	43	NA	63	4.5	586	910	146	16	0.49	0.64	5.8	5	829
5	13	NA	34	0.7	177	267	338	50	0.04	0.03	0.1	8	830
28	24	0.1	153	0.2	169	92	211	52	0.05	0.26	0.3	1	831
0	55	3.3	28	1.6	83	479	35	4	0.18	0.14	1.8	2	832
21	48	0.0	207	0.6	395	182	221	57	0.06	0.30	1.1	2	833
44	29	NA	324	1.3	240	784	1,161	186	0.08	0.42	1.9	1	834
68	48	NA	185	3.5	353	939	432	97	0.46	0.42	4.2	3	835
0	34	3.0	12	0.7	586	168	0	0	0.07	0.03	2.4	10	836
0	53	4.7	19	1.0	923	265	0	0	0.11	0.05	3.8	16	837
0	67	5.9	24	1.3	1,164	335	0	0	0.14	0.07	4.8	20	838
37	29	NA	189	2.2	605	882	456	70	0.13	0.33	1.5	2	839
103	39	NA	92	5.5	527	742	54	4	0.34	0.41	6.7	1	840
30	34	2.3	126	2.7	251	534	74	10	0.29	0.24	3.9	2	841
122	40	NA	102	5.9	570	791	102	11	0.36	0.38	7.6	1	842
87	40	NA	96	4.9	480	824	312	33	0.41	0.37	7.3	3	843
44	18	NA	24	2.3	143	670	0	0	0.24	0.27	3.6	TR	844
51	31	NA	19	3.3	166	480	58	6	0.22	0.40	3.7	3	845
79	56	NA	102	6.2	263	973	207	37	0.28	0.70	4.2	0	846
135	35	NA	69	1.4	188	965	94	27	0.00	0.02	2.0	0	847

Food No.	Food Description	Measure of Edible Portion	Weight (g)	Water (%)	Calories (kcal)	Protein (g)	Total Fat (g)	Fatty Acids Saturated (g)	Mono-unsaturated (g)	Poly-unsaturated (g)
MIXED DISHES AND FAST FOODS (CONTINUED)										
848	MASHED POTATOES	1/3 CUP	80	79	66	2	1	0.4	0.3	0.2
849	NACHOS, WITH CHEESE SAUCE	6–8 NACHOS	113	40	346	9	19	7.8	8.0	2.2
850	ONION RINGS, BREADED AND FRIED	8–9 RINGS	83	37	276	4	16	7.0	6.7	0.7
	PIZZA (SLICE = 1/8 OF 12" PIZZA)									
851	CHEESE	1 SLICE	63	48	140	8	3	1.5	1.0	0.5
852	MEAT AND VEGETABLES	1 SLICE	79	48	184	13	5	1.5	2.5	0.9
853	PEPPERONI	1 SLICE	71	47	181	10	7	2.2	3.1	1.2
854	ROAST BEEF SANDWICH, PLAIN	1 SANDWICH	139	49	346	22	14	3.6	6.8	1.7
855	SALAD, TOSSED, WITH CHICKEN, NO DRESSING	1 1/2 CUPS	218	87	105	17	2	0.6	0.7	0.6
856	SALAD, TOSSED, WITH EGG, CHEESE, NO DRESSING	1 1/2 CUPS	217	90	102	9	6	3.0	1.8	0.5
	SHAKE									
857	CHOCOLATE	16 FL OZ	333	72	423	11	12	7.7	3.6	0.5
858	VANILLA	16 FL OZ	333	75	370	12	10	6.2	2.9	0.4
859	SHRIMP, BREADED AND FRIED	6–8 SHRIMP	164	48	454	19	25	5.4	17.4	0.6
	SUBMARINE SANDWICH (6" LONG), WITH OIL AND VINEGAR									
860	COLD CUTS (WITH LETTUCE, CHEESE, SALAMI, HAM, TOMATO, ONION)	1 SANDWICH	228	58	456	22	19	6.8	8.2	2.3
861	ROAST BEEF (WITH TOMATO, LETTUCE, MAYO)	1 SANDWICH	216	59	410	29	13	7.1	1.8	2.6
862	TUNA SALAD (WITH MAYO, LETTUCE)	1 SANDWICH	256	54	584	30	28	5.3	13.4	7.3
863	TACO, BEEF	1 SMALL	171	58	369	21	21	11.4	6.6	1.0
864		1 LARGE	263	58	568	32	32	17.5	10.1	1.5
865	TACO SALAD (WITH GROUND BEEF, CHEESE, TACO SHELL)	1 1/2 CUPS	198	72	279	13	15	6.8	5.2	1.7
	TOSTADA (WITH CHEESE, TOMATO, LETTUCE)									
866	WITH BEANS AND BEEF	1 TOSTADA	225	70	333	16	17	11.5	3.5	0.6
867	WITH GUACAMOLE	1 TOSTADA	131	73	181	6	12	5.0	4.3	1.5
POULTRY AND POULTRY PRODUCTS										
	CHICKEN									
	FRIED IN VEGETABLE SHORTENING, MEAT WITH SKIN									
	BATTER DIPPED									
868	BREAST, 1/2 BREAST (5.6 OZ WITH BONES)	1/2 BREAST	140	52	364	35	18	4.9	7.6	4.3
869	DRUMSTICK (3.4 OZ WITH BONES)	1 DRUMSTICK	72	53	193	16	11	3.0	4.6	2.7
870	THIGH	1 THIGH	86	52	238	19	14	3.8	5.8	3.4
871	WING	1 WING	49	46	159	10	11	2.9	4.4	2.5
	FLOUR-COATED									
872	BREAST, 1/2 BREAST (4.2 OZ WITH BONES)	1/2 BREAST	98	57	218	31	9	2.4	3.4	1.9
873	DRUMSTICK (2.6 OZ WITH BONES)	1 DRUMSTICK	49	57	120	13	7	1.8	2.7	1.6
	FRIED, MEAT ONLY									
874	DARK MEAT	3 OZ	85	56	203	25	10	2.7	3.7	2.4
875	LIGHT MEAT	3 OZ	85	60	163	28	5	1.3	1.7	1.1
	ROASTED, MEAT ONLY									
876	BREAST, 1/2 BREAST (4.2 OZ WITH BONE AND SKIN)	1/2 BREAST	86	65	142	27	3	0.9	1.1	0.7
877	DRUMSTICK (2.9 OZ WITH BONE AND SKIN)	1 DRUMSTICK	44	67	76	12	2	0.7	0.8	0.6

Cholesterol (mg)	Carbo-hydrate (g)	Total Dietary Fiber (g)	Calcium (mg)	Iron (mg)	Potassium (mg)	Sodium (mg)	Vitamin A (IU)	(RE)	Thiamine (mg)	Ribo-flavin (mg)	Niacin (mg)	Ascorbic Acid (mg)	Food No.
2	13	NA	17	0.4	235	182	33	8	0.07	0.04	1.0	TR	848
18	36	NA	272	1.3	172	816	559	92	0.19	0.37	1.5	1	849
14	31	NA	73	0.8	129	430	8	1	0.08	0.10	0.9	1	850
9	21	NA	117	0.6	110	336	382	74	0.18	0.16	2.5	1	851
21	21	NA	101	1.5	179	382	524	101	0.21	0.17	2.0	2	852
14	20	NA	65	0.9	153	267	282	55	0.13	0.23	3.0	2	853
51	33	NA	54	4.2	316	792	210	21	0.38	0.31	5.9	2	854
72	4	NA	37	1.1	447	209	935	96	0.11	0.13	5.9	17	855
98	5	NA	100	0.7	371	119	822	115	0.09	0.17	1.0	10	856
43	68	2.7	376	1.0	666	323	310	77	0.19	0.82	0.5	1	857
37	60	1.3	406	0.3	579	273	433	107	0.15	0.61	0.6	3	858
200	40	NA	84	3.0	184	1,446	120	36	0.21	0.90	0.0	0	859
36	51	NA	189	2.5	394	1,651	424	80	1.00	0.80	5.5	12	860
73	44	NA	41	2.8	330	845	413	50	0.41	0.41	6.0	6	861
49	55	NA	74	2.6	335	1,293	187	41	0.46	0.33	11.3	4	862
56	27	NA	221	2.4	474	802	855	147	0.15	0.44	3.2	2	863
87	41	NA	339	3.7	729	1,233	1,315	226	0.24	0.68	4.9	3	864
44	24	NA	192	2.3	416	762	588	77	0.10	0.36	2.5	4	865
74	30	NA	189	2.5	491	871	1,276	173	0.09	0.50	2.9	4	866
20	16	NA	212	0.8	326	401	879	109	0.07	0.29	1.0	2	867
119	13	0.4	28	1.8	281	385	94	28	0.16	0.20	14.7	0	868
62	6	0.2	12	1.0	134	194	62	19	0.08	0.15	3.7	0	869
80	8	0.3	15	1.2	165	248	82	25	0.10	0.20	4.9	0	870
39	5	0.1	10	0.6	68	157	55	17	0.05	0.07	2.6	0	871
87	2	0.1	16	1.2	254	74	49	15	0.08	0.13	13.5	0	872
44	1	TR	6	0.7	112	44	41	12	0.04	0.11	3.0	0	873
82	2	0.0	15	1.3	215	82	67	20	0.08	0.21	6.0	0	874
77	TR	0.0	14	1.0	224	69	26	8	0.06	0.11	11.4	0	875
73	0	0.0	13	0.9	220	64	18	5	0.06	0.10	11.8	0	876
41	0	0.0	5	0.6	108	42	26	8	0.03	0.10	2.7	0	877

Food No.	Food Description	Measure of Edible Portion	Weight (g)	Water (%)	Calories (kcal)	Protein (g)	Total Fat (g)	Fatty Acids Saturated (g)	Mono-unsaturated (g)	Poly-unsaturated (g)
POULTRY AND POULTRY PRODUCTS (CONTINUED)										
878	THIGH	1 THIGH	52	63	109	13	6	1.6	2.2	1.3
879	STEWED, MEAT ONLY, LIGHT AND DARK MEAT, CHOPPED OR DICED	1 CUP	140	56	332	43	17	4.3	5.7	4.0
880	CHICKEN GIBLETS, SIMMERED, CHOPPED	1 CUP	145	68	228	37	7	2.2	1.7	1.6
881	CHICKEN LIVER, SIMMERED	1 LIVER	20	68	31	5	1	0.4	0.3	0.2
882	CHICKEN NECK, MEAT ONLY, SIMMERED	1 NECK	18	67	32	4	1	0.4	0.5	0.4
883	DUCK, ROASTED, FLESH ONLY	1/2 DUCK	221	64	444	52	25	9.2	8.2	3.2
	TURKEY									
	ROASTED, MEAT ONLY									
884	DARK MEAT	3 OZ	85	63	159	24	6	2.1	1.4	1.8
885	LIGHT MEAT	3 OZ	85	66	133	25	3	0.9	0.5	0.7
886	LIGHT AND DARK MEAT, CHOPPED OR DICED	1 CUP	140	65	238	41	7	2.3	1.4	2.0
	GROUND, COOKED									
887	PATTY, FROM 4 OZ RAW	1 PATTY	82	59	193	22	11	2.8	4.0	2.6
888	CRUMBLED	1 CUP	127	59	298	35	17	4.3	6.2	4.1
889	TURKEY GIBLETS, SIMMERED, CHOPPED	1 CUP	145	65	242	39	7	2.2	1.7	1.7
890	TURKEY NECK, MEAT ONLY, SIMMERED	1 NECK	152	65	274	41	11	3.7	2.5	3.3
	POULTRY FOOD PRODUCTS									
	CHICKEN									
891	CANNED, BONELESS	5 OZ	142	69	234	31	11	3.1	4.5	2.5
892	FRANKFURTER (10 PER 1-LB PKG)	1 FRANK	45	58	116	6	9	2.5	3.8	1.8
893	ROLL, LIGHT MEAT (6 SLICES PER 6-OZ PKG)	2 SLICES	57	69	90	11	4	1.1	1.7	0.9
	TURKEY									
894	GRAVY AND TURKEY, FROZEN	5-OZ PACKAGE	142	85	95	8	4	1.2	1.4	0.7
895	PATTIES, BREADED OR BATTERED, FRIED (2.25 OZ)	1 PATTY	64	50	181	9	12	3.0	4.8	3.0
896	ROAST, BONELESS, FROZEN, SEASONED, LIGHT AND DARK MEAT, COOKED	3 OZ	85	68	132	18	5	1.6	1.0	1.4
SOUPS, SAUCES, AND GRAVIES										
	SOUPS									
	CANNED, CONDENSED									
	PREPARED WITH EQUAL VOLUME OF WHOLE MILK									
897	CLAM CHOWDER, NEW ENGLAND	1 CUP	248	85	164	9	7	3.0	2.3	1.1
898	CREAM OF CHICKEN	1 CUP	248	85	191	7	11	4.6	4.5	1.6
899	CREAM OF MUSHROOM	1 CUP	248	85	203	6	14	5.1	3.0	4.6
900	TOMATO	1 CUP	248	85	161	6	6	2.9	1.6	1.1
	PREPARED WITH EQUAL VOLUME OF WATER									
901	BEAN WITH PORK	1 CUP	253	84	172	8	6	1.5	2.2	1.8
902	BEEF BROTH, BOUILLON, CONSOMME	1 CUP	241	96	29	5	0	0.0	0.0	0.0
903	BEEF NOODLE	1 CUP	244	92	83	5	3	1.1	1.2	0.5
904	CHICKEN NOODLE	1 CUP	241	92	75	4	2	0.7	1.1	0.6
905	CHICKEN AND RICE	1 CUP	241	94	60	4	2	0.5	0.9	0.4
906	CLAM CHOWDER, MANHATTAN	1 CUP	244	92	78	2	2	0.4	0.4	1.3
907	CREAM OF CHICKEN	1 CUP	244	91	117	3	7	2.1	3.3	1.5
908	CREAM OF MUSHROOM	1 CUP	244	90	129	2	9	2.4	1.7	4.2
909	MINESTRONE	1 CUP	241	91	82	4	3	0.6	0.7	1.1
910	PEA, GREEN	1 CUP	250	83	165	9	3	1.4	1.0	0.4
911	TOMATO	1 CUP	244	90	85	2	2	0.4	0.4	1.0

Cholesterol (mg)	Carbo-hydrate (g)	Total Dietary Fiber (g)	Calcium (mg)	Iron (mg)	Potassium (mg)	Sodium (mg)	Vitamin A (IU)	Vitamin A (RE)	Thiamine (mg)	Ribo-flavin (mg)	Niacin (mg)	Ascorbic Acid (mg)	Food No.
49	0	0.0	6	0.7	124	46	34	10	0.04	0.12	3.4	0	878
116	0	0.0	18	2.0	283	109	157	46	0.16	0.39	9.0	0	879
570	1	0.0	17	9.3	229	84	10,775	3,232	0.13	1.38	5.9	12	880
126	TR	0.0	3	1.7	28	10	3,275	983	0.03	0.35	0.9	3	881
14	0	0.0	8	0.5	25	12	22	6	0.01	0.05	0.7	0	882
197	0	0.0	27	6.0	557	144	170	51	0.57	1.04	11.3	0	883
72	0	0.0	27	2.0	247	67	0	0	0.05	0.21	3.1	0	884
59	0	0.0	16	1.1	259	54	0	0	0.05	0.11	5.8	0	885
106	0	0.0	35	2.5	417	98	0	0	0.09	0.25	7.6	0	886
84	0	0.0	21	1.6	221	88	0	0	0.04	0.14	4.0	0	887
130	0	0.0	32	2.5	343	136	0	0	0.07	0.21	6.1	0	888
606	3	0.0	19	9.7	290	86	8,752	2,603	0.07	1.31	6.5	2	889
185	0	0.0	56	3.5	226	85	0	0	0.05	0.29	2.6	0	890
88	0	0.0	20	2.2	196	714	166	48	0.02	0.18	9.0	3	891
45	3	0.0	43	0.9	38	617	59	17	0.03	0.05	1.4	0	892
28	1	0.0	24	0.5	129	331	46	14	0.04	0.07	3.0	0	893
26	7	0.0	20	1.3	87	787	60	18	0.03	0.18	2.6	0	894
40	10	0.3	9	1.4	176	512	24	7	0.06	0.12	1.5	0	895
45	3	0.0	4	1.4	253	578	0	0	0.04	0.14	5.3	0	896
22	17	1.5	186	1.5	300	992	164	40	0.07	0.24	1.0	3	897
27	15	0.2	181	0.7	273	1,047	714	94	0.07	0.26	0.9	1	898
20	15	0.5	179	0.6	270	918	154	37	0.08	0.28	0.9	2	899
17	22	2.7	159	1.8	449	744	848	109	0.13	0.25	1.5	68	900
3	23	8.6	81	2.0	402	951	888	89	0.09	0.03	0.6	2	901
0	2	0.0	10	0.5	154	636	0	0	0.02	0.03	0.7	1	902
5	9	0.7	15	1.1	100	952	630	63	0.07	0.06	1.1	TR	903
7	9	0.7	17	0.8	55	1,106	711	72	0.05	0.06	1.4	TR	904
7	7	0.7	17	0.7	101	815	660	65	0.02	0.02	1.1	TR	905
2	12	1.5	27	1.6	188	578	964	98	0.03	0.04	0.8	4	906
10	9	0.2	34	0.6	88	986	561	56	0.03	0.06	0.8	TR	907
2	9	0.5	46	0.5	100	881	0	0	0.05	0.09	0.7	1	908
2	11	1.0	34	0.9	313	911	2,338	234	0.05	0.04	0.9	1	909
0	27	2.8	28	2.0	190	918	203	20	0.11	0.07	1.2	2	910
0	17	0.5	12	1.8	264	695	688	68	0.09	0.05	1.4	66	911

Food No.	Food Description	Measure of Edible Portion	Weight (g)	Water (%)	Calories (kcal)	Protein (g)	Total Fat (g)	Fatty Acids Saturated (g)	Mono-unsaturated (g)	Poly-unsaturated (g)
SOUPS, SAUCES, AND GRAVIES (CONTINUED)										
912	VEGETABLE BEEF	1 CUP	244	92	78	6	2	0.9	0.8	0.1
913	VEGETARIAN VEGETABLE	1 CUP	241	92	72	2	2	0.3	0.8	0.7
	CANNED, READY TO SERVE, CHUNKY									
914	BEAN WITH HAM	1 CUP	243	79	231	13	9	3.3	3.8	0.9
915	CHICKEN NOODLE	1 CUP	240	84	175	13	6	1.4	2.7	1.5
916	CHICKEN AND VEGETABLE	1 CUP	240	83	166	12	5	1.4	2.2	1.0
917	VEGETABLE	1 CUP	240	88	122	4	4	0.6	1.6	1.4
	CANNED, READY TO SERVE, LOW FAT, REDUCED SODIUM									
918	CHICKEN BROTH	1 CUP	240	97	17	3	0	0.0	0.0	0.0
919	CHICKEN NOODLE	1 CUP	237	92	76	6	2	0.4	0.6	0.4
920	CHICKEN AND RICE	1 CUP	241	88	116	7	3	0.9	1.3	0.7
921	CHICKEN AND RICE WITH VEGETABLES	1 CUP	239	91	88	6	1	0.4	0.5	0.5
922	CLAM CHOWDER, NEW ENGLAND	1 CUP	244	89	117	5	2	0.5	0.7	0.4
923	LENTIL	1 CUP	242	88	126	8	2	0.3	0.8	0.2
924	MINESTRONE	1 CUP	241	87	123	5	3	0.4	0.9	1.0
925	VEGETABLE	1 CUP	238	91	81	4	1	0.3	0.4	0.3
	DEHYDRATED UNPREPARED									
926	BEEF BOUILLON	1 PACKET	6	3	14	1	1	0.3	0.2	TR
927	ONION	1 PACKET	39	4	115	5	2	0.5	1.4	0.3
	PREPARED WITH WATER									
928	CHICKEN NOODLE	1 CUP	252	94	58	2	1	0.3	0.5	0.4
929	ONION	1 CUP	246	96	27	1	1	0.1	0.3	0.1
	HOME PREPARED, STOCK									
930	BEEF	1 CUP	240	96	31	5	TR	0.1	0.1	TR
931	CHICKEN	1 CUP	240	92	86	6	3	0.8	1.4	0.5
932	FISH	1 CUP	233	97	40	5	2	0.5	0.5	0.3
	SAUCES HOME RECIPE									
933	CHEESE	1 CUP	243	67	479	25	36	19.5	11.5	3.4
934	WHITE, MEDIUM, MADE WITH WHOLE MILK	1 CUP	250	75	368	10	27	7.1	11.1	7.2
	READY TO SERVE									
935	BARBECUE	1 TBSP	16	81	12	TR	TR	TR	0.1	0.1
936	CHEESE	1/4 CUP	63	71	110	4	8	3.8	2.4	1.6
937	HOISIN	1 TBSP	16	44	35	1	1	0.1	0.2	0.3
938	NACHO CHEESE	1/4 CUP	63	70	119	5	10	4.2	3.1	2.1
939	PEPPER OR HOT	1 TSP	5	90	1	TR	TR	TR	TR	TR
940	SALSA	1 TBSP	16	90	4	TR	TR	TR	TR	TR
941	SOY	1 TBSP	16	69	9	1	TR	TR	TR	TR
942	SPAGHETTI/MARINARA/PASTA	1 CUP	250	87	143	4	5	0.7	2.2	1.8
943	TERIYAKI	1 TBSP	18	68	15	1	0	0.0	0.0	0.0
944	TOMATO CHILI	1/4 CUP	68	68	71	2	TR	TR	TR	0.1
945	WORCESTERSHIRE	1 TBSP	17	70	11	0	0	0.0	0.0	0.0
	GRAVIES, CANNED									
946	BEEF	1/4 CUP	58	87	31	2	1	0.7	0.6	TR
947	CHICKEN	1/4 CUP	60	85	47	1	3	0.8	1.5	0.9
948	COUNTRY SAUSAGE	1/4 CUP	62	75	96	3	8	2.0	2.9	2.2
949	MUSHROOM	1/4 CUP	60	89	30	1	2	0.2	0.7	0.6
950	TURKEY	1/4 CUP	60	89	31	2	1	0.4	0.5	0.3

Cholesterol (mg)	Carbo-hydrate (g)	Total Dietary Fiber (g)	Calcium (mg)	Iron (mg)	Potassium (mg)	Sodium (mg)	Vitamin A (IU)	Vitamin A (RE)	Thiamine (mg)	Ribo-flavin (mg)	Niacin (mg)	Ascorbic Acid (mg)	Food No.
5	10	0.5	17	1.1	173	791	1,891	190	0.04	0.05	1.0	2	912
0	12	0.5	22	1.1	210	822	3,005	301	0.05	0.05	0.9	1	913
22	27	11.2	78	3.2	425	972	3,951	396	0.15	0.15	1.7	4	914
19	17	3.8	24	1.4	108	850	1,222	122	0.07	0.17	4.3	0	915
17	19	NA	26	1.5	367	1,068	5,990	600	0.04	0.17	3.3	6	916
0	19	1.2	55	1.6	396	1,010	5,878	588	0.07	0.06	1.2	6	917
0	1	0.0	19	0.6	204	554	0	0	TR	0.03	1.6	1	918
19	9	1.2	19	1.1	209	460	920	95	0.11	0.11	3.4	1	919
14	14	0.7	22	1.0	422	482	2,010	202	0.05	0.13	5.0	2	920
17	12	0.7	24	1.2	275	459	1,644	165	0.12	0.07	2.6	1	921
5	20	1.2	17	0.9	283	529	244	59	0.05	0.09	0.9	5	922
0	20	5.6	41	2.7	336	443	951	94	0.11	0.09	0.7	1	923
0	20	1.2	39	1.7	306	470	1,357	135	0.15	0.08	1.0	1	924
5	13	1.4	31	1.5	290	466	3,196	319	0.08	0.07	1.8	1	925
1	1	0.0	4	0.1	27	1,019	3	TR	TR	0.01	0.3	0	926
2	21	4.1	55	0.6	260	3,493	8	1	0.11	0.24	2.0	1	927
10	9	0.3	5	0.5	33	578	15	5	0.20	0.08	1.1	0	928
0	5	1.0	12	0.1	64	849	2	0	0.03	0.06	0.5	TR	929
0	3	0.0	19	0.6	444	475	0	0	0.08	0.22	2.1	0	930
7	8	0.0	7	0.5	252	343	0	0	0.08	0.20	3.8	TR	931
2	0	0.0	7	TR	336	363	0	0	0.08	0.18	2.8	TR	932
92	13	0.2	756	0.9	345	1,198	1,473	389	0.11	0.59	0.5	1	933
18	23	0.5	295	0.8	390	885	1,383	138	0.17	0.46	1.0	2	934
0	2	0.2	3	0.1	28	130	139	14	TR	TR	0.1	1	935
18	4	0.3	116	0.1	19	522	199	40	TR	0.07	TR	TR	936
TR	7	0.4	5	0.2	19	258	2	TR	TR	0.03	0.2	TR	937
20	3	0.5	118	0.2	20	492	128	32	TR	0.08	TR	TR	938
0	TR	0.1	TR	TR	7	124	14	1	TR	TR	TR	4	939
0	1	0.3	5	0.2	34	69	96	10	0.01	0.01	0.1	2	940
0	1	0.1	3	0.3	64	871	0	0	0.01	0.03	0.4	0	941
0	21	4.0	55	1.8	738	1,030	938	95	0.14	0.10	2.7	20	942
0	3	TR	5	0.3	41	690	0	0	0.01	0.01	0.2	0	943
0	17	4.0	14	0.5	252	910	462	46	0.06	0.05	1.1	11	944
0	3	0.0	18	0.9	136	167	18	2	0.01	0.02	0.1	2	945
2	3	0.2	3	0.4	47	325	0	0	0.02	0.02	0.4	0	946
1	3	0.2	12	0.3	65	346	221	67	0.01	0.03	0.3	0	947
13	4	0.4	4	0.3	48	236	0	0	0.10	0.04	0.7	TR	948
0	3	0.2	4	0.4	64	342	0	0	0.02	0.04	0.4	0	949
1	3	0.2	2	0.4	65	346	0	0	0.01	0.05	0.8	0	950

Food No.	Food Description	Measure of Edible Portion	Weight (g)	Water (%)	Calories (kcal)	Protein (g)	Total Fat (g)	Fatty Acids Saturated (g)	Mono-unsaturated (g)	Poly-unsaturated (g)
SUGARS AND SWEETS										
	CANDY									
951	BUTTERFINGER									
	(NESTLE)	1 FUN SIZE BAR	7	2	34	1	1	0.7	0.4	0.2
	CARAMEL									
952	PLAIN	1 PIECE	10	9	39	TR	1	0.7	0.1	TR
953	CHOCOLATE-FLAVORED ROLL	1 PIECE	7	7	25	TR	TR	TR	0.1	0.1
954	CAROB	1 OZ	28	2	153	2	9	8.2	0.1	0.1
	CHOCOLATE, MILK									
955	PLAIN	1 BAR (1.55 OZ)	44	1	226	3	14	8.1	4.4	0.5
956	WITH ALMONDS	1 BAR (1.45 OZ)	41	2	216	4	14	7.0	5.5	0.9
957	WITH PEANUTS, MR. GOODBAR									
	(HERSHEY)	1 BAR (1.75 OZ)	49	1	267	5	17	7.3	5.7	2.4
958	WITH RICE CEREAL, NESTLÉ CRUNCH	1 BAR (1.55 OZ)	44	1	230	3	12	6.7	3.8	0.4
	CHOCOLATE CHIPS									
959	MILK	1 CUP	168	1	862	12	52	31.0	16.7	1.8
960	SEMISWEET	1 CUP	168	1	805	7	50	29.8	16.7	1.6
961	WHITE	1 CUP	170	1	916	10	55	33.0	15.5	1.7
962	CHOCOLATE COATED PEANUTS	10 PIECES	40	2	208	5	13	5.8	5.2	1.7
963	CHOCOLATE COATED RAISINS	10 PIECES	10	11	39	TR	1	0.9	0.5	0.1
964	FRUIT LEATHER, PIECES	1 OZ	28	12	97	TR	2	0.3	0.9	0.8
965	FRUIT LEATHER, ROLLS	1 LARGE	21	11	74	TR	1	0.1	0.3	0.1
966	FUDGE, PREPARED	1 SMALL	14	11	49	TR	TR	0.1	0.2	0.1
	FROM RECIPE									
	CHOCOLATE									
967	PLAIN	1 PIECE	17	10	65	TR	1	0.9	0.4	0.1
968	WITH NUTS	1 PIECE	19	7	81	1	3	1.1	0.8	1.0
	VANILLA									
969	PLAIN	1 PIECE	16	11	59	TR	1	0.5	0.2	TR
970	WITH NUTS	1 PIECE	15	8	62	TR	2	0.6	0.5	0.8
	GUMDROPS/GUMMY CANDIES									
971	GUMDROPS (3/4″ DIA)	1 CUP	182	1	703	0	0	0.0	0.0	0.0
972		1 MEDIUM	4	1	16	0	0	0.0	0.0	0.0
973	GUMMY BEARS	10 BEARS	22	1	85	0	0	0.0	0.0	0.0
974	GUMMY WORMS	10 WORMS	74	1	286	0	0	0.0	0.0	0.0
975	HARD CANDY	1 PIECE	6	1	24	0	TR	0.0	0.0	0.0
976		1 SMALL PIECE	3	1	12	0	TR	0.0	0.0	0.0
977	JELLY BEANS	10 LARGE	28	6	104	0	TR	TR	0.1	TR
978		10 SMALL	11	6	40	0	TR	TR	TR	TR
979	KIT KAT (HERSHEY)	1 BAR (1.5 OZ)	42	2	216	3	11	6.8	3.1	0.3
	MARSHMALLOWS									
980	MINIATURE	1 CUP	50	16	159	1	TR	TR	TR	TR
981	REGULAR	1 REGULAR	7	16	23	TR	TR	TR	TR	TR
	M&M'S (M&M MARS)									
982	PEANUT	1/4 CUP	43	2	222	4	11	4.4	4.7	1.8
983		10 PIECES	20	2	103	2	5	2.1	2.2	0.8
984	PLAIN	1/4 CUP	52	2	256	2	11	6.8	3.6	0.3
985		10 PIECES	7	2	34	TR	1	0.9	0.5	TR
986	MILKY WAY									
	(M&M MARS)	1 FUN SIZE BAR	18	6	76	1	3	1.4	1.1	0.1
987		1 BAR (2.15 OZ)	61	6	258	3	10	4.8	3.7	0.4
988	REESE'S PEANUT BUTTER CUP									
	(HERSHEY)	1 MINIATURE CUP	7	2	38	1	2	0.8	0.9	0.4

Cholesterol (mg)	Carbo-hydrate (g)	Total Dietary Fiber (g)	Calcium (mg)	Iron (mg)	Potassium (mg)	Sodium (mg)	Vitamin A (IU)	Vitamin A (RE)	Thiamine (mg)	Ribo-flavin (mg)	Niacin (mg)	Ascorbic Acid (mg)	Food No.
TR	5	0.2	2	0.1	27	14	0	0	0.01	TR	0.2	0	951
1	8	0.1	14	TR	22	25	3	1	TR	0.02	TR	TR	952
0	6	TR	2	TR	7	6	1	TR	TR	0.01	TR	TR	953
1	16	1.1	86	0.4	179	30	7	2	0.03	0.05	0.3	TR	954
10	26	1.5	84	0.6	169	36	81	24	0.03	0.13	0.1	TR	955
8	22	2.5	92	0.7	182	30	30	6	0.02	0.18	0.3	TR	956
4	25	1.7	53	0.6	219	73	70	18	0.08	0.12	1.6	TR	957
6	29	1.1	74	0.2	151	59	30	9	0.15	0.25	1.7	TR	958
37	99	5.7	321	2.3	647	138	311	92	0.13	0.51	0.5	1	959
0	106	9.9	54	5.3	613	18	35	3	0.09	0.15	0.7	0	960
36	101	0.0	338	0.4	486	153	60	2	0.11	0.48	1.3	1	961
4	20	1.9	42	0.5	201	16	0	0	0.05	0.07	1.7	0	962
TR	7	0.4	9	0.2	51	4	4	1	0.01	0.02	TR	TR	963
0	22	1.0	5	0.2	46	114	33	3	0.01	0.03	TR	16	964
0	18	0.8	7	0.2	62	13	24	3	0.01	TR	TR	1	965
0	12	0.5	4	0.1	41	9	16	2	0.01	TR	TR	1	966
2	14	0.1	7	0.1	18	11	32	8	TR	0.01	TR	TR	967
3	14	0.2	10	0.1	30	11	38	9	0.01	0.02	TR	TR	968
3	13	0.0	6	TR	8	11	33	8	TR	0.01	TR	TR	969
2	11	0.1	7	0.1	17	9	30	7	0.01	0.01	TR	TR	970
0	180	0.0	5	0.7	9	80	0	0	0.00	TR	TR	0	971
0	4	0.0	TR	TR	TR	2	0	0	0.00	TR	TR	0	972
0	22	0.0	1	0.1	1	10	0	0	0.00	TR	TR	0	973
0	73	0.0	2	0.3	4	33	0	0	0.00	TR	TR	0	974
0	6	0.0	TR	TR	TR	2	0	0	TR	TR	TR	0	975
0	3	0.0	TR	TR	TR	1	0	0	TR	TR	TR	0	976
0	26	0.0	1	0.3	10	7	0	0	0.00	0.00	0.0	0	977
0	10	0.0	TR	0.1	4	3	0	0	0.00	0.00	0.0	0	978
3	27	0.8	69	0.4	122	32	68	20	0.07	0.23	1.1	TR	979
0	41	0.1	2	0.1	3	24	1	0	TR	TR	TR	0	980
0	6	TR	TR	TR	TR	3	TR	0	TR	TR	TR	0	981
4	26	1.5	43	0.5	149	21	40	10	0.04	0.07	1.6	TR	982
2	12	0.7	20	0.2	69	10	19	5	0.02	0.03	0.7	TR	983
7	37	1.3	55	0.6	138	32	106	28	0.03	0.11	0.1	TR	984
1	5	0.2	7	0.1	19	4	14	4	TR	0.01	TR	TR	985
3	13	0.3	23	0.1	43	43	19	6	0.01	0.04	0.1	TR	986
9	44	1.0	79	0.5	147	146	66	20	0.02	0.14	0.2	1	987
TR	4	0.2	5	0.1	25	22	5	1	0.02	0.01	0.3	TR	988

Food No.	Food Description	Measure of Edible Portion	Weight (g)	Water (%)	Calories (kcal)	Protein (g)	Total Fat (g)	Fatty Acids Satu-rated (g)	Mono-unsatu-rated (g)	Poly-unsatu-rated (g)
SUGARS AND SWEETS (CONTINUED)										
989		1 PACKAGE (CONTAINS 2)	45	2	243	5	14	5.0	5.9	2.5
990	SNICKERS BAR (M&M MARS)	1 FUN SIZE BAR	15	5	72	1	4	1.3	1.6	0.7
991		1 KING SIZE BAR (4 OZ)	113	5	541	9	28	10.2	11.8	5.6
992		1 BAR (2 OZ)	57	5	273	5	14	5.1	6.0	2.8
993	SPECIAL DARK SWEET CHOCOLATE (HERSHEY)	1 MINIATURE	8	1	46	TR	3	1.7	0.9	0.1
994	STARBURST FRUIT CHEWS (M&M MARS)	1 PIECE	5	7	20	TR	TR	0.1	0.2	0.2
995		1 PACKAGE (2.07 OZ)	59	7	234	TR	5	0.7	2.1	1.8
	FROSTING, READY TO EAT									
996	CHOCOLATE	1/12 PACKAGE	38	17	151	TR	7	2.1	3.4	0.8
997	VANILLA	1/12 PACKAGE	38	13	159	TR	6	1.9	3.3	0.9
	FROZEN DESSERTS (NONDAIRY)									
998	FRUIT AND JUICE BAR	1 BAR (2.5 FL OZ)	77	78	63	1	TR	0.0	0.0	TR
999	ICE POP	1 BAR (2 FL OZ)	59	80	42	0	0	0.0	0.0	0.0
1000	ITALIAN ICES	1/2 CUP	116	86	61	TR	TR	0.0	0.0	0.0
1001	FRUIT BUTTER, APPLE	1 TBSP	17	56	29	TR	0	0.0	0.0	0.0
	GELATIN DESSERT, PREPARED WITH GELATIN DESSERT POWDER AND WATER									
1002	REGULAR	1/2 CUP	135	85	80	2	0	0.0	0.0	0.0
1003	REDUCED CALORIE (WITH ASPARTAME)	1/2 CUP	117	98	8	1	0	0.0	0.0	0.0
1004	HONEY, STRAINED OR EXTRACTED	1 TBSP	21	17	64	TR	0	0.0	0.0	0.0
1005		1 CUP	339	17	1,031	1	0	0.0	0.0	0.0
1006	JAMS AND PRESERVES	1 TBSP	20	30	56	TR	TR	TR	TR	0.0
1007		1 PACKET (0.5 OZ)	14	30	39	TR	TR	TR	TR	0.0
1008	JELLIES	1 TBSP	19	29	54	TR	TR	TR	TR	TR
1009		1 PACKET (0.5 OZ)	14	29	40	TR	TR	TR	TR	TR
	PUDDINGS									
	PREPARED WITH DRY MIX AND 2% MILK									
	CHOCOLATE									
1010	INSTANT	1/2 CUP	147	75	150	5	3	1.6	0.9	0.2
1011	REGULAR (COOKED)	1/2 CUP	142	74	151	5	3	1.8	0.8	0.1
	VANILLA									
1012	INSTANT	1/2 CUP	142	75	148	4	2	1.4	0.7	0.1
1013	REGULAR (COOKED)	1/2 CUP	140	76	141	4	2	1.5	0.7	0.1
	READY TO EAT									
	REGULAR									
1014	CHOCOLATE	4 OZ	113	69	150	3	5	0.8	1.9	1.6
1015	RICE	4 OZ	113	68	184	2	8	1.3	3.6	3.2
1016	TAPIOCA	4 OZ	113	74	134	2	4	0.7	1.8	1.5
1017	VANILLA	4 OZ	113	71	147	3	4	0.6	1.7	1.5
	FAT FREE									
1018	CHOCOLATE	4 OZ	113	76	107	3	TR	0.3	0.1	TR
1019	TAPIOCA	4 OZ	113	77	98	2	TR	0.1	TR	TR
1020	VANILLA	4 OZ	113	76	105	2	TR	0.1	TR	TR

Cholesterol (mg)	Carbo-hydrate (g)	Total Dietary Fiber (g)	Calcium (mg)	Iron (mg)	Potassium (mg)	Sodium (mg)	Vitamin A (IU)	(RE)	Thiamine (mg)	Ribo-flavin (mg)	Niacin (mg)	Ascorbic Acid (mg)	Food No.
2	25	1.4	35	0.5	158	143	33	9	0.11	0.08	2.1	TR	989
2	9	0.4	14	0.1	49	40	23	6	0.01	0.02	0.6	TR	990
15	67	2.8	106	0.9	366	301	172	44	0.11	0.17	4.7	1	991
7	34	1.4	54	0.4	185	152	87	22	0.06	0.09	2.4	TR	992
TR	5	0.4	2	0.2	25	1	3	TR	TR	0.01	TR	0	993
0	4	0.0	TR	TR	TR	3	0	0	TR	TR	TR	3	994
0	50	0.0	2	0.1	1	33	0	0	TR	TR	TR	31	995
0	24	0.2	3	0.5	74	70	249	75	TR	0.01	TR	0	996
0	26	TR	1	TR	14	34	283	86	0.00	TR	TR	0	997
0	16	0.0	4	0.1	41	3	22	2	0.01	0.01	0.1	7	998
0	11	0.0	0	0.0	2	7	0	0	0.00	0.00	0.0	0	999
0	16	0.0	1	0.1	7	5	194	0	0.01	0.01	0.8	1	1000
0	7	0.3	2	0.1	15	1	20	2	TR	TR	TR	TR	1001
0	19	0.0	3	TR	1	57	0	0	0.00	TR	TR	0	1002
0	1	0.0	2	TR	0	56	0	0	0.00	TR	TR	0	1003
0	17	TR	1	0.1	11	1	0	0	0.00	0.01	TR	TR	1004
0	279	0.7	20	1.4	176	14	0	0	0.00	0.13	0.4	2	1005
0	14	0.2	4	0.1	15	6	2	TR	0.00	TR	TR	2	1006
0	10	0.2	3	0.1	11	4	2	TR	0.00	TR	TR	1	1007
0	13	0.2	2	TR	12	5	3	TR	TR	TR	TR	TR	1008
0	10	0.1	1	TR	9	4	2	TR	TR	TR	TR	TR	1009
9	28	0.6	153	0.4	247	417	253	56	0.05	0.21	0.1	1	1010
10	28	0.4	160	0.5	240	149	253	68	0.05	0.21	0.2	1	1011
9	28	0.0	146	0.1	185	406	241	64	0.05	0.20	0.1	1	1012
10	26	0.0	153	0.1	193	224	252	70	0.04	0.20	0.1	1	1013
3	26	1.1	102	0.6	203	146	41	12	0.03	0.18	0.4	2	1014
1	25	0.1	59	0.3	68	96	129	40	0.02	0.08	0.2	1	1015
1	22	0.1	95	0.3	110	180	0	0	0.02	0.11	0.4	1	1016
8	25	0.1	99	0.1	128	153	24	7	0.02	0.16	0.3	0	1017
2	23	0.9	89	0.6	235	192	174	52	0.02	0.12	0.1	TR	1018
1	23	0.1	76	0.2	99	251	121	36	0.02	0.09	0.1	TR	1019
1	24	0.1	86	TR	123	241	174	52	0.02	0.10	0.1	TR	1020

Food No.	Food Description	Measure of Edible Portion	Weight (g)	Water (%)	Calories (kcal)	Protein (g)	Total Fat (g)	Fatty Acids Saturated (g)	Fatty Acids Mono-unsaturated (g)	Fatty Acids Poly-unsaturated (g)
SUGARS AND SWEETS (CONTINUED)										
	SUGAR									
	BROWN									
1021	PACKED	1 CUP	220	2	827	0	0	0.0	0.0	0.0
1022	UNPACKED	1 CUP	145	2	545	0	0	0.0	0.0	0.0
1023		1 TBSP	9	2	34	0	0	0.0	0.0	0.0
	WHITE									
1024	GRANULATED	1 PACKET	6	0	23	0	0	0.0	0.0	0.0
1025		1 TSP	4	0	16	0	0	0.0	0.0	0.0
1026		1 CUP	200	0	774	0	0	0.0	0.0	0.0
1027	POWDERED, UNSIFTED	1 TBSP	8	TR	31	0	TR	TR	TR	TR
1028		1 CUP	120	TR	467	0	TR	TR	TR	0.1
	SYRUP									
	CHOCOLATE-FLAVORED SYRUP OR TOPPING									
1029	THIN TYPE	1 TBSP	19	31	53	TR	TR	0.1	0.1	TR
1030	FUDGE TYPE	1 TBSP	19	22	67	1	2	0.8	0.7	0.1
1031	CORN, LIGHT	1 TBSP	20	23	56	0	0	0.0	0.0	0.0
1032	MAPLE	1 TBSP	20	32	52	0	TR	TR	TR	TR
1033	MOLASSES, BLACKSTRAP	1 TBSP	20	29	47	0	0	0.0	0.0	0.0
1034		1 CUP	328	29	771	0	0	0.0	0.0	0.0
	TABLE BLEND, PANCAKE									
1035	REGULAR	1 TBSP	20	24	57	0	0	0.0	0.0	0.0
1036	REDUCED CALORIE	1 TBSP	15	55	25	0	0	0.0	0.0	0.0
VEGETABLES AND VEGETABLE PRODUCTS										
1037	ALFALFA SPROUTS, RAW	1 CUP	33	91	10	1	TR	TR	TR	0.1
1038	ARTICHOKES, GLOBE OR FRENCH, COOKED, DRAINED	1 CUP	168	84	84	6	TR	0.1	TR	0.1
1039		1 MEDIUM	120	84	60	4	TR	TR	TR	0.1
	ASPARAGUS, GREEN									
	COOKED, DRAINED									
1040	FROM RAW	1 CUP	180	92	43	5	1	0.1	TR	0.2
1041		4 SPEARS	60	92	14	2	TR	TR	TR	0.1
1042	FROM FROZEN	1 CUP	180	91	50	5	1	0.2	TR	0.3
1043		4 SPEARS	60	91	17	2	TR	0.1	TR	0.1
1044	CANNED, SPEARS, ABOUT 5″ LONG, DRAINED	1 CUP	242	94	46	5	2	0.4	0.1	0.7
1045		4 SPEARS	72	94	14	2	TR	0.1	TR	0.2
1046	BAMBOO SHOOTS, CANNED, DRAINED	1 CUP	131	94	25	2	1	0.1	TR	0.2
	BEANS									
	LIMA, IMMATURE SEEDS, FROZEN, COOKED, DRAINED									
1047	FORD HOOKS	1 CUP	170	74	170	10	1	0.1	TR	0.3
1048	BABY LIMAS	1 CUP	180	72	189	12	1	0.1	TR	0.3
	SNAP, CUT									
	COOKED, DRAINED									
	FROM RAW									
1049	GREEN	1 CUP	125	89	44	2	TR	0.1	TR	0.2
1050	YELLOW	1 CUP	125	89	44	2	TR	0.1	TR	0.2
	FROM FROZEN									
1051	GREEN	1 CUP	135	91	38	2	TR	0.1	TR	0.1
1052	YELLOW	1 CUP	135	91	38	2	TR	0.1	TR	0.1
	CANNED, DRAINED									

Cholesterol (mg)	Carbo-hydrate (g)	Total Dietary Fiber (g)	Calcium (mg)	Iron (mg)	Potassium (mg)	Sodium (mg)	Vitamin A (IU)	(RE)	Thiamine (mg)	Ribo-flavin (mg)	Niacin (mg)	Ascorbic Acid (mg)	Food No.
0	214	0.0	187	4.2	761	86	0	0	0.02	0.02	0.2	0	1021
0	141	0.0	123	2.8	502	57	0	0	0.01	0.01	0.1	0	1022
0	9	0.0	8	0.2	31	4	0	0	TR	TR	TR	0	1023
0	6	0.0	TR	TR	TR	TR	0	0	0.00	TR	0.0	0	1024
0	4	0.0	TR	TR	TR	TR	0	0	0.00	TR	0.0	0	1025
0	200	0.0	2	0.1	4	2	0	0	0.00	0.04	0.0	0	1026
0	8	0.0	TR	TR	TR	TR	0	0	0.00	0.00	0.0	0	1027
0	119	0.0	1	0.1	2	1	0	0	0.00	0.00	0.0	0	1028
0	12	0.3	3	0.4	43	14	6	1	TR	0.01	0.1	TR	1029
TR	12	0.5	15	0.2	69	66	3	1	0.01	0.04	0.1	TR	1030
0	15	0.0	1	TR	1	24	0	0	TR	TR	TR	0	1031
U	13	0.0	13	0.2	41	2	0	0	TR	TR	TR	0	1032
0	12	0.0	172	3.5	498	11	0	0	0.01	0.01	0.2	0	1033
0	199	0.0	2,821	57.4	8,174	180	0	0	0.11	0.17	3.5	0	1034
0	15	0.0	TR	TR	TR	17	0	0	TR	TR	TR	0	1035
0	7	0.0	TR	TR	TR	30	0	0	TR	TR	TR	0	1036
0	1	0.8	11	0.3	26	2	51	5	0.03	0.04	0.2	3	1037
0	19	9.1	76	2.2	595	160	297	30	0.11	0.11	1.7	17	1038
0	13	6.5	54	1.5	425	114	212	22	0.08	0.08	1.2	12	1039
0	8	2.9	36	1.3	288	20	970	97	0.22	0.23	1.9	19	1040
0	3	1.0	12	0.4	96	7	323	32	0.07	0.08	0.6	6	1041
0	9	2.9	41	1.2	392	7	1,472	148	0.12	0.19	1.9	44	1042
0	3	1.0	14	0.4	131	2	491	49	0.04	0.06	0.6	15	1043
0	6	3.9	39	4.4	416	695	1,285	128	0.15	0.24	2.3	45	1044
0	2	1.2	12	1.3	124	207	382	38	0.04	0.07	0.7	13	1045
0	4	1.8	10	0.4	105	9	10	1	0.03	0.03	0.2	1	1046
0	32	9.9	37	2.3	694	90	323	32	0.13	0.10	1.8	22	1047
0	35	10.8	50	3.5	740	52	301	31	0.13	0.10	1.4	10	1048
0	10	4.0	58	1.6	374	4	833	84	0.09	0.12	0.8	12	1049
0	10	4.1	58	1.6	374	4	101	10	0.09	0.12	0.8	12	1050
0	9	4.1	66	1.2	170	12	541	54	0.05	0.12	0.5	6	1051
0	9	4.1	66	1.2	170	12	151	15	0.05	0.12	0.5	6	1052

Food No.	Food Description	Measure of Edible Portion	Weight (g)	Water (%)	Calories (kcal)	Protein (g)	Total Fat (g)	Fatty Acids Saturated (g)	Fatty Acids Mono-unsaturated (g)	Fatty Acids Poly-unsaturated (g)
VEGETABLES AND VEGETABLE PRODUCTS (CONTINUED)										
1053	GREEN	1 CUP	135	93	27	2	TR	TR	TR	0.1
1054	YELLOW	1 CUP	135	93	27	2	TR	TR	TR	0.1
	BEANS, DRY. SEE LEGUMES.									
	BEAN SPROUTS (MUNG)									
1055	RAW	1 CUP	104	90	31	3	TR	TR	TR	0.1
1056	COOKED, DRAINED	1 CUP	124	93	26	3	TR	TR	TR	TR
	BEETS									
	COOKED, DRAINED									
1057	SLICES	1 CUP	170	87	75	3	TR	TR	0.1	0.1
1058	WHOLE BEET, 2″ DIA	1 BEET	50	87	22	1	TR	TR	TR	TR
	CANNED, DRAINED									
1059	SLICES	1 CUP	170	91	53	2	TR	TR	TR	0.1
1060	WHOLE BEET	1 BEET	24	91	7	TR	TR	TR	TR	TR
1061	BEET GREENS, LEAVES AND STEMS, COOKED, DRAINED, 1″ PIECES	1 CUP	144	89	39	4	TR	TR	0.1	0.1
	BLACK-EYED PEAS, IMMATURE SEEDS, COOKED, DRAINED									
1062	FROM RAW	1 CUP	165	75	160	5	1	0.2	0.1	0.3
1063	FROM FROZEN	1 CUP	170	66	224	14	1	0.3	0.1	0.5
	BROCCOLI									
	RAW									
1064	CHOPPED OR DICED	1 CUP	88	91	25	3	TR	TR	TR	0.1
1065	SPEAR, ABOUT 5″ LONG	1 SPEAR	31	91	9	1	TR	TR	TR	0.1
1066	FLOWER CLUSTER	1 FLOWERET	11	91	3	TR	TR	TR	TR	TR
	COOKED, DRAINED									
	FROM RAW									
1067	CHOPPED	1 CUP	156	91	44	5	1	0.1	TR	0.3
1068	SPEAR, ABOUT 5″ LONG	1 SPEAR	37	91	10	1	TR	TR	TR	0.1
1069	FROM FROZEN, CHOPPED	1 CUP	184	91	52	6	TR	TR	TR	0.1
	BRUSSELS SPROUTS, COOKED, DRAINED									
1070	FROM RAW	1 CUP	156	87	61	4	1	0.2	0.1	0.4
1071	FROM FROZEN	1 CUP	155	87	65	6	1	0.1	TR	0.3
	CABBAGE, COMMON VARIETIES, SHREDDED									
1072	RAW	1 CUP	70	92	18	1	TR	TR	TR	0.1
1073	COOKED, DRAINED	1 CUP	150	94	33	2	1	0.1	TR	0.3
	CABBAGE, CHINESE, SHREDDED, COOKED, DRAINED									
1074	PAK CHOI OR BOK CHOY	1 CUP	170	96	20	3	TR	TR	TR	0.1
1075	PE TSAI	1 CUP	119	95	17	2	TR	TR	TR	0.1
1076	CABBAGE, RED, RAW, SHREDDED	1 CUP	70	92	19	1	TR	TR	TR	0.1
1077	CABBAGE, SAVOY, RAW, SHREDDED	1 CUP	70	91	19	1	TR	TR	TR	TR
1078	CARROT JUICE, CANNED	1 CUP	236	89	94	2	TR	0.1	TR	0.2
	CARROTS									
	RAW									
1079	WHOLE, 7 1/2″ LONG	1 CARROT	72	88	31	1	TR	TR	TR	0.1
1080	GRATED	1 CUP	110	88	47	1	TR	TR	TR	0.1
1081	BABY	1 MEDIUM	10	90	4	TR	TR	TR	TR	TR
	COOKED, SLICED, DRAINED									
1082	FROM RAW	1 CUP	156	87	70	2	TR	0.1	TR	0.1
1083	FROM FROZEN	1 CUP	146	90	53	2	TR	TR	TR	0.1
1084	CANNED, SLICED, DRAINED	1 CUP	146	93	37	1	TR	0.1	TR	0.1

Cholesterol (mg)	Carbo-hydrate (g)	Total Dietary Fiber (g)	Calcium (mg)	Iron (mg)	Potassium (mg)	Sodium (mg)	Vitamin A (IU)	(RE)	Thiamine (mg)	Ribo-flavin (mg)	Niacin (mg)	Ascorbic Acid (mg)	Food No.
0	6	2.6	35	1.2	147	354	471	47	0.02	0.08	0.3	6	1053
0	6	1.8	35	1.2	147	339	142	15	0.02	0.08	0.3	6	1054
0	6	1.9	14	0.9	155	6	22	2	0.09	0.13	0.8	14	1055
0	5	1.5	15	0.8	125	12	17	1	0.06	0.13	1.0	14	1056
0	17	3.4	27	1.3	519	131	60	7	0.05	0.07	0.6	6	1057
0	5	1.0	8	0.4	153	39	18	2	0.01	0.02	0.2	2	1058
0	12	2.9	26	3.1	252	330	19	2	0.02	0.07	0.3	7	1059
0	2	0.4	4	0.4	36	47	3	TR	TR	0.01	TR	1	1060
0	8	4.2	164	2.7	1,309	347	7,344	734	0.17	0.42	0.7	36	1061
0	34	8.3	211	1.8	690	7	1,305	130	0.17	0.24	2.3	4	1062
0	40	10.9	39	3.6	638	9	128	14	0.44	0.11	1.2	4	1063
0	5	2.6	42	0.8	286	24	1,357	136	0.06	0.10	0.6	82	1064
0	2	0.9	15	0.3	101	8	478	48	0.02	0.04	0.2	29	1065
0	1	0.3	5	0.1	36	3	330	33	0.01	0.01	0.1	10	1066
0	8	4.5	72	1.3	456	41	2,165	217	0.09	0.18	0.9	116	1067
0	2	1.1	17	0.3	108	10	514	51	0.02	0.04	0.2	28	1068
0	10	5.5	94	1.1	331	44	3,481	348	0.10	0.15	0.8	74	1069
0	14	4.1	56	1.9	495	33	1,122	112	0.17	0.12	0.9	97	1070
0	13	6.4	37	1.1	504	36	913	91	0.16	0.18	0.8	71	1071
0	4	1.6	33	0.4	172	13	93	9	0.04	0.03	0.2	23	1072
0	7	3.5	47	0.3	146	12	198	20	0.09	0.08	0.4	30	1073
0	3	2.7	158	1.8	631	58	4,366	437	0.05	0.11	0.7	44	1074
0	3	3.2	38	0.4	268	11	1,151	115	0.05	0.05	0.6	19	1075
0	4	1.4	36	0.3	144	8	28	3	0.04	0.02	0.2	40	1076
0	4	2.2	25	0.3	161	20	700	70	0.05	0.02	0.2	22	1077
0	22	1.9	57	1.1	689	68	25,833	2,584	0.22	0.13	0.9	20	1078
0	7	2.2	19	0.4	233	25	20,253	2,025	0.07	0.04	0.7	7	1079
0	11	3.3	30	0.6	355	39	30,942	3,094	0.11	0.06	1.0	10	1080
0	1	0.2	2	0.1	28	4	1,501	150	TR	0.01	0.1	1	1081
0	16	5.1	48	1.0	354	103	38,304	3,830	0.05	0.09	0.8	4	1082
0	12	5.1	41	0.7	231	86	25,845	2,584	0.04	0.05	0.6	4	1083
0	8	2.2	37	0.9	261	353	20,110	2,010	0.03	0.04	0.8	4	1084

Food No.	Food Description	Measure of Edible Portion	Weight (g)	Water (%)	Calories (kcal)	Protein (g)	Total Fat (g)	Saturated (g)	Monounsaturated (g)	Polyunsaturated (g)
								Fatty Acids		
	VEGETABLES AND VEGETABLE PRODUCTS (CONTINUED)									
	CAULIFLOWER									
1085	RAW	1 FLOWERET	13	92	3	TR	TR	TR	TR	TR
1086		1 CUP	100	92	25	2	TR	TR	TR	0.1
	COOKED, DRAINED, 1" PIECES									
1087	FROM RAW	1 CUP	124	93	29	2	1	0.1	TR	0.3
1088		3 FLOWERETS	54	93	12	1	TR	TR	TR	0.1
1089	FROM FROZEN	1 CUP	180	94	34	3	TR	0.1	TR	0.2
	CELERY									
	RAW									
1090	STALK, 7 1/2" TO 8" LONG	1 STALK	40	95	6	TR	TR	TR	TR	TR
1091	PIECES, DICED	1 CUP	120	95	19	1	TR	TR	TR	0.1
	COOKED, DRAINED									
1092	STALK, MEDIUM	1 STALK	38	94	7	TR	TR	TR	TR	TR
1093	PIECES, DICED	1 CUP	150	94	27	1	TR	0.1	TR	0.1
1094	CHIVES, RAW, CHOPPED	1 TBSP	3	91	1	TR	TR	TR	TR	TR
1095	CILANTRO, RAW	1 TSP	2	92	TR	TR	TR	TR	TR	TR
1096	COLESLAW, HOME PREPARED	1 CUP	120	82	83	2	3	0.5	0.8	1.6
	COLLARDS, COOKED, DRAINED, CHOPPED									
1097	FROM RAW	1 CUP	190	92	49	4	1	0.1	TR	0.3
1098	FROM FROZEN	1 CUP	170	88	61	5	1	0.1	TR	0.4
	CORN, SWEET, YELLOW									
	COOKED, DRAINED									
1099	FROM RAW, KERNELS ON COB	1 EAR	77	70	83	3	1	0.2	0.3	0.5
	FROM FROZEN									
1100	KERNELS ON COB	1 EAR	63	73	59	2	TR	0.1	0.1	0.2
1101	KERNELS	1 CUP	164	77	131	5	1	0.1	0.2	0.3
	CANNED									
1102	CREAM STYLE	1 CUP	256	79	184	4	1	0.2	0.3	0.5
1103	WHOLE KERNEL, VACUUM PACK	1 CUP	210	77	166	5	1	0.2	0.3	0.5
1104	CORN, SWEET, WHITE, COOKED, DRAINED	1 EAR	77	70	83	3	1	0.2	0.3	0.5
	CUCUMBER									
	PEELED									
1105	SLICED	1 CUP	119	96	14	1	TR	TR	TR	0.1
1106	WHOLE, 8 1/4" LONG	1 LARGE	280	96	34	2	TR	0.1	TR	0.2
	UNPEELED									
1107	SLICED	1 CUP	104	96	14	1	TR	TR	TR	0.1
1108	WHOLE, 8 1/4" LONG	1 LARGE	301	96	39	2	TR	0.1	TR	0.2
1109	DANDELION GREENS, COOKED, DRAINED	1 CUP	105	90	35	2	1	0.2	TR	0.3
1110	DILL WEED, RAW	5 SPRIGS	1	86	TR	TR	TR	TR	TR	TR
1111	EGGPLANT, COOKED, DRAINED	1 CUP	99	92	28	1	TR	TR	TR	0.1
1112	ENDIVE, CURLY (INCLUDING SCAROLE), RAW, SMALL PIECES	1 CUP	50	94	9	1	TR	TR	TR	TR
1113	GARLIC, RAW	1 CLOVE	3	59	4	TR	TR	TR	TR	TR
1114	HEARTS OF PALM, CANNED	1 PIECE	33	90	9	1	TR	TR	TR	0.1
1115	JERUSALEM ARTICHOKE, RAW, SLICED	1 CUP	150	78	114	3	TR	0.0	TR	TR
	KALE, COOKED, DRAINED, CHOPPED									
1116	FROM RAW	1 CUP	130	91	36	2	1	0.1	TR	0.3
1117	FROM FROZEN	1 CUP	130	91	39	4	1	0.1	TR	0.3
1118	KOHLRABI, COOKED, DRAINED, SLICES	1 CUP	165	90	48	3	TR	TR	TR	0.1
1119	LEEKS, BULB AND LOWER LEAF PORTION, CHOPPED OR DICED, COOKED, DRAINED	1 CUP	104	94	32	1	TR	TR	TR	0.1

*White varieties contain only a trace amount of vitamin A; other nutrients are the same.

Cholesterol (mg)	Carbo-hydrate (g)	Total Dietary Fiber (g)	Calcium (mg)	Iron (mg)	Potassium (mg)	Sodium (mg)	Vitamin A (IU)	Vitamin A (RE)	Thiamine (mg)	Ribo-flavin (mg)	Niacin (mg)	Ascorbic Acid (mg)	Food No.
0	1	0.3	3	0.1	39	4	2	TR	0.01	0.01	0.1	6	1085
0	5	2.5	22	0.4	303	30	19	2	0.06	0.06	0.5	46	1086
0	5	3.3	20	0.4	176	19	21	2	0.05	0.06	0.5	55	1087
0	2	1.5	9	0.2	77	8	9	1	0.02	0.03	0.2	24	1088
0	7	4.9	31	0.7	250	32	40	4	0.07	0.10	0.6	56	1089
0	1	0.7	16	0.2	115	35	54	5	0.02	0.02	0.1	3	1090
0	4	2.0	48	0.5	344	104	161	16	0.06	0.05	0.4	8	1091
0	2	0.6	16	0.2	108	35	50	5	0.02	0.02	0.1	2	1092
0	6	2.4	63	0.6	426	137	198	20	0.06	0.07	0.5	9	1093
0	TR	0.1	3	TR	9	TR	131	13	TR	TR	TR	2	1094
0	TR	TR	1	TR	8	1	98	10	TR	TR	TR	1	1095
10	15	1.8	54	0.7	217	28	762	98	0.08	0.07	0.3	39	1096
0	9	5.3	226	0.9	494	17	5,945	595	0.08	0.20	1.1	35	1097
0	12	4.8	357	1.9	427	85	10,168	1,017	0.08	0.20	1.1	45	1098
0	19	2.2	2	0.5	192	13	167	17	0.17	0.06	1.2	5	1099
0	14	1.8	2	0.4	158	3	133*	13*	0.11	0.04	1.0	3	1100
0	32	3.9	7	0.6	241	8	361*	36*	0.14	0.12	2.1	5	1101
0	46	3.1	8	1.0	343	730	248*	26*	0.06	0.14	2.5	12	1102
0	41	4.2	11	0.9	391	571	506*	50*	0.09	0.15	2.5	17	1103
0	19	2.1	2	0.5	192	13	0	0	0.17	0.06	1.2	5	1104
0	3	0.8	17	0.2	176	2	88	8	0.02	0.01	0.1	3	1105
0	7	2.0	39	0.4	414	6	207	20	0.06	0.03	0.3	8	1106
0	3	0.8	15	0.3	150	2	224	22	0.02	0.02	0.2	6	1107
0	8	2.4	42	0.8	433	6	647	63	0.07	0.07	0.7	16	1108
0	7	3.0	147	1.9	244	46	12,285	1,229	0.14	0.18	0.5	19	1109
0	TR	TR	2	0.1	7	1	77	8	TR	TR	TR	1	1110
0	7	2.5	6	0.3	246	3	63	6	0.08	0.02	0.6	1	1111
0	2	1.6	26	0.4	157	11	1,025	103	0.04	0.04	0.2	3	1112
0	1	0.1	5	0.1	12	1	0	0	0.01	TR	TR	1	1113
0	2	0.8	19	1.0	58	141	0	0	TR	0.02	0.1	3	1114
0	26	2.4	21	5.1	644	6	30	3	0.30	0.09	2.0	6	1115
0	7	2.6	94	1.2	296	30	9,620	962	0.07	0.09	0.7	53	1116
0	7	2.6	179	1.2	417	20	8,260	826	0.06	0.15	0.9	33	1117
0	11	1.8	41	0.7	561	35	58	7	0.07	0.03	0.6	89	1118
0	8	1.0	31	1.1	90	10	48	5	0.03	0.02	0.2	4	1119

Food No.	Food Description	Measure of Edible Portion	Weight (g)	Water (%)	Calories (kcal)	Protein (g)	Total Fat (g)	Fatty Acids Saturated (g)	Mono-unsaturated (g)	Poly-unsaturated (g)
VEGETABLES AND VEGETABLE PRODUCTS (CONTINUED)										
	LETTUCE, RAW									
	BUTTERHEAD, AS BOSTON TYPES									
1120	LEAF	1 MEDIUM LEAF	8	96	1	TR	TR	TR	TR	TR
1121	HEAD, 5″ DIA	1 HEAD	163	96	21	2	TR	TR	TR	0.2
	CRISPHEAD, AS ICEBERG									
1122	LEAF	1 MEDIUM	8	96	1	TR	TR	TR	TR	TR
1123	HEAD, 6″ DIA	1 HEAD	539	96	65	5	1	0.1	TR	0.5
1124	PIECES, SHREDDED OR CHOPPED	1 CUP	55	96	7	1	TR	TR	TR	0.1
	LOOSELEAF									
1125	LEAF	1 LEAF	10	94	2	TR	TR	TR	TR	TR
1126	PIECES, SHREDDED	1 CUP	56	94	10	1	TR	TR	TR	0.1
	ROMAINE OR COS									
1127	INNERLEAF	1 LEAF	10	95	1	TR	TR	TR	TR	TR
1128	PIECES, SHREDDED	1 CUP	56	95	8	1	TR	TR	TR	0.1
	MUSHROOMS									
1129	RAW, PIECES OR SLICES	1 CUP	70	92	18	2	TR	TR	TR	0.1
1130	COOKED, DRAINED, PIECES	1 CUP	156	91	42	3	1	0.1	TR	0.3
1131	CANNED, DRAINED, PIECES	1 CUP	156	91	37	3	TR	0.1	TR	0.2
	MUSHROOMS, SHIITAKE									
1132	COOKED PIECES	1 CUP	145	83	80	2	TR	0.1	0.1	TR
1133	DRIED	1 MUSHROOM	4	10	11	TR	TR	TR	TR	TR
1134	MUSTARD GREENS, COOKED, DRAINED	1 CUP	140	94	21	3	TR	TR	0.2	0.1
	OKRA, SLICED, COOKED, DRAINED									
1135	FROM RAW	1 CUP	160	90	51	3	TR	0.1	TR	0.1
1136	FROM FROZEN	1 CUP	184	91	52	4	1	0.1	0.1	0.1
	ONIONS									
	RAW									
1137	CHOPPED	1 CUP	160	90	61	2	TR	TR	TR	0.1
1138	WHOLE, MEDIUM, 2 1/2″ DIA	1 WHOLE	110	90	42	1	TR	TR	TR	0.1
1139	SLICE, 1/8″ THICK	1 SLICE	14	90	5	TR	TR	TR	TR	TR
1140	COOKED (WHOLE OR SLICED), DRAINED	1 CUP	210	88	92	3	TR	0.1	0.1	0.2
1141		1 MEDIUM	94	88	41	1	TR	TR	TR	0.1
1142	DEHYDRATED FLAKES	1 TBSP	5	4	17	TR	TR	TR	TR	TR
	ONIONS, SPRING, RAW, TOP AND BULB									
1143	CHOPPED	1 CUP	100	90	32	2	TR	TR	TR	0.1
1144	WHOLE, MEDIUM, 4 1/8″ LONG	1 WHOLE	15	90	5	TR	TR	TR	TR	TR
1145	ONION RINGS, 2–3″ DIA, BREADED, PAR FRIED, FROZEN, OVEN HEATED	10 RINGS	60	29	244	3	16	5.2	6.5	3.1
1146	PARSLEY, RAW	10 SPRIGS	10	88	4	TR	TR	TR	TR	TR
1147	PARSNIPS, SLICED, COOKED, DRAINED	1 CUP	156	78	126	2	TR	0.1	0.2	0.1
	PEAS, EDIBLE POD, COOKED, DRAINED									
1148	FROM RAW	1 CUP	160	89	67	5	TR	0.1	TR	0.2
1149	FROM FROZEN	1 CUP	160	87	83	6	1	0.1	0.1	0.3
	PEAS, GREEN									
1150	CANNED, DRAINED	1 CUP	170	82	117	8	1	0.1	0.1	0.3
1151	FROZEN, BOILED, DRAINED	1 CUP	160	80	125	8	TR	0.1	TR	0.2
	PEPPERS									
	HOT CHILI, RAW									
1152	GREEN	1 PEPPER	45	88	18	1	TR	TR	TR	TR
1153	RED	1 PEPPER	45	88	18	1	TR	TR	TR	TR

Cholesterol (mg)	Carbo-hydrate (g)	Total Dietary Fiber (g)	Calcium (mg)	Iron (mg)	Potassium (mg)	Sodium (mg)	Vitamin A (IU)	Vitamin A (RE)	Thiamine (mg)	Ribo-flavin (mg)	Niacin (mg)	Ascorbic Acid (mg)	Food No.
0	TR	0.1	2	TR	19	TR	73	7	TR	TR	TR	1	1120
0	4	1.6	52	0.5	419	8	1,581	158	0.10	0.10	0.5	13	1121
0	TR	0.1	2	TR	13	1	26	3	TR	TR	TR	TR	1122
0	11	7.5	102	2.7	852	49	1,779	178	0.25	0.16	1.0	21	1123
0	1	0.8	10	0.3	87	5	182	18	0.03	0.02	0.1	2	1124
0	TR	0.2	7	0.1	26	1	190	19	0.01	0.01	TR	2	1125
0	2	1.1	38	0.8	148	5	1,064	106	0.03	0.04	0.2	10	1126
0	TR	0.2	4	0.1	29	1	260	26	0.01	0.01	0.1	2	1127
0	1	1.0	20	0.6	162	4	1,456	146	0.06	0.06	0.3	13	1128
0	3	0.8	4	0.7	259	3	0	0	0.06	0.30	2.8	2	1129
0	8	3.4	9	2.7	555	3	0	0	0.11	0.47	7.0	6	1130
0	8	3.7	17	1.2	201	663	0	0	0.13	0.03	2.5	0	1131
0	21	3.0	4	0.6	170	6	0	0	0.05	0.25	2.2	TR	1132
0	3	0.4	TR	0.1	55	TR	0	0	0.01	0.05	0.5	TR	1133
0	3	2.8	104	1.0	283	22	4,243	424	0.06	0.09	0.6	35	1134
0	12	4.0	101	0.7	515	8	920	93	0.21	0.09	1.4	26	1135
0	11	5.2	177	1.2	431	6	946	94	0.18	0.23	1.4	22	1136
0	14	2.9	32	0.4	251	5	0	0	0.07	0.03	0.2	10	1137
0	9	2.0	22	0.2	173	3	0	0	0.05	0.02	0.2	7	1138
0	1	0.3	3	TR	22	TR	0	0	0.01	TR	TR	1	1139
0	21	2.9	46	0.5	349	6	0	0	0.09	0.05	0.3	11	1140
0	10	1.3	21	0.2	156	3	0	0	0.04	0.02	0.2	5	1141
0	4	0.5	13	0.1	81	1	0	0	0.03	0.01	TR	4	1142
0	7	2.6	72	1.5	276	16	385	39	0.06	0.08	0.5	19	1143
0	1	0.4	11	0.2	41	2	58	6	0.01	0.01	0.1	3	1144
0	23	0.8	19	1.0	77	225	135	14	0.17	0.08	2.2	1	1145
0	1	0.3	14	0.6	55	6	520	52	0.01	0.01	0.1	13	1146
0	30	6.2	58	0.9	573	16	0	0	0.13	0.08	1.1	20	1147
0	11	4.5	67	3.2	384	6	210	21	0.20	0.12	0.9	77	1148
0	14	5.0	94	3.8	347	8	267	27	0.10	0.19	0.9	35	1149
0	21	7.0	34	1.6	294	428	1,306	131	0.21	0.13	1.2	16	1150
0	23	8.8	38	2.5	269	139	1,069	107	0.45	0.16	2.4	16	1151
0	4	0.7	8	0.5	153	3	347	35	0.04	0.04	0.4	109	1152
0	4	0.7	8	0.5	153	3	4,838	484	0.04	0.04	0.4	109	1153

Food No.	Food Description	Measure of Edible Portion	Weight (g)	Water (%)	Calories (kcal)	Protein (g)	Total Fat (g)	Fatty Acids Saturated (g)	Mono-unsaturated (g)	Poly-unsaturated (g)
VEGETABLES AND VEGETABLE PRODUCTS (CONTINUED)										
1154	JALAPENO, CANNED, SLICED, SOLIDS AND LIQUIDS	1/4 CUP	26	89	7	TR	TR	TR	TR	0.1
	SWEET (2 3/4″ LONG, 2 1/2″ DIA)									
	RAW									
	GREEN									
1155	CHOPPED	1 CUP	149	92	40	1	TR	TR	TR	0.2
1156	RING (1/4″ THICK)	1 RING	10	92	3	TR	TR	TR	TR	TR
1157	WHOLE (2 3/4″ × 2 1/2″)	1 PEPPER	119	92	32	1	TR	TR	TR	0.1
	RED									
1158	CHOPPED	1 CUP	149	92	40	1	TR	TR	TR	0.2
1159	WHOLE (2 3/4″ × 2 1/2″)	1 PEPPER	119	92	32	1	TR	TR	TR	0.1
	COOKED, DRAINED, CHOPPED									
1160	GREEN	1 CUP	136	92	38	1	TR	TR	TR	0.1
1161	RED	1 CUP	136	92	38	1	TR	TR	TR	0.1
1162	PIMENTO, CANNED	1 TBSP	12	93	3	TR	TR	TR	TR	TR
	POTATOES									
	BAKED (2 1/3″ × 3 1/4″)									
1163	WITH SKIN	1 POTATO	202	71	220	5	TR	0.1	TR	0.1
1164	FLESH ONLY	1 POTATO	156	75	145	3	TR	TR	TR	0.1
1165	SKIN ONLY	1 SKIN	58	47	115	2	TR	TR	TR	TR
	BOILED (2 1/2″ DIA)									
1166	PEELED AFTER BOILING	1 POTATO	136	77	118	3	TR	TR	TR	0.1
1167	PEELED BEFORE BOILING	1 POTATO	135	77	116	2	TR	TR	TR	0.1
1168		1 CUP	156	77	134	3	TR	TR	TR	0.1
	POTATO PRODUCTS, PREPARED									
	AU GRATIN									
1169	FROM DRY MIX, WITH WHOLE MILK, BUTTER	1 CUP	245	79	228	6	10	6.3	2.9	0.3
1170	FROM HOME RECIPE, WITH BUTTER	1 CUP	245	74	323	12	19	11.6	5.3	0.7
1171	FRENCH FRIED, FROZEN, OVEN HEATED	10 STRIPS	50	57	100	2	4	0.6	2.4	0.4
	HASHED BROWN									
1172	FROM FROZEN (ABOUT 3″ × 1 1/2″ × 1/2″)	1 PATTY	29	56	63	1	3	1.3	1.5	0.4
1173	FROM HOME RECIPE	1 CUP	156	62	326	4	22	8.5	9.7	2.5
	MASHED									
1174	FROM DEHYDRATED FLAKES (WITHOUT MILK); WHOLE MILK, BUTTER, AND SALT ADDED	1 CUP	210	76	237	4	12	7.2	3.3	0.5
	FROM HOME RECIPE									
1175	WITH WHOLE MILK	1 CUP	210	78	162	4	1	0.7	0.3	0.1
1176	WITH WHOLE MILK AND MARGARINE	1 CUP	210	76	223	4	9	2.2	3.7	2.5
1177	POTATO PANCAKES, HOME PREPARED	1 PANCAKE	76	47	207	5	12	2.3	3.5	5.0
1178	POTATO PUFFS, FROM FROZEN	10 PUFFS	79	53	175	3	8	4.0	3.4	0.6
1179	POTATO SALAD, HOME PREPARED	1 CUP	250	76	358	7	21	3.6	6.2	9.3
	SCALLOPED									
1180	FROM DRY MIX, WITH WHOLE MILK, BUTTER	1 CUP	245	79	228	5	11	6.5	3.0	0.5
1181	FROM HOME RECIPE, WITH BUTTER	1 CUP	245	81	211	7	9	5.5	2.5	0.4
	PUMPKIN									
1182	COOKED, MASHED	1 CUP	245	94	49	2	TR	0.1	TR	TR
1183	CANNED	1 CUP	245	90	83	3	1	0.4	0.1	TR
1184	RADISHES, RAW (3/4″ TO 1″ DIA)	1 RADISH	5	95	1	TR	TR	TR	TR	TR
1185	RUTABAGAS, COOKED, DRAINED, CUBES	1 CUP	170	89	66	2	TR	TR	TR	0.2
1186	SAUERKRAUT, CANNED, SOLIDS AND LIQUID	1 CUP	236	93	45	2	TR	0.1	TR	0.1

Cholesterol (mg)	Carbo-hydrate (g)	Total Dietary Fiber (g)	Calcium (mg)	Iron (mg)	Potassium (mg)	Sodium (mg)	Vitamin A (IU)	Vitamin A (RE)	Thiamine (mg)	Ribo-flavin (mg)	Niacin (mg)	Ascorbic Acid (mg)	Food No.
0	1	0.7	6	0.5	50	434	442	44	0.01	0.01	0.1	3	1154
0	10	2.7	13	0.7	264	3	942	94	0.10	0.04	0.8	133	1155
0	1	0.2	1	TR	18	TR	63	6	0.01	TR	0.1	9	1156
0	8	2.1	11	0.5	211	2	752	75	0.08	0.04	0.6	106	1157
0	10	3.0	13	0.7	264	3	8,493	849	0.10	0.04	0.8	283	1158
0	8	2.4	11	0.5	211	2	6,783	678	0.08	0.04	0.6	226	1159
0	9	1.6	12	0.6	226	3	805	80	0.08	0.04	0.6	101	1160
0	9	1.6	12	0.6	226	3	5,114	511	0.08	0.04	0.6	233	1161
0	1	0.2	1	0.2	19	2	319	32	TR	0.01	0.1	10	1162
0	51	4.8	20	2.7	844	16	0	0	0.22	0.07	3.3	26	1163
0	34	2.3	8	0.5	610	8	0	0	0.16	0.03	2.2	20	1164
0	27	4.6	20	4.1	332	12	0	0	0.07	0.06	1.8	8	1165
0	27	2.4	7	0.4	515	5	0	0	0.14	0.03	2.0	18	1166
0	27	2.4	11	0.4	443	7	0	0	0.13	0.03	1.8	10	1167
0	31	2.8	12	0.5	512	8	0	0	0.15	0.03	2.0	12	1168
37	31	2.2	203	0.8	537	1,076	522	76	0.05	0.20	2.3	8	1169
56	28	4.4	292	1.6	970	1,061	647	93	0.16	0.28	2.4	24	1170
0	16	1.6	4	0.6	209	15	0	0	0.06	0.01	1.0	5	1171
0	8	0.6	4	0.4	126	10	0	0	0.03	0.01	0.7	2	1172
0	33	3.1	12	1.3	501	37	0	0	0.12	0.03	3.1	9	1173
29	32	4.8	103	0.5	489	697	378	44	0.23	0.11	1.4	20	1174
4	37	4.2	55	0.6	628	636	40	13	0.18	0.08	2.3	14	1175
4	35	4.2	55	0.5	607	620	355	42	0.18	0.08	2.3	13	1176
73	22	1.5	18	1.2	597	386	109	11	0.10	0.13	1.6	17	1177
0	24	2.5	24	1.2	300	589	13	2	0.15	0.06	1.7	5	1178
170	28	3.3	48	1.6	635	1,323	523	83	0.19	0.15	2.2	25	1179
27	31	2.7	88	0.9	497	835	363	51	0.05	0.14	2.5	8	1180
29	26	4.7	140	1.4	926	821	331	47	0.17	0.23	2.6	26	1181
0	12	2.7	37	1.4	564	2	2,651	265	0.08	0.19	1.0	12	1182
0	20	7.1	64	3.4	505	12	54,037	5,405	0.06	0.13	0.9	10	1183
0	TR	0.1	1	TR	10	1	TR	TR	TR	TR	TR	1	1184
0	15	3.1	82	0.9	554	34	954	95	0.14	0.07	1.2	32	1185
0	10	5.9	71	3.5	401	1,560	42	5	0.05	0.05	0.3	35	1186

Food No.	Food Description	Measure of Edible Portion	Weight (g)	Water (%)	Calories (kcal)	Protein (g)	Total Fat (g)	Fatty Acids Saturated (g)	Monounsaturated (g)	Polyunsaturated (g)
VEGETABLES AND VEGETABLE PRODUCTS (CONTINUED)										
	SEAWEED									
1187	KELP, RAW	2 TBSP	10	82	4	TR	TR	TR	TR	TR
1188	SPIRULINA, DRIED	1 TBSP	1	5	3	1	TR	TR	TR	TR
1189	SHALLOTS, RAW, CHOPPED	1 TBSP	10	80	7	TR	TR	TR	TR	TR
1190	SOYBEANS, GREEN, COOKED, DRAINED	1 CUP	180	69	254	22	12	1.3	2.2	5.4
	SPINACH									
	RAW									
1191	CHOPPED	1 CUP	30	92	7	1	TR	TR	TR	TR
1192	LEAF	1 LEAF	10	92	2	TR	TR	TR	TR	TR
	COOKED, DRAINED									
1193	FROM RAW	1 CUP	180	91	41	5	TR	0.1	TR	0.2
1194	FROM FROZEN (CHOPPED OR LEAF)	1 CUP	190	90	53	6	TR	0.1	TR	0.2
1195	CANNED, DRAINED	1 CUP	214	92	49	6	1	0.2	TR	0.4
	SQUASH									
	SUMMER (ALL VARIETIES), SLICED									
1196	RAW	1 CUP	113	94	23	1	TR	TR	TR	0.1
1197	COOKED, DRAINED	1 CUP	180	94	36	2	1	0.1	TR	0.2
1198	WINTER (ALL VARIETIES), BAKED, CUBES	1 CUP	205	89	80	2	1	0.3	0.1	0.5
1199	WINTER, BUTTERNUT, FROZEN, COOKED, MASHED	1 CUP	240	88	94	3	TR	TR	TR	0.1
	SWEET POTATOES									
	COOKED (2″ DIA, 5″ LONG RAW)									
1200	BAKED, WITH SKIN	1 POTATO	146	73	150	3	TR	TR	TR	0.1
1201	BOILED, WITHOUT SKIN	1 POTATO	156	73	164	3	TR	0.1	TR	0.2
1202	CANDIED (2 1/2″ × 2 PIECE)	1 PIECE	105	67	144	1	3	1.4	0.7	0.2
	CANNED									
1203	SYRUP PACK, DRAINED	1 CUP	196	72	212	3	1	0.1	TR	0.3
1204	VACUUM PACK, MASHED	1 CUP	255	76	232	4	1	0.1	TR	0.2
1205	TOMATILLOS, RAW	1 MEDIUM	34	92	11	TR	TR	TR	0.1	0.1
	TOMATOES									
	RAW, YEAR-ROUND AVERAGE									
1206	CHOPPED OR SLICED	1 CUP	180	94	38	2	1	0.1	0.1	0.2
1207	SLICE, MEDIUM, 1/4″ THICK	1 SLICE	20	94	4	TR	TR	TR	TR	TR
	WHOLE									
1208	CHERRY	1 CHERRY	17	94	4	TR	TR	TR	TR	TR
1209	MEDIUM, 2 3/5″ DIA	1 TOMATO	123	94	26	1	TR	0.1	0.1	0.2
1210	CANNED, SOLIDS AND LIQUID	1 CUP	240	94	46	2	TR	TR	TR	0.1
	SUN DRIED									
1211	PLAIN	1 PIECE	2	15	5	TR	TR	TR	TR	TR
1212	PACKED IN OIL, DRAINED	1 PIECE	3	54	6	TR	TR	0.1	0.3	0.1
1213	TOMATO JUICE, CANNED, WITH SALT ADDED	1 CUP	243	94	41	2	TR	TR	TR	0.1
	TOMATO PRODUCTS, CANNED									
1214	PASTE	1 CUP	262	74	215	10	1	0.2	0.2	0.6
1215	PUREE	1 CUP	250	87	100	4	TR	0.1	0.1	0.2
1216	SAUCE	1 CUP	245	89	74	3	TR	0.1	0.1	0.2
	SPAGHETTI/MARINARA/PASTA SAUCE. SEE SOUPS, SAUCES, AND GRAVIES.									
1217	STEWED	1 CUP	255	91	71	2	TR	TR	0.1	0.1

*For product with no salt added: If salt added, consult the nutrition label for sodium value.

Cholesterol (mg)	Carbo-hydrate (g)	Total Dietary Fiber (g)	Calcium (mg)	Iron (mg)	Potassium (mg)	Sodium (mg)	Vitamin A (IU)	Vitamin A (RE)	Thiamine (mg)	Ribo-flavin (mg)	Niacin (mg)	Ascorbic Acid (mg)	Food No.
0	1	0.1	17	0.3	9	23	12	1	0.01	0.02	TR	TR	1187
0	TR	TR	1	0.3	14	10	6	1	0.02	0.04	0.1	TR	1188
0	2	0.2	4	0.1	33	1	119	12	0.01	TR	TR	1	1189
0	20	7.6	261	4.5	970	25	281	29	0.47	0.28	2.3	31	1190
0	1	0.8	30	0.8	167	24	2,015	202	0.02	0.06	0.2	8	1191
0	TR	0.3	10	0.3	56	8	672	67	0.01	0.02	0.1	3	1192
0	7	4.3	245	6.4	839	126	14,742	1,474	0.17	0.42	0.9	18	1193
0	10	5.7	277	2.9	566	163	14,790	1,478	0.11	0.32	0.8	23	1194
0	7	5.1	272	4.9	740	58	18,781	1,879	0.03	0.30	0.8	31	1195
0	5	2.1	23	0.5	220	2	221	23	0.07	0.04	0.6	17	1196
0	8	2.5	49	0.6	346	2	517	52	0.00	0.07	0.9	10	1197
0	18	5.7	29	0.7	896	2	7,292	730	0.17	0.05	1.4	20	1198
0	24	2.2	46	1.4	319	5	8,014	802	0.12	0.09	1.1	8	1199
0	35	4.4	41	0.7	508	15	31,860	3,186	0.11	0.19	0.9	36	1200
0	38	2.8	33	0.9	287	20	26,604	2,660	0.08	0.22	1.0	27	1201
8	29	2.5	27	1.2	198	74	4,398	440	0.02	0.04	0.4	7	1202
0	50	5.9	33	1.9	378	76	14,028	1,403	0.05	0.07	0.7	21	1203
0	54	4.6	56	2.3	796	135	20,357	2,035	0.09	0.15	1.9	67	1204
0	2	0.6	2	0.2	91	TR	39	4	0.01	0.01	0.6	4	1205
0	8	2.0	9	0.8	400	16	1,121	112	0.11	0.09	1.1	34	1206
0	1	0.2	1	0.1	44	2	125	12	0.01	0.01	0.1	4	1207
0	1	0.2	1	0.1	38	2	106	11	0.01	0.01	0.1	3	1208
0	6	1.4	6	0.6	273	11	766	76	0.07	0.06	0.8	23	1209
0	10	2.4	72	1.3	530	355	1,428	144	0.11	0.07	1.8	34	1210
0	1	0.2	2	0.2	69	42	17	2	0.01	0.01	0.2	1	1211
0	1	0.2	1	0.1	47	8	39	4	0.01	0.01	0.1	3	1212
0	10	1.0	22	1.4	535	877	1,351	136	0.11	0.08	1.6	44	1213
0	51	10.7	92	5.1	2,455	231	6,406	639	0.41	0.50	8.4	111	1214
0	24	5.0	43	3.1	1,065	85*	3,188	320	0.18	0.14	4.3	26	1215
0	18	3.4	34	1.9	909	1,482	2,399	240	0.16	0.14	2.8	32	1216
0	17	2.6	84	1.9	607	564	1,380	138	0.12	0.09	1.8	29	1217

Food No.	Food Description	Measure of Edible Portion	Weight (g)	Water (%)	Calories (kcal)	Protein (g)	Total Fat (g)	Fatty Acids Saturated (g)	Fatty Acids Mono-unsaturated (g)	Fatty Acids Poly-unsaturated (g)
VEGETABLES AND VEGETABLE PRODUCTS (CONTINUED)										
1218	TURNIPS, COOKED, CUBES	1 CUP	156	94	33	1	TR	TR	TR	0.1
	TURNIP GREENS, COOKED, DRAINED									
1219	FROM RAW (LEAVES AND STEMS)	1 CUP	144	93	29	2	TR	0.1	TR	0.1
1220	FROM FROZEN (CHOPPED)	1 CUP	164	90	49	5	1	0.2	TR	0.3
1221	VEGETABLE JUICE COCKTAIL, CANNED	1 CUP	242	94	46	2	TR	TR	TR	0.1
	VEGETABLES, MIXED									
1222	CANNED, DRAINED	1 CUP	163	87	77	4	TR	0.1	TR	0.2
1223	FROZEN, COOKED, DRAINED	1 CUP	182	83	107	5	TR	0.1	TR	0.1
1224	WATERCHESTNUTS, CANNED, SLICES, SOLIDS AND LIQUIDS	1 CUP	140	86	70	1	TR	TR	TR	TR
MISCELLANEOUS ITEMS										
1225	BACON BITS, MEATLESS	1 TBSP	7	8	31	2	2	0.3	0.4	0.9
	BAKING POWDERS FOR HOME USE DOUBLE ACTING									
1226	SODIUM ALUMINUM SULFATE	1 TSP	5	5	2	0	0	0.0	0.0	0.0
1227	STRAIGHT PHOSPHATE	1 TSP	5	4	2	TR	0	0.0	0.0	0.0
1228	LOW SODIUM	1 TSP	5	6	5	TR	TR	TR	TR	TR
1229	BAKING SODA	1 TSP	5	TR	0	0	0	0.0	0.0	0.0
1230	BEEF JERKY	1 LARGE PIECE	20	23	81	7	5	2.1	2.2	0.2
1231	CATSUP	1 CUP	240	67	250	4	1	0.1	0.1	0.4
1232		1 TBSP	15	67	16	TR	TR	TR	TR	TR
1233		1 PACKET	6	67	6	TR	TR	TR	TR	TR
1234	CELERY SEED	1 TSP	2	6	8	TR	1	TR	0.3	0.1
1235	CHILI POWDER	1 TSP	3	8	8	TR	TR	0.1	0.1	0.2
	CHOCOLATE, UNSWEETENED, BAKING									
1236	SOLID	1 SQUARE	28	1	148	3	16	9.2	5.2	0.5
1237	LIQUID	1 OZ	28	1	134	3	14	7.2	2.6	3.0
1238	CINNAMON	1 TSP	2	10	6	TR	TR	TR	TR	TR
1239	COCOA POWDER, UNSWEETENED	1 CUP	86	3	197	17	12	6.9	3.9	0.4
1240		1 TBSP	5	3	12	1	1	0.4	0.2	TR
1241	CREAM OF TARTAR	1 TSP	3	2	8	0	0	0.0	0.0	0.0
1242	CURRY POWDER	1 TSP	2	10	7	TR	TR	TR	0.1	0.1
1243	GARLIC POWDER	1 TSP	3	6	9	TR	TR	TR	TR	TR
1244	HORSERADISH, PREPARED	1 TSP	5	85	2	TR	TR	TR	TR	TR
1245	MUSTARD, PREPARED, YELLOW	1 TSP OR 1 PACKET	5	82	3	TR	TR	TR	0.1	TR
	OLIVES, CANNED									
1246	PICKLED, GREEN	5 MEDIUM	17	78	20	TR	2	0.3	1.6	0.2
1247	RIPE, BLACK	5 LARGE	22	80	25	TR	2	0.3	1.7	0.2
1248	ONION POWDER	1 TSP	2	5	7	TR	TR	TR	TR	TR
1249	OREGANO, GROUND	1 TSP	2	7	5	TR	TR	TR	TR	0.1
1250	PAPRIKA	1 TSP	2	10	6	TR	TR	TR	TR	0.2
1251	PARSLEY, DRIED	1 TBSP	1	9	4	TR	TR	TR	TR	TR
1252	PEPPER, BLACK	1 TSP	2	11	5	TR	TR	TR	TR	TR
	PICKLES, CUCUMBER									
1253	DILL, WHOLE, MEDIUM (3 3/4″ LONG)	1 PICKLE	65	92	12	TR	TR	TR	TR	0.1
1254	FRESH (BREAD AND BUTTER PICKLES), SLICES 1 1/2″ DIA, 1/4″ THICK	3 SLICES	24	79	18	TR	TR	TR	TR	TR
1255	PICKLE RELISH, SWEET	1 TBSP	15	62	20	TR	TR	TR	TR	TR

Cholesterol (mg)	Carbo-hydrate (g)	Total Dietary Fiber (g)	Calcium (mg)	Iron (mg)	Potassium (mg)	Sodium (mg)	Vitamin A (IU)	Vitamin A (RE)	Thiamine (mg)	Ribo-flavin (mg)	Niacin (mg)	Ascorbic Acid (mg)	Food No.
0	8	3.1	34	0.3	211	78	0	0	0.04	0.04	0.5	18	1218
0	6	5.0	197	1.2	292	42	7,917	792	0.06	0.10	0.6	39	1219
0	8	5.6	249	3.2	367	25	13,079	1,309	0.09	0.12	0.8	36	1220
0	11	1.9	27	1.0	467	653	2,831	283	0.10	0.07	1.8	67	1221
0	15	4.9	44	1.7	474	243	18,985	1,899	0.07	0.08	0.9	8	1222
0	24	8.0	46	1.5	308	64	7,784	779	0.13	0.22	1.5	6	1223
0	17	3.5	6	1.2	165	11	6	0	0.02	0.03	0.5	2	1224
0	2	0.7	7	0.1	10	124	0	0	0.04	TR	0.1	TR	1225
0	1	TR	270	0.5	1	488	0	0	0.00	0.00	0.0	0	1226
0	1	TR	339	0.5	TR	363	0	0	0.00	0.00	0.0	0	1227
0	2	0.1	217	0.4	505	5	0	0	0.00	0.00	0.0	0	1228
0	0	0.0	0	0.0	0	1,259	0	0	0.00	0.00	0.0	0	1229
10	2	0.4	4	1.1	118	438	0	0	0.03	0.03	0.3	0	1230
0	65	3.1	46	1.7	1,154	2,846	2,438	245	0.21	0.18	3.3	36	1231
0	4	0.2	3	0.1	72	178	152	15	0.01	0.01	0.2	2	1232
0	2	0.1	1	TR	29	71	61	6	0.01	TR	0.1	1	1233
0	1	0.2	35	0.9	28	3	1	TR	0.01	0.01	0.1	TR	1234
0	1	0.9	7	0.4	50	26	908	91	0.01	0.02	0.2	2	1235
0	8	4.4	21	1.8	236	4	28	3	0.02	0.05	0.3	0	1236
0	10	5.1	15	1.2	331	3	3	TR	0.01	0.08	0.6	0	1237
0	2	1.2	28	0.9	11	1	6	1	TR	TR	TR	1	1238
0	47	28.6	110	11.9	1,311	18	17	2	0.07	0.21	1.9	0	1239
0	3	1.8	7	0.7	82	1	1	TR	TR	0.01	0.1	0	1240
0	2	TR	TR	0.1	495	2	0	0	0.00	0.00	0.0	0	1241
0	1	0.7	10	0.6	31	1	20	2	0.01	0.01	0.1	TR	1242
0	2	0.3	2	0.1	31	1	0	0	0.01	TR	TR	1	1243
0	1	0.2	3	TR	12	16	TR	0	TR	TR	TR	1	1244
0	TR	0.2	4	0.1	8	56	7	1	TR	TR	TR	TR	1245
0	TR	0.2	10	0.3	9	408	51	5	0.00	0.00	TR	0	1246
0	1	0.7	19	0.7	2	192	89	9	TR	0.00	TR	TR	1247
0	2	0.1	8	0.1	20	1	0	0	0.01	TR	TR	TR	1248
0	1	0.6	24	0.7	25	TR	104	10	0.01	TR	0.1	1	1249
0	1	0.4	4	0.5	49	1	1,273	127	0.01	0.04	0.3	1	1250
0	1	0.4	19	1.3	49	6	303	30	TR	0.02	0.1	2	1251
0	1	0.6	9	0.6	26	1	4	TR	TR	0.01	TR	TR	1252
0	3	0.8	6	0.3	75	833	214	21	0.01	0.02	TR	1	1253
0	4	0.4	8	0.1	48	162	34	3	0.00	0.01	0.0	2	1254
0	5	0.2	TR	0.1	4	122	23	2	0.00	TR	TR	TR	1255

Food No.	Food Description	Measure of Edible Portion	Weight (g)	Water (%)	Calories (kcal)	Protein (g)	Total Fat (g)	Fatty Acids		
								Satu-rated (g)	Mono-unsatu-rated (g)	Poly-unsatu-rated (g)
MISCELLANEOUS ITEMS (CONTINUED)										
1256	PORK SKINS/RINDS, PLAIN	1 OZ	28	2	155	17	9	3.2	4.2	1.0
	POTATO CHIPS									
	REGULAR									
	PLAIN									
1257	SALTED	1 OZ	28	2	152	2	10	3.1	2.8	3.5
1258	UNSALTED	1 OZ	28	2	152	2	10	3.1	2.8	3.5
1259	BARBECUE FLAVOR	1 OZ	28	2	139	2	9	2.3	1.9	4.6
1260	SOUR CREAM AND ONION FLAVOR	1 OZ	28	2	151	2	10	2.5	1.7	4.9
1261	REDUCED FAT	1 OZ	28	1	134	2	6	1.2	1.4	3.1
1262	FAT FREE, MADE WITH OLESTRA	1 OZ	28	2	75	2	TR	TR	0.1	0.1
	MADE FROM DRIED POTATOES									
1263	PLAIN	1 OZ	28	1	158	2	11	2.7	2.1	5.7
1264	SOUR CREAM AND ONION FLAVOR	1 OZ	28	2	155	2	10	2.7	2.0	5.3
1265	REDUCED FAT	1 OZ	28	1	142	2	7	1.5	1.7	3.8
1266	SALT	1 TSP	6	TR	0	0	0	0.0	0.0	0.0
	TRAIL MIX									
1267	REGULAR, WITH RAISINS, CHOCOLATE CHIPS, SALTED NUTS AND SEEDS	1 CUP	146	7	707	21	47	8.9	19.8	16.5
1268	TROPICAL	1 CUP	140	9	570	9	24	11.9	3.5	7.2
1269	VANILLA EXTRACT	1 TSP	4	53	12	TR	TR	TR	TR	TR
	VINEGAR									
1270	CIDER	1 TBSP	15	94	2	0	0	0.0	0.0	0.0
1271	DISTILLED	1 TBSP	17	95	2	0	0	0.0	0.0	0.0
	YEAST, BAKER'S									
1272	DRY, ACTIVE	1 PKG	7	8	21	3	TR	TR	0.2	TR
1273		1 TSP	4	8	12	2	TR	TR	0.1	TR
1274	COMPRESSED	1 CAKE	17	69	18	1	TR	TR	0.2	TR

Cholesterol (mg)	Carbo-hydrate (g)	Total Dietary Fiber (g)	Calcium (mg)	Iron (mg)	Potassium (mg)	Sodium (mg)	Vitamin A		Thiamine (mg)	Ribo-flavin (mg)	Niacin (mg)	Ascorbic Acid (mg)	Food No.
							(IU)	(RE)					
27	0	0.0	9	0.2	36	521	37	11	0.03	0.08	0.4	TR	1256
0	15	1.3	7	0.5	361	168	0	0	0.05	0.06	1.1	9	1257
0	15	1.4	7	0.5	361	2	0	0	0.05	0.06	1.1	9	1258
0	15	1.2	14	0.5	357	213	62	6	0.06	0.06	1.3	10	1259
2	15	1.5	20	0.5	377	177	48	6	0.05	0.06	1.1	11	1260
0	19	1.7	6	0.4	494	139	0	0	0.06	0.08	2.0	7	1261
0	17	1.1	10	0.4	366	185	1,469	441	0.10	0.02	1.3	8	1262
0	14	1.0	7	0.4	286	186	0	0	0.06	0.03	0.9	2	1263
1	15	0.3	18	0.4	141	204	214	28	0.05	0.03	0.7	3	1264
0	18	1.0	10	0.4	285	121	0	0	0.05	0.02	1.2	3	1265
0	0	0.0	1	TR	TR	2,325	0	0	0.00	0.00	0.0	0	1266
6	66	8.8	159	4.9	946	177	64	7	0.60	0.33	6.4	2	1267
0	92	10.6	80	3.7	993	14	69	7	0.63	0.16	2.1	11	1268
0	1	0.0	TR	TR	6	TR	0	0	TR	TR	TR	0	1269
0	1	0.0	1	0.1	15	TR	0	0	0.00	0.00	0.0	0	1270
0	1	0.0	0	0.0	2	TR	0	0	0.00	0.00	0.0	0	1271
0	3	1.5	4	1.2	140	4	TR	0	0.17	0.38	2.8	TR	1272
0	2	0.8	3	0.7	80	2	TR	0	0.09	0.22	1.6	TR	1273
0	3	1.4	3	0.6	102	5	0	0	0.32	0.19	2.1	TR	1274

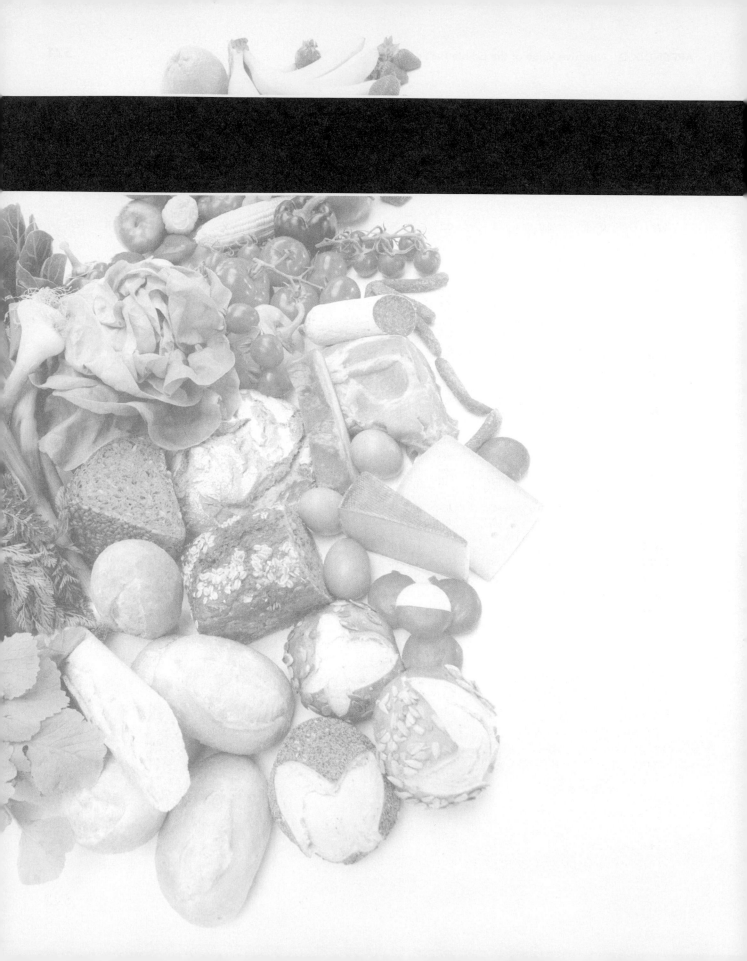

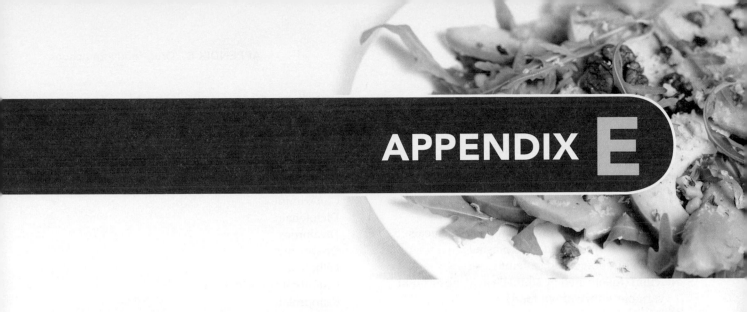

DRUG-FOOD INTERACTIONS

From *Delmar Nurse's Drug Handbook 2009 Edition,* by G. R. Spratto and A. L. Woods, 2009. Clifton Park, NY: Delmar Cengage Learning.

A. DRUGS THAT SHOULD BE TAKEN WHILE FASTING

Alendronate
Ampicillin
AzoGantanol/Gantrisin
Bacampicillin
Bethanechol (may experience N&V)
Bisacodyl
Calcium carbonate
Captopril
Carbenicillin
Castor oil
Chloramphenicol
Claritin
Cyclosporine gel caps only (avoid fatty meals)
Demeclocycline (avoid high calcium foods/dairy products)
Dicloxacillin
Digitalis preparations (not with high fiber foods)
Digoxin (avoid high fiber cereals and oatmeal)
Disopyramide
Erythromycin base/estolate
Etidronate
Ferrous salts (not with tea, coffee, egg, cereals, fiber, or milk)
Fexofenadine
Flavoxate
Furosemide
Isoniazid
Isosorbide dinitrate
Ketoprofen (if Gl distress occurs, may take with food)

Lansoprazole

Levodopa (not with high protein foods; meals delay absorption and peak plasma concentration; avoid caffeine)

Lisinopril

Lomustine (empty stomach will reduce nausea)

Methotrexate (milk, cream, or yogurt may decrease absorption)

Methyldopa (not with high protein foods; meals delay absorption and peak plasma concentration; avoid caffeine)

Nafcillin (inactivated by stomach acid; absorption variable with/without food)

Nalidixic acid

Naltrexone

Norfloxacin (milk, cream, or yogurt may decrease absorption)

Oxytetracycline (avoid dairy products and foods high in calcium)

Penicillamine (antacids, iron and food decreases absorption)

Penicillin

Phenytoin (if GI distress occurs, may take with food; food effect depends on preparation)

Propantheline

Rifampicin

Sotalol

Sulfamethoxazole

Terbutaline sulfate

Tetracycline (avoid dairy products and foods high in calcium)

Theophylline (absorption of controlled release varies by preparation)

Thyroid hormone preparations (limit foods containing goitrogens)

Trientine (antacids, iron, and food reduces absorption)

Trimethoprim

Zyrtec

B. DRUGS THAT SHOULD BE TAKEN WITH FOOD

Allopurinol (after meal)

Amiodarone

Aspirin

Atovaquone

Augmentin

Baclofen

Bromocriptine

Buspirone

Carbamazepine (erratic absorption)

Carvedilol

Cefpodoxime

Chloroquine

Chlorothiazide

Cimetidine

Clofazimine

Diclofenac

Divalproex

Doxycyline

Felbamate

Fenofibrate (TriCor)

Fenoprofen

Fiorinal

Fludrocortisone

Gemfibrozil

Glyburide

Griseofulvin (high fat meals)

Hydrocortisone

Hydroxychloroquine (Plaquenil)

Indomethacin

Iron products

Isotretinoin

Itraconazole capsules

Ketorolac

Labetalol

Lithium

Lovastatin

Mebendazole

Methenamine

Methylprednisolone

Metoprolol

Metronidazole

Misoprostol

Naltrexone

Naproxen

Nelfinavir (Viracept)

Niacin

Nifedipine (grapefruit juice increases bioavailability)

Nitrofurantoin

Olsalazine

Oxcarbazepine

Pentoxifylline

Pergolide

Piroxicam

Potassium salts

Prednisone

Probucol (high fat meals)

Procainamide
Propranolol
Ritonavir
Salsalate
Saquinavir
Sevelamer
Spironolactone
Sulfasalazine
Sulfinpyrazone
Sulindac
Ticlopidine
Tolmetin
Trazodone
Verapamil SR (absorption varies by manufacturer; too rapid absorption may cause heart block)

C. CONSTIPATING AGENTS
Antacids
Anticholinergic drugs
Anticonvulsants
Antihistamines
Antiparkinsonian drugs
BP meds (calcium channel blockers)
Clonidine
Corticosteroids
Diuretics
Ganglionic blocking agents
Iron supplements
Laxatives (when abused)
Lithium
MAO Inhibitors
Muscle relaxants
NSAIDs
Octreotide
Opioids
Phenothiazines
Prostaglandin synthesis inhibitors
Tranquilizers
Tricyclic antidepressants

D. DIARRHEAL AGENTS
Adrenergic neuron blockers: reserpine, guanethidine
Antacids (Mg containing) H_2 receptor antagonists (i.e., ranitidine) PPIs (i.e, Omeprazole)
Antiarrhythmics (i.e., quinidine)
Antibiotics (especially broad spectrum agents)

Antihypertensives (beta blockers, ACE Inhibitors)
Anti-inflammatory drugs (NSAIDs, colchicine)
Chemotherapy agents
Cholinergic agonists and cholinesterase inhibitors
Glucophage
Metoclopramide
Misoprostol
Osmotic and stimulant laxatives
Theophylline

E. TYRAMINE CONTAINING FOODS
Moderate amounts of tyramine:
Banana peel
Broad beans
Cheese (all except cream cheese and cottage cheese)
Chianti, vermouth
Concentrated yeast extracts/Brewer's yeast
Fermented cabbage products: sauerkraut, kimchee
Fermented soy products: fermented bean curd, soya bean paste, miso soup
Hydrolyzed protein extracts for sauces, soups, gravies
Imitation cheese
Liquid and powdered protein supplements
Meat extracts
Nonalcoholic beers
Prepared meats (sausage, chopped liver, pate, salami, mortadella)
Raspberries
Some non-United States brands of beer
Yeast products

Significant amounts of tyramine:
Avocado
Chocolate
Cream from fresh pasteurized milk
Distilled spirits
Peanuts
Red and white wines, port wines
Soy sauce
Yogurt

F. FOODS CONTAINING GOITROGENS
Asparagus
Brocolli
Brussels sprouts
Cabbage

Cauliflower
Kale
Lettuce
Millet
Mustard
Other leafy green vegetables
Peaches
Peanuts
Peas
Radishes
Rutabaga
Soy beans
Spinach
Strawberries
Turnip greens
Watercress

G. COUMARIN ANTICOAGULANTS AND DIETARY EFFECTS

Consumption of vitamin K-enriched foods may counteract the effects of anticoagulants since the drugs act through antagonism of vitamin K. Advise client on anticoagulants to maintain a steady, consistent intake of vitamin K-containing foods. The drug monograph for warfarin clearly lists these foods. Additionally, certain herbal teas (green tea, buckeye, horse chestnut, Woodruff, tonka beans, melitot) contain natural coumarins that can potentiate the effects of coumadin and should be avoided. Large amounts of avocado also potentiate the drug's effects. Brussels sprouts, broccoli, spinach, kale, turnip greens, and other cruciferous vegetables increase the catabolism of warfarin thereby decreasing its anticoagulant activities. Caffeinated beverages (i.e., cola, coffee, tea, hot chocolate, chocolate milk) can affect therapy. Alcohol intake of more than three drinks per day can affect clotting times. Herbal supplements can also affect bleeding time: Coenzyme Q10 is structurally similar to vitamin K, feverfew, garlic, and ginseng. Avoid herbal medications while on warfarin therapy.

H. GENERAL DRUG CLASS RECOMMENDATIONS

ACE inhibitors: Take captopril and moexipril 1 hr before or 2 hr after meals; food decreases absorption. Avoid high potassium foods as ACE increases K^+.

Analgesic/Antipyretic: Take on an empty stomach as food may slow the absorption.

Antacids: Take 1 hr after or between meals. Avoid dairy foods as the protein in them can increase stomach acid.

Anti-anxiety agents: Caffeine may cause excitability, nervousness, and hyperactivity lessening the anti-anxiety drug effects.

Antibiotics: Penicillin generally should be taken on an empty stomach; may take with food if Gl upset occurs. Do not mix with acidic foods: coffee, citrus fruits, and tomatoes; the acid interferes with absorption of penicillin, ampicillin, erythromycin and cloxacillin.

Anticoagulants: High vitamin K produces blood-clotting substance and may reduce drug effectiveness. Vitamin E >400 IU may prolong clotting time and increase bleeding risk.

Antidepressant drugs: May be taken with or without food.

Antifungals: Avoid taking with dairy products; avoid alcohol.

Antihistamines: Take on an empty stomach to increase effectiveness.

Bronchodilators with theophylline: High-fat meals may increase bioavailability while high-carbohydrate meals may decrease it. Food increases absorption of Theo-24 and Uniphyl which may cause increased N&V, headache and irritability.

Cephalosporins: Take on an empty stomach 1 hr before or 2 hr after meals. May take with food if Gl upset occurs.

Diuretics: Vary in interactions; some cause loss of potassium, calcium, and magnesium. Avoid salty food and natural black licorice as these increase K and Mg losses. Large doses of vitamin D can elevate blood pressure.

H_2 blockers: May take with or without regard to food.

HMG-CoA reductase inhibitors: Take lovastatin with the evening meal to enhance absorption.

Laxatives: Avoid dairy foods as calcium can decrease absorption.

Macrolides: Take on an empty stomach 1 hr before or 2 hr after meals. May take with food for GI upset.

MAO inhibitors: Have many dietary restrictions, so follow dietary guidelines as prescribed. Foods or alcoholic beverages containing tyramine may cause a fatal increase in BP.

Narcotic analgesics: Avoid alcohol as it may increase sedative effects.

Nitroimadazole (metronidazole): Avoid alcohol or food prepared with alcohol for at least three days after finishing the medicine. Alcohol may cause nausea, abdominal cramps, vomiting, headaches, and flushing.

NSAIDs: Take with food or milk to prevent irritation of the stomach.

Quinolones: Take on an empty stomach 1 hr before or 2 hr after meals. May take with food for GI upset but avoid calcium containing foods such as milk, yogurt, vitamins/minerals containing iron and antacids because they decrease drug concentrations. Caffeine containing products may lead to excitability and nervousness.

Sulfonamides: Take on an empty stomach 1 hr before or 2 hr after meals. May take with food if GI upset occurs.

Tetracyclines: Take on an empty stomach 1 hr before or 2 hr after meals. May take with food but avoid dairy products, antacids, and vitamins containing iron with tetracycline.

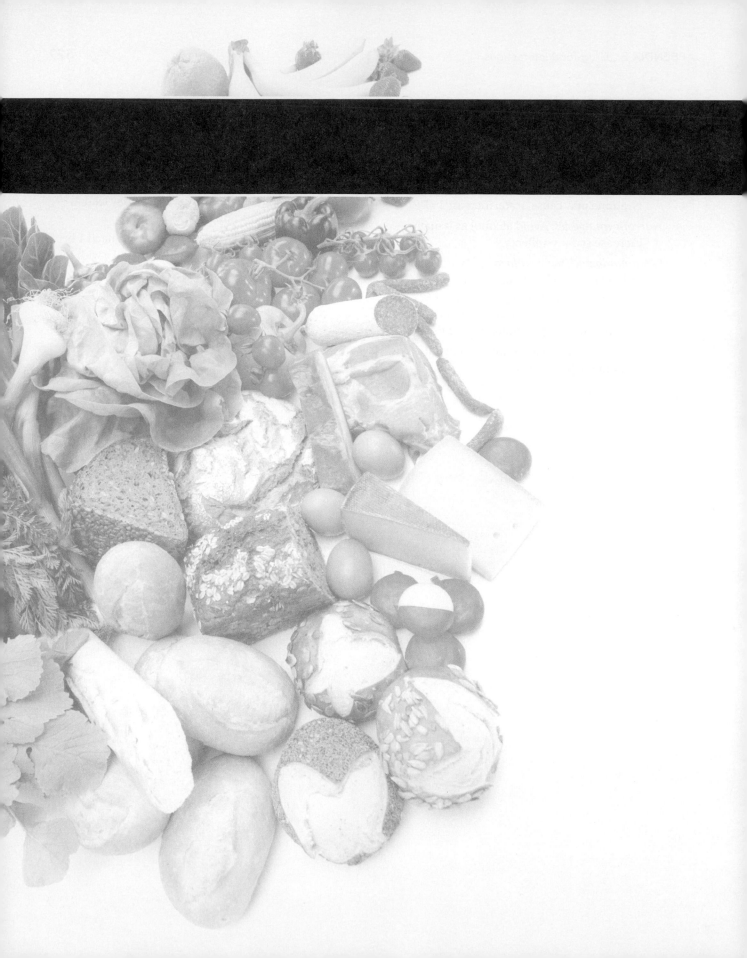

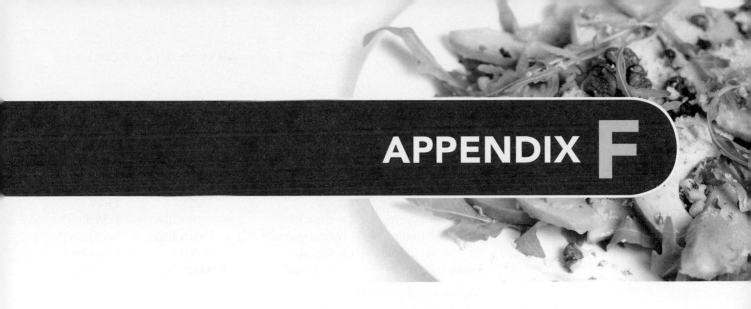

ENGLISH AND METRIC UNITS AND CONVERSIONS

Units of Measure in the English System

Unit	Abbreviation	Equivalent
dash		less than 1/8 teaspoon
few grains	f.g.	less than 1/8 teaspoon
drop		—
15 drops		—
1 teaspoon	tsp	1/3 tablespoon
1 tablespoon	Tbsp	3 teaspoons
1 fluid ounce	oz	2 tablespoons
1 cup	c	8 fluid ounces or 16 tablespoons
1 pint	pt	2 cups
1 quart	qt	2 pints or 4 cups
1 gallon	gal	4 quarts
1 peck	pk	2 gallons
1 bushel	bu	4 pecks
1 pound	lb	16 ounces

Units of Measure in the Metric System

Basic unit of *weight* is the *gram* (g)
Basic unit of *volume* is the *liter* (l)
Basic unit of *length* is the *meter* (m)
***Temperature* is measured in degrees *Celsius* (°C)**

kilo: (*key*-low) = 1,000
deci: (*dess*-ee) = 0.1 (1/10)
centi: (*sent*-ee) = 0.01 (1/100)
milli: (*mill*-ee) = 0.001 (1/1000)

Unit Relationships within the Metric System

Weight			Volume		
1,000 grams	=	1 *kilo*gram	1000 liters	=	1 *kilo*liter*
100 grams	=	1 *hecto*gram*	100 liters	=	1 *hecto*liter*
10 grams	=	1 *deka*gram*	10 liters	=	1 *deka*liter*
		1 gram			1 liter
0.1 gram	=	1 *deci*gram*	0.1 liter	=	1 *deci*liter*
0.01 gram	=	1 *centi*gram*	0.01 liter	=	1 *centi*liter*
0.001 gram	=	1 *milli*gram	0.001 liter	=	1 *milli*liter
0.000001 gram	=	1 *micro*gram*	0.000001 liter	=	1 *micro*liter*

*Units not commonly used.

Converting from the English System to the Metric System

Convert to Metric	When You Know	Multiply By	To Find
Weight	ounces (oz)	28	grams (g)
	pounds (lb)	0.45	kilograms (kg)
	teaspoons (tsp)	5	milliliters (ml)
	tablespoons (Tbsp)	15	milliliters
	fluid ounces (fl oz)	30	milliliters
	cups (c)	0.24	liters (l)
Volume	pints (pt)	0.47	liters
	quarts (qt)	0.95	liters
	gallons (gal)	3.8	liters
	cubic feet (ft^3)	0.03	cubic meters (m^3)
	cubic yards (yd^3)	0.76	cubic meters
Temperature	Fahrenheit (°F) temperature	5/9 (after subtracting 32)	Celsius (°C) temperature

Source: Adapted from "Some References on Metric Information" by U.S. Department of Commerce, National Bureau of Standards.

Converting from the Metric System to the English System

Convert to Metric	When You Know	Multiply By	To Find
Weight	grams (g)	0.035	ounces (oz)
	kilograms (kg)	2.2	pounds (lb)
	metric tons (1,000 kg)	1.1	short tons
	milliliters (ml)	0.03	fluid ounces (fl oz)
	liters (l)	2.1	pints (pt)
	liters	1.06	quarts (qt)
Volume	liters	0.26	gallons (gal)
	cubic meters (m^3)	35	cubic feet (ft^3)
	cubic meters	1.3	cubic yards (yd^3)
Temperature	Celsius (°C) temperature	9/5 (then add 32)	Fahrenheit (°F) temperature

Source: Adapted from "Some References on Metric Information" by U.S. Department of Commerce, National Bureau of Standards.

Weight Equivalents

	Milligram	Gram	Kilogram	Grain	Ounce	Pound
1 microgram (mg)	0.001	0.000001				
1 milligram (mg)	1.0	0.001		0.0154		
1 gram (g)	1,000.0	1.0	0.001	15.4	0.035	0.0022
1 kilogram (kg)	1,000,000.0	1,000.0	1.0	15,400.0	35.2	2.2
1 grain (gr)	64.8	0.065		1.0		
1 ounce (oz)		28.3		437.5	1.0	0.063
1 pound (lb)		453.6	0.454		16.0	1.0

Volume Equivalents

	Cubic Millimeter	Cubic Centimeter	Liter	Fluid Ounce	Pint	Quart
1 cubic millimeter (mm^3)	1.0	0.001				
1 cubic centimeter (cm^3)	1,000.0	1.0	0.001			
1 liter (l)	1,000,000.0	1,000.0	1.0	33.8	2.1	1.06
1 fluid ounce (fl oz)		30.(29.57)	0.03	1.0		
1 pint (pt)		473.0	0.473	16.0	1.0	
1 quart (qt)		946.0	0.946	32.0	2.0	1.0

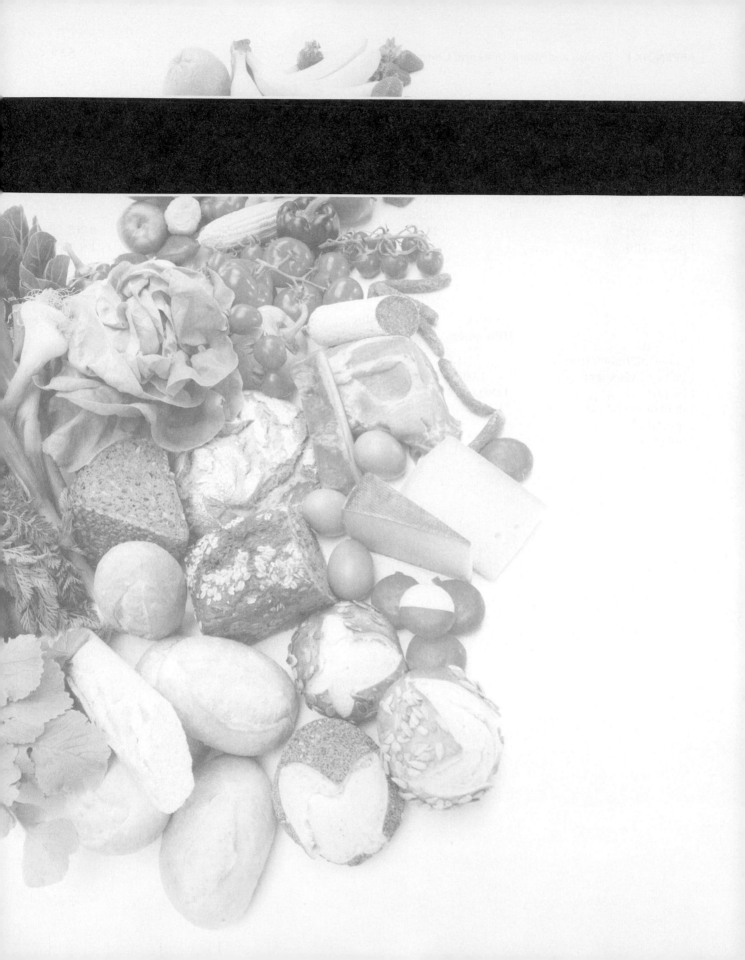

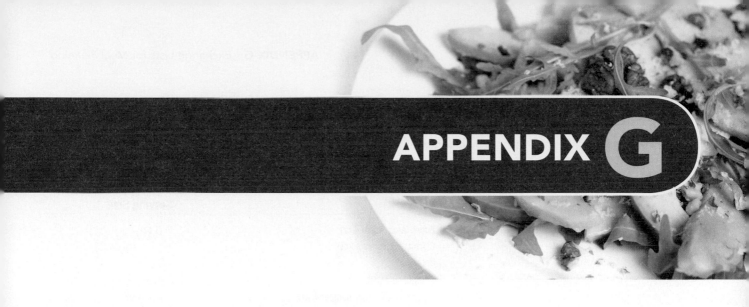

APPENDIX G

EXCHANGE LISTS FOR MEAL PLANNING

Balanced Energy: A healthy weight is the result of balancing energy in and energy out of the body. You get energy from the food you eat. Energy is measured in calories. You use energy when you breathe, sit, walk, and move. You stay at the same weight when energy in—the food you eat—is the same as the energy you use. You gain weight when you take in more energy (calories) than your body uses. This extra energy is stored as unwanted weight. You can lose weight by taking in fewer calories than your body needs or burning off more than you take in. Then your body uses stored energy to meet your needs. Ask your RD to estimate how much energy your body needs. When you balance energy from food and energy used for exercise, you can maintain a healthy weight.

Starch

One starch exchange equals 15 g carbohydrate, 3 g protein, 0–1 g fat, and 80 calories

Bread

	Food	Serving Size
	Bagel, large (about 4 oz)	¼ (1 oz)
⚠	Biscuit, 2½ inches across	1
	Bread	
☺	reduced-calorie	2 slices (1½ oz)
	with, whole-grain, pumpernickel, rye, unfrosted raisin	1 slice (1 oz)
	Chapatti, small, 6 inches across	1
⚠	Cornbread, 1¾ inch cube	1 (1½ oz)
	English muffin	½
	Hot dog bun or hamburger bun	½ (1 oz)
	Naan, 8 inches by 2 inches	¼
	Pancake, 4 inches across, ¼ inch thick	1
	Pita, 6 inches across	½
	Roll, plain, small	1 (1 oz)
⚠	Stuffing, bread	⅓ cup
⚠	Taco shell, 5 inches across	2
	Tortilla, corn, 6 inches across	1
	Tortilla, flour, 6 inches across	1
	Tortilla, flour, 10 inches across	⅓ tortilla
⚠	Waffle, 4-inch square or 4 inches across	1

Source: Reproduction of the Exchange Lists in whole or part, without permission of the American Dietetic Association or the American Diabetes Association, Inc., is a violation of federal law. This material has been modified from Choose Your Foods: Exchange Lists for Diabetes, which is the basis of a meal planning system designed by a committee of the American Diabetes Association and the American Dietetic Association. While designed primarily for people with diabetes and others who must follow special diets, the Exchange Lists are based on principles of good nutrition that apply to everyone. Copyright © 2008 by the American Diabetes Association and Academy of Nutrition and Dietetics (formerly American Dietetic Association)

Cereals and Grains

	Food	Serving Size
	Barley, cooked	⅓ cup
	Bran, dry	
☺	oat	¼ cup
☺	wheat	½ cup

(continues)

☺ = More than 3 grams of dietary fiber per serving.

⚠ = Extra fat, or prepared with added fat (Count as 1 starch + fat.).

Cereals and Grains (*continued*)

	Food	Serving Size
☺	Bulgur (cooked)	½ cup
	Cereals	
☺	bran	½ cup
	cooked (oats, oatmeal)	½ cup
	puffed	1½ cups
	shredded wheat, plain	½ cup
	sugar-coated	½ cup
	unsweetened, ready-to-eat	¾ cup
	Couscous	⅓ cup
	Granola	
	low-fat	¼ cup
⚠	regular	¼ cup
	Grits, cooked	½ cup
	Kasha	½ cup
	Millet, cooked	⅓ cup
	Muesli	¼ cup
	Pasta, cooked	⅓ cup
	Polenta, cooked	⅓ cup
	Quinoa, cooked	⅓ cup
	Rice, white or brown, cooked	⅓ cup
	Tabbouleh (tabouli), prepared	½ cup
	Wheat germ, dry	3 Tbsp
	Wild rice, cooked	½ cup

Tip: An open handful is equal to about 1 cup or 1 to 2 oz of snack food.

Source: Reproduction of the Exchange Lists in whole or part, without permission of the American Dietetic Association or the American Diabetes Association, Inc., is a violation of federal law. This material has been modified from Choose Your Foods: Exchange Lists for Diabetes, which is the basis of a meal planning system designed by a committee of the American Diabetes Association and the American Dietetic Association. While designed primarily for people with diabetes and others who must follow special diets, the Exchange Lists are based on principles of good nutrition that apply to everyone. Copyright © 2008 by the American Diabetes Association and Academy of Nutrition and Dietetics (formerly American Dietetic Association)

Crackers and Snacks

	Food	Serving Size
	Animal crackers	8
	Crackers	
⚠	round-butter type	6
	saltine-type	6
⚠	sandwich-style, cheese or peanut butter filling	3
⚠	whole-wheat regular	2–5 (¾ oz)
☺	whole-wheat lower fat or crispbreads	2–5 (¾ oz)

(continues)

☺ = More than 3 grams of dietary fiber per serving.

⚠ = Extra fat, or prepared with added fat.

Crackers and Snacks (*continued*)

Food	Serving Size
Graham cracker, 2½-inch square	3
Matzoh	¾ oz
Melba toast, about 2-inch by 4-inch piece	4 pieces
Oyster crackers	20
Popcorn	3 cups
⚠ with butter	3 cups
☺ no fat added	3 cups
☺ lower fat	3 cups
Pretzels	¾ oz
Rice cakes, 4 inches across	2
Snack chips	
fat-free or baked (tortilla, potato), baked pita chips	15–20 (¾ oz)
⚠ regular (tortilla, potato)	9–13 (¾ oz)

Note: For other snacks, see the **Sweets, Desserts, and Other Carbohydrates**.

Source: Reproduction of the Exchange Lists in whole or part, without permission of the American Dietetic Association or the American Diabetes Association, Inc., is a violation of federal law. This material has been modified from Choose Your Foods: Exchange Lists for Diabetes, which is the basis of a meal planning system designed by a committee of the American Diabetes Association and the American Dietetic Association. While designed primarily for people with diabetes and others who must follow special diets, the Exchange Lists are based on principles of good nutrition that apply to everyone. Copyright © 2008 by the American Diabetes Association and Academy of Nutrition and Dietetics (formerly American Dietetic Association)

Fruits

Fruit

The weight listed includes skin, core, seeds, and rind.

Food	Serving Size
Apple, unpeeled, small	1 (4 oz)
Apples, dried	4 rings
Applesauce, unsweetened	½ cup
Apricots	
canned	½ cup
dried	8 halves
☺ fresh	4 whole (5½ oz)
Banana, extra small	1 (4 oz)
☺ Blackberries	¾ cup
Blueberries	¾ cup
Cantaloupe, small	⅓ melon or 1 cup cubed (11 oz)
Cherries	
sweet, canned	½ cup
sweet fresh	12 (3 oz)

(continues)

☺ = More than 3 grams of dietary fiber per serving.

⚠ = Extra fat, or prepared with added fat.

Fruit (*continued*)

	Food	Serving Size
	Dates	3
	Dried fruits (blueberries, cherries, cranberries, mixed fruit, raisins)	2 Tbsp
	Figs	
	dried	1½
☺	fresh	1½ large or 2 medium (3½ oz)
	Fruit cocktail	½ cup
	Grapefruit	
	large	½ (11 oz)
	sections, canned	¾ cup
	Grapes, small	17 (3 oz)
	Honeydew melon	1 slice or 1 cup cubed (10 oz)
☺	Kiwi	1 (3½ oz)
	Mandarin oranges, canned	¾ cup
	Mango, small	½ fruit (5½ oz) or ½ cup
	Nectarine, small	1 (5 oz)
☺	Orange, small	1 (6½ oz)
	Papaya	½ fruit or 1 cup cubed (8 oz)
	Peaches	
	canned	½ cup
	fresh, medium	1 (6 oz)
	Pears	
	canned	½ cup
	fresh, large	½ (4 oz)
	Pineapple	
	canned	½ cup
	fresh	¾ cup
	Plums	
	canned	⅛ cup
	dried (prunes)	3
	small	2 (5 oz)
☺	Raspberries	1 cup
☺	Strawberries	1¼ cup whole berries
☺	Tangerines, small	2 (8 oz)
	Watermelon	1 slice or 1¼ cups cubes (13½ oz)

☺ = More than 3 grams of dietary fiber per serving.

Fruit Juice

Food	Serving Size
Apple juice/cider	½ cup
Fruit juice blends, 100% juice	⅓ cup
Grape juice	⅓ cup
Grapefruit juice	½ cup
Orange juice	½ cup
Pineapple juice	½ cup
Prune juice	⅓ cup

Source: Reproduction of the Exchange Lists in whole or part, without permission of the American Dietetic Association or the American Diabetes Association, Inc., is a violation of federal law. This material has been modified from Choose Your Foods: Exchange Lists for Diabetes, which is the basis of a meal planning system designed by a committee of the American Diabetes Association and the American Dietetic Association. While designed primarily for people with diabetes and others who must follow special diets, the Exchange Lists are based on principles of good nutrition that apply to everyone. Copyright © 2008 by the American Diabetes Association and Academy of Nutrition and Dietetics (formerly American Dietetic Association)

Milk
Milk and Yogurts

Food	Serving Size	Count as
Fat-free or low-fat (1%)		
Milk, buttermilk, acidophilus milk, Lactaid	1 cup	1 fat-free milk
Evaporated milk	½ cup	1 fat-free milk
Yogurt, plain or flavored with an artificial sweetener	⅔ cup (6 oz)	1 fat-free milk
Reduced-fat (2%)		
Milk, acidophilus milk, kefir, Lactaid	1 cup	1 reduced-fat milk
Yogurt, plain	⅔ cup (6 oz)	1 reduced-fat milk
Whole		
Milk, buttermilk, goat's milk	1 cup	1 whole milk
Evaporated milk	½ cup	1 whole milk
Yogurt, plain	8 oz	1 whole milk

Source: Reproduction of the Exchange Lists in whole or part, without permission of the American Dietetic Association or the American Diabetes Association, Inc., is a violation of federal law. This material has been modified from Choose Your Foods: Exchange Lists for Diabetes, which is the basis of a meal planning system designed by a committee of the American Diabetes Association and the American Dietetic Association. While designed primarily for people with diabetes and others who must follow special diets, the Exchange Lists are based on principles of good nutrition that apply to everyone. Copyright © 2008 by the American Diabetes Association and Academy of Nutrition and Dietetics (formerly American Dietetic Association)

Dairy-like Foods

Food	Serving Size	Count as
Chocolate milk		
fat-free	1 cup	1 fat-free milk + 1 carbohydrate
whole	1 cup	1 whole milk + 1 carbohydrate
Eggnog, whole milk	½ cup	1 carbohydrate + 2 fats
Rice drink		
flavored, low-fat	1 cup	2 carbohydrates
plain, fat-free	1 cup	1 carbohydrate
Smoothies, flavored, regular	10 oz	1 fat-free milk + 2½ carbohydrates
Soy milk		
light	1 cup	1 carbohydrate + ½ fat
regular, plain	1 cup	1 carbohydrate + 1 fat
Yogurt		
and juice blends	1 cup	1 fat-free milk + 1 carbohydrate
low carbohydrate (less than 6 grams carbohydrate per choice)	⅔ cup (6 oz)	½ fat-free milk
with fruit, low-fat	⅔ cup (6 oz)	1 fat-free milk + 1 carbohydrate

Note: Coconut milk is on the **Fats** list

Source: Reproduction of the Exchange Lists in whole or part, without permission of the American Dietetic Association or the American Diabetes Association, Inc., is a violation of federal law. This material has been modified from Choose Your Foods: Exchange Lists for Diabetes, which is the basis of a meal planning system designed by a committee of the American Diabetes Association and the American Dietetic Association. While designed primarily for people with diabetes and others who must follow special diets, the Exchange Lists are based on principles of good nutrition that apply to everyone. Copyright © 2008 by the American Diabetes Association and Academy of Nutrition and Dietetics (formerly American Dietetic Association)

Sweets, Desserts, and other Carbohydrates

Beverages, Soda, and Energy/Sports Drinks

Food	Serving Size	Count as
Cranberry juice cocktail	½ cup	1 carbohydrate
Energy drink	1 can (8.3 oz)	2 carbohydrates
Fruit drink or lemonade	1 cup (8 oz)	2 carbohydrates
Hot chocolate		
regular	1 envelope added to 8 oz water	1 carbohydrate + 1 fat
sugar-free or light	1 envelope added to 8 oz water	1 carbohydrate
Soft drink (soda), regular	1 can (12 oz)	2½ carbohydrates
Sports drink	1 cup (8 oz)	1 carbohydrate

Source: Reproduction of the Exchange Lists in whole or part, without permission of the American Dietetic Association or the American Diabetes Association, Inc., is a violation of federal law. This material has been modified from Choose Your Foods: Exchange Lists for Diabetes, which is the basis of a meal planning system designed by a committee of the American Diabetes Association and the American Dietetic Association. While designed primarily for people with diabetes and others who must follow special diets, the Exchange Lists are based on principles of good nutrition that apply to everyone. Copyright © 2008 by the American Diabetes Association and Academy of Nutrition and Dietetics (formerly American Dietetic Association)

Brownies, Cake, Cookies, Gelatin, Pie, and Pudding

Food	Serving Size	Count as
Brownie, small, unfrosted	1¼-inch square, ⅔ inch high (about 1 oz)	1 carbohydrate + 1 fat
Cake		
angel food, unfrosted	1½ of cake (about 2 oz)	2 carbohydrates
frosted	2-inch square (about 2 oz)	2 carbohydrates + 1 fat
unfrosted	2-inch square (about 2 oz)	1 carbohydrate + 1 fat
Cookies		
chocolate chip	2 cookies (2¼ inches across)	1 carbohydrate + 2 fats
gingersnap	3 cookies	1 carbohydrate
sandwich, with crème filling	2 small (about ⅔ oz)	1 carbohydrate + 1 fat
sugar-free	3 small or 1 large (¾–1 oz)	1 carbohydrate + 1–2 fats
vanilla wafer	5 cookies	1 carbohydrate + 1 fat
Cupcake, frosted	1 small (about 1¾ oz)	2 carbohydrates + 1–1½ fats
Fruit cobbler	½ cup (3½ oz)	3 carbohydrates + 1 fat
Gelatin, regular	½ cup	1 carbohydrate
Pie		
commercially prepared fruit, 2 crusts	⅛ of 8-inch pie	3 carbohydrates + 2 fats
pumpkin or custard	⅛ of 8-inch pie	1½ carbohydrates + 1½ fats
Pudding		
regular (made with reduced-fat milk)	½ cup	2 carbohydrates
sugar-free or sugar- and fat-free (made with fat-free milk)	½ cup	1 carbohydrate

Candy, Spreads, Sweets, Sweeteners, Syrups, and Toppings

Food	Serving Size	Count as
Candy bar, chocolate/peanut	2 "fun size" bars (1 oz)	1½ carbohydrates + 1½ fats
Candy, hard	3 pieces	1 carbohydrate
Chocolate "kisses"	5 pieces	1 carbohydrate + 1 fat
Coffee creamer		
dry, flavored	4 tsp	½ carbohydrate + ½ fat
liquid, flavored	2 Tbsp	1 carbohydrate
Fruit snacks, chewy (pureed fruit concentrate)	1 roll (¾ oz)	1 carbohydrate
Fruit spreads, 100% fruit	1½ Tbsp	1 carbohydrate
Honey	1 Tbsp	1 carbohydrate

(continues)

Candy, Spreads, Sweets, Sweeteners, Syrups, and Toppings (*continued*)

Food	Serving Size	Count as
Jam or jelly, regular	1 Tbsp	1 carbohydrate
Sugar	1 Tbsp	1 carbohydrate
Syrup		
chocolate	2 Tbsp	2 carbohydrates
light (pancake type)	2 Tbsp	1 carbohydrate
regular (pancake type)	1 Tbsp	1 carbohydrate

Source: Reproduction of the Exchange Lists in whole or part, without permission of the American Dietetic Association or the American Diabetes Association, Inc., is a violation of federal law. This material has been modified from Choose Your Foods: Exchange Lists for Diabetes, which is the basis of a meal planning system designed by a committee of the American Diabetes Association and the American Dietetic Association. While designed primarily for people with diabetes and others who must follow special diets, the Exchange Lists are based on principles of good nutrition that apply to everyone. Copyright © 2008 by the American Diabetes Association and Academy of Nutrition and Dietetics (formerly American Dietetic Association)

Condiments and Sauces

Food	Serving Size	Count as
Barbeque sauce	3 Tbsp	1 carbohydrate
Cranberry sauce, jellied	¼ cup	1½ carbohydrates
🧂 Gravy, canned or bottled	½ cup	½ carbohydrate + ½ fat
Salad dressing, fat-free, low-fat, cream-based	3 Tbsp	1 carbohydrate
Sweet and sour sauce	3 Tbsp	1 carbohydrate

Source: Reproduction of the Exchange Lists in whole or part, without permission of the American Dietetic Association or the American Diabetes Association, Inc., is a violation of federal law. This material has been modified from Choose Your Foods: Exchange Lists for Diabetes, which is the basis of a meal planning system designed by a committee of the American Diabetes Association and the American Dietetic Association. While designed primarily for people with diabetes and others who must follow special diets, the Exchange Lists are based on principles of good nutrition that apply to everyone. Copyright © 2008 by the American Diabetes Association and Academy of Nutrition and Dietetics (formerly American Dietetic Association)

Doughnuts, Muffins, Pastries, and Sweet Breads

Food	Serving Size	Count as
Banana nut bread	1-inch slice (1 oz)	2 carbohydrates + 1 fat
Doughnut		
cake, plain	1 medium (1½ oz)	1½ carbohydrates + 2 fats
yeast type, glazed	3¾ inches across (2 oz)	2 carbohydrates + 2 fats
Muffin (4 oz)	¼ muffin (1 oz)	1 carbohydrate + ½ fat
Sweet roll or Danish	1 (2½ oz)	2½ carbohydrates + 2 fats

(continues)

🧂 = 480 milligrams or more of sodium per serving.

Doughnuts, Muffins, Pastries, and Sweet Breads (*continued*)

Note: You can also check the **Fats** list and **Free Foods** list for other condiments.

Source: Reproduction of the Exchange Lists in whole or part, without permission of the American Dietetic Association or the American Diabetes Association, Inc., is a violation of federal law. This material has been modified from Choose Your Foods: Exchange Lists for Diabetes, which is the basis of a meal planning system designed by a committee of the American Diabetes Association and the American Dietetic Association. While designed primarily for people with diabetes and others who must follow special diets, the Exchange Lists are based on principles of good nutrition that apply to everyone. Copyright © 2008 by the American Diabetes Association and Academy of Nutrition and Dietetics (formerly American Dietetic Association)

Frozen Bars, Frozen Desserts, Frozen Yogurt, and Ice Cream

Food	Serving Size	Count as
Frozen pops	1	½ carbohydrate
Fruit, juice bars, frozen, 100% juice	1 bar (3 oz)	1 carbohydrate
Ice cream		
fat-free	½ cup	1½ carbohydrates
light	½ cup	1 carbohydrate + 1 fat
no sugar added	½ cup	1 carbohydrate + 1 fat
regular	½ cup	1 carbohydrate + 2 fats
Sherbet, sorbet	½ cup	2 carbohydrates
Yogurt, frozen		
fat-free	⅓ cup	1 carbohydrate
regular	½ cup	1 carbohydrate + 0–1 fat

Source: Reproduction of the Exchange Lists in whole or part, without permission of the American Dietetic Association or the American Diabetes Association, Inc., is a violation of federal law. This material has been modified from Choose Your Foods: Exchange Lists for Diabetes, which is the basis of a meal planning system designed by a committee of the American Diabetes Association and the American Dietetic Association. While designed primarily for people with diabetes and others who must follow special diets, the Exchange Lists are based on principles of good nutrition that apply to everyone. Copyright © 2008 by the American Diabetes Association and Academy of Nutrition and Dietetics (formerly American Dietetic Association)

Granola Bars, Meal Replacement Bars/Shakes, and Trail Mix

Food	Serving Size	Count as
Granola or snack bar, regular or low-fat	1 bar (1 oz)	1½ carbohydrates
Meal replacement bar	1 bar (1⅓ oz)	1½ carbohydrates + 0–1 fat
Meal replacement bar	1 bar (2 oz)	2 carbohydrates + 1 fat
Meal replacement shake, reduced calorie	1 can (10–11 oz)	1½ carbohydrates + 0–1 fat
Trail mix		
candy/nut-based	1 oz	1 carbohydrate + 2 fats
dried fruit–based	1 oz	1 carbohydrate + 1 fat

(continues)

Granola Bars, Meal Replacement Bars/Shakes, and Trail Mix (*continued*)

Vegetables

Beans, Peas, and Lentils

The choices on this list count as 1 starch + 1 lean meat.

Food	Serving Size
☺ Baked beans	⅓ cup
☺ Beans, cooked (black, garbanzo, kidney, lima, navy, pinto, white)	½ cup
☺ Lentils, cooked (brown, green, yellow)	½ cup
☺ Peas, cooked (black-eyed, split)	½ cup
🧂 ☺ Refried beans, canned	½ cup

Starchy Vegetables

Food	Serving Size
Cassava	⅓ cup
Corn	½ cup
on cob, large	½ cob (5 oz)
☺ Hominy, canned	¾ cup
☺ Mixed vegetables with corn, peas, or pasta	1 cup
☺ Parsnips	½ cup
☺ Peas, green	½ cup
Plantain, ripe	⅓ cup

(continues)

 = More than 3 grams of dietary fiber per serving.

🧂 = 480 milligrams or more of sodium per serving.

Starchy Vegetables (*continued*)

Food	Serving Size
Potato	
baked with skin	¼ large (3 oz)
boiled, all kinds	½ cup or ½ medium (3 oz)
▽! mashed, with milk and fat	½ cup
French fried (oven-baked)	1 cup (2 oz)
☺ Pumpkin, canned, no sugar added	1 cup
Spaghetti/pasta sauce	½ cup
☺ Squash, winter (acorn, butternut)	1 cup
☺ Succotash	½ cup
Yam, sweet potato, plain	½ cup

Source: Reproduction of the Exchange Lists in whole or part, without permission of the American Dietetic Association or the American Diabetes Association, Inc., is a violation of federal law. This material has been modified from Choose Your Foods: Exchange Lists for Diabetes, which is the basis of a meal planning system designed by a committee of the American Diabetes Association and the American Dietetic Association. While designed primarily for people with diabetes and others who must follow special diets, the Exchange Lists are based on principles of good nutrition that apply to everyone. Copyright © 2008 by the American Diabetes Association and Academy of Nutrition and Dietetics (formerly American Dietetic Association)

Nonstarchy Vegetables

Amaranth or Chinese spinach
Artichoke
Artichoke hearts
Asparagus
Baby corn
Bamboo shoots
Bean sprouts
Beans (green, wax, Italian)
Beets
🔲 Borscht
Broccoli
☺ Brussels sprouts
Cabbage (green, bok choy, Chinese)
☺ Carrots
Cauliflower
Celery
☺ Chayote
Coleslaw, packaged, no dressing
Cucumber
Eggplant
Gourds (bitter, bottle, luffa, bitter melon)
Green onions or scallions
Greens (collard, kale, mustard, turnip)
Hearts of palm
Jicama
Kohlrabi

Leeks
Mixed vegetables (without corn, peas, or pasta)
Mung bean sprouts
Mushrooms, all kinds, fresh
Okra
Onions
Oriental radish or daikon
Pea pods
☺ Peppers (all varieties)
Radishes
Rutabaga
🔲 Sauerkraut
Soybean sprouts
Spinach
Squash (summer, crookneck, zucchini)
Sugar pea snaps
☺ Swiss chard
Tomato
🔲 Tomato sauce
Tomatoes, canned
▽! Tomato/vegetable juice
Turnips
Water chestnuts
Yard-long beans

(continues)

☺ = More than 3 grams of dietary fiber per serving.

▽! = Extra fat, or prepared with added fat.

🔲 = 480 milligrams or more of sodium per serving.

Nonstarchy Vegetables (*continued*)

Note: Salad greens (like chicory, endive, escarole, lettuce, romaine, spinach, arugula, radicchio, watercress) are on the **Free Foods**.

Source: Reproduction of the Exchange Lists in whole or part, without permission of the American Dietetic Association or the American Diabetes Association, Inc., is a violation of federal law. This material has been modified from Choose Your Foods: Exchange Lists for Diabetes, which is the basis of a meal planning system designed by a committee of the American Diabetes Association and the American Dietetic Association. While designed primarily for people with diabetes and others who must follow special diets, the Exchange Lists are based on principles of good nutrition that apply to everyone. Copyright © 2008 by the American Diabetes Association and Academy of Nutrition and Dietetics (formerly American Dietetic Association)

Meat and Meat Substitutes

	Carbohydrate (grams)	Protein (grams)	Fat (grams)	Calories
Lean meat	—	7	0–3	45
Medium-fat meat	—	7	4–7	75
High-fat meat	—	7	8+	100
Plant-based protein	varies	7	varies	varies

Source: Reproduction of the Exchange Lists in whole or part, without permission of the American Dietetic Association or the American Diabetes Association, Inc., is a violation of federal law. This material has been modified from Choose Your Foods: Exchange Lists for Diabetes, which is the basis of a meal planning system designed by a committee of the American Diabetes Association and the American Dietetic Association. While designed primarily for people with diabetes and others who must follow special diets, the Exchange Lists are based on principles of good nutrition that apply to everyone. Copyright © 2008 by the American Diabetes Association and Academy of Nutrition and Dietetics (formerly American Dietetic Association)

Portion Sizes: Portion size is an important part of meal planning. The **Meat and Meat Substitute** list is based on cooked weight (4 oz of raw meat is equal to 3 oz of cooked meat) after bone and fat have been removed. Try using the following comparisons to help estimate portion sizes:

- 1 oz cooked meat, poultry, or fish is about the size of a matchbox.
- 3 oz cooked meat, poultry, or fish is about the size of a deck of playing cards.
- 2 Tbsp peanut butter is about the size of a golf ball.
- The palm of a woman's hand is about 3 to 4 oz of cooked, boneless meat. The palm of a man's hand is a larger serving.
- 1 oz cheese is about the size of 4 dice.

Lean Meats and Meat Substitutes

Food	Amount
Beef: Select or Choice grades trimmed of fat: ground round, roast (chuck, rib, rump), round, sirloin, steak (cubed, flank, porterhouse, T-bone), tenderloin	1 oz
Beef jerky	1 oz
Cheeses with 3 grams of fat or less per oz	1 oz
Cottage cheese	¼ cup
Egg substitutes, plain	¼ cup
Egg whites	2
Fish, fresh or frozen, plain: catfish, cod, flounder, haddock, halibut, orange roughy, salmon, tilapia, trout, tuna	1 oz
Fish, smoked: herring or salmon (lox)	1 oz
Game: buffalo, ostrich, rabbit, venison	1 oz
Hot dog with 3 grams of fat or less per oz (8 dogs per 14 oz package) *Note: May be high in carbohydrate*	1
Lamb: chop, leg, or roast	1 oz
Organ meats: heart, kidney, liver *Note: May be high in cholesterol*	1 oz
Oysters, fresh or frozen	6 medium
Pork, lean	
Canadian bacon	1 oz
rib or loin chop/roast, ham, tenderloin	1 oz
Poultry, without skin: Cornish hen, chicken, domestic duck or goose (well drained of fat), turkey	1 oz
Processed sandwich meats with 3 grams of fat or less per oz: chipped beef, deli thin-sliced meats, turkey ham, turkey kielbasa, turkey pastrami	1 oz
Salmon, canned	1 oz
Sardines, canned	2 medium
Sausage with 3 grams of fat or less per oz	1 oz
Shellfish: clams, crab, imitation shellfish, lobster, scallops, shrimp	1 oz
Tuna, canned in water or oil, drained	1 oz
Veal, lean chop, roast	1 oz

Source: Reproduction of the Exchange Lists in whole or part, without permission of the American Dietetic Association or the American Diabetes Association, Inc., is a violation of federal law. This material has been modified from Choose Your Foods: Exchange Lists for Diabetes, which is the basis of a meal planning system designed by a committee of the American Diabetes Association and the American Dietetic Association. While designed primarily for people with diabetes and others who must follow special diets, the Exchange Lists are based on principles of good nutrition that apply to everyone. Copyright © 2008 by the American Diabetes Association and Academy of Nutrition and Dietetics (formerly American Dietetic Association)

 = 480 milligrams or more of sodium per serving (based on the sodium content of a typical 3-oz serving of meat, unless 1 or 2 oz is the normal serving size).

Medium-Fat Meat and Meat Substitutes

Food	Amount
Beef: corned beef, ground beef, meatloaf, Prime grades trimmed of fat (prime rib), short ribs, tongue	1 oz
Cheeses with 4–7 grams of fat per oz: feta, mozzarella, pasteurized processed cheese spread, reduced-fat cheeses, string	1 oz
Egg	1
Note: High in cholesterol, so limit to 3 per week	
Fish, any fried product	1 oz
Lamb: ground, rib roast	1 oz
Pork: cutlet, shoulder roast	1 oz
Poultry: chicken with skin; dove, pheasant, wild duck, or goose; fried chicken; ground turkey	1 oz
Ricotta cheese	2 oz or ¼ cup
Sausage with 4–7 grams of fat per oz	1 oz
Veal, cutlet (no breading)	1 oz

Source: Reproduction of the Exchange Lists in whole or part, without permission of the American Dietetic Association or the American Diabetes Association, Inc., is a violation of federal law. This material has been modified from Choose Your Foods: Exchange Lists for Diabetes, which is the basis of a meal planning system designed by a committee of the American Diabetes Association and the American Dietetic Association. While designed primarily for people with diabetes and others who must follow special diets, the Exchange Lists are based on principles of good nutrition that apply to everyone. Copyright © 2008 by the American Diabetes Association and Academy of Nutrition and Dietetics (formerly American Dietetic Association)

High-Fat Meat and Meat Substitutes

These foods are high in saturated fat, cholesterol, and calories and may raise blood cholesterol levels if eaten on a regular basis. Try to eat 3 or fewer servings from this group per week.

Food	Amount
Bacon	
pork	2 slices (16 slices per lb or 1 oz each, before cooking)
turkey	3 slices (½ oz each before cooking)
Cheese, regular: American, bleu, brie, cheddar, hard goat, Monterey jack, queso, and Swiss	1 oz
Hot dog: beef, pork, or combination (10 per lb-sized package)	1
Hot dog: turkey or chicken (10 per lb-sized package)	1
Pork: ground, sausage, spareribs	1 oz

(continues)

= Extra fat, or prepared with added fat. (Add an additional fat choice to this food.)

= 480 milligrams or more of sodium per serving (based on the sodium content of a typical 3-oz serving of meat, unless 1 or 2 oz is the normal serving size).

High-Fat Meat and Meat Substitutes (*continued*)

Food	Amount
Processed sandwich meats with 8 grams of fat or more per oz: bologna, pastrami, hard salami	1 oz
Ⓢ Sausage with 8 grams fat or more per oz: bratwurst, chorizo, Italian, knockwurst, Polish, smoked, summer	1 oz

Source: Reproduction of the Exchange Lists in whole or part, without permission of the American Dietetic Association or the American Diabetes Association, Inc., is a violation of federal law. This material has been modified from Choose Your Foods: Exchange Lists for Diabetes, which is the basis of a meal planning system designed by a committee of the American Diabetes Association and the American Dietetic Association. While designed primarily for people with diabetes and others who must follow special diets, the Exchange Lists are based on principles of good nutrition that apply to everyone. Copyright © 2008 by the American Diabetes Association and Academy of Nutrition and Dietetics (formerly American Dietetic Association)

Plant-Based Proteins

Because carbohydrate content varies among plant-based proteins, you should read the food label.

	Food	Amount	Count as
	"Bacon" strips, soy-based	3 strips	1 medium-fat meat
☺	Baked beans	⅓ cup	1 starch + 1 lean meat
☺	Beans, cooked: black, garbanzo, kidney, lima, navy, pinto, white	½ cup	1 starch + 1 lean meat
☺	"Beef" or "sausage" crumbles, soy-based	2 oz	½ carbohydrate + 1 lean meat
	"Chicken" nuggets, soy-based	2 nuggets (1½ oz)	½ carbohydrate + 1 medium-fat meat
☺	Edamame	½ cup	½ carbohydrate + 1 lean meat
	Falafel (spiced chickpea and wheat patties)	3 patties (about 2 inches across)	1 carbohydrate + 1 high-fat meat
	Hot dog, soy-based	1 (1½ oz)	½ carbohydrate + 1 lean meat
☺	Hummus	⅓ cup	1 carbohydrate + 1 high-fat meat
☺	Lentils, brown, green, or yellow	½ cup	1 carbohydrate + 1 lean meat
☺	Meatless burger, soy-based	3 oz	½ carbohydrate + 2 lean meats
☺	Meatless burger, vegetable- and starch-based	1 patty (about 2½ oz)	1 carbohydrate + 2 lean meats
	Nut spreads: almond butter, cashew butter, peanut butter, soy nut butter	1 Tbsp	1 high-fat meat
☺	Peas, cooked: black-eyed and split peas	½ cup	1 starch + 1 lean meat
☺	Refried beans, canned	½ cup	1 starch + 1 lean meat
	"Sausage" patties, soy-based	1 (1½ oz)	1 medium-fat meat

(continues)

☺ = More than 3 grams of dietary fiber per serving.

Ⓢ = 480 milligrams or more of sodium per serving (based on the sodium content of a typical 3-oz serving of meat, unless 1 or 2 oz is the normal serving size).

Plant-Based Proteins (*continued*)

Food	Amount	Count as
Soy nuts, unsalted	¾ oz	½ carbohydrate + 1 medium-fat meat
Tempeh	¼ cup	1 medium-fat meat
Tofu	4 oz (½ cup)	1 medium-fat meat
Tofu, light	4 oz (½ cup)	1 lean meat

Note: Beans, peas, and lentils are also found on the **Starch** list. Nut butters in smaller amounts are found in the **Fats** list.

Source: Reproduction of the Exchange Lists in whole or part, without permission of the American Dietetic Association or the American Diabetes Association, Inc., is a violation of federal law. This material has been modified from Choose Your Foods: Exchange Lists for Diabetes, which is the basis of a meal planning system designed by a committee of the American Diabetes Association and the American Dietetic Association. While designed primarily for people with diabetes and others who must follow special diets, the Exchange Lists are based on principles of good nutrition that apply to everyone. Copyright © 2008 by the American Diabetes Association and Academy of Nutrition and Dietetics (formerly American Dietetic Association)

Fats

1 fat choice equals:

- 1 teaspoon of regular margarine, vegetable oil, butter
- 1 tablespoon of regular salad dressing

Unsaturated Fats—Monounsaturated Fats

Food	Serving Size
Avocado, medium	2 Tbsp (1 oz)
Nut butters (trans fat-free): almond butter, cashew butter, peanut butter (smooth or crunchy)	1½ tsp
Nuts	
almonds	6 nuts
Brazil	2 nuts
cashews	6 nuts
filberts (hazelnuts)	5 nuts
macadamia	3 nuts
mixed (50% peanuts)	6 nuts
peanuts	10 nuts
pecans	4 halves
pistachios	16 nuts
Oil: canola, olive, peanut	1 tsp
Olives	
black (ripe)	8 large
green, stuffed	10 large

Polyunsaturated Fats

Food	Serving Size
Margarine: lower-fat spread (30%–50% vegetable oil, *trans* fat-free)	1 Tbsp
Margarine: stick, tub (*trans* fat-free), or squeeze (*trans* fat-free)	1 tsp
Mayonnaise	
reduced-fat	1 Tbsp
regular	1 tsp
Mayonnaise-style salad dressing	
reduced-fat	1 Tbsp
regular	2 tsp
Nuts	
Pignolia (pine nuts)	1 Tbsp
walnuts, English	4 halves
Oil: corn, cottonseed, flaxseed, grape seed, safflower, soybean, sunflower	1 tsp
Oil: made from soybean and canola oil—Enova	1 tsp
Plant stanol esters	
light	1 Tbsp
regular	2 tsp
Salad dressing	
reduced-fat	2 Tbsp
Note: May be high in carbohydrate.	
regular	1 Tbsp
Seeds	
flaxseed, whole	1 Tbsp
pumpkin, sunflower	1 Tbsp
sesame seeds	1 Tbsp
Tahini or sesame paste	2 tsp

Source: Reproduction of the Exchange Lists in whole or part, without permission of the American Dietetic Association or the American Diabetes Association, Inc., is a violation of federal law. This material has been modified from Choose Your Foods: Exchange Lists for Diabetes, which is the basis of a meal planning system designed by a committee of the American Diabetes Association and the American Dietetic Association. While designed primarily for people with diabetes and others who must follow special diets, the Exchange Lists are based on principles of good nutrition that apply to everyone. Copyright © 2008 by the American Diabetes Association and Academy of Nutrition and Dietetics (formerly American Dietetic Association)

Saturated Fats

Food	Serving Size
Bacon, cooked, regular or turkey	1 slice
Butter	
reduced-fat	1 Tbsp
stick	1 tsp
whipped	2 tsp

(continues)

 = 480 milligrams or more of sodium per serving.

Saturated Fats (*continued*)

Food	Serving Size
Butter blends made with oil	
reduced-fat or light	1 Tbsp
regular	1½ tsp
Chitterlings, boiled	2 Tbsp (½ oz)
Coconut, sweetened, shredded	2 Tbsp
Coconut milk	
light	⅓ cup
regular	1½ Tbsp
Cream	
half and half	2 Tbsp
heavy	1 Tbsp
light	1½ Tbsp
whipped	2 Tbsp
whipped, pressurized	¼ cup
Cream cheese	
reduced-fat	1½ Tbsp (¾ oz)
regular	1 Tbsp (½ oz)
Lard	1 tsp
Oil: coconut, palm, palm kernel	1 tsp
Salt pork	¼ oz
Shortening, solid	1 tsp
Sour cream	
reduced-fat or light	3 Tbsp
regular	2 Tbsp

Source: Reproduction of the Exchange Lists in whole or part, without permission of the American Dietetic Association or the American Diabetes Association, Inc., is a violation of federal law. This material has been modified from Choose Your Foods: Exchange Lists for Diabetes, which is the basis of a meal planning system designed by a committee of the American Diabetes Association and the American Dietetic Association. While designed primarily for people with diabetes and others who must follow special diets, the Exchange Lists are based on principles of good nutrition that apply to everyone. Copyright © 2008 by the American Diabetes Association and Academy of Nutrition and Dietetics (formerly American Dietetic Association)

Free Foods

Selection Tips

- Most foods on this list should be limited to 3 servings (as listed here) per day.
- Food and drink choices listed here without a serving size can be eaten whenever you like.

Low Carbohydrate Foods

Food	Serving Size
Cabbage, raw	½ cup
Candy, hard (regular or sugar-free)	1 piece
Carrots, cauliflower, or green beans, cooked	¼ cup
Cranberries, sweetened with sugar substitute	½ cup
Cucumber, sliced	½ cup
Gelatin	
dessert, sugar-free	
unflavored	
Gum	
Jam or jelly, light or no sugar added	2 tsp
Rhubarb, sweetened with sugar substitute	½ cup
Salad greens	
Sugar substitutes (artificial sweeteners)	
Syrup, sugar-free	2 Tbsp

Source: Reproduction of the Exchange Lists in whole or part, without permission of the American Dietetic Association or the American Diabetes Association, Inc., is a violation of federal law. This material has been modified from Choose Your Foods: Exchange Lists for Diabetes, which is the basis of a meal planning system designed by a committee of the American Diabetes Association and the American Dietetic Association. While designed primarily for people with diabetes and others who must follow special diets, the Exchange Lists are based on principles of good nutrition that apply to everyone. Copyright © 2008 by the American Diabetes Association and Academy of Nutrition and Dietetics (formerly American Dietetic Association)

Modified Fat Foods with Carbohydrate

Food	Serving Size
Cream cheese, fat-free	1 Tbsp (½ oz)
Creamers	
nondairy, liquid	1 Tbsp
nondairy, powdered	2 tsp
Margarine spread	
fat-free	1 Tbsp
reduced-fat	1 tsp
Mayonnaise	
fat-free	1 Tbsp
reduced-fat	1 tsp
Mayonnaise-style salad dressing	
fat-free	1 Tbsp
reduced-fat	1 tsp
Salad dressing	
fat-free or low-fat	1 Tbsp
fat-free, Italian	2 Tbsp

(continues)

Modified Fat Foods with Carbohydrate (*continued*)

Food	Serving Size
Sour cream, fat-free or reduced-fat	1 Tbsp
Whipped topping	
light or fat-free	2 Tbsp
regular	1 Tbsp

Source: Reproduction of the Exchange Lists in whole or part, without permission of the American Dietetic Association or the American Diabetes Association, Inc., is a violation of federal law. This material has been modified from Choose Your Foods: Exchange Lists for Diabetes, which is the basis of a meal planning system designed by a committee of the American Diabetes Association and the American Dietetic Association. While designed primarily for people with diabetes and others who must follow special diets, the Exchange Lists are based on principles of good nutrition that apply to everyone. Copyright © 2008 by the American Diabetes Association and Academy of Nutrition and Dietetics (formerly American Dietetic Association)

Condiments

Food	Serving Size
Barbecue sauce	2 tsp
Catsup (ketchup)	1 Tbsp
Honey mustard	1 Tbsp
Horseradish	
Lemon juice	
Miso	1½ tsp
Mustard	
Parmesan cheese, freshly grated	1 Tbsp
Pickle relish	1 Tbsp
Pickles	
dill	1½ medium
sweet, bread and butter	2 slices
sweet, gherkin	¾ oz
Salsa	¼ cup
Soy sauce, light or regular	1 Tbsp
Sweet and sour sauce	2 tsp
Sweet chili sauce	2 tsp
Taco sauce	1 Tbsp
Vinegar	
Yogurt, any type	2 Tbsp

Source: Reproduction of the Exchange Lists in whole or part, without permission of the American Dietetic Association or the American Diabetes Association, Inc., is a violation of federal law. This material has been modified from Choose Your Foods: Exchange Lists for Diabetes, which is the basis of a meal planning system designed by a committee of the American Diabetes Association and the American Dietetic Association. While designed primarily for people with diabetes and others who must follow special diets, the Exchange Lists are based on principles of good nutrition that apply to everyone. Copyright © 2008 by the American Diabetes Association and Academy of Nutrition and Dietetics (formerly American Dietetic Association)

= 480 milligrams or more of sodium per serving.

Free Food List

A *free food* is any food or drink that contains less than 20 calories or less than 5 g of carbohydrate per serving. Foods with a serving size listed should be limited to three servings per day. Be sure to spread them out throughout the day. Eating all three servings at one time could affect your blood glucose level. Foods listed without a serving size can be eaten as often as you like.

Artificial Sweeteners: Sugar substitutes, alternatives, or replacements that are approved by the Food and Drug Administration (FDA) are safe to use. Common brand names include:

- Equal and Nutrasweet (aspartame)
- Splenda (sucralose)
- Sugar Twin, Sweet-10, Sweet'N Low, and Sprinkle Sweet (saccharin)
- Sweet One (acesulfame K)

Although each sweetener is tested for safety before it can be marketed and sold, use a variety of sweeteners and in moderate amounts.

Fat-Free or Reduced-Fat Foods

Cream cheese, fat-free	1 Tbsp
Creamers, nondairy, liquid	1 Tbsp
Creamers, nondairy, powdered	2 tsp
Mayonnaise, fat-free	1 Tbsp
Mayonnaise, reduced fat	1 tsp
Margarine, fat-free	4 Tbsp
Margarine, reduced fat	1 tsp
Miracle Whip, nonfat	1 Tbsp
Miracle Whip, reduced fat	1 tsp
Nonstick cooking spray	
Salad dressing, fat-free	1 Tbsp
Salad dressing, fat-free, Italian	2 Tbsp
Salsa	¼ cup
Sour cream, fat-free, reduced fat	1 Tbsp
Whipped topping, regular light	2 Tbsp

Sugar-Free or Low-Sugar Foods

Candy, hard, sugar-free	1 candy
Gelatin dessert, sugar-free	
Gelatin, unflavored	
Gum, sugar-free	
Jam or jelly, low-sugar or light	2 tsp
Syrup, sugar-free	2 Tbsp
Sugar substitutes, alternatives, or replacements that are approved by the Food and Drug Administration (FDA) are safe to use. Common brand names include:	

   Equal (aspartame)
   Sprinkle Sweet (saccharin)
   Sweet One (acesulfame K)
   Sweet-10 (saccharin)
   Sugar Twin (saccharin)
   Sweet'N Low (saccharin)

Drinks

Bouillon, broth, consommé*

Bouillon or broth, low sodium

Carbonated or mineral water

Club soda

Cocoa powder, unsweetened   1 Tbsp

Coffee

Diet soft drinks, sugar-free

Drink mixes, sugar-free

Tea

Tonic water, sugar-free

* = 400 milligrams or more of sodium per exchange.

Source: Reproduction of the Exchange Lists in whole or part, without permission of the American Dietetic Association or the American Diabetes Association, Inc., is a violation of federal law. This material has been modified from Choose Your Foods: Exchange Lists for Diabetes, which is the basis of a meal planning system designed by a committee of the American Diabetes Association and the American Dietetic Association. While designed primarily for people with diabetes and others who must follow special diets, the Exchange Lists are based on principles of good nutrition that apply to everyone. Copyright © 2008 by the American Diabetes Association and Academy of Nutrition and Dietetics (formerly American Dietetic Association)

Condiments

Catsup	1 Tbsp
Horseradish	
Lemon juice	
Lime juice	
Mustard	
Pickles, dill,*	1½ large
Soy sauce, regular or light*	
Taco sauce	1 Tbsp
Vinegar	

Source: Reproduction of the Exchange Lists in whole or part, without permission of the American Dietetic Association or the American Diabetes Association, Inc., is a violation of federal law. This material has been modified from Choose Your Foods: Exchange Lists for Diabetes, which is the basis of a meal planning system designed by a committee of the American Diabetes Association and the American Dietetic Association. While designed primarily for people with diabetes and others who must follow special diets, the Exchange Lists are based on principles of good nutrition that apply to everyone. Copyright © 2008 by the American Diabetes Association and Academy of Nutrition and Dietetics (formerly American Dietetic Association)

Drinks/Mixes

Any food on this list—without a serving size listed—can be consumed in any moderate amount.

- Bouillon, broth, consomme
- Bouillon or broth, low-sodium
- Carbonated or mineral water
- Club soda
- Cocoa powder, unsweetened (1 Tbsp)
- Coffee, unsweetened or with sugar substitute
- Diet soft drinks, sugar-free
- Drink mixes, sugar-free
- Tea, unsweetened or with sugar substitute
- Tonic water, diet
- Water
- Water, flavored, carbohydrate-free

Source: Reproduction of the Exchange Lists in whole or part, without permission of the American Dietetic Association or the American Diabetes Association, Inc., is a violation of federal law. This material has been modified from Choose Your Foods: Exchange Lists for Diabetes, which is the basis of a meal planning system designed by a committee of the American Diabetes Association and the American Dietetic Association. While designed primarily for people with diabetes and others who must follow special diets, the Exchange Lists are based on principles of good nutrition that apply to everyone. Copyright © 2008 by the American Diabetes Association and Academy of Nutrition and Dietetics (formerly American Dietetic Association)

Seasonings

Any food on this list can be consumed in any moderate amount.

- Flavoring extracts (for example, vanilla, almond, peppermint)
- Garlic
- Herbs, fresh or dried
- Nonstick cooking spray
- Pimento
- Spices
- Hot pepper sauce
- Wine, used in cooking
- Worcestershire sauce

 Be careful with seasonings that contain sodium or are salts, such as garlic salt, celery salt, and lemon pepper.

(continues)

 = 480 milligrams or more of sodium per serving.

Seasonings (*continued*)

Read the label, and choose those seasonings that do not contain sodium or salt.

Basil (fresh)	Garlic	Onion powder
Celery seeds	Garlic powder	Oregano
Cinnamon	Herbs	Paprika
Chili powder	Hot pepper sauce	Pepper
Chives	Lemon	Pimento
Curry	Lemon juice	Spices
Dill	Lemon pepper	Soy sauce
Flavoring extracts	Lime	Soy sauce, low sodium ("lite")
(vanilla, almond, walnut, peppermint,	Lime juice	Wine, used in cooking (¼ cup)
lemon, butter, etc.)	Mint	Worcestershire sauce

Source: Reproduction of the Exchange Lists in whole or part, without permission of the American Dietetic Association or the American Diabetes Association, Inc., is a violation of federal law. This material has been modified from Choose Your Foods: Exchange Lists for Diabetes, which is the basis of a meal planning system designed by a committee of the American Diabetes Association and the American Dietetic Association. While designed primarily for people with diabetes and others who must follow special diets, the Exchange Lists are based on principles of good nutrition that apply to everyone. Copyright © 2008 by the American Diabetes Association and Academy of Nutrition and Dietetics (formerly American Dietetic Association)

Combination Foods

Entrees

	Food	Serving Size	Count as
🧂	Casserole type (tuna noodle, lasagna, spaghetti with meatballs, chili with beans, macaroni and cheese)	1 cup (8 oz)	2 carbohydrates + 2 medium-fat meats
🧂	Stews (beef/other meats and vegetables)	1 cup (8 oz)	1 carbohydrate + 1 medium-fat meat + 0–3 fats
	Tuna salad or chicken salad	½ cup (3½ oz)	½ carbohydrate + 2 lean meats + 1 fat

Source: Reproduction of the Exchange Lists in whole or part, without permission of the American Dietetic Association or the American Diabetes Association, Inc., is a violation of federal law. This material has been modified from Choose Your Foods: Exchange Lists for Diabetes, which is the basis of a meal planning system designed by a committee of the American Diabetes Association and the American Dietetic Association. While designed primarily for people with diabetes and others who must follow special diets, the Exchange Lists are based on principles of good nutrition that apply to everyone. Copyright © 2008 by the American Diabetes Association and Academy of Nutrition and Dietetics (formerly American Dietetic Association)

Frozen Meals/Entrees

	Food	Serving Size	Count as
🧂 😃	Burrito (beef and bean)	1 (5 oz)	3 carbohydrates + 1 lean meat + 2 fats
🧂	Dinner-type meal	generally 14–17 oz	3 carbohydrates + 3 medium-fat meats + 3 fats
🧂	Entree or meal with less than 340 calories	about 8–11 oz	2–3 carbohydrates + 1–2 lean meats
	Pizza		
🧂	cheese/vegetarian, thin crust	¼ of a 12 inch (4½–5 oz)	2 carbohydrates + 2 medium-fat meats
🧂	meat topping, thin crust	¼ of a 12 inch (5 oz)	2 carbohydrates + 2 medium-fat meats + 1½ fats
🧂	Pocket sandwich	1 (4½ oz)	3 carbohydrates + 1 lean meat + 1–2 fats
🧂	Pot pie	1 (7 oz)	2½ carbohydrates + 1 medium-fat meat + 3 fats

(continues)

😃 = More than 3 grams of dietary fiber per serving.

 = 600 milligrams or more of sodium per serving (for fast food main dishes/meals).

Frozen Meals/Entrees (*continued*)

Source: Reproduction of the Exchange Lists in whole or part, without permission of the American Dietetic Association or the American Diabetes Association, Inc., is a violation of federal law. This material has been modified from Choose Your Foods: Exchange Lists for Diabetes, which is the basis of a meal planning system designed by a committee of the American Diabetes Association and the American Dietetic Association. While designed primarily for people with diabetes and others who must follow special diets, the Exchange Lists are based on principles of good nutrition that apply to everyone. Copyright © 2008 by the American Diabetes Association and Academy of Nutrition and Dietetics (formerly American Dietetic Association)

	Salads (Deli-Style) Food	Serving Size	Count as
	Coleslaw	½ cup	1 carbohydrate + 1½ fats
	Macaroni/pasta salad	½ cup	2 carbohydrates + 3 fats
	Potato salad	½ cup	1½–2 carbohydrates + 1–2 fats

Source: Reproduction of the Exchange Lists in whole or part, without permission of the American Dietetic Association or the American Diabetes Association, Inc., is a violation of federal law. This material has been modified from Choose Your Foods: Exchange Lists for Diabetes, which is the basis of a meal planning system designed by a committee of the American Diabetes Association and the American Dietetic Association. While designed primarily for people with diabetes and others who must follow special diets, the Exchange Lists are based on principles of good nutrition that apply to everyone. Copyright © 2008 by the American Diabetes Association and Academy of Nutrition and Dietetics (formerly American Dietetic Association)

Soups

	Food	Serving Size	Count as
	Bean, lentil, or split pea	1 cup	1 carbohydrate + 1 lean meat
	Chowder (made with milk)	1 cup (8 oz)	1 carbohydrate + 1 lean meat + 1½ fats
	Cream (made with water)	1 cup (8 oz)	1 carbohydrate + 1 fat
	Instant	6 oz prepared	1 carbohydrate
	with beans or lentils	8 oz prepared	2½ carbohydrates + 1 lean meat
	Miso soup	1 cup	½ carbohydrate + 1 fat
	Oriental noodle	1 cup	2 carbohydrates + 2 fats
	Rice (congee)	1 cup	1 carbohydrate
	Tomato (made with water)	1 cup (8 oz)	1 carbohydrate
	Vegetable beef, chicken noodle, or other broth type	1 cup (8 oz)	1 carbohydrate

Source: Reproduction of the Exchange Lists in whole or part, without permission of the American Dietetic Association or the American Diabetes Association, Inc., is a violation of federal law. This material has been modified from Choose Your Foods: Exchange Lists for Diabetes, which is the basis of a meal planning system designed by a committee of the American Diabetes Association and the American Dietetic Association. While designed primarily for people with diabetes and others who must follow special diets, the Exchange Lists are based on principles of good nutrition that apply to everyone. Copyright © 2008 by the American Diabetes Association and Academy of Nutrition and Dietetics (formerly American Dietetic Association)

Fast Foods

The choices in the **Fast Foods** list are not specific fast-food meals or items, but are estimates based on popular foods. You can get specific nutrition information for almost every fast-food or restaurant chain. Ask the restaurant or check its website for nutrition information about your favorite fast foods.

 = 600 milligrams or more of sodium per serving (for fast food main dishes/meals).

Breakfast Sandwiches

	Food	Serving Size	Count as
(s)	Egg, cheese, meat, English muffin	1 sandwich	2 carbohydrates + 2 medium-fat meats
(s)	Sausage biscuit sandwich	1 sandwich	2 carbohydrates + 2 high-fat meats + 3½ fats

Source: Reproduction of the Exchange Lists in whole or part, without permission of the American Dietetic Association or the American Diabetes Association, Inc., is a violation of federal law. This material has been modified from Choose Your Foods: Exchange Lists for Diabetes, which is the basis of a meal planning system designed by a committee of the American Diabetes Association and the American Dietetic Association. While designed primarily for people with diabetes and others who must follow special diets, the Exchange Lists are based on principles of good nutrition that apply to everyone. Copyright © 2008 by the American Diabetes Association and Academy of Nutrition and Dietetics (formerly American Dietetic Association)

Main Dishes/Entrees

	Food	Serving Size	Count as
(s) ☺	Burrito (beef and beans)	1 (about 8 oz)	3 carbohydrates + 3 medium-fat meats + 3 fats
	Chicken breast, breaded and fried	1 (about 5 oz)	1 carbohydrate + 4 medium-fat meats
	Chicken drumstick, breaded and fried	1 (about 2 oz)	2 medium-fat meats
(s)	Chicken nuggets	6 (about 3½ oz)	1 carbohydrate + 2 medium-fat meats + 1 fat
(s)	Chicken thigh, breaded and fried	1 (about 4 oz)	½ carbohydrate + 3 medium-fat meats + 1½ fats
(s)	Chicken wings, hot	6 (5 oz)	5 medium-fat meats + 1½ fats

Source: Reproduction of the Exchange Lists in whole or part, without permission of the American Dietetic Association or the American Diabetes Association, Inc., is a violation of federal law. This material has been modified from Choose Your Foods: Exchange Lists for Diabetes, which is the basis of a meal planning system designed by a committee of the American Diabetes Association and the American Dietetic Association. While designed primarily for people with diabetes and others who must follow special diets, the Exchange Lists are based on principles of good nutrition that apply to everyone. Copyright © 2008 by the American Diabetes Association and Academy of Nutrition and Dietetics (formerly American Dietetic Association)

Oriental

	Food	Serving Size	Count as
(s)	Beef/chicken/shrimp with vegetables in sauce	1 cup (about 5 oz)	1 carbohydrate + 1 lean meat + 1 fat
(s)	Egg roll, meat	1 (about 3 oz)	1 carbohydrate + 1 lean meat + 1 fat
	Fried rice, meatless	½ cup	1½ carbohydrates + 1½ fats
(s)	Meat and sweet sauce (orange chicken)	1 cup	3 carbohydrates + 3 medium-fat meats + 2 fats
(s) ☺	Noodles and vegetables in sauce (chow mein, lo mein)	1 cup	2 carbohydrates + 1 fat

Source: Reproduction of the Exchange Lists in whole or part, without permission of the American Dietetic Association or the American Diabetes Association, Inc., is a violation of federal law. This material has been modified from Choose Your Foods: Exchange Lists for Diabetes, which is the basis of a meal planning system designed by a committee of the American Diabetes Association and the American Dietetic Association. While designed primarily for people with diabetes and others who must follow special diets, the Exchange Lists are based on principles of good nutrition that apply to everyone. Copyright © 2008 by the American Diabetes Association and Academy of Nutrition and Dietetics (formerly American Dietetic Association)

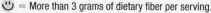 = More than 3 grams of dietary fiber per serving.

 = 600 milligrams or more of sodium per serving (for fast food main dishes/meals).

Pizza

	Food	Serving Size	Count as
🧂	Pizza		
	cheese, pepperoni, regular crust	½ of a 14 inch (about 4 oz)	2½ carbohydrates + 1 medium-fat meat + 1½ fats
🧂	cheese/vegetarian, thin crust	¼ of a 12 inch (about 6 oz)	2½ carbohydrates + 2 medium-fat meats + 1½ fats

Source: Reproduction of the Exchange Lists in whole or part, without permission of the American Dietetic Association or the American Diabetes Association, Inc., is a violation of federal law. This material has been modified from Choose Your Foods: Exchange Lists for Diabetes, which is the basis of a meal planning system designed by a committee of the American Diabetes Association and the American Dietetic Association. While designed primarily for people with diabetes and others who must follow special diets, the Exchange Lists are based on principles of good nutrition that apply to everyone. Copyright © 2008 by the American Diabetes Association and Academy of Nutrition and Dietetics (formerly American Dietetic Association)

Sandwiches

	Food	Serving Size	Count as
🧂	Chicken sandwich, grilled	1	3 carbohydrates + 4 lean meats
🧂	Chicken sandwich, crispy	1	3½ carbohydrates + 3 medium-fat meats + 1 fat
	Fish sandwich with tartar sauce	1	2½ carbohydrates + 2 medium-fat meats + 2 fats
	Hamburger		
🧂	large with cheese	1	2½ carbohydrates + 4 medium-fat meats + 1 fat
🧂	regular	1	2 carbohydrates + 1 medium-fat meat + 1 fat
🧂	Hot dog with bun	1	1 carbohydrate + 1 high-fat meat + 1 fat
	Submarine sandwich		
🧂	less than 6 grams fat	6-inch sub	3 carbohydrates + 2 lean meats
🧂	regular	6-inch sub	3½ carbohydrates + 2 medium-fat meats + 1 fat
	Taco, hard or soft shell (meat and cheese)	1 small	1 carbohydrate + 1 medium-fat meat + 1½ fats

Source: Reproduction of the Exchange Lists in whole or part, without permission of the American Dietetic Association or the American Diabetes Association, Inc., is a violation of federal law. This material has been modified from Choose Your Foods: Exchange Lists for Diabetes, which is the basis of a meal planning system designed by a committee of the American Diabetes Association and the American Dietetic Association. While designed primarily for people with diabetes and others who must follow special diets, the Exchange Lists are based on principles of good nutrition that apply to everyone. Copyright © 2008 by the American Diabetes Association and Academy of Nutrition and Dietetics (formerly American Dietetic Association)

Salads

	Food	Serving Size	Count as
🧂 😋	Salad, main dish (grilled chicken type, no dressing or croutons)	Salad	1 carbohydrate + 4 lean meats
	Salad, side, no dressing or cheese	Small (about 5 oz)	1 vegetable

Source: Reproduction of the Exchange Lists in whole or part, without permission of the American Dietetic Association or the American Diabetes Association, Inc., is a violation of federal law. This material has been modified from Choose Your Foods: Exchange Lists for Diabetes, which is the basis of a meal planning system designed by a committee of the American Diabetes Association and the American Dietetic Association. While designed primarily for people with diabetes and others who must follow special diets, the Exchange Lists are based on principles of good nutrition that apply to everyone. Copyright © 2008 by the American Diabetes Association and Academy of Nutrition and Dietetics (formerly American Dietetic Association)

 = Extra fat, or prepared with added fat.

 = 600 milligrams or more of sodium per serving (for fast food main dishes/meals).

Sides/Appetizers

	Food	Serving Size	Count as
⚠	French fries, restaurant style	small	3 carbohydrates + 3 fats
		medium	4 carbohydrates + 4 fats
		large	5 carbohydrates + 6 fats
Ⓢ	Nachos with cheese	Small (about 4½ oz)	2½ carbohydrates + 4 fats
Ⓢ	Onion rings	1 serving (about 3 oz)	2½ carbohydrates + 3 fats

Source: Reproduction of the Exchange Lists in whole or part, without permission of the American Dietetic Association or the American Diabetes Association, Inc., is a violation of federal law. This material has been modified from Choose Your Foods: Exchange Lists for Diabetes, which is the basis of a meal planning system designed by a committee of the American Diabetes Association and the American Dietetic Association. While designed primarily for people with diabetes and others who must follow special diets, the Exchange Lists are based on principles of good nutrition that apply to everyone. Copyright © 2008 by the American Diabetes Association and Academy of Nutrition and Dietetics (formerly American Dietetic Association)

Desserts

Food	Serving Size	Count as
Milkshake, any flavor	12 oz	6 carbohydrates + 2 fats
Soft-serve ice cream cone	1 small	2½ carbohydrates + 1 fat

Note: See the **Starch** list and **Sweets, Desserts, and Other Carbohydrates** list for foods such as bagels and muffins.

Source: Reproduction of the Exchange Lists in whole or part, without permission of the American Dietetic Association or the American Diabetes Association, Inc., is a violation of federal law. This material has been modified from Choose Your Foods: Exchange Lists for Diabetes, which is the basis of a meal planning system designed by a committee of the American Diabetes Association and the American Dietetic Association. While designed primarily for people with diabetes and others who must follow special diets, the Exchange Lists are based on principles of good nutrition that apply to everyone. Copyright © 2008 by the American Diabetes Association and Academy of Nutrition and Dietetics (formerly American Dietetic Association)

Alcohol

Food	Serving Size	Count as
Beer		
light (4.2%)	12 fl oz	1 alcohol equivalent + ½ carbohydrate
regular (4.9%)	12 fl oz	1 alcohol equivalent + 1 carbohydrate
Distilled spirits: vodka, rum, gin, whiskey 80 or 86 proof	1½ fl oz	1 alcohol equivalent
Liqueur, coffee (53 proof)	1 fl oz	1 alcohol equivalent + 1 carbohydrate
Sake	1 fl oz	½ alcohol equivalent

(continues)

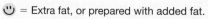

☺ = Extra fat, or prepared with added fat.

Ⓢ = 600 milligrams or more of sodium per serving (for fast-food main dishes/meals).

Alcohol (*continued*)

Food	Serving Size	Count as
Wine		
dessert (sherry)	3½ fl oz	1 alcohol equivalent + 1 carbohydrate
dry, red or white (10%)	5 fl oz	1 alcohol equivalent

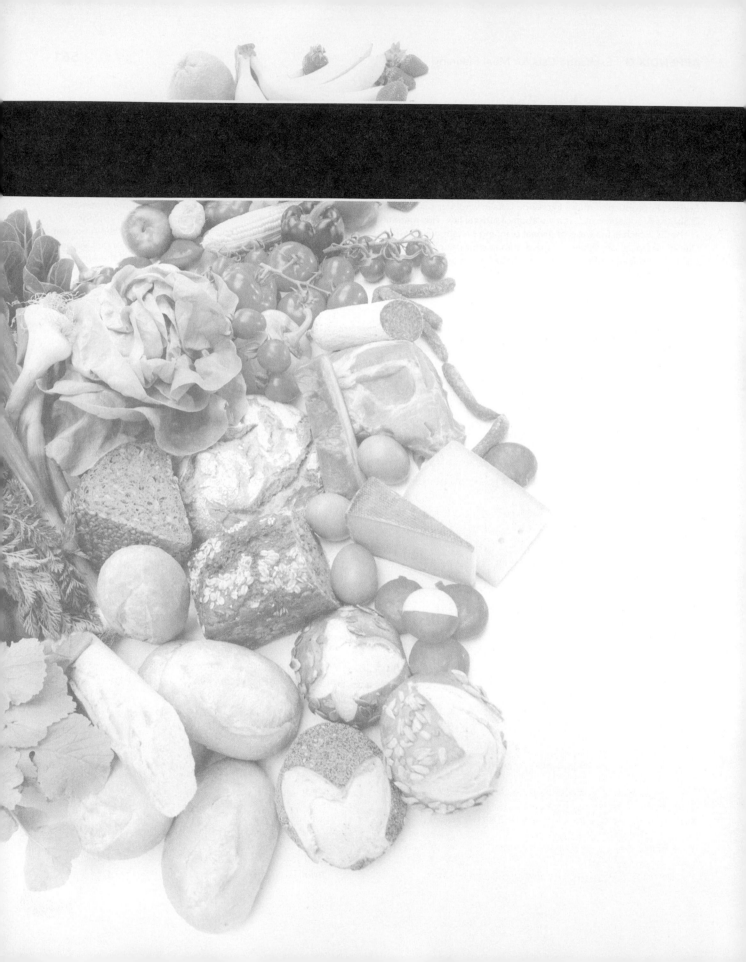

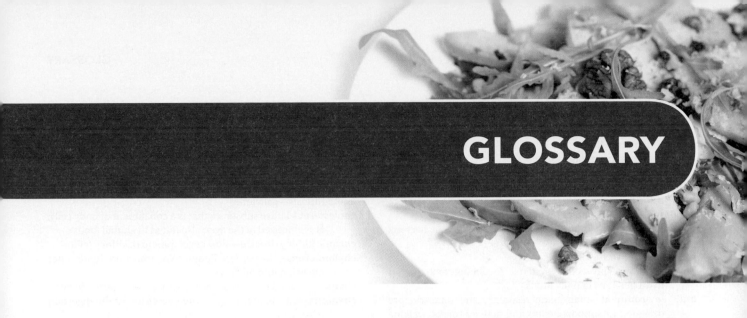

GLOSSARY

24-hour recall—listing the types, amounts, and preparation of all foods eaten in the past 24 hours

A

A1c—a blood test to determine how well blood glucose has been controlled for the last 3 months

absorption—taking up of nutrients in the intestines

abstinence—avoidance

acid-base balance—the regulation of hydrogen ions in body fluids

acidosis—condition in which excess acids accumulate or there is a loss of base in the body

acquired immune deficiency syndrome (AIDS)—caused by the human immunodeficiency virus (HIV) which weakens the body's immune system, leaving it susceptible to fatal infections

acute renal failure (ARF)—suddenly occurring failure of the kidneys

adipose tissue—fatty tissue

adjustable gastric band—surgical reduction of stomach, but to lesser degree than bypass

adolescent—person between the ages of 13 and 20

aerobic metabolism—combining nutrients with oxygen within the cell; also called oxidation

albumin—protein that occurs in blood plasma

alcoholism—chronic and excessive use of alcohol

alkaline—base; capable of neutralizing acids

alkalosis—condition in which excess base accumulates in, or acids are lost from, the body

allergens—substance causing an allergic reaction

allergic reactions—adverse physical reactions to specific substances

allergy—sensitivity to specific substance(s)

amenorrhea—the stoppage of the monthly menstrual flow

amino acids—nitrogen-containing chemical compounds of which protein is composed

amniocentesis—a test to determine the status of the fetus in utero

amniotic fluid—fluid that surrounds fetus in the uterus

anabolism—the creation of new compounds during metabolism

anaerobic metabolism—reduces fats without the use of oxygen

anemia—condition caused by insufficient number of red blood cells, hemoglobin, or blood volume

anencephaly—absence of the brain

angina pectoris—pain in the heart muscle due to inadequate blood supply

anorexia—loss of appetite, especially as a result of disease

anorexia nervosa—psychologically induced lack of appetite

anthropometric measurements—measurements of height, weight, head, skinfold

antibodies—substances produced by the body in reaction to foreign substance; neutralize toxins from foreign bodies

antioxidant—substance preventing damage from oxygen

anxiety—apprehension

arteriosclerosis—generic term for thickened arteries

arthritis—chronic disease involving the joints

ascites—abnormal collection of fluid in the abdomen

ascorbic acid—vitamin C

aspartame—artificial sweetener made from two amino acids; does not require insulin for metabolism

aspirated—inhaled or suctioned

atherosclerosis—a form of arteriosclerosis affecting the intima (inner lining) of the artery walls

autoimmune disease—an illness that occurs when the body tissues are attacked by its own immune system

avitaminosis—without vitamins

B

balanced diet—one that includes all the essential nutrients in appropriate amounts

basal metabolism rate (BMR)—the rate at which energy is needed for body maintenance

beriberi—deficiency disease caused by a lack of vitamin B1 (thiamine)

bile—secretion of the liver, stored in the gallbladder, essential for the digestion of fats

bioavailable—ability of a nutrient to be readily absorbed and used by the body

biochemical tests—involving biology and chemistry

biotin—a B vitamin; necessary for metabolism

body mass index (BMI)—number calculated from a person's weight and height; fairly reliable indicator of body fatness for most people

bolus—food in the mouth that is ready to be swallowed

bomb calorimeter—device used to scientifically determine the caloric value of foods

bonding—emotional attachment

botulism—deadliest of food poisonings; caused by the bacteria *Clostridium botulinum*

bran—outer covering of grain kernels

buffer systems—protective systems regulating amounts of hydrogen ions in body fluids

built environment—man-made resources and infrastructure designed to support health and activity (parks, walking and bike paths, access to healthy foods, etc.)

bulimia—condition in which client alternately binges and purges

C

cachexia—severe malnutrition and body wasting caused by chronic disease

caliper—mechanical device used to measure percentage of body fat by skinfold measurement

calorie—also known as kcal or kilocalorie; represents the amount of heat needed to raise the temperature of one kilogram of water by 1 degree Celsius (C)

calorie requirements—numbers of calories required daily to meet energy needs

capillaries—tiny blood vessels connecting veins and arteries

carbohydrates (CHO)—the nutrient providing the major source of energy in the average diet

carboxypeptidase—pancreatic enzyme necessary for protein digestion

carcinogens—cancer-causing substances

cardiac sphincter—the muscle at the base of the esophagus that prevents gastric reflux from moving into the esophagus

cardiomyopathy—damage to the heart muscle caused by infection, alcohol, or drug abuse

cardiovascular—pertaining to the heart and entire circulatory system

cardiovascular disease (CVD)—disease affecting heart and blood vessels

carotenoids—plant pigments, some of which yield vitamin A

carriers—those who are capable of transmitting an infectious organism

catabolism—the breakdown of compounds during metabolism

catalyst—a substance that causes another substance to react

celiac disease—a disorder of the gastrointestinal tract characterized by malabsorption; also called gluten sensitivity

cellular edema—swelling of body cells caused by inadequate amount of sodium in extracellular fluid

cellulose—indigestible carbohydrate; provides fiber in the diet

cerebrovascular accident (CVA)—either a blockage or bursting of blood vessel leading to the brain

chemical digestion—chemical changes in foods during digestion caused by hydrolysis

chemotherapy—treatment of diseased tissue with chemicals

cholecystectomy—removal of the gallbladder

cholecystitis—inflammation of the gallbladder

cholecystokinin (CCK)—the hormone that triggers the gallbladder to release bile

cholelithiasis—gallstones

cholesterol—fatlike substance that is a constituent of body cells; is synthesized in the liver; also found in animal foods

chronic kidney disease—slow development of kidney failure

chylomicrons—the largest lipoprotein; transport lipids after digestion into the body

chyme—the food mass as it has been mixed with gastric juices

chymotrypsin—pancreatic enzyme necessary for the digestion of proteins

circulation—the body process whereby the blood is moved throughout the body

cirrhosis—generic term for liver disease characterized by cell loss

clinical examination—physical observation

coagulation—thickening

cobalamin—organic compound known as vitamin B12

coenzymes—an active part of an enzyme

collagen—protein substance that holds body cells together

colon—the large intestine

colostomy—opening from colon to abdomen surface

coma—state of unconsciousness

compensated heart disease—heart disease in which the heart is able to maintain circulation to all body parts

complementary proteins—incomplete proteins that when combined provide all nine essential amino acids

complete proteins—proteins that contain all nine essential amino acids

congestive heart failure (CHF)—a form of decompensated heart disease

coronary artery disease (CAD)—severe narrowing of the arteries that supply blood to the heart

creatinine—an end (waste) product of protein metabolism

Crohn's disease—a chronic progressive disorder that causes inflammation, ulcers, and thickening of intestinal walls, sometimes causing obstruction

cumulative effects—results of something done repeatedly over many years

cystine—a nonessential amino acid

cysts—growths

D

daily values—represent percentage per serving of each nutritional item listed on new food labels based on daily intake of 2,000 calories

decompensated heart disease—heart disease in which the heart cannot maintain circulation to all body parts

deficiency diseases—disease caused by the lack of a specific nutrient

dehydrated—having lost large amounts of water

dehydration—loss of water

demineralization—loss of mineral or minerals

dentition—arrangement, type, and number of teeth

depression—an indentation; or feelings of extreme sadness

dermatitis—inflammation of the skin

descriptors—terms used to describe something

desensitized—having gradually reduced the body's sensitivity (allergic reaction) to specific items

diabetes mellitus—chronic disease in which the body lacks the normal ability to metabolize glucose

dialysis—mechanical filtration of the blood; used when the kidneys are no longer able to perform normally

diaphragm—thin membrane or partition

dietary fiber—indigestible parts of plants; absorbs water in large intestine, helping to create soft, bulky stool; some is believed to bind cholesterol in the colon, helping to rid cholesterol from the body; some is believed to lower blood glucose levels

Dietary Guidelines for Americans—general goals for optimal nutrient intake

dietary laws—rules to be followed in meal planning in some religions

Dietary Reference Intakes (DRIs)—combines the Recommended Dietary Allowances, Adequate Intake, Estimated Average Requirements, and Tolerable Upper Intake Levels for individuals into one value representative of the average daily nutrient intake of individuals over time

dietary-social history—evaluations of food habits, including client's ability to buy and prepare foods

dietitian—a professional trained to assess nutrition status and recommend appropriate diet therapy

digestion—breakdown of food in the body in preparation for absorption

disaccharides—double sugars that are reduced by hydrolysis to monosaccharides; examples are sucrose, maltose, and lactose

diuretics—substances used to increase the amount of urine excreted

diverticulitis—inflammation of the diverticula

diverticulosis—intestinal disorder characterized by little pockets forming in the sides of the intestines; pockets are called diverticula

dumping syndrome—nausea and diarrhea caused by food moving too quickly from the stomach to the small intestine

duodenal ulcer—ulcer occurring in the duodenum

duodenum—first (and smallest) section of the small intestine

dysentery—disease caused by microorganism; characterized by diarrhea

dyslipidemia—increased lipids in the blood

dyspepsia—gastrointestinal discomfort of vague origin

dysphagia—difficulty swallowing

E

eclamptic stage—convulsive stage of toxemia

edema—the abnormal retention of fluid by the body

electrolytes—chemical compounds that dissolves in water break up into electrically charged atoms called ions

elemental formulas—those formulas containing products of digestion of proteins, carbohydrates, and fats; also called hydrolyzed formulas

elimination—evacuation of wastes

elimination diet—limited diet in which only certain foods are allowed; intended to find the food allergen causing reaction

endocardium—lining of the heart

endogenous insulin—insulin produced within the body

endometrium—mucous membrane of the uterus

endosperm—the inner part of the kernel of grain; contains the carbohydrate

end-stage renal disease (ESRD)—the stage at which the kidneys have lost most or all of their ability to function

energy balance—occurs when the caloric value of food ingested equals the kcal expended

energy imbalance—eating either too much or too little for the amount of energy expended

energy requirement—number of calories required by the body each day

enriched foods—foods to which nutrients, usually B vitamins and iron, have been added to improve their nutritional value

enteral nutrition—feeding by tube directly into the client's digestive tract

enterotoxins—toxins affecting mucous membranes

enzymes—organic substances that causes changes in other substances

esophagitis—inflammation of mucosal lining of esophagus

esophagus—tube leading from the mouth to the stomach; part of the gastrointestinal system

essential hypertension—high blood pressure with unknown cause; also called primary hypertension

essential nutrients—nutrients found only in food

estrogen—hormone secreted by the ovaries

etiology—cause

exchange lists—lists of foods with interchangeable nutrient and kcal contents; used in specific forms of diet therapy

exogenous insulin—insulin produced outside the body

extracellular—outside the cell

extracellular fluid (ECF)—water outside the cells; approximately 35% of total body fluid

F

fat cell theory—belief that fat cells have a natural drive to regain any weight lost

fats (lipids)—highest caloric-value nutrient

fat soluble—can be dissolved in fat

fatty acids—a component of fats that determines the classification of the fat

feces—solid waste from the large intestine

fermentation—changing of sugars and starches to alcohol

fetal alcohol syndrome (FAS)—subnormal physical and mental development caused by mother's excessive use of alcohol during pregnancy

fetal malformations—physical abnormalities of the fetus

fetus—infant in utero

fibrosis—development of tough, stringy tissue

flatulence—gas in the intestinal tract

flavonoids—naturally occurring water-soluble plant pigments that act as antioxidants

folate/folic acid—a form of vitamin B, also called folacin; essential for metabolism

food customs—food habits

food diary—written record of all food and drink ingested in a specified period

food faddists—people who have certain beliefs about particular foods or diets

food poisoning—foodborne illness

foodways—the food traditions or customs of a group of people

free radicals—atoms or groups of atoms with an odd (unpaired) number of electrons; can be formed when oxygen interacts with certain molecules

fructose—the simple sugar (monosaccharide) found in fruit and honey

fundus (of the stomach)—upper part of the stomach

fusion—a style of cooking that combines ingredients and techniques from different cultures or countries

G

galactose—the simple sugar (monosaccharide) to which lactose is broken down during digestion

galactosemia—inherited error in metabolism that prevents normal metabolism of galactose

galactosuria—galactose in the urine

gastric juices—the digestive secretions of the stomach

gastric ulcer—ulcer in the stomach

gastrin—hormone released by the stomach

gastroesophageal reflux (GER)—backflow of stomach contents into the esophagus

gastrointestinal (GI) tract—pertaining to the stomach and intestines

gastrostomy—opening created by the surgeon directly into the stomach for enteral nutrition

genetic predisposition—inherited tendency

geriatrics—the branch of medicine involved with diseases of the elderly

germ—embryo or tiny life center of each kernel of grain

gerontology—the study of aging

gestational diabetes—diabetes occurring during pregnancy; usually disappears after delivery of the infant

ghrelin—a hormone from the stomach that signals the brain it's time to eat

glomerular filtration rate (GFR)—the rate at which the kidneys filter the blood

glomerulonephritis—inflammation of the glomeruli of the kidneys

glomerulus—filtering unit in the kidneys

glucagon—hormone from alpha cells of pancreas; helps cells release energy

glucose—the simple sugar to which carbohydrate must be broken down for absorption; also known as *dextrose*

gluten—protein found in grains

glycerol—a component of fat; derived form a water-soluble carbohydrate

glycogen—glucose as stored in the liver and muscles

glycogen loading (carb-loading)—process in which the muscle store of glycogen is maximized; also called carb-loading

glycosuria—excess sugar in the urine

goiter—enlarged tissue of the thyroid gland due to a deficiency of iodine

growth spurt—significant rapid gain in size near the onset of adolescence

H

Heliobacter pylori—bacteria that can cause peptic ulcer

heme iron—part of hemoglobin molecule in animal foods

hemicellulose—dietary fiber found in whole grains

hemodialysis—cleansing the blood of wastes by circulating the blood through a machine that contains tubing of semipermeable membranes

hemolysis—the destruction of red blood cells

hemorrhage—unusually heavy bleeding

hepatitis—inflammation of the liver caused by viruses, drugs, and alcohol

hiatal hernia—condition wherein part of the stomach protrudes through the diaphragm into the chest cavity

high-density lipoproteins (HDLs)—lipoproteins that carry cholesterol from cells to the liver for eventual excretion

homeostasis—state of physical balance; stable condition

hormones—chemical messengers secreted by a variety of glands

human immunodeficiency virus (HIV)—a virus that weakens the body's immune system and ultimately leads to AIDS

hydrogenation—the combining of fat with hydrogen, thereby making it a saturated fat and solid at room temperature

hydrolysis—the addition of water resulting in the breakdown of the molecule

hydrolyzed formulas—contain products of digestion of proteins, carbohydrates, and fats; also called elemental formulas; used for clients who have difficulty digesting food

hypercholesterolemia—unusually high levels of cholesterol in blood; also known as high serum cholesterol

hyperemesis gravidarum—nausea so severe as to be life-threatening

hyperglycemia—excessive amounts of sugar in the blood

hyperkalemia—excessive amounts of potassium in the blood

hyperlipidemia—excessive amounts of fats in the blood

hypermetabolic—higher than normal rate of metabolism

hypersensitivity—abnormally strong sensitivity to certain substance(s)

hypertension—higher than normal blood pressure

hyperthyroidism—condition in which the thyroid gland secretes too much thyroxine and T3; the body's rate of metabolism is unusually high

hypervitaminosis—condition caused by excessive ingestion of one or more vitamins

hypoalbuminemia—abnormally low amounts of protein in the blood

hypoglycemia—subnormal levels of blood sugar

hypokalemia—low level of potassium in the blood

hypothalamus—area at base of brain that regulates appetite and thirst

hypothyroidism—condition in which the thyroid gland secretes too little thyroxine and T3; body metabolism is slower than normal

I

iatrogenic malnutrition—caused by treatment or diagnostic procedures

ileostomy—opening from ileum to abdomen surface

ileum—last part of the small intestine

immunity—ability to resist certain diseases

inborn errors of metabolism—congenital disabilities preventing normal metabolism

incomplete proteins—proteins that do not contain all of the nine essential amino acids

infarct—dead tissue resulting from blocked artery

inflammatory bowel diseases (IBDs)—chronic conditions causing inflammation in the gastrointestinal tract

insecticides—agents that destroy insects

insulin—secretion of the islets of Langerhans in the pancreas gland; essential for the proper metabolism of glucose

insulin reaction—hypoglycemia leading to insulin coma caused by too much insulin or too little food

internationals units (IUs)—unit of measurement of some vitamins; 5 mcg = 200 international units

interstitial fluid—fluid between cells

intracellular—within the cell

intracellular fluid (ICF)—water within cells; approximately 65% of total body fluid

intrinsic factor—secretion of stomach mucosa essential for B12 absorption

invisible fats—fats that are not immediately noticeable, such as those in egg yolk, cheese, cream, and salad dressings

iodized salt—salt that has the mineral iodine added for the prevention of goiter

ions—electrically charged atoms resulting from chemical reactions

iron deficiency—intake of iron is adequate, but the body has no extra iron stored

iron-deficiency anemia—condition resulting from inadequate amount of iron in the diet, reducing the amount of oxygen carried by the blood to the cells

ischemia—reduced blood flow causing inadequate supply of nutrients and oxygen to, and wastes from, tissues

islets of Langerhans—part of the pancreas from which insulin is secreted

isoleucine—an amino acid

J

jaundice—yellow cast of the skin and eyes

jejunostomy—opening created by the surgeon in the intestine for enteral nutrition

jejunum—the middle section comprising about two-fifths of the small intestine

K

Kaposi's sarcoma—type of cancer common to individuals with AIDS

kcal—the unit used to measure the fuel value of foods

Keshan disease—condition causing abnormalities in the heart muscle

ketoacidosis—condition in which ketones collect in the blood; caused by insufficient glucose available for energy

ketonemia—ketones collected in the blood

ketones—substances to which fatty acids are broken down in the liver

ketonuria—ketone bodies in the urine

kilocalorie—*see* kcal

Krebs cycle—a series of enzymatic reactions that serve as the main source of cellular energy

kwashiorkor—deficiency disease caused by extreme lack of protein

L

lactase—enzyme secreted by the small intestine for the digestion of lactose

lactation—the period during which the mother is nursing the baby

lactation specialist—expert on breastfeeding

lacteals—lymphatic vessels in the small intestine that absorb fatty acids and glycerol

lacto ovo vegetarians—vegetarians who will eat dairy products and eggs but no meat, poultry, or fish

lactose—the sugar in milk; a disaccharide

lactose intolerance—inability to digest lactose because of a lack of the enzyme lactase; causes abdominal cramps and diarrhea

lacto-vegetarians—vegetarians who eat dairy products

lean body mass—mass percentage of muscle tissue

lecithin—fatty substance found in plant and animal foods; a natural emulsifier that helps transport fats in the bloodstream; used commercially to make food products smooth

legumes—plant food that is grown in a pod; for example, beans or peas

leptin—a belief that fat cells have a natural drive to regain any weight lost

leucine—an amino acid

lignins—dietary fiber found in the woody parts of vegetables

linoleic acid—fatty acid essential for humans; cannot be synthesized by the body

linolenic acid—one of three fatty acids needed by the body; cannot be synthesized by the body

lipids—fats

lipoproteins—carriers of fat in the blood

Lofenalac—commercial infant formula with 95% of phenylalanine removed

longevity—length of life

low-density lipoproteins (LDLs)—carry blood cholesterol to the cells

lumen—the hollow area in a tube

lymphatic system—transports fat-soluble substances from the small intestine to the vascular system

M

macrosomia—birth weight over 9 pounds

malignant—life-threatening

malnutrition—poor nutrition

maltase—enzyme secreted by the small intestine essential for the digestion of maltose

maltose—the double sugar (disaccharide) occurring as a result of the digestion of grain

maple syrup urine disease (MSUD)—disease caused by an inborn error of metabolism in which the body cannot metabolize certain amino acids

marasmus—severe wasting caused by lack of protein and all nutrients or faulty absorption; PEM

masa harina—traditional flour made from field corn

mechanical digestion—the part of digestion that requires certain mechanical movement such as chewing, swallowing, and peristalsis

megadoses—extraordinarily large amount

megaloblastic anemia—anemia in which the red blood cells are unusually large and are not completely mature

menopause—the end of menstruation

menses—another term for menstruation

mental retardation—below-normal intellectual capacity

metabolism—the use of food by the body after digestion which results in energy

metastasize—spread of cancer cells from one organ to another

milliequivalents—the concentrations of electrolytes in a solution

minerals—one of many inorganic substances essential to life and classified generally as minerals

mirin—rice wine with 40–50% sugar

miso—a thick fermented paste made from soy beans

modular formulas—made by combining specific nutrients

mold—a type of fungus

monosaccharides—simplest carbohydrates; sugars that cannot be further reduced by hydrolysis; examples are glucose, fructose, and galactose

monosodium glutamate (MSG)—a form of flavor enhancer containing large amounts of sodium

monounsaturated fats—fats that are neither saturated nor polyunsaturated and are thought to play little part in atherosclerosis

morning sickness—early morning nausea common to some pregnancies

mucilage—gel-forming dietary fiber

mutations—changes in the genes

myelin—lipoprotein essential for the protection of nerves

myocardial infarction (MI)—heart attack; caused by the blockage of an artery leading to the heart

myocardium—heart muscle

myoglobin—protein compound in muscle that provides oxygen to cells

MyPlate—outline for making selections based on *Dietary Guidelines for America, 2010;* from the U.S. Department of Agriculture

N

nasogastric (NG) tube—tube leading from the nose to the stomach for tube feeding

necrosis—tissue death due to lack of blood supply

negative nitrogen balance—more nitrogen lost than taken in

neophobic—a fear of new things or experiences

neoplasia—abnormal development of cells

neoplasm—abnormal growth of new tissue

nephritis—inflammatory disease of the kidneys

nephrolithiasis—kidney, or renal, stones

nephrons—unit of the kidney containing a glomerulus

nephropathy—damage to the kidneys

nephrosclerosis—hardening of renal arteries

neural tube defects (NTDs)—congenital malformation of brain and/or spinal column due to failure of neural tube to close during embryonic development

neuropathy—nerve damage

neurotoxins—toxins affecting the nervous system

niacin—B vitamin

niacin equivalent (NE)—unit for measuring niacin; 1 NE equals 1 mg niacin or 60 mg tryptophan

nitrogen—chemical element found in protein; essential to life

nitrogen balance—when nitrogen intake equals nitrogen excreted

nonheme iron—iron from animal foods that is not part of the hemoglobin molecule; and all iron from plant foods

nourishing—foods or beverages that provide substantial amounts of essential nutrients

nutrients—chemical substance found in food that is necessary for good health

nutrient density—nutrient value of foods compared with number of calories

nutrient requirements—amounts of specific nutrient needed by the body

nutrition—the result of those processes whereby the body takes in and uses food for growth, development, and the maintenance of health

nutritional status—one's physical condition as determined by diet

nutrition assessment—evaluation of nutritional status

nutritious—foods or beverages containing substantial amounts of essential nutrients

O

obesity—excessive body fat, 20% above average

obstetricians—doctors who care for mothers during pregnancy and delivery

occlusions—blockages

oliguria—decreased output of urine to less than 500 ml a day

omega-3 fatty acids—polyunsaturated fatty acids found in fish oil; may contribute to reduction of coronary artery disease

oncologist—doctor specializing in the study of cancer

oncology—the study of cancer

on demand—feeding infants as they desire

opportunistic infections—caused by microorganisms that are present but that do not normally affect people with healthy immune systems

oral diabetes medications—oral hypoglycemic agents; medications that may be given to type 2 diabetics to lower blood glucose

osmolality—number of particles per kilogram of solution; solutions with high osmolality exert more pressure than do those with fewer particles

osmosis—movement of a substance through a semipermeable membrane

osteomalacia—a condition in which bones become soft, usually in adult women, because of calcium loss

osteoporosis—condition in which bones become brittle because there have been insufficient mineral deposits, especially calcium

P

pancreas—gland that secretes enzymes essential for digestion and insulin, which is essential for glucose metabolism

pancreatic amylase—the enzyme secreted by the pancreas that is essential for the digestion of starch

pancreatic lipase—the enzyme secreted by the pancreas that is essential for the digestion of fat

pancreatic proteases—enzymes secreted by the pancreas that are essential for the digestion of protein

pancreatitis—inflammation of the pancreas

pantothenic acid—B vitamin

parenteral nutrition—nutrition provided via a vein

pathogens—disease-causing agents

pectin—edible thickening agent

peer pressure—pressure of one's friends and colleagues of the same age

peers—people who are approximately one's own age

pellagra—deficiency disease caused by a lack of niacin

pepsin—an enzyme secreted by the stomach that is essential for the digestion of proteins

peptic ulcers—ulcer of the stomach or duodenum

peptidases—enzymes secreted by the small intestine that are essential for the digestion of protein

pericardium—outer covering of the heart

periodontal disease—disease of the mouth and gums

peripheral vascular disease (PVD)—narrowed arteries some distance from the heart

peripheral vein—a vein that is near the surface of the skin

peristalsis—rhythmical movement of the intestinal tract; moves the chyme along

peritoneal dialysis—removal of waste products from the blood by injecting the flushing solution into the abdomen and using the client's peritoneum as the semipermeable membrane

pernicious anemia—severe, chronic anemia caused by a deficiency of vitamin B12; usually due to the body's inability to absorb B12

pH—symbol for the degree of acidity or alkalinity of a solution

phenylalanine—an amino acid

phenylalanine hydroxylase—liver enzyme necessary to metabolize the amino acid phenylalanine

phenylketonuria (PKU)—condition caused by an inborn error of metabolism in which the infant lacks an enzyme necessary to metabolize the amino acid phenylalanine

phlebitis—inflammation of a vein

physical trauma—extreme physical stress

physiological—relating to bodily functions

phytochemicals—substances occurring naturally in plant foods

pica—abnormal craving for nonfood substance

placenta—organ in the uterus that links blood supplies of mother and infant

plaque—fatty deposit on interior of artery walls

plateau period—period in which there is no change

polycystic kidney disease—rare, hereditary kidney disease causing cysts or growths on the kidneys that can ultimately cause kidney failure in middle age

polydipsia—abnormal thirst

polymeric formulas—commercially prepared formulas for tube feedings that contain intact proteins, carbohydrates, and fats that require digestion

polypeptides—10 or more amino acids bonded together

polyphagia—excess hunger

polysaccharides—complex carbohydrates containing combinations of monosaccharides; examples include starch, dextrin, cellulose, and glycogen

polyunsaturated fats—fats whose carbon atoms contain only limited amounts of hydrogen

polyuria—excessive urination

positive nitrogen balance—nitrogen intake exceeds outgo

precursor—something that comes before something else; in vitamins it is also called a provitamin, something from which the body can synthesize the specific vitamin

pregnancy-induced hypertension (PIH)—typically occurs during late pregnancy; characterized by high blood pressure, albumin in the urine, and edema

pressure ulcers—bedsores

primary hypertension—high blood pressure resulting from an unknown cause

prohormone—substance that precedes the hormone and from which the body can synthesize the hormone

proteins—the only one of six essential nutrients containing nitrogen

protein energy malnutrition (PEM)—marasmus and kwashiorkor

proteinuria—protein in the urine

provitamin—a precursor of a vitamin

psychosocial development—relating to both psychological and social development

purines—end products of nucleoprotein metabolism

pylorus—the end of the stomach nearest the intestine

R

regurgitation—vomiting

renal stones—kidney stones

renal threshold—kidneys' capacity

resection—reduction

respiration—breathing

resting energy expenditure (REE)—*see* basal metabolism rate

retardation—slowing

retinol—the preformed vitamin A

retinol equivalent (RE)—the equivalent of 3.33 IU of vitamin A

retinopathy—damage to small blood vessels in the eyes

riboflavin—the name for vitamin B2

rickets—deficiency disease caused by the lack of vitamin D; causes malformed bones and pain in infants

S

saliva—secretion of the salivary glands

salivary amylase—also called ptyalin; the enzyme secreted by the salivary glands to act on starch

Salmonella—an infection caused by the *Salmonella* bacteria

satiety—feeling of satisfaction; fullness

saturated fats—fats whose carbon atoms contain all of the hydrogen atoms they can; considered a contributory factor in atherosclerosis

scurvy—a deficiency disease caused by a lack of vitamin C

secondary hypertension—high blood pressure caused by another condition such as kidney disease

secretin—the hormone that causes the pancreas to release sodium bicarbonate to neutralize acidity of the chyme

self-esteem—feelings of self-worth

sepsis—infection of the blood

serum cholesterol—cholesterol in the blood

set point theory—belief that everyone has a natural weight ("set point") at which the body is most comfortable

skeletal system—body's bone structure

skin tests—allergy tests using potential allergens on scratches on the skin

solute—the substance dissolved in a solution

solvent—liquid part of a solution

spina bifida—spinal cord or spinal fluid bulge through the back

spontaneous abortion—occurring naturally; miscarriage

Staphylococcus (staph)—genus of bacteria causing food poisoning called "staph" or "staphylococcal poisoning"

starch—polysaccharide found in grains and vegetables

stasis—stoppage or slowing

steatorrhea—abnormal amounts of fat in the feces

sterile—free of infectious organisms

stoma—surgically created opening in the abdominal wall

subcutaneous fat—fat stored directly under the skin

sucralose—a sweetener made from molecule of sugar

sucrase—enzyme secreted by the small intestine to aid in digestion of sucrose

sucrose—a double sugar or disaccharide; examples are granulated, powdered, and brown sugar

T

tastant—a chemical that stimulates the sensory cells in the taste bud

tetany—involuntary muscle movement

thiamine—vitamin B1

thrombosis—blockage, as a blood clot

thrombus—blood clot

thrush—a yeast infection of the mucus membrane lining the mouth and tongue

tocopherols—a form of vitamin E

tocotrienols—a form of vitamin E

total parenteral nutrition—*see* TPN

toxicity—state of being poisonous

TPN—total parenteral nutrition; process of providing all nutrients intravenously

trans-fatty acids (TFAs)—produced by adding hydrogen atoms to a liquid fat, making it a solid

transferase—a liver enzyme necessary for the metabolism of galactose

trichinosis—disease caused by the parasitic roundworm *Trichinella spiralis*; can be transmitted through undercooked pork

triglycerides—combinations of fatty acids and glycerol

trimester—3-month period; commonly used to denote periods of pregnancy

trypsin—pancreatic enzyme; helps digest proteins

tube feeding (TF)—feeding by tube directly into the stomach or intestine

type 1 diabetes—diabetes occurring suddenly between the ages of 1 and 40; clients secrete little, if any, insulin and require insulin injections and a carefully controlled diet

type 2 diabetes—diabetes occurring after age 40; onset is gradual, and production of insulin gradually diminishes; can usually be controlled by diet and exercise

U

ulcerative colitis—disease characterized by inflammation and ulceration of the colon, rectum, and sometimes entire large intestine

urea—chief nitrogenous waste product of protein metabolism

uremia—condition in which protein wastes are circulating in the blood

ureters—tubes leading from the kidneys to the bladder

uric acid—one of the nitrogenous waste products of protein metabolism

urticaria—hives; common allergic reaction

V

valine—an amino acid

vascular disease—disease of the blood vessels

vascular osmotic pressure—high concentration of electrolytes in the blood; low blood volume or blood pressure

vascular system—circulatory system

vegans—vegetarians who avoid all animal foods

very-low-density lipoproteins (VLDLs)—lipoproteins made by the liver to transport lipids throughout the body

villi—the tiny, hairlike structures in the small intestines through which nutrients are absorbed

visceral fat—fat stored within the abdominal cavity

visible fats—fats in foods that are purchased and used as fats, such as butter or margarine

vitamins—organic substances necessary for life although they do not, independently, provide energy

vitamin supplements—concentrated forms of vitamins; may be in tablet or liquid form

W

wasabi—Japanese horseradish

water—major constituent of all living cells; composed of hydrogen and oxygen

water soluble—can be dissolved in water

weaning—training an infant to drink from the cup instead of the nipple

wellness—a way of life that integrates body, mind, and spirit

whey—the liquid part of milk that separates from the curd (solid part) during the making of hard cheese

X

xerophthalmia—serious eye disease characterized by dry mucous membranes of the eye, caused by a deficiency of vitamin A

xerostomia—sore, dry mouth caused by a reduction of salivary secretions; may be caused by radiation for treatment of cancer

Y

yo-yo effect—when a dieters' weight goes up and down over short periods due to swings in eating (from strict dieting to overconsumption)

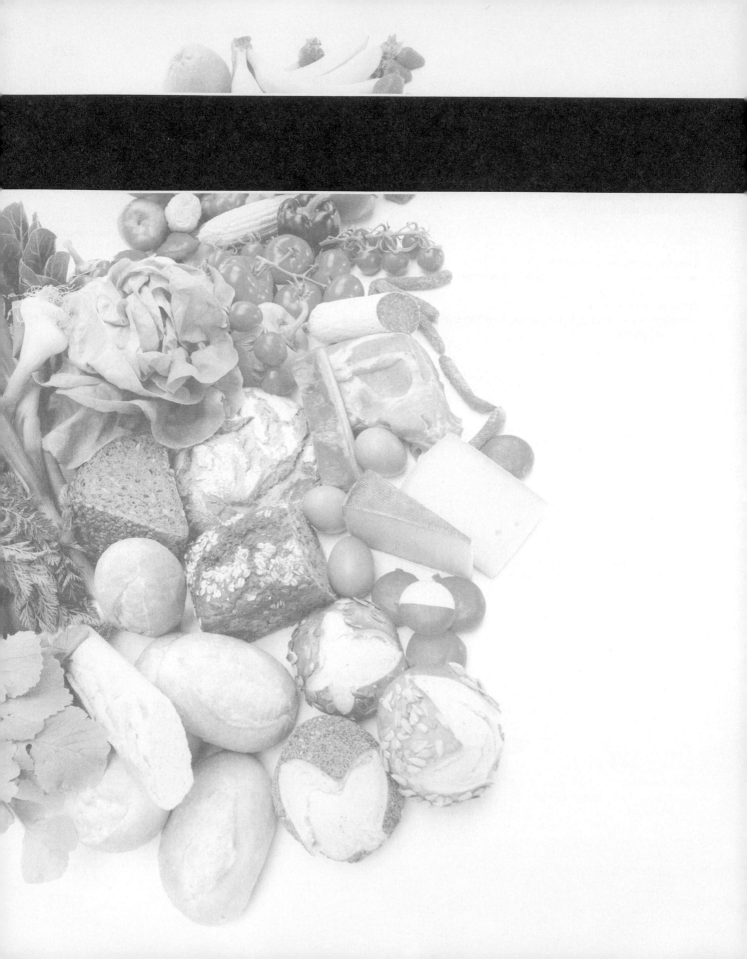

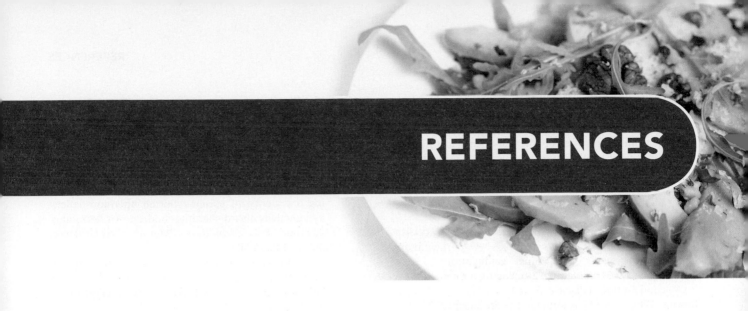

Adolfsson, Arnold. (2006). *Behavioral approaches to treating obesity.* City: Alexandria, Virgina

American Academy of Nutrition and Dietetics. (2012). *Eating right during menopause.* Accessed April 21 from http://www.eatright.org/Public/content.aspx?id=6809

American Academy of Pediatrics. (2003, June). Diagnosing, treating and managing food allergies in children. *Pediatrics* (Supplement). Accessed January 19, 2005 from http://pediatrics.aapublications.org

American Academy of Pediatrics. (2003, June). *Pediatrics, 111*(6) Suppl. Accessed January 19, 2005 from http://pediatrics.aapublications.org/content/vol1111/issue6/index/shtml#suppLS2.

American Association of Clinical Endocrinologists Board of Directors and American College of Endocrinologist Board of Trustees. (2010, March/April). American Association of Clinical Endocrinologists/American College of Endocrinology statement on the use of the hemoglobin A1c for the diagnosis of diabetes. *Endocrine Practice 16*(2), 155.

American Cancer Society. (2003). *Resolve to reduce your risk of cancer.* Accessed June 14, 2006 from http://www.cancer.org/docroot/NWS/content/NWS_2_1x_Resolve_to_Reduce_Your_Risk_of_Cancer.asp

American Cancer Society 2006 Nutrition, Physical Activity and Cancer Survivorship Advisory Committee. (2006, November/December). Nutrition and physical activity during and after cancer treatment: An American Cancer Society guide for informed choices. *CA: A Cancer Journal for Clinicians.* http://onlinelibrary.wiley.com/doi/10.3322/canjclin.56.6.323/abstract

The American Cancer Society. (2011). *Karposi sarcoma.* Accessed November 2, 2011 from http://www.cancer.org/Cancer/KaposiSarcoma/DetailedGuide/kaposi-sarcoma-what-is-kaposi-sarcoma

American Diabetes Association. (2011, June). Guidelines and recommendations for laboratory analysis in the diagnosis and management of diabetes mellitus. *Diabetes Care 34*, e61–e99.

American Diabetes Association. (2012). Standards of medical care in diabetes—2012. *Diabetes Care 35* (Suppl. 1), S11–S49.

American Diabetes Association. *Pop star Nick Jonas speaks out about diabetes.* Accessed June 26, 2008 from http://www.diabetes.org

American Diabetes Association. *Total prevalence of diabetes and pre-diabetes.* Accessed June 24, 2009 from https://www.diabetes.org/diabetes-statistics/prevalence.jsp

American Diabetes Association and the American Dietetic Association. (1995). *Exchange list for meal planning.* Alexandria, VA: American Diabetes Association.

American Dietetic Association. *Childhood overweight evidence analysis project.* http://www.adaevidencelibrary.com/topic.cfm?cat=1046 (requires password to access).

American Heart Association. *High-protein diets.* Accessed January 2009 from http://www.americanheart.org

Anorexia. http://medical-dictionary.thefreedictionary.com/anorexia

Atlanta Journal-Constitution. *Obesity.* Accessed June 15, 2006 from http://www.ajc.com

Aubrey, A. (2012, January 12). For kids with ADHD, some foods may complement treatment. The Salt, National Public Radio's Food Blog.

Bailey, D.A. et al. (2000). Calcium accretion in girls and boys during puberty: A longitudinal analysis. *Journal of Bone and Mineral Research 15*(11), 2245–2250.

Bakalar, N. (2005). Healthful benefits seen in teen diets with zinc. *New York Times*, April 7.

Bakalar, Nicholas. (2011, December 12). Patterns: Coffee may help cut cancer risk in women. *The New York Times.* Accessed December 14, 2011 from www.nytimes.com

Bakalar, Nicholas. (2012, January 2). Nutrition: 4 vitamins that strengthen older brains. *The New York Times.* www.nytimes.com

Baker, R.D., and Greer, F.R. (2010). Committee on Nutrition, American Academy of Pediatrics. Diagnosis and prevention of iron deficiency and iron-deficiency anemia in infants and young children (0-3 years of age). *Pediatrics 126*(5), 1040–1050.

The benefits of eating eggs for breakfast. (2009, April 20). RedOrbit. Accessed December 14, 2011 from www.redorbit.com/news/health/1673141/the_benefits_of_eating_eggs_for_breakfast/

Binge eating in children. (2011, December). Accessed December 2011 from http://www.kidshealth.org/parent/growth/feeding/binge_eating.html

Bitomsky, M. (2001, September 29). Yogurt, fermented drinks good for bowel disease. *Reuters Health.*

Bittman, Mark. (2011). Is junk food really cheaper? *The New York Times.* Accessed December 26, 2011 from http://www.nytimes.com/2011/09/25/opinion/sunday/is-junk-food-really-cheaper.html?pagewanted=all

Body Recomposition. (2008). *How many carbohydrates do you need?* http://www.bodyrecomposition.com/nutrition/how-many-carbohydrates-do-you-need.html

Breastfeeding-mom.com. (2010). *How long to breastfeed.* Accessed January 11, 2012 from http://www.breastfeeding-mom.com/how-long-to-breastfeed.html

Briefel, R.R., Wilson, A., and Gleason, P.M. (2009). Consumption of low-nutrient, energy-dense foods and beverages at school, home, and other locations among school lunch participants and nonparticipants. *Journal of the American Dietetic Association, 109*(Suppl 2), S79–S90.

Brody, J. (2005). What's good for the heart is good for the head. *New York Times*, March 22.

Burn patients: Review of nutrition. (2011). Accessed January 26, 2012 from http://rd411.com/index.php?option=com_content&view=article&id=395:burn-patients:-review-of-nutrition&catid=105:professional-refreshers&Itemid=400

California bans soda in public high schools. (n.d.). *MSNBC News.* Accessed January 19, 2006 from http://www.msnbc.msn.com/id/9355436

Carbohydrate loading diet. Accessed December 2011 from www.mayoclinic.com/health/carbohydrate-loading/MY00223

Cardoni, Salvatore. (2011, December 6). *Conference room cardio: Firm stands behind walking meetings.* Accessed January 2012 from http://www.takepart.com/article/2011/12/06/conference-room-cardio-minnesota-firm-stands-firm-behind-walking-meetings

Carlson, J.J., Eisenmann, J.C., Norman, G.J., Ortiz, K.A., and Young, P.C. (2011). Dietary fiber and nutrient density are inversely associated with the metabolic syndrome in U.S. adolescents. *Journal of the American Dietetic Association 111*, 1688–1695

Center for Disease Control. (2011). *National diabetes fact sheet.* http://www.cdc.gov/diabetes/pubs/pdf/ndfs_2011.pdf

Center for Disease Control and Prevention. (2011). *National diabetes fact sheet.* http://www.cdc.gov/diabetes/pubs/pdf/ndfs_2011.pdf

Center for Disease Control and Prevention. U.S. obesity trends, PowerPoint slide 5. http://www.cdc.gov/obesity/data/trends.html

Centers for Disease Control and Prevention. (2010). Increasing prevalence of parent-reported attention-deficit/hyperactivity disorder among children—United States, 2003 and 2007. *Morbidity and Mortality Weekly Report 59*(44), 1439–1443

Centers for Disease Control and Prevention. (2010, November). *Parasites: Crytosporidium.* Accessed January 9, 2012 from http://www.cdc.gov/parasites/crypto/gen_info/infect.html

Centers for Disease Control and Prevention. (2010). State-specific trends in fruit and vegetable consumption among adults—United States, 2000–2009. *Morbidity and Mortality Weekly Report 59*(35), 1125–1130.

Centers for Disease Control and Prevention. (2011, April). *Calcium and bone health.* Accessed February 10, 2012 from http://www.cdc.gov/nutrition/everyone/basics/vitamins/calcium.html

Centers for Disease Control and Prevention. (2012, January 12). *Estimates of foodborne illness in the United States.* Accessed December 16, 2011 from http://www.cdc.gov/foodborneburden/index.html

Centers for Disease Control and Prevention. *Alcohol and drug use.* Accessed December 2011 from http://www.cdc.gov/healthyyouth/alcoholdrug/index

Centers for Disease Control and Prevention, Division of Birth Defects, National Center on Birth Defects and Developmental Disabilities. (2009, October 7). *Folic acid.* Accessed January 2009 from http://www.cdc.gov

Centers for Disease Control and Prevention. Incidence of anemia: National Health and Nutrition Examination Survey (NHANES) 2003-2006. http://www.cdc.gov

Centers for Disease Control and Prevention. Overweight and Obesity. (2011, July). *Adult obesity.* Accessed December 2011 from http://www.cdc.gov/obesity/data/adult.html

Centers for Disease Control and Prevention. National Center for Chronic Disease Prevention and Health Promotion. Division for Heart Disease and Stroke Prevention. (2010). *Sodium: The facts.* Accessed January 3, 2011 from www.cdc.gov/salt/pdfs/sodium_fact_sheet.pdf

Centers for Disease Control and Prevention, National Center for Health Statistics. (2010, June). *Prevalence of overweight, obesity, and extreme obesity among adults: United States, trends 1960-1962 through 2007-2008, NHANES.* http://www.cdc.gov/nchs/data/hestat/obesity_adult_07_08/obesity_adult_07_08.pdf

Centers for Disease Control and Prevention, National Center for Health Statistics, in collaboration with the National Center for Chronic Disease Prevention and Health Promotion. (2000/2005). *2000 CDC growth charts: United States.* Accessed June 23, 2009 from http://www.cdc.gov/growthcharts

Centers for Disease Control and Prevention, National Center for Health Statistics in collaboration with the National Center for Chronic Disease Prevention and Health Promotion. (2000/2009, November 1). *CDC growth charts: United States.* http://www.cdc.gov/growthcharts

Chait, J. (2003, February). Siblings of African American with diabetes often have kidney problems, too. *Diabetes Health Magazine—American Journal of Kidney Diseases.* Accessed June 19, 2009 from http://www.diabeteshealth.com.

The Cleveland Clinic. *Nutrition-cholesterol guidelines.* Accessed November 5, 2011 from http://my.clevelandclinic.org/heart/prevention/nutrition/atp3.aspx

Cornell Food & Brand Lab. (2009, March 2). Eat your vegetables: Preschoolers love vegetables with catchy names like "x-ray vision carrots" and "tomato bursts." *ScienceDaily.*

Correll, C. et al. (2009). Cardiometabolic risk of second-generation antipsychotic medications during first-time use in children and adolescents. *JAMA 302*(16), 1765–1773

Cost of obesity approaching $300 billion a year, Robert Preidt Health Day. (2011, January 21). *USA Today.* http://www.usatoday.com/yourlife/health/medical/2011-01-12-obesity-costs-300-bilion_N.htm

Current trends in diabetes management: A guide for healthcare professionals. (2008). Franklin, TN: Healthways, Inc.

Curry, Andrew. (2009, September). Team type 1: Serious competition. *Diabetes Forecast Magazine.* http://www.forecast.diabetes.org

Dallas, Mary Elizabeth. (2011). *Regular teeth cleanings could cut heart attack risk: Study.* Accessed January 2, 2012 from http://news.health.com/2011/11/13/regular-teeth-cleanings-could-cut-heart-attack-risk-study/

DaVita. (2012). *Can children do peritoneal dialysis?* Accessed February 9, 2012 from http://www.davita.com/treatment-options/home-peritoneal-dialysis/what-is-peritoneal-disease-/can-children-do-peritoneal-dialysis?/t/5484

Definition of tastant. http://www.medilexicon.com/medicaldictionary.php?t=89750

Department of Health and Human Services. Administration on Aging. (2011). Aging statistics. Accessed November 2011 from http://www.aoa.gov/aoaroot/aging_statistics/index.aspx

De Zwaan, M. et al. (2008, August 21). Weight loss maintenance in a population-based sample of German adults. *Obesity 16*(11), 2535–2540.

Dietary Recommendations for Children and Adolescents: A Guide for Practitioners. (2005). Consensus statement from the American Heart Association. *Circulation 112,* 2061–2075

Dietary Reference Intakes: Recommended Intakes for Individuals, National Academy of Sciences. (2011). Institute of Medicine, Food and Nutrition Board. Accessed December 2011 from URLhttp://www.iom.eduURL

Encinosa, W. et al. (2009). Recent improvements in bariatric surgery outcomes. *Medical Care 47*(5), 531–535. doi:10.1097/MLR.0b013e31819434c6

Falkenstein, D. (2010, May 30). *Clostridium perfringens*: Information and Statistics. *Food Poison Journal.* Accessed December 26, 2011 from http://www.foodpoisonjournal.com/foodborne-illness-outbreaks/clostridium-perfringens-information-and-statistics/

Farshchi, H., Taylor, M., and Macdonald, I. (2005, February). Deleterious effects of omitting breakfast on insulin sensitivity and fasting lipid profiles in healthy lean women. *American Journal of Clinical Nutrition 81,* 388–396.

Fasano, A. et al. (2003). University of Maryland Center for Celiac Research. Prevalence of celiac disease in at-risk and not-at-risk groups in the United States: A large multicenter study.*Achieves of Internal Medicine 163*(3), 286–292. http://www.celiaccenter.org

Finkelstei, E.A., Trogdon, J.G., Cohen, J.W., and Dietz, W. (2009). Annual medical spending attributable to obesity: Payer- and service-specific estimates. *Health Affairs 28*(5), w822–w831.

Fontenot, Beth. (2012). *A gluten-free diet reality check.* Accessed January 10, 2012 from www.theatlantic.com/health/archive/2012/01/a-gluten-free-diet-reality-check/250750/

Food and Nutrition Board, Institute of Medicine, & National Academies of Science. (2002). *Dietary reference intakes for energy, carbohydrates, fiber, fat, fatty acids, cholesterol, protein, and amino acids.* Accessed June 15, 2006 from http://www.iom.edu/?id=4340&redirect=0

Food and Nutrition Board, Institute of Medicine of the National Academies. (2005). *Dietary reference intakes for energy, carbohydrate, fiber, fat, fatty acids, cholesterol, protein, and amino acids.* Washington, DC: National Academy Press.

Food and Nutrition Board, National Academies of Sciences, & Institute of Medicine. (2001). *Dietary reference intakes for vitamin A, vitamin K, arsenic, boron, chromium, copper, iodine, iron, manganese, molybdenum, nickel, silicon, vanadium, and zinc.* Accessed June 15, 2006 from http://www.iom.edu/CMS/3788/4574/8521.aspx

Food and Nutrition Service, U.S. Department of Agriculture. (1990). *Meal pattern requirements and offer verses serve manual.* Adapted from Publication FNS-265. Accessed June 23, 2009 from http://www.fns.usda.gov/fns/search "fns-265"

Food and Nutrition Service, U.S. Department of Agriculture, Centers for Disease Control and Prevention, U.S. Department of Education. (2005, January). *Making it happen! School nutrition success stories.* Accessed May 4, 2006 from http://apps.nccd.cdc.gov/MIH/MainPage.aspx

Franks, P.W., Hanson, R.L., Knowler, W.C., Sievers, M.L., Bennett, P.H., and Looker, H.C. (2010). Childhood obesity, other cardiovascular risk factors, and premature death. *New England Journal of Medicine 362*, 485–493.

Fulgoni, V.L., Keast, D.R, Bailey, R.L., and Dwyer, J. (2011, October). Food, fortificants, and supplements: Where do Americans get their nutrients? *Journal of Nutrition 141*, 1847–1854.

Gardner, Amanda. (2011, December 21). *Taste for salt may be shaped during infancy.* Accessed December 26, 2011 from http://www.cnn.com/2011/12/21/health/salt-preferences-determined-early/index.html

Gebhardt, S.E., and Thomas, R.G. (2002). Nutritive value of foods. *Agricultural Research Home and Garden Bulletin 72*, 14–89.

Grever, John. (2011, November 30). Medicare to pay for obesity counseling. Med Page Today. *ABC News.* Accessed January 2012 from http://abcnews.go.com/Health/w_DietAndFitnessNews/medicare-pay-obesity-counseling/story?id=15055422#.TyVkklxWq8A

Gupta, R. et al. (2011, June 20). *The prevalence, severity, and distribution of childhood food allergy in the United States.* doi: 10.1542/peds 2011-0204.

Haney, E.M. et al. (2007). Screening and treatment for lipid disorders in children and adolescents: Systematic evidence review for the U.S. Preventive Services Task Force. *Pediatrics 120*, e189–e214.

Harmon, Christine. (2010, September). *Teen snacking habits present opportunity to improve youth diets.* Accessed December 2011 from http://www.examiner.com

Harris, J.H., and Benedict, F. (1919). *A biometric study of basal metabolism in man.* Washington, DC: Carnegie Institute of Washington.

Hopkins, Katy. (2011, July 7). Colleges that offer courses, choices for vegetarians. *U.S. News.* http://www.usnews.com

Hoyert, D.L., Kung, H.C., and Smith, B.L. (2005). Deaths: Preliminary data for 2003. *National Vital Statistics Reports, 53*(15). Hyattsville, MD: National Center for Health Statistics.

The importance of family dinners VI. (2010, September). The National Center on Addiction and Substance Abuse. New York, NY: Columbia University.

Indian Country: Today Media Network. (2012, January 17). *Paula Deen announces she has type 2 diabetes, cooking not to blame.* ICTMN Staff.

Adapted from Institute of Medicine. Report Brief. (2010, November). *Dietary Reference Intakes for calcium and vitamin D.* Accessed November 10, 2011 from http://www.iom.edu

International Osteoporosis Foundation. (2011). *Facts and statistics about osteoporosis and its impact.* Accessed December 2011 from http://www.iofbonehealth.org/facts-and-statistics.html

Jaslow, Ryan. (2012, January 4). Calories count more than protein for weight loss. *CBS News.* Accessed January 5, 2012 from http://www.cbsnews.com/8301-504763_162-57352169-10391704/calories-count-more-than-protein-for-weight-loss/?tag=mncol;lst;1

Johnston, L.D., O'Malley, P.M., Bachman, J.G., and Schulenberg, J.E. (2011, December 14). *Marijuana use continues to rise among U.S. teens, while alcohol use hits historic lows.* Ann Arbor, MI: University of Michigan News Service.

The Journal Gazette. (2011, November 24). Food habits begin in womb, researchers say. *Washington Post.* Accessed December 14, 2011 from http://www.journalgazette.net/article/20111124/NEWS12/311249949/1180/NEWS12

Jovanovic, L., Nathan, D., Greene, M., and Barss, V. (2011, September 26). *Glycemic control in women with type 1 and type 2 diabetes mellitus during pregnancy.* http://www.uptodate.com/contents/glycemic-control-in-women-with-type-1-and-type-2-diabetes-mellitus-during-pregnancy?source=search_result&search=glycemic+control+in+women+with+type+1+and+type+2+diabetes+mellitus+during+pregnancy&selectedTitle=1%7E150

Kaiser, L., and Allen, L.H. (2008, March). Position of the American Dietetic Association: Nutrition and lifestyle for a healthy pregnancy outcome. *Journal of the American Dietetic Association 108*, 553–561.

Karfonta, K. et al. (2010). Chocolate milk enhances glycogen replenishment after endurance exercise in moderately trained males. *Medicine & Science in Sports and Exercise 42*, S64

Khosia, S. et al. (2003). Incidence of childhood distal forearm fractures over 30 years—A population based study. *JAMA 290*(11), 1479–1485

KidsHealth. (2012). *Kids and exercise.* Accessed February 13, 2012 from http://kidshealth.org

Kilham, Chris. (2011, December 21). Herbs to improve digestion. *Fox News.* Accessed January 4, 2012 from http://www.foxnews.com

Kliff, Sarah. (2011, October 4). Will a fat tax make Denmark healthier? *The Washington Post.* Accessed January 5, 2012 from http://www.washingtonpost.com/blogs/ezra-klein/post/will-a-fat-tax-make-denmark-healthier/2011/10/04/gIQA3D5nKL_blog.html

Larson, N.I. et al. (2007). Family meals during adolescence are associated with higher diet quality and healthful meal patterns during young adulthood. *Journal of the American Dietetic Association 107*, 1502–1510.

Liquid candy—How soft drinks are harming our health. Accessed January 2012 from http://www.cspinet.org/new/pdf/sdtaxes_obesity_factsheet.pdf

Machowsky, Jason. (2010, December). *Sports drinks and vitamin waters: Are they right for me?* Accessed January 5, 2012 from http://www.rd411.com

Mayo Clinic. (2011, February 2). *New dietary guidelines: How to make smart choices.* Accessed November 5, 2011 from http://www.mayoclinic.com/health/dietary-guidelines/MY01594/NSECTIONGROUP=2

Mayo Foundation for Medical Education and Research. (2010). *Artificial sweeteners: Understanding these and other sugar substitutes.* Accessed February 1, 2012 from http://www.mayoclinic.com/health/artificial-sweeteners/MY00073

McCulloch, D., Nathan, D., Fletcher, S., and Mulder, J. (2011, July 21). *Screening for diabetes mellitus.* http://www.uptodate.com/contents/screening-for-diabetes-mellitus?source=search_result&search=screening+for+diabetes+mellitus&selectedTitle=1%7E150

McQueen, Courtney. (2012). Early treatment adherence decreases risk of treatment failure in HIV-positive adults. *The AIDS Beacon.* Accessed January 10, 2012 from http://www.aidsbeacon.com

McMichael, William. (2009, November 3). *Most U.S youths unfit to serve, data show.* Accessed January 2012 from http://www.armytimes.com/news/2009/11/military_unfityouths_recruiting_110309w/

The Medical News. (2004, May). *Protein in human milk reduces risk of obesity.* Accessed June 23, 2009 from http://www.news-medical.net/news/2004/05/03/1173.aspx

Mensing, C., Cypress, M., Halstenson, C., McLaughlin, S., and Walker, E. (2006). *The art and science of diabetes self-management education.* Chicago IL: American Association of Diabetes Educators.

Monsivais, P., and Drewnowski, A. (2007). The rising cost of low-energy-density foods. *Journal of the American Dietetic Association 107*(12), 2071–2076.

Nanney, M.S. et al. (2004). Rationale for a consistent "powerhouse" approach to vegetable and fruit messages. *Journal of the American Dietetic Association 104*(3), 352.

Narayan, K. et al. (2003). Lifetime risk for diabetes mellitus in the United States. *JAMA 290*, 1884–1890.

National Academy of Sciences. (1998). *DRI report.* http://www.nap.edu.

National Academy of Sciences. (2001). *Adequate intakes for selected minerals.* Washington, DC: National Academy Press.

National Academy of Sciences. (2006, August). *Dietary reference intakes: The essential guide to nutrient requirements.* Washington, DC: National Academy Press.

National Academy of Sciences. (2011). *Dietary reference intakes for calcium and vitamin D.* Washington, DC: National Academy Press.

National Center for Complementary and Alternative Medicine, National Institutes of Health. (2008). *An introduction to probiotics.* Accessed June 24, 2009 from http://nccam.nih.gov/health/probiotics/#effects

National Center for Health Statistics in collaboration with the National Center for Chronic Disease Prevention and Health Promotion. (2000). *Growth charts.* http://www.cdc.gov/growthcharts

National Diabetes Education Program, National Institutes of Health. *Lifestyle changes especially effective at preventing type 2 diabetes in adults aged 60 and older.* Data compiled December 2, 2005, from http://ndep.nih.gov

National Glycohemoglobin Stabilization Program. (2010). *2010 consensus statement on the worldwide standardization of HbA1c.* http://www.ngsp.org/news.asp

National Heart Lung and Blood Institute, U.S. Department of Health and Human Services. (2011). *Who is at risk for iron-deficiency anemia?* Accessed February 10, 2012 from http://www.nhlbi.nih.gov/health/health-topics/topics/ida/atrisk.html

National Institute of Allergy and Infectious Diseases, Department of Health and Human Services, National Institutes of Health. (2010, March). *Food allergy quick facts.* Accessed January 2, 2012 from http://www.niaid.nih.gov/topics/foodallergy/understanding/pages/quickfacts.aspx

National Institute of Arthritis and Musculoskeletal and Skin Diseases, National Institutes of Health. *Osteoporosis overview.* Accessed June 2009 from http://www.niams.nih.gov/Health_Info/Bone/Osteoporosis/default.asp

National Institute of Child Health and Human Development. (2012). *Why are tween and teen years so critical?* Accessed February 13, 2012 from http://www.nichd.nih.gov/milk/prob/critical.cfm

National Institutes of Health. (2005). *Lifestyle changes especially effective at preventing type 2 diabetes in adults aged 60 and older.* Data complied and retrieved December 2, 2005, from http://www.ndep.nih.gov/campaigns/tools.htm

National Institutes of Health, Osteoporosis and Related Bone Diseases Resource Center. (2000, October). *Osteoporosis overview.* Accessed June 15, 2006 from http://www.osteo.org/osteo.html

The National Institutes of Health, The Office of Dietary Supplements. (2011, June). *Dietary supplement fact sheet: Vitamin D.* Accessed November 15, 2011 from http://ods.od.nih.gov/factsheets/VitaminD-HealthProfessional/

National Kidney Foundation. (2009, December). *Ten facts about African Americans and kidney disease.* Accessed January 3, 2012 from http://www.kidney.org/news/newsroom/fs_new/10factsaboutaframerkd.cfm

National Kidney Foundation. (2012). *Diet and kidney stones.* Accessed February 2, 2012 from http://www.kidney.org/atoz/content/diet.cfm

Nelson, J.K., Moxness, K.E., Gastineau, C.F., and Jenson, M.D. (1994). *Mayo Clinic diet manual: A handbook of nutrition practices* (7th ed.). St. Louis, MO: Mosby.

NIH Osteoporosis and Related Bone Diseases National Resource Center. National Institute of Arthritis and Musculoskeletal and Skin Diseases. (2010, June). *Osteoporosis and Hispanic women.* Accessed February 15, 2012 from http://www.niams.nih.gov/Health_Info/Bone/Osteoporosis/Background/hispanic_women.asp

NIH Osteoporosis and Related Bone Diseases National Resource Center. National Institute of Arthritis and Musculoskeletal and Skin Diseases. (2011, January). *Osteoporosis and men.* Accessed February 15, 2012 from http://www.niams.nih.gov/Health_Info/Bone/Osteoporosis/men.asp

Nutrition 411. *Estimating energy requirements for an obese patient professional refresher.* http://www.rd411.com/professional-learning/professional-refreshers/item/405-estimating-energy-requirements-for-the-obese-patients

Nutrition and athletic performance; Nutrition Stand. (2009). *Medicine & Science in Sports and Exercise 41*(3), 709–731.

Obesity. (2005). *Atlanta Journal-Constitution.* Retrieved June 15, 2006 from http://www.ajc.com/health/healthfd/shared/health/adam/ency/article/003101.html

O'Connor, Anahad. (2011, December 12). Beware of raw cookie dough. *The New York Times.* Accessed December 14, 2011 from http://well.blogs.nytimes.com/2011/12/12/beware-of-raw-cookie-dough/

Ogden, C., and Carroll, M. (2010). National Center for Health Statistic (NCHS) Health E-Stat. *Prevalence of obesity among children and adolescents: United States, trends 1963-1965 through 2007-2008.* http://www.cdc.gov/nchs/data/hestat/obesity_child_07_08/obesity_child_07_08.htm

Olshansky, S.J. et al. (2005). A potential decline in life expectancy in the United States in the 21st century. *New England Journal of Medicine 352,* 1138–1145

Partnership for Food Safety Education. (2006, April). *Fight foodborne bacteria: Four simple steps to food safety* [brochure]. http://www.fightbac.org

Perry, Arthur. (2011). Surgery and obesity: The deadly risks. *The Dr. Oz Show.* Accessed January 26, 2012 from http://www.doctoroz.com/blog/arthur-perry-md-facs/surgery- and- obesity-deadly-risks

Pifer, Angela. (2011). *Protein.* Nutrition Northwest. Accessed January 30, 2012 from www.nutritionnorthwest.com/Protein-Requirements.pdf

Picot, J. et al. (2009). The clinical effectiveness and cost-effectiveness of bariatric (weight loss) surgery for obesity: A systematic review and economic evaluation. *Health Technology Assessment 13*(41), iii–iv, 1–190, 215–357.

Protein in human milk reduces risk of obesity. (2004, May). *Medical Study News.* Accessed June 15, 2006 from http://www.news-medical.net/?id=1173.

Prout, Linda. (2011). Yin-yang balance and food choice. *Acufinder Magazine.* Accessed October 12, 2011 from https://www.acufinder.com/Acupuncture+Information/Detail/Yin-Yang+Balance+and+Food+Choice

Raw Food Explained.com. *Lesson 85: The dangers of a high protein diet. The problems with protein.* Accessed November 15, 2011 from http://www.rawfoodexplained.com/the-dangers-of-a-high-protein-diet/the-problems-with-protein.html

RD411. (2010, June). *Breastfeeding and nutrition.* Accessed January 9, 2012 from http://www.rd411.com/index.php?option=com_content&view=article&id=1415:breastfeeding-and-nutrition&catid=100:miscellaneous-topics&Itemid=394

RD411. (2011, April). *Eating for two? Good nutrition during pregnancy and lactation.* Accessed January 7, 2012 from http://www.rd411.com/index.php?option=com_content&view=article&id=592:eating-for-two&catid=100:miscellaneous-topics&Itemid=394

Reinberg, Steven. (2010). *1 in 4 U.S. teens and young adults binge drink.* Accessed January 2012 from http://www.usatoday.com/yourlife/parenting-family/teen-ya/2010-10-08-binge-drinking_N.htm

Robertson, Laura. (2011, June 20). *The most and least active cities in America. Where sit happens.* Accessed December 2011 from http://www.menshealth.com/health/most-active-cities

Rosenberg, K.D., Gelow, J.M., and Sandoval, A.P. (2004, May). Pregnancy intendedness and the use of periconceptual folic acid. *Pediatrics, 111*(5), 1142–1145.

The Rudd Center for Food Policy and Obesity. (2010). *Evaluating fast food nutrition and marketing to youth.* http://www.yaleruddcenter.org/newsletter/issue.aspx?id=27

Sacks, D., Arnold, M., Bakris, G., Bruns, D., Horvath, A., Kirkman, M. et al. (2011, June). Guidelines and recommendations for laboratory analysis in the diagnosis and management of diabetes mellitus. *Diabetes Care 34,* e61–e99.

Saint Louis University. (2004, March 19). *Aging successfully* [newsletter].

Salahi, Laura. (2010). Staying fit: Majority of older adults struggle with weight. *ABC News.* Accessed December 30, 2011 from http://abcnews.go.com

Satter, E. (1999). *Secrets of feeding a healthy family.* Madison, WI: Kelcy Press.

Schmitt, B.D. (2010). *Solid (strained) foods.* Children's Physician Network. Accessed October 21, 2011 from http://www.cpnonline.org/CRS/CRS/pa_solidfoo_hhg.htm

Schwimmer, J. et al. (2003, April). Health-related quality of life of severely obese children and adolescents. *JAMA 289,* 1813–1819

Simon, Nissa. (2011). Fish reduces Alzheimer's risk. *AARP Bulletin.* Accessed December 27, 2011 from http://www.aarp.org/health/brain-health/info-11-2011/fish-reduces-alzheimers-risk-health-discovery.html

Sloane, Matt. (2009, November 5). Obesity responsible for 100,000 cancer cases annually. *CNN Medical News.* Accessed November 3, 2011 from http://www.cnn.com/2009/HEALTH/11/05/obesity.cancer.link/index.html?iref=allsearch

Spratto, G.R., and Woods, A.L. (2006). *PDR nurse's drug handbook.* Clifton Park, NY: Delmar Cengage Learning and Medical Economics of Thomson Healthcare.

Study: Some low-carb diets up cancer, death risk. (2010, September 7). *CBS News.* Accessed January 5, 2012 from http://www.cbsnews.com/stories/2010/09/07/earlyshow/health/main6841541.shtml

Terrie, Y.C. (2009, January 1). Multivitamins for the senior population. *Pharmacy Times.* Accessed February 15, 2012 from http://www.pharmacytimes.com/publications/issue/2009/2009-01/2009-01-5384

Texas Heart Institute, Texas Heart Institute Information Center. (2008, August). *Tips for reducing salt intake.* Accessed June 24, 2009 from http://www.texasheartinstitute.org/HIC/Topics/HSmart/saltips.cfm

Tobacco use statistics. Accessed January 2012 from http://www.cdc.gov/tobacco/data_statistics/fact_sheets/youth_data/tobacco_use/index.htm

Trecroci, D. (2005, November). Mark Consuelos encourages Type 2s and their loved ones to take "diabetes freedom" pledge. *Diabetes Health.* Accessed June 15, 2006 from http://www.diabeteshealth.com/read,1038,4443.html

Trends in the prevalence of alcohol use National YRBS: 1991—2009. Accessed December 2011 from http://www.cdc.gov/healthyyouth/yrbs/pdf/us_alcohol_trend_yrbs.pdf

Troiano, R.P., Berrigan, D., Dodd, K.W., Mâsse, L.C., Tilert, T., and McDowell, M. (2008). Physical activity in the United States measured by accelerometer. *Medicine & Science in Sports and Exercise 40*(1), 181–188.

U.S. Department of Agriculture. (2002). Nutritive values of foods. *Home and Garden Bulletin 72* (Rev. ed.).

U.S. Department of Agriculture. (2009, April). *The quality of children's diets in 2003-04 as measured by the Healthy Eating Index-2005.* Washington, DC: The Center for Nutrition Policy and Promotion.

U.S. Department of Agriculture. (2011). *How many grain foods are needed daily.* Accessed November 11, 2011 from www.choosemyplate.gov/foodgroups/grains_amount_table.html

U.S. Department of Agriculture. (2011). *Sample menus for a 2000 calorie food pattern.* Accessed November 2011 from www.choosemyplate.gov/food-groups/downloads/sample_menu-MyPyramid.pdf

U.S. Department of Agriculture, Agricultural Research Service. (2005). *USDA national nutrient database for standard reference, release 18.* Accessed June 13, 2006 from http://www.ars.usda.gov/ba/bhnrc/ndl.

U.S. Department of Agriculture, Agricultural Research Service. (2010). *Snacking patterns of U.S. adolescents: What we eat in America,* NHANES 2005-2006. http://www.ars.usda.gov/Services/docs.htm?docid=19476

U.S. Department of Agriculture, Center for Nutrition Policy and Promotion. (2005, April). Publication CNPP-XX. Washington, DC: Author.

U.S. Department of Agriculture, Center for Nutrition Policy and Promotions. (2011). *MyPlate.* http://www.choosemyplate.gov

U.S. Department of Agriculture, Center for Nutrition Policy and Promotions. (2011). *MyPlate Food Intake Patterns.* http://www.choosemyplate.gov/professionals/pdf_food_intake.html

U.S. Department of Agriculture, Food Safety and Inspection Service. (2011, May). *Foodborne illness: What consumers need to know.* Accessed January 9, 2012 from http://www.fsis.usda.gov

U.S. Department of Agriculture. SuperTracker and BMI calculator. http://www.choosemyplate.gov

U.S. Department of Health and Human Services, National Institutes of Health, National Institutes of Child Health and Human Development. (2006, January). *Lactose intolerance: Information for health care providers.* NIH Publication No. 05-5305B. Accessed October 2011 from www.nichd.nih.gov

U.S. Department of Health and Human Services. National Institute of Diabetes and Digestive and Kidney Diseases. National Institute of Health. (2007). Celiac disease: National Digestive Diseases Information Clearinghouse. Accessed December 2011 from www.digestive.niddk.nih.gov

U.S. Department of Health and Human Services. National Institutes of Health. National Center for Complementary and Alternative Medicine. (2011, March). *Get the facts: Using dietary supplements wisely.* Accessed December 16, 2011 from http://nccam.nih.gov/health/supplements/wiseuse.htm

U.S. Department of Health and Human Services. National Institutes of Health. National Heart, Lung, and Blood Institute. (2005). *Your guide to lowering your cholesterol with TLC.* NIH Publication No. 06-5235. Accessed December 2011 from www.nhlbi.nih.gov/health/public/heart/chol/chol_tlc.pdf

Adapted from the U.S. Department of Health and Human Services and U.S. Department of Agriculture. *Dietary Guidelines for Americans, 2010* (7th ed.). Accessed December 2011 from http://www.cnpp.usda.gov/DGAs2010-PolicyDocument.htm

Adapted from U.S. Department of Health and Human Services. (2008). *2008 physical activity guidelines for Americans.* Washington, DC: U.S. Department of Health and Human Services. ODPHP Publication No. U0036. http://www.health.gov/paguidelines. Accessed December 2011

University of Iowa Hospitals and Clinics. (2001). *Viruses and cancer.* Accessed November 2, 2011 from http://www.uihealthcare.com/topics/medicaldepartments/cancercenter/cancertips/viruses.html

U.S. Department of Health and Human Services, U.S. Food and Drug Administration. (2009, October). Requirements for health claims made in labeling. *Food 11,* Appendix C: Health Claims. Accessed October 12, 2011 from http://www.fda.gov

U.S. National Library of Medicine. (2011). Thrush. *A.D.A.M. Medical Encyclopedia.* Accessed January 30, 2012 from http://www.ncbi.nlm.nih.gov/pubmedhealth/PMH0001650/

U.S. National Library of Medicine. National Institutes of Health. (2010). Medline Plus. *Low-residue fiber diet.* Accessed November 2, 2011 from http://www.nlm.nih.gov/medlineplus/ency/patientinstructions/000200.htm

U.S. weight loss market work $60.9 billion. (2011, May 5). RedOrbit. Accessed January 2012 from http://www.redorbit.com/news/health/2045046/us_weight_loss_market_worth_609_billion/

WebMD. (2010). *7 nutrients your diet may be missing.* Accessed April 20, 2012 from http://www.webmd.com/diet/guide/7-nutrients-your-diet-may-be-missing

Web MD. (2010). *Rheumatoid arthritis health center.* Accessed November 11, 2011 from http://www.webmd.com/rheumatoid-arthritis/guide/can-your-diet-help-relieve-rheumatoid-arthritis?page=2

Wheat Foods Council. (2005). Twists and turns of fad diets. http://www.wheatfoods.org.

White, L. (2005). *Foundations of adult health nursing* (2nd ed.). Clifton Park, NY: Delmar Cengage Learning.

Williams, D. et al. (2008). *Prevalence of pre-diabetes in youth.* Presented at 68th Scientific Session 2008, American Diabetes Association (NHANES data 2005-2006).

Wilson, Margaret-Mary (Ed.). (2007). *The Merck manual. Overview of nutrition.* Accessed January 10, 2012 from http://www.merckmanuals.com/professional/nutritional_disorders/nutrition_general_considerations/overview_of_nutrition.html#v881783

Wing, R.R., and Phelan, S. (2005). Long term weight loss maintenance. *The American Journal of Clinical Nutrition 82* (1 Suppl), 222S–225S.

World Health Organization. (2002, August). *Botulism.* Accessed December 20, 2011 from http://www.who.int/mediacentre/factsheets/fs270/en/

www.cdc.gov/NCHS/data/hestat/obesity_adult_07_08/obesity_adult_07_08.p

Young athletes and energy drink—A bad mix? (2011, December 5). *USA Today/Sports.* http://www.usatoday.com

Zelman, Kathleen. (2011, August 28). *Know the difference between fat- and water-soluble nutrients.* Accessed December 13, 2011 from http://www.webmd.com/vitamins-and-supplements/nutrition-vitamins-11/fat-water-nutrient

BIBLIOGRAPHY

BOOKS

Abdominal fat and what to do about it—The Harvard Medical School family health guide. Accessed January 2012 from http://www.health.harvard.edu/fhg/updates/Abdominal-fat-and-what-to-do-about-it.shtml

American Dietetic Association. (2007). How to spot a food fad. http://www.eatright.org

Anderson, J. et al. (2000). Health advantages and disadvantages of weight-reducing diets: A computer analysis and critical review. *Journal of the American College of Nutrition 19*(5), 578–590

Barlow, S.E., and Dietz, W.H. (1998). Obesity evaluation and treatment: Expert committee recommendations. *Pediatrics 102*, E29.

Brown, J.E. et al. (2007). *Nutritions through the life cycle* (3rd ed.). Belmont, CA: Wadsworth Publishing Company.

Cataldo, C.B. (2003). *Nutrition and diet therapy* (6th ed.). Belmont, CA: Wadsworth Publishing Company.

Centers for Disease Control and Prevention. (2011, October). Healthy weight—It's not a diet, it's a lifestyle. Tips for parents—Ideas to help children maintain a healthy weight. Accessed December 2011 from http://www.cdc.gov/healthyweight/children/

Centers for Disease Control and Prevention. Physical activity for everyone. Accessed January 2012 from http://www.cdc.gov/physicalactivity/everyone/guidelines/adults.html

Centers for Disease Control, Obesity and Genetics. Accessed January 2012 from http://www.cdc.gov/Features/Obesity/

Cepeda, Esther. (2012, January). Obesity crisis far from over; Trust for America's Health. *Washington Post.* Accessed January 21, 2012 from http://healthyamericans.org/newsroom/news/?newsid=2359

Daniels, S.R., Arnett, D.K., Eckel, R.H. et al. (2005). Overweight in children and adolescents: Pathophysiology, consequences, prevention, and treatment. *Circulation 111*, 1999–2012.

Escott-Stump, S., (2007). *Nutrition and diagnosis—related care* (6th ed.). Philadelphia, PA: Lippincott.

Fletcher, A. (2003). *Thin for life: 10 keys to success from people who have lost weight and kept it off.* New York, NY: Houghton Mifflin Harcourt.

Grodner, M., Long, S., and DeYoung, S. (2004). *Foundations and clinical applications of nutrition: A nursing approach* (3rd ed.). St. Louis, MO: Mosby.

Hadley, A. et al. (2010, July). What works for the prevention and treatment of obesity among children. Child Trends Fact Sheet. http://www.childtrends.org

Healthy Hunger Free Kids Act 2010: http://www.fns.usda.gov/cnd/governance/legislation/cnr_2010.htm

Kegan, R. (1994). *In over our heads: The mental demands of modern life.* Cambridge, MA: Harvard University Press.

Lutz, C.A., and Rutherford, K.P. (2006). *Nutrition and diet therapy* (4th ed.). Philadelphia, PA: Davis.

Mahan, L.K., and Escott-Stump, S. (2007). *Krause's food nutrition and diet therapy* (11th ed.). Philadelphia, PA: Saunders.

Mitchell, M.K. (2002). *Nutrition across the life span* (2nd ed.). Philadelphia, PA: Saunders.

National Cholesterol Education Program, National Institute of Health, Expert Panel on Blood Cholesterol Panels in Children and Adolescents. (1992). *Pediatrics 89*, 525–584.

National Institute for Drug Abuse, NIDA for Teens. Marijuana. Accessed December 2011 from www.teens.drugabuse.gov/facts/facts_mji.php

The National Weight Control Registry, Brown Medical School/The Miriam Hospital Weight Control & Diabetes Research Center. http://www.nwcr.ws/

Nestle, M., and Jacobson, M. (2000, Jan/Feb). Halting the obesity epidemic: A public health policy approach. *Public Health Reports 115*, 12–22.

NIH, NHLBI Obesity Education Initiative. Clinical Guidelines on the Identification, Evaluation, and Treatment of Overweight and Obesity in Adults. http://www.nhlbi.nih.gov/guidelines/obesity/ob_gdlns.pdf

581

Patel, Alpa V. et al. (2010). Leisure time spent sitting in relation to total mortality in a prospective cohort of U.S. adults. *American Journal of Epidemiology 172*(4), 419–429. doi: 10.1093/aje/kwq155

Pronnsky, Z.M. (2008). *Food—medication interactions* (15th ed.). Birchrunville, PA: Publisher.

Robert Wood Johnson Foundation. (2011, July). F as in fat: How obesity threatens America's future; Trust for America's Health. Accessed December 2011 from http://healthyamericans.org/assets/files/TFAH2011FasInFat10.pdf

Roizen, M., and Oz, M. (2006). *You, on a diet: The owner's manual for waist management.* City: Free Press.

Rolls, B. (2007). *The volumetric eating plan—Techniques and recipes for feeling fuller on fewer calories.* New York, NY: Harper.

Samour, P. (2009). *Pediatric nutrition handbook* (6th ed.). Boston, MA: Jones and Bartlett Inc.

Satter, E. (1987). *How to get your kid to eat . . . But not too much.* Boulder, CO: Bull Publishing.

Satter, E. (2000). *Child of mine* (3rd ed.). Boulder, CO: Bull Publishing.

Satter, Ellyn. (2000). *Child of mine: Feeding with love and good sense.* Boulder, CO: Bull Publishing Company.

Savage, Jennifer S., Orlet Fisher, Jennifer, and Birch, Leann L. (2007). Parental influence on eating behavior, conception to adolescence. *The Journal of Law, Medicine, and Ethics 35*(1), 22–34. Accessed January 2012 from NIH author manuscript at http://www.ncbi.nlm.nih.gov/pmc/articles/PMC2531152/

Sizer, S., and Whitney, E. (2007). *Nutrition: Concepts and controversies* (11th ed.). Salt Lake City, UT: Brooks Cole Publishing Company.

Skin and Acanthosis Nigricans. Accessed December 2011 from http://www.webmd.com/skin-problems-and-treatments/acanthosis-nigricans-overview

Straub, Richard. (2006). *Health psychology: A biopsychosocial approach* (2nd ed.). New York, NY: W.H. Freeman.

The Surgeon General's Call to Action to Prevent and Decrease Overweight and Obesity. http://www.surgeongeneral.gov/topics/obesity/calltoaction/fact_adolescents.htm

Swartz, M.B., and Puhl, R. (2003). Childhood obesity: A societal problem to solve. *Obesity Reviews 4*(1), 57–71.

Trahms, C.M., and Pipes P. (2001). *Nutrition in infancy and childhood* (7th ed.). New York, NY: McGraw-Hill.

U.S. News and World Report. Health, best diet rankings 2012. Accessed January 2012 from http://health.usnews.com/best-diet

Wansink, Brian. (2007). *Mindless eating—Why we eat more than we think.* New York, NY: Bantam Publishing.

Weight Control & Diabetes Research Center. http://www.nwcr.ws/

Weight-Control Information Network, National Heart Lung and Blood Institute. Economic costs of overweight and obesity. Accessed January 2012 from http://win.niddk.nih.gov/statistics/#econ

Weight-Control Information Network, National Heart Lung Blood Institute. Facts about healthy weight. Accessed January 2012 from http://www.nhlbi.nih.gov/health/prof/heart/obesity/aim_kit/healthy_wt_facts.htm

Weight-Control Information Network, National Heart Lung Blood Institute. Prescription medicines for the treatment of obesity. Accessed January 2012 from http://win.niddk.nih.gov/publications/prescription.htm

Weight loss: Choosing a diet that's right for you. Accessed January 2012 from http://www.mayoclinic.com/health/weight-loss/NU00616

Whitaker, R.C., Wright, J.A., Pepe, M.S., Seidel, K.D., and Dietz, W.H. (1997). Predicting obesity in young adulthood from childhood and parental obesity. *New England Journal of Medicine 37*, 869–873.

Whitney, E.N., DeBruyne, L.K., Pinna, K., and Rolfes, S.R. (2007). *Nutrition for health & health care* (3rd ed.). Belmont, CA: Wadsworth Publishing Company.

Whitney, E.N., and Rolfes, S.R. (2005). *Understanding nutrition* (10th ed.). Belmont, CA: Wadsworth Publishing Company.

Williams, S.R. (2005). *Basic nutrition and diet therapy* (12th ed.). St. Louis, MO: Mosby.

Worthington-Roberts, B.S., and Williams, S.R. (Eds.). (2000). *Nutrition throughout the life cycle.* New York, NY: McGraw-Hill.

Xuemei, S. (2007). Cardiorespiratory fitness and adiposity as mortality predictors in older adults. *JAMA 298*(21), 2507–2516. doi:10.1001/jama.298.21.2507

PERIODICALS AND PUBLICATIONS

American Dietetic Association. (2007). How to spot a food fad. http://www.eatright.org

American Heart Association. (2005). AHA Scientific Statement. Dietary recommendations for children and adolescents. *Circulation 112*, 1061–1075.

Amylin Pharmaceuticals. (n.d.). First-in-class, incretin mimetic. http://www.Byetta.com

Barclay, L. (2005). American Heart Association updates guidelines for children. Accessed April 4, 2006 from http://www.medscape.com/viewarticle/513792

Browning, R., and Kram, R. (2005, May). Energetic cost and preferred speed of walking in obese vs. normal weight women. *Obesity Research 13*, 891–899.

Centers for Disease Control and Prevention. (2005). Overweight and obesity: Home. Accessed April 12, 2005 from http://www.cdc.gov

Centers for Disease Control and Prevention. (2006). BMI—Body mass index: BMI for children and teens. Accessed June 8, 2006 from http://www.cdc.gov/nccdphp/dnpa/bmi/childrens_BMI/about_childrens_BMI.htm

Collins, N. (2001, March/April). Tube feeding and pressure ulcers. *Advances in Skin and Wound Care.*

Diabetic-Lifestyle Online Magazine. (2004, December). Diabetes and osteoporosis. http://www.diabetic-lifestyle.com

Eyre, C. (2007). Orange juice flavonoids fight disease? http://beveragedaily.com.

Food & Nutrition Board, Institute of Medicine. (1997). *Dietary reference intakes of calcium, phosphorus, magnesium, vitamin D, and fluoride.* Washington, DC: National Academy Press.

Food & Nutrition Board, Institute of Medicine. (2000). *Dietary reference intakes for vitamin C, vitamin E, selenium, and carotenoids.* Washington, DC: National Academy Press.

Food & Nutrition Board, Institute of Medicine. (2001). *Dietary reference intakes for vitamin A, vitamin K, arsenic, boron, chromium, copper, iodine, iron, manganese, molybdenum, nickel, silicon, vanadium, and zinc.* Washington, DC: National Academy Press.

Food & Nutrition Board, Institute of Medicine. (2004). *Dietary reference intakes for water, potassium, sodium, chloride, and sulfate.* Washington, DC: National Academy Press.

Food & Nutrition Board, Institute of Medicine. (2005). *Dietary reference intakes for energy, carbohydrate, fiber, fat, fatty acids, cholesterol, protein, and amino acids (macronutrients).* Washington, DC: National Academy Press.

Food insight: Current topics in food safety and nutrition. (2001, July/August). *IACP ON Tour: Exploring the Issues of Food Biotechnology,* 2–3.

Greene, A. (2008). Healthy eating. http://www.drgreene.com

Greene, A. (2008). Vitamins and children. http://www.drgreene.com

Gutzin, S.J. et al. (2003). The safety of oral hypoglycemic agents in the first trimester of pregnancy: A meta analysis. *Canadian Journal of Pharmacology* 42(4), 303–313.

Hamvas, J., Schwab, R., and Pap, A. (2001). Jejunal feeding in chronic pancreatitis with severe necrosis. *Journal of Pancreas* (Online), 2(3), 112–116. [Full text]. http://www.jcplink.net/prev/200105/200105_5.pdf

Hellwig, J. (2009). Improving nutrition in the elderly. http://www.tufts-nemc.org.

Horbul, B.A. (2008). Diet and cancer. http://www.porcupinehu.on.ca/Nutrition/2008/DietandCancer.com

Iannelli, V. (2008). Food portion sizes. http://www.pediatrics.about.com.

Lakdawalla, D., Goldman, D., and Shang, B. (2005, September 26). The health and cost consequences of obesity among the elderly. *Health Affair.*

Lockyear, P.L.B. (2004). Childhood eating behaviors: Developmental and sociocultural consideration. *Medscape OB/GYN & Women's Health* 9(1). Accessed April 4, 2005 from http://www.medscape.com/viewarticle/467523_print

Morey, M.C. (2009). Diet and exercise intervention helps older, overweight cancer survivors reduce functional decline. http://www.pubs.ama-assn.org

Mukherjee, S., Anlonarakis, E., Asadvzzaman, S., and Peters, J. (2005). Acute psychological stress-induced water intoxication. *International Journal of Psychiatry in Clinical Practice* 9(2), 142–144.

National Kidney Foundation. (2009). Diet and kidney stones. http://www.kidney.org.

Nordqvist, Christian. (2007). Organic tomatoes better for heart and blood pressure. http://www.medicalnewstoday.com.

Nutrition in the elderly. (2009). Nursing Care Guide. http://www.nursingcareguide.com.

Office of Dietary Supplements, National Institute of Health. (2007). Dietary supplements fact sheet: Vitamin B6. http://www.ods.od.nih.gov.

Pearce, C.B., and Duncan, H.D. (2002). Enteral feeding, nasogastric, nasojejunal, percutaneous endoscopic, gastrostomy vs. jejunostomy; its indications and limitations. *Postgraduate Medical Journal* 78, 198–204.

Regions Hospital. Coming to the burn center. Accessed December 2005 from http://www.regionshospital.com/Regions/Menu/0,11369,00.html

Rhodes, M. (2009). Facts about fat: The good, the bad, and the ugly. http://www.food-facts.suite101.com.

Rose, S. (2008). How much do you know about triglycerides? http://www.tufts-nemc.org.

Schoenstadt, A. (2008). Calcium deficiency. http://www.osteoporosis.emedtv.com.

Schroeder-Kassel, K. (2008). Eating a diet moderate in protein-rich foods. http://www.tufts-nemc.org.

Schroeder-Kassel, K. (2008). Limiting potassium in your diet. http://www.tufts-nemc.org.

Science News. (2009). Key regulations of fat cell development discoveries. http://www.siencedaily.com.

Shashidhar, H.R. (2009). Malnutrition. http://www.emedicine.medscape.com.

Stroud, M., Duncan, H., and Nightingale, J. (2003). Guidelines for enteral feeding in adult hospital patients. *Gut* 52, vii1–vii12.

Tangpricha, V. (2008). Vitamin D deficiency and related disorders. http://emedicine.medscape.com.

University of Maryland Medical Center. (2005). How can gallstones and gallbladder disease be prevented? Accessed September 19, 2006 from http://www.umm.edu/patiented/articles/how_can_gallstones_gallbladder_disease_be_prevented

U.S. Department of Health & Human Services. (2005). Citing "dangerous increase" in deaths, HHS launches new strategies against overweight epidemic. Accessed June 12, 2005 from http://www.hhs.gov http://www.hhs/news/2004 pres/20040309.html

U.S. National Library of Medicine. (2005). Gastric bypass (Medline). Accessed September 19, 2005 from http://www.nlm.nih.gov/medlineplus/print/ency/article/009199.htm

INTERNET SITES

http://www.aarp.org
http://www.asiarecipe.com
http://www.cbsnews.com
http://www.chinese-food-info.com
http://www.chinesefood-recipes.com
http://www.choosemyplate.gov
http://www.cnn.com
http://www.content.karger.com
http://www.countriesandcities.com
http://www.davita.com
http://www.foodbycountry.com
http://www.globalgourmet.com
http://www.goeasterneurope.com
http://www.iexplore.com
http://www.indianfoodgourmet.com
http://www.indigoguide.com
http://www.japan-guide.com
http://www.jn.nutrition.org
http://www.journalgazette.net
http://www.kidshealth.org
http://www.localhistories.org
http://www.mayoclinic.com
http://www.medterms.com
http://www.myannardot.com
http://www.my.clevelandclinic.org
http://www.nal.usda.gov
http://www.Native-languages.org
http://news.health.com
http://www.nicemeal.com
http://www.norway.hel.com
http://www.nytimes.com
http://www.outreachworld.org
http://www.puntacana-information-guide.com
http://www.ra.com
http://www.rd411.com
http://www.recipes.howstuffworks.com
http://www.southeastasianfoods.about.com
http://www.spicecuisine.com
http://www.strenafoods.com
http://www.theatlantic.com
http://www.topuertorico.org
http://www.uniteam-travel-myanmar.com
http://www.usatoday.com
http://www.usnews.com
http://www.wanogakkou.com
http://www.webmd.com
Academy of Nutrition and Dietetics, http://www.eatright.org
Action for Healthy Kids, http://www.actionforhealthykids.org
Administration on Aging, http://www.aoa.gov
Agricultural Research Service, http://www.ars.usda.gov
AIDS.Org, http://www.aids.org

Alliance for a Healthier Generation, http://www.healthiergeneration.org
American Academy of Pediatrics, http://www.aap.org
American Cancer Society, http://www.cancer.org
American Diabetes Association, http://www.diabetes.org
American Heart Association, http://www.americanheart.com
American Obesity Association, http://www.obesity.org
American Society for Gastrointestinal Endoscopy, http://www.asge.org
American Society for Parenteral and Enteral Nutrition, http://www.clinnutr.org
Arthritis Foundation, http://www.arthritis.org
Cancer Supportive Care, http://www.cancersupportivecare.com
Cycling Performance Tips, http://www.cptips.com
Food Allergy and Anaphylaxis Network, http://www.foodallergy.org
HeartInfo.Org, http://www.heartinfo.org
Institute of Medicine, http://www.iom.edu
International Osteoporosis Foundation, http://www.iofbonehealth.org
La Leche League International, http://www.lalecheleague.org
March of Dimes Birth Defects Foundation, http://www.marchofdimes.org
Mayo Foundation for Medical Education and Research, http://www.mayoclinic.com
McDonald's, http://www.mcdonalds.com
Medical College of Wisconsin, http://www.healthlink.mcw.edu
National Digestive Diseases Information Clearinghouse, http://www.digestive.niddk.nih.gov
National Eating Disorder Association, http://www.nationaleatingdisorders.org
National Heart, Lung, and Blood Institute, http://www.nhlbi.nib.gov
National Institute of Diabetes & Digestive & Kidney Diseases, http://www.niddk.nih.gov
National Institute for Drug Abuse, http://www.drugabuse.gov
National Institutes of Health, http://www.nih.gov
National Kidney Foundation, http://www.kidney.org
National Library of Medicine, http://www.nlm.nih.gov
National Osteoporosis Foundation, http://www.nof.org
New York Times, http://www.nytimes.com
Pennington Biomedical Research Center, http://www.pbrc.edu
People Living with Cancer, http://www.plwc.org
Personal MD, http://www.personalmd.com
U.S. Centers for Disease Control and Prevention, http://www.cdc.gov
U.S. Department of Agriculture, http://www.usda.gov

U.S. Department of Agriculture Food Safety and Inspection Service, http://www.fsis.usda.gov

U.S. Department of Health & Human Services, http://www.hhs.gov

U.S. Food and Drug Administration, http://www.fda.gov

U.S. National Agricultural Library, http://www.nal.usda.gov

U.S. National Institute of Allergy and Infectious Disease, http://www.niaid.nih.gov

U.S. National Institutes of Health, http://www.nih.gov

U.S. National Library of Medicine, http://www.nlm.nih.gov

World Health Organization, http://www.who.int/

WorldWide Anaesthetist, http://www.anaesthetist.com

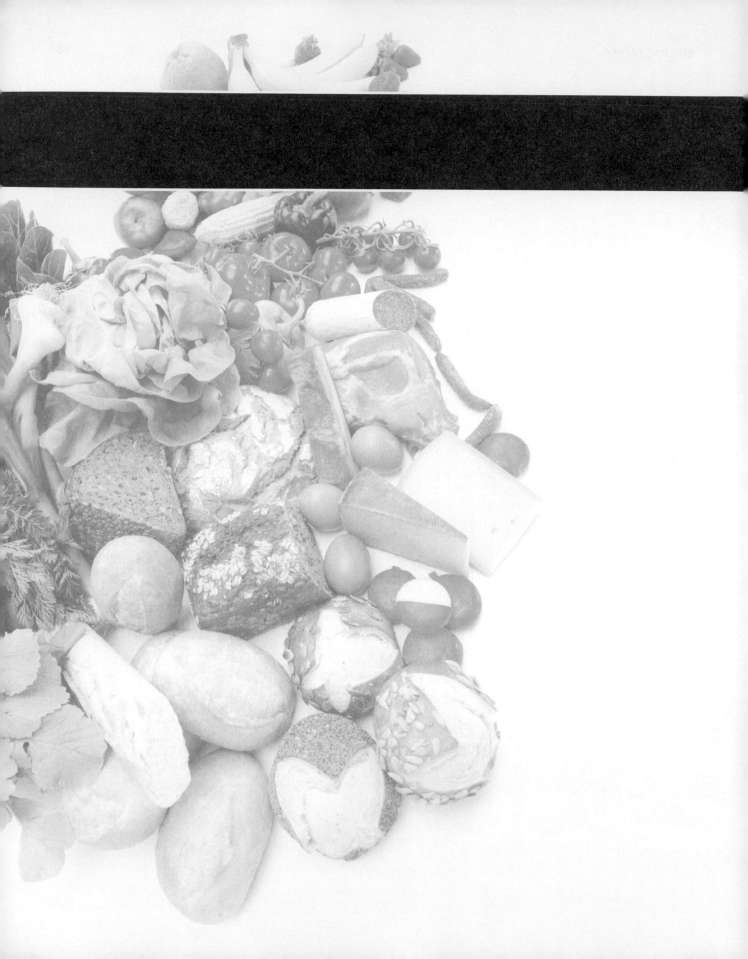

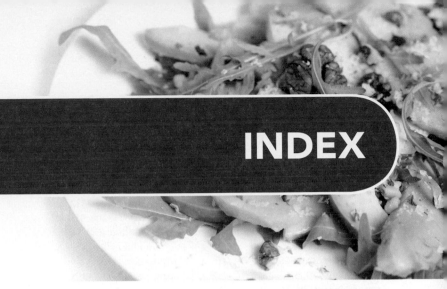

INDEX

A

A1c, 328
Abdominal fat, 299
Absorption, 62–64
  carbohydrates, 83
  case studies, 71–73
  fats (lipids), 98–99
  health care professionals,
    considerations for, 69
  iron and, 163
  large intestine, 63–64
  proteins, 110
  small intestine, 62
Abstinence, 200
Acanthosis nigricans, 253
Accessory organ disorders,
    379–382
ACE inhibitors, 534
Acid-base balance, 179
Acidosis, 159, 179
Acne, 255
Active lifestyles, calorie needs related
    to, 68, 437–438
Acute renal failure (ARF), 361
Adequate Intake (AI)
  calcium, 156
  chloride, 161
  Dietary Guidelines for Americans,
    20–21
  fiber, 247
  fluoride, 167
  magnesium, 161
  nutrients, 20
  phosphorus, 157
  potassium, 161
  pregnancy and lactation, 207
  sodium, 161

  trace minerals, 154
  water, 175
Adipose tissue, 67
Adjustable gastric band (AGB), 309
Adolescents, 255–265
  alcohol and, 29, 261
  anorexia nervosa and, 256–257
  appetites of, 252, 255
  as athletes, 263–265
  bulimia and, 257–258
  calcium, 156, 256
  calorie recommendations for, 33
  calorie requirements, 256, 437–438
  case studies, 268–269
  cocaine use by, 262
  dairy recommendations for, 35
  definition, 206
  diabetes and, 254
  dietary fiber needs of, 246–247
  Dietary Guidelines for Americans, 24
  dietary requirements of, 256
  drug use by, 261–262
  energy drinks and, 262–263
  fast food and, 259, 260
  fluoride and, 167
  food habits, 255
  growth spurts, 255
  health care professionals,
    considerations for, 265
  inhalants and, 262
  marijuana, use of, 261
  nutritional intake problems of, 7
  obesity in, 258–259
  overweight, 258–259
  phosphorus, 157
  physical activity recommendations
    for, 24
  pregnancy and, 210, 213–214

  tobacco and, 262
  trace minerals needs of, 154
  vitamins, 123
  weight and self-esteem in, 258–259
  weight management, 22
Adult rickets. *See* Osteomalacia
Adults
  calcium, 156
  calorie recommendations for, 33
  calorie requirements, 274, 276,
    437–438
  case studies, 279–280
  chloride, 161
  dairy recommendations for, 35
  Dietary Guidelines for Americans, 24
  dietary recommendations, 23
  dietary requirements, 273–274
  energy requirements for, 272–273
  fluoride, 167
  food habits, 274
  health care professionals,
    considerations for, 277
  height and weight chart, 69
  nutrient requirements, 273
  nutrition concerns for, 274–275
  phosphorus, 157
  physical activity recommendations
    for, 22
  protein intake, 112
  sodium, 161
  trace minerals needs, 156
  vitamins, 123
  water, 175
  weight control/management, 275–276
  weight management, 275–276
  See also Older adults
Aerobic metabolism, 64
Aflatoxin, 194

587